Handbook of

Geriatric Care Management

Third Edition

Edited by
Cathy Jo Cress, MSW
Cress GCM Consult
Santa Cruz, California

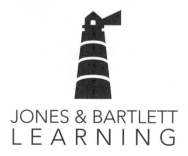

JONES & BARTLETT
LEARNING

World Headquarters

Jones & Bartlett Learning
40 Tall Pine Drive
Sudbury, MA 01776
978-443-5000
info@jblearning.com
www.jblearning.com

Jones & Bartlett Learning
Canada
6339 Ormindale Way
Mississauga, Ontario L5V 1J2
Canada

Jones & Bartlett Learning
International
Barb House, Barb Mews
London W6 7PA
UK

Jones & Bartlett Learning books and products are available through most bookstores and online booksellers. To contact Jones & Bartlett Learning directly, call 800-832-0034, fax 978-443-8000, or visit our website, www.jblearning.com.

Substantial discounts on bulk quantities of Jones & Bartlett Learning publications are available to corporations, professional associations, and other qualified organizations. For details and specific discount information, contact the special sales department at Jones & Bartlett Learning via the above contact information or send an email to specialsales@jblearning.com.

The authors, editor, and publisher have made every effort to provide accurate information. However, they are not responsible for errors, omissions, or for any outcomes related to the use of the contents of this book and take no responsibility for the use of the products and procedures described. Treatments and side effects described in this book may not be applicable to all people; likewise, some people may require a dose or experience a side effect that is not described herein. Drugs and medical devices are discussed that may have limited availability controlled by the Food and Drug Administration (FDA) for use only in a research study or clinical trial. Research, clinical practice, and government regulations often change the accepted standard in this field. When consideration is being given to use of any drug in the clinical setting, the health care provider or reader is responsible for determining FDA status of the drug, reading the package insert, and reviewing prescribing information for the most up-to-date recommendations on dose, precautions, and contraindications, and determining the appropriate usage for the product. This is especially important in the case of drugs that are new or seldom used.

Production Credits

Publisher: Kevin Sullivan
Acquisitions Editor: Amanda Harvey
Editorial Assistant: Rachel Shuster
Production Manager: Carolyn Rogers
Marketing Manager: Meagan Norlund
V.P., Manufacturing and Inventory Control:
  Therese Connell
Composition: Laurel Muller, Cohographics
Cover Design: Kate Ternullo
Cover Image: © Monkey Business Images/
  ShutterStock, Inc.
Printing and Binding: Malloy, Inc.
Cover Printing: Malloy, Inc.

Library of Congress Cataloging-in-Publication Data
Handbook of geriatric care management / [edited by] Cathy Cress. — 3rd ed.
    p. ; cm.
  Includes bibliographical references and index.
  ISBN: 978-0-7637-9026-4 (casebound)
  1. Geriatrics—Handbooks, manuals, etc. 2. Older people—Medical care—
Management—Handbooks, manuals, etc.   I. Cress, Cathy.
  [DNLM: 1. Health Services for the Aged—organization & administration. 2. Geriatrics.
3. Practice Management—organization & administration.   WT 31 H236 2007]
  RC952.55.C74 2011
  362.198′97—dc22
                                    2010026639
6048

Printed in the United States of America
15 14 13 12 11 10 9 8 7 6 5 4 3 2 1

Contents

Foreword

America is heading toward the crest of an "age wave": 70 million baby boomers are turning 65—the fastest growing population in the United States. By 2030, there will be over 72 million people who are 65 and older.

The demand for professional geriatric care managers is increasing. The profession provides valuable services and products that allow the aging population options for living a comfortable, independent, and dignified lifestyle.

At the same time, healthcare issues emerge, as we struggle to take care of those afflicted by diseases such as Alzheimer's, Parkinson's, and dementia. In addition, assisted care living facilities, nursing homes, and continuing care communities are vying for clientele. Financial concerns have taken on increased importance as elders are faced with a volatile economy, increasing healthcare costs, and decreasing insurance and government benefits. Finally, independence and autonomy are a major concern as elders struggle to remain in their own homes while maintaining a high quality of life.

If you are thinking about becoming a geriatric care manager (GCM), or starting your own business, or if you are a family member trying to figure out how to work with a care manager, you have found the right book.

Cathy Jo Cress has assembled the nation's premier care managers to write chapters for this book that contain real-life situations and solutions. The first and second editions of the *Handbook of Geriatric Care Management* were a resounding success that provided guidance on how to build, manage, and market a care management practice. It is recognized by care managers and aging network advocates across the country as a "must have" reference book. Now, the third edition goes one step further in offering more information in each of these areas, as well as updated and expanded resources for use in a rapidly changing society.

Care, compassion, and concern, coupled with an extensive knowledge of the aging network, are the professional hallmarks of a great GCM. This book explores the training needed, the skills to be obtained, and the traits of a GCM. It takes a special person to make this 24/7 job a career, but it comes with some of the greatest rewards in knowing you are improving the quality of life of each client you touch.

GCMs are professionally trained to assist the elderly in a variety of circumstances and to become active advocates for their clients. Often, GCMs are called in to handle a crisis: Mom has fallen and broken her hip, Dad has Alzheimer's and can no longer live at home, there has been a death in the family, or there are immediate financial problems. GCMs are usually available 24 hours a day, 7 days a week. They are the lifesavers who are onsite immediately—looking out for the best interests of older adults. They are the ones with an emergency evacuation plan in place before the hurricane or tornado hits, the ones who can intervene with physicians when there are drug complications, the ones who can discuss documents needed and forms to be filed to ensure that all benefits can be accessed appropriately.

Creating, marketing, building, and maintaining a geriatric care management business has its own unique challenges. This is a business that provides highly personalized care and requires employees who are well trained and supported in working with ill, frail, and often lonely seniors. No aspect of the business is easy, and you will, no doubt, find yourself referring back to this book for answers to your business and clinical dilemmas.

Kaaren Boothroyd
Executive Director
National Association of Professional
Geriatric Care Managers

Linda Fodrini-Johnson, MA, MFT, CMC
Past President
National Association of Professional
Geriatric Care Managers

Introduction

Since the first edition of the *Handbook of Geriatric Care Management* was published in 2000, the urgency of families seeking solutions for care of their aging parents has continued to explode. An estimated 65 million family members now care for older or disabled relatives in the United States. This backbreaking job assumed by kin now costs $275 billion in informal care that is not reimbursed by the federal government. This loving load of elder care has shattered caregiving families and made the geriatric care manager an even more urgent lifesaver compared to its role in the year 2000 when this book was first published.

Geriatric care management was born at the end of the 1900s to oversee the ballooning, illusive, and many times, unreachable aging continuum of care. This new profession was a beacon of hope for desperate family caregivers.

Geriatric care managers (GCMs) are now one of the central points of entry for baby boomers who remain lost in the mystifying maze of aging services. By 2010, GCMs had climbed to the level of national experts, as evidenced by numerous national news stories and books discussing the merits of the profession. Gail Sheehy's new book in her Passages series, *Passages in Caregiving* (Harper Collins, 2010), devotes a section to GCMs. Sheehy labels GCMs as the real "fixers" in the long-term care system, giving the direction that desperate caregiving families need.

Why did GCM climb to this level of public recognition? Because GCMs are the GPS to navigate the convoluted, fractional web of senior services. They are the fixers, as Sheehy says, who locate the correct services and a premium care plan for each older client, giving relief and peace of mind to their harried caregivers, like Sheehy, who cared for her husband Clay Felker.

GCMs ensure that care is right for the individual client, delivered by the right person at the right time. The third edition of the *Handbook of Geriatric Care Management* is being published at a time when geriatric care management is exploding nationally and internationally. Although the field has existed for more than 35 years, it is just coming into its own.

Geriatric care management originated as a cutting-edge addition to case management. But as the profession matured, it mainstreamed and separated from case management. Geriatric care management bridges larger businesses such as elder law, banking, trust departments, accounting, the assisted living industry, senior real estate business, home health care and the ballooning U.S. medical care system that ministers to the chronic care needs of older people. Geriatric care managers are both salient guides to all these senior industries and the grease that helps all work better and in tandem, like a well-run machine. The geriatric care management profession's growth is reflected in its increasing inclusion in the portfolios of very large for-profit and nonprofit healthcare businesses and the emergence of large nationwide geriatric care management corporations.

Geriatric care management continues to bridge several educational domains such as nursing, social work, physical therapy, occupational therapy, and gerontology. The new field ¬synthesizes theory and pedagogical frameworks from all of these disciplines to create a new field, with its own academic degrees and certificates, reflected in the many emerging academic programs at universities all over the country.

Why has this new profession grown so quickly, spread so far, and created an academic place of its own? What created it in the first place? Quite simply, the field evolved out of a genuine gap in aging services that still exists today. It began in the 1980s as a result of astounding demographics—the fastest-growing segment of US population was over age 85. This burgeoning population of middle- and upper-income elders needed community and healthcare services to remain in their homes. Their needs were not being met. Their adult children were trying to raise their own family while working as dual earners and were already overpowered by their load. Many adult children had moved long distances from their aging parents. When aging mothers, fathers, aunts, and uncles called out to their adult children for help in the early 1980s, the "call" sent shock waves in baby boomers children. All of these demographic, economic, and family system factors converged to launch the field of geriatric care management, answering the needs of both adult children and their older family members who wished to remain in their homes.

What did not evolve was a training program for GCMs, a large gap that this book aims to fill. The *Handbook of Geriatric Care Management, Third Edition,* delivers an expand-ing training program to the growing number of colleges and universities offering geriatric care management programs. This textbook is a great choice for schools that form the frontline for geriatric care management education, including those that have programs in social welfare, nursing, gerontology, physical therapy, sociology and geriatric care management itself. This book gives educators throughout the United States and the world a text to add to classes that addresses the multiple needs of aging adults and their families. This handbook of GCM is a critical tool to use in health, social services, and business curricula in undergraduate and graduate courses. This textbook can also be used as an additional reading resource in introductory aging issues classes and can augment courses in related fields, such as physical therapy, occupational therapy, law, insurance, banking, medicine, and real estate, when instructors want to provide a bridge to help their particular profession solve the problems of aging families.

As the vocation of geriatric care management has grown, so has a much-needed GCM credentialing process. This book discusses the many credentialing choices and the credentialing process in general. Why is the credentialing process important? It is a stamp of approval for consumers—families and older people seeking a skilled and professionally trained GCM. The credentialing process is also helpful to GCMs, giving them credibility with the public, thus helping to build their practice. This book can help aspiring and experienced GCMs choose the right credentials to pursue.

The *Handbook of Geriatric Care Management, Third Edition,* can help beginning GCMs get their sea legs and seasoned GCMs grow as professionals. Because geriatric care management is a business, whether nonprofit or for-profit, this book covers critical aspects of running, adding to, and making a profit while operating a geriatric care management practice. The book covers launching the business, promoting the business, running a fiscally sound business, making money, and expanding the business.

This textbook covers critical new clinical issues, like working with aging families and how a GCM can use mediation as an accidental mediator and when to refer to a professional mediator. It also pilots GCMs through clinical work such as coaching and problem solving with normal but highly stressed aging families and intervening in dysfunctional aging families. It gives readers therapeutic interventions to help families function as a unit to solve the myriad problems of their older parents or relatives.

This third edition offers three substantial new chapters that cover assessing and supporting aging in place through technology, combining a home care agency with a GCM practice, and mediation and the GCM as the accidental mediator.

Because after 35 years the public is still unclear why they should buy the product of geriatric care management, marketing geriatric care management services can be difficult. This book offers clear guidance to define geriatric care management as a business product to sell, get new customers, and make a profit. This information is helpful to beginning GCMs, experienced GCMs, nonprofit agencies and home care agencies and anyone offering geriatric care management services. This includes large healthcare corporations that want to add GCM into their menu of services, or law or real estate businesses that want to add GCM to their practices.

This handbook also offers an entire chapter on the ethics of geriatric care management. GCMs try to ensure that senior services are not only highly individualized, appropriate, and coordinated, but also ethical. GCM providers help seniors and their families make very difficult decisions. GCMs have also developed a code of ethics for all practitioners to follow. Consumers should know to choose only GCMs who abide by this code of ethics.

An updated chapter on working with clients from different cultural and ethnic backgrounds continues to be a landmark chapter in broadening the scope of practice of GCMs and giving GCMs of multiethnic and cultural backgrounds tools to appropriately assess the needs of elders from different cultures.

The handbook will also serve as a tool for the business world. The chapters in Part III, The Business of Geriatric Care Management, include thoroughly updated information on how to begin or add a geriatric care management business, grow a mature or seasoned geriatric care management business, add a geriatric care management practice to a nonprofit business, and sell GCM services and gain customers thereby critically making money in all of these business arenas. Business owners wishing to integrate geriatric care management into their business or portfolio of businesses (e.g., accountants, elder-law attorneys, persons who work in a trust department or large national healthcare corporation) will learn all they need to know through this book.

Intended as a practical guide, the *Handbook of Geriatric Care Management, Third Edition*, includes sample forms and letters. We have added websites in every chapter as an excellent technological guide for students and practitioners. And because this book is intended as a teaching tool, it contains many case examples. Instructors working with this textbook can use the examples to explain some of the how-to techniques mentioned and give students a good sense of the problems likely to arise and how they can be solved. The textbook also offers multiple assessment tools critical to the field, which can assist instructors in helping students learn to appraise the problems of older people and their stressed families.

This textbook is a manual to a stage of life finally addressed in the annals of how-to books of the 21st century. Whole series of classes have been developed for the study of babies and preschoolers. Entire curricula have been developed through schools of nursing and social work to instruct the family facing adolescents and their prospective problems. Yet guidebooks for the difficulties of the midlife family, a distinct new stage of life, are scanty at best. Recently retired baby boomers facing the continued support of their own adult children are now additionally affected by the needs and crises of their aging parents. The textbooks for them are just beginning to be codified and accepted into academia. A flurry of "how to deal with our aging parents" books are just hitting the bookstores in volumes. This textbook is a major contribution to this needed body of literature that addresses this new developmental stage not identified until the last few decades.

Geriatric care management in the not-so-distant year 2030 may be completely different from geriatric care management today. This handbook gives a sense of the metamorphosis the field is likely to undergo in the next few decades.

The *Handbook of Geriatric Care Management, Third Edition,* is meant as a rich resource discussing this incredibly complex and interesting field. I hope that it will serve you well, and help you become a better GCM, integrate geriatric care management into your business, learn more about aging, and help these midlife families and their aging parents function as successful and loving systems of care.

Cathy Jo Cress

Acknowledgments

I would like to thank the authors who contributed to this book: Their immense professional expertise in the field of geriatric care management fill these pages. In this emerging national field, some of these authors are the founding mothers and fathers of the profession. Many are rising stars whose new perspectives have already changed the practical tool box and academic knowledge of geriatric care management.

I would like to dedicate this book to my grandparents Anna Mae and Ike Cress whose unconditional love gave me the foundation to be the writer I am today.

I would also like to dedicate it to my daughter Kali Cress Peterson, a fellow gerontologist and cowriter of the "Working with Aging Siblings" chapter in *Care Managers: Working with the Aging Family* (Jones & Bartlett Learning, 2009), and *Mom Loves You Best: Forgiving and Forging Sibling Relationships* (New Horizon, 2010). She will eclipse my star and create her own universe.

And to my daughter Jill Paul Gallo, a great artist whose step-parenting has taught me so much about the aging family.

And finally, to my grandchildren, Julia Gallo, Joseph Gallo, Emory Peterson, Alexa Haskell, Ellie Nestaval, Benjamin Peterson, Jacob Peterson, Hannah Peterson, and Taryn De Mars. They will spawn their own, staggeringly bright, alternative universe.

Cathy Jo Cress

Contributors

Carolyn Barber, MSN, PHN, CMC

Liz Barlowe, MA, CMC
CEO, Innovative Today, LLC
Clearwater, FL

Phyllis Mensh Brostoff, CISW, CMC
CEO, Stowell Associates
SelectStaff, Inc.
Milwaukee, WI

Dana Curtis, MA, JD
Director, Elder Mediation Group
Sausalito, CA

Jack Herndon, MBA
Managing Partner, Sage Eldercare Solutions,
    LLC
Millbrae, CA

Nina Pflumm Herndon, MA, CMC, CLPF
Principal, Sage Eldercare Solutions
Millbrae, CA

Nancy Hikoyeda, DrPH, MPH
Consultant, Health, Aging, and Diversity
San Jose, CA

Erica Karp, MSW, LCSW, CCM, RG-NGF
Principal and Director
Northshore Eldercare Management, Inc.
Evanston, IL

Angela Koenig, MA
Freelance Writer
Chicago, IL

Stephne Lencioni, MSW, CMC
Geriatric Care Manager
Palo Alto, CA

Kathleen J. McConnell, LCSW
Palo Alto VA Hospital
Geriatric Research Education and Clinical
    Center (GRFCC)
Palo Alto, CA

Julie Menack, MA, CLPF, CAPS
21st Century Care Solutions
Oakland, CA

Christina E. Miyawaki, MA, MSW
Director of Programs and Administration
Japanese American Services of the East Bay,
    Inc. (JASEB)
Berkley, CA

Barbara Morano, LCSW, MSW
Geriatric Research Education Clinical Center
    (GRECC)
James J. Peters VA Medical Center
Bronx, NY

Carmen L. Morano, PhD, LCSW
Associate Professor
Hunter College
School of Social Work
New York, NY

Deborah Newquist, PhD, MSW, CMC
Director of Geriatric Services
ResCare, Inc.
Costa Mesa, CA

Leonie Nowitz, LCSW, BCD
Director
Center for Lifelong Growth
New York, NY

Merrily Orsini, MSSW
Managing Director, corecubed
Louisville, KY

Robert E. O'Toole, MSW, LICSW
President, Informed Eldercare Decisions, Inc.
Dedham, MA

Cathie Ramey, MA
Walnut Creek, CA

Connie Rosenberg, MPS, RN, CMC
President, Services and Resources for Seniors
Morristown, NJ

Anne Rosenthal, PhD, MFT, CMC
Geriatric Care Manager
Eldercare Services
Walnut Creek, CA

Emily B. Saltz, LICSW, CMC
Director
Elder Resources
Newton, MA

Victoria Thorpe, MEd
Sage Elder Care Solutions
Millbrae, CA

Monika White, PhD
President/CEO
Monika White Consulting
Adjunct Associate Professor
University of Southern California
Schools of Social Work & Gerontology
Los Angeles, CA

Cheryl M. Whitman, BSN, MS, CMC
Director NACCM
Colchester, CT

PART 1

Introduction to Geriatric Care Management

Chapter 1

Overview and History of Geriatric Care Management

Cathy Jo Cress

What is geriatric care management? It is a series of steps taken by a professional geriatric care manager (GCM) to help solve older people's problems. A GCM, who may be a social worker, a nurse, a gerontologist, or another human service professional, serves older people and their families. The GCM usually steps in when the older person or family is in crisis. Geriatric care management is also a preventative service rendered on demand, increasing the quality of an older person's life, managing all the players rendering services to the older person, and offering assurance and peace of mind to the adult children of the older individual. How does the GCM solve these problems and render these services? The GCM uses classic social work and nursing tools, including client assessment, care planning, service coordination, and referral and monitoring.

What is a professional GCM? Geriatric care manager's jobs are similar to the role of case managers, and GCMs use all the classic tools of case management. But unlike other case managers, GCMs specialize in serving adults aged 65 and older and offer very personalized services. GCMs historically have had much smaller caseloads than case managers have (especially those in public case management settings), giving GCMs great flexibility in delivering highly individualized services to their older clients. Unlike many case man-

agers in public case management settings, GCMs are generally available 24 hours a day, 7 days a week, 365 days a year. They respond to client needs at the convenience of the client, which enables the GCM to cross the line from public-sector human services into the for-profit service business. The GCM's product is service, and that product must be available at all times to be useful to older people, their families, and third parties such as trust departments and conservators, who are willing to buy the product if it is offered in this manner.[1]

The GCM is not just the classic anonymous public-sector case manager delivering impersonal services. In fact, the GCM is a kind of surrogate family member with special expertise in the phases and tasks of care management and a long-standing and personal relationship with clients. GCMs deliver the kind of old-fashioned good service that many older clients nostalgically remember. GCMs not only respond to clients' demands, but they are proactive as well, always maintaining a positive attitude.

In addition, GCMs deliver the level of service that older clients' and adult children expect. These children are usually baby boomers from two-income families who are accustomed to purchasing services (housecleaning, day care, after-school transportation, tax assistance) to help make their busy lives easier. Purchasing geriatric care management services to assist with the problems of their older family members, who frequently live far away, seems logical to these adult children. The GCM is providing time and expertise, neither of which the adult child has. The GCM also sells peace of mind. Most baby boomers do not want to get up in the middle of the night to respond to an older person's crisis, but the GCM will. The adult child may not have enough vacation time to fly to the parent's home to arrange services once the older person gets out of hospital, but the GCM does this. Many adult children want the assurance that the older family member is cared for and safe, without having to solve the problem themselves. So, the personalized services of the GCM, a surrogate family member, appeal to adult children.[2]

In addition to handling client assessment, care planning, service coordination, and referral and monitoring, the GCM keeps track of the giant web of senior services that makes up the continuum of care. GCMs are like Charlotte, the friendly spider in Charlotte's Web. They run back and forth across the web, linking services, repairing gaps, spinning new solutions to problems, and coordinating answers. At their root, GCMs are problem solvers.

This chapter offers an overview of what a GCM does and discusses the history of the profession.

■ HISTORY OF GERIATRIC CARE MANAGEMENT

GCMs are now relatively familiar participants in the world of senior services and health care. But what conditions led to the rise of geriatric care management? This section discusses the history of this important profession.

The Origins of Case Management

In a seminal study of geriatric care management, Secord and Parker note that case management itself, the root of geriatric care management, has its foundation in the social services for new immigrants and other poor people that emerged in the late 1800s.[3] At that time, urbanization and industrialization had left so many people poor and homeless that churches and local communities were paralyzed and unable to care for everyone in need. Social service bureaucracies began to arise, which led to the beginning of case management. Secord and Parker hypothesize that the core elements of today's case management were born by "helping the client find the least costly, most appropriate services to meet his or her needs."[3(p4)] Since then, community agencies, social workers, hospital discharge planners, and case coordinators have provided what we now call case management.

No one group or movement was solely responsible for the emergence of case management. In the arena of early social services, in 1833 Joseph Tuckerman organized a group of churches to help needy families. The Settlement House movement at the turn of the 20th century is another example of early case management. The Settlement House movement established institutions called settlement houses that tried to improve living conditions in city neighborhoods. Most settlement houses had social workers on staff. Many charity organizations and societies coordinated assistance for children and families; a case management program was set up by the Massachusetts Board of Charities in the mid-1800s. The roots of case management can also be found in early workers' compensation programs of the 1940s.[4]

In the medical world, case management appeared in the treatment of chronically ill and long-term care populations, including children, people with disabilities, substance abusers, and people with acquired immune deficiency syndrome. As acute care costs skyrocketed in the United States after World War II, case management techniques developed to lower costs. Case managers appeared in institutional settings and followed patients into the community to coordinate care for high-cost, high-risk individuals. At the same time, private medical case managers appeared in order to respond to the needs of patients, insurers, and medical providers by helping these constituents make difficult decisions (e.g., Is a medical procedure appropriate? Is there a less costly alternative? Can a patient spend recovery time at home?). Today, the medical case manager makes a path for the patient through the maze of the healthcare delivery system, coordinates a plan of care, and offers support from family agencies, suppliers of health care, and healthcare entities.[5]

Growth of Case Management for Older People

According to Parker and Secord, case management for older people emerged because of two factors. The first was the rapid growth of the older population in the United States. The second was the increased cost of health care, especially Medicare, in the United States. At the time of their study in 1987, Secord and Parker reported that Medicare expenditures totaled $83 billion in 1981 and were projected to increase to $200 billion in the year 2000.[3]

When healthcare costs exploded in the 1950s and 1960s, and the number of older people grew, a national effort was made to stem the fiscal bloodletting. This was true especially with nursing home expenditures, which ate up a large part of public funds, mostly through Medicaid payments for older people. In the 1970s and 1980s, many states developed nursing home preadmission screening programs in an attempt to reduce nursing home placement. In other states, a moratorium was placed on nursing home bed construction. People realized that nursing home placement was not only costly but often unnecessary or inappropriate; many older Americans could be cared for in their own homes.

In addition, services for older people were expanding. This growth was driven (after World War II) by five major federal programs with mandates to finance gerontological services: Title VIII of the Social Security Act (Medicare), Title XIX of the Social Security Act (Medicaid), Title XX of the Social Security Act, the Older Americans Act, and the Department of Veterans Affairs.[6]

As a result of these developments, in the 1960s and 1970s a plethora of senior programs blossomed in the United States. These services included home care, homemaker services, chore services, housing alternatives, transportation services, adult day care, and in-home meals. These senior services, all of which helped keep seniors in their own homes, were not coordinated. Some services emerged from states, some from the federal government, and some from the local community. Because this fragmented system was difficult to navigate, it did not serve older people well.

To help with this fragmentation and lack of a single point of entry into the web of senior programs, many public and private programs developed aspects of case management. In the 1970s, Medicare funded a number of Medicare waiver programs to find out whether older people could remain more independent when provided with community-based coordinated care. Case managers guided older people through the complex web of senior services and decided which services were appropriate for each individual.

A case manager might help in the following way: Suppose an older person who lives alone at home and is very lonely becomes depressed enough to stop eating on a regular basis. The nutritional deficit can lead to confusion, which makes it more likely that the older person will not take needed medications. If these medications, say, are for high blood pressure, the unmedicated older person may have a stroke and need to be hospitalized, and then placed in a nursing home. This eventual nursing home placement could be avoided if the older person had a case manager who knew that depression might lead to this outcome and who understood that a regular friendly visitor could allay the depression. The case manager might also suggest regular visits to a senior center as a way for this person to reenter the world. The case manager might talk to some of the older person's friends and encourage them to visit more frequently or for them to have a weekly meal together so that the older person has company and something to look forward to each week. The case manager might also arrange for the older person to visit his or her physician so medications can be monitored and arrange for prepared meals to be dropped off daily by Meals on Wheels. Thus, the case manager could help avoid an unnecessary nursing home placement by helping the older person navigate the very confusing continuum of care.

The emerging Medicare waiver programs of the 1970s included Connecticut Triage on the East Coast, the Multipurpose Senior Services Project on the West Coast, the National Long-Term Care Channeling Project, the 2176 Medicaid Waiver Programs, and the Community Nursing and Home Health programs. Case management was viewed as central to these Medicare waiver programs. In addition, these programs allowed older people to purchase items they normally would not be able to buy through Medicare, such as medications and eyeglasses. This was done on an experimental basis to see what mix of services would help keep older people out of nursing homes and in the community.

Out of these very experimental programs of the 1970s and 1980s emerged the classic model of case management.[7]

The Emergence of Professional Geriatric Care Management

The frail elderly have historically been the prime consumers of case management services. They experience functional and cogni-tive impairments that demand a wide array of informal and formal services. Case managers are expert in brokering these services. The publicly funded case management programs of the 1970s and 1980s demonstrated that case management was an ideal tool in brokering these formal and informal services and in helping older people remain in the community. Years of studies showed that older people wanted to stay at home and that they could remain at home with coordinated in-home and community-based services. The key was case management. Many factors came together to encourage the development of geriatric care management, which was at first a specialized form of case management.

One factor that contributed to the rise of geriatric care management was the emergence of a new pool of qualified professional case managers interested in pursuing a slightly different type of work. Many case managers from public case management programs burned themselves out by working in the public system. They wanted more independence in their jobs while still doing good and working with older people. Others from the helping professions (nurses and social workers) had not worked in public case management programs but had experienced burnout and wanted a different, perhaps more exciting, career path where they would still be helping others.

At the same time, the voluminous and very fragmented web of senior services continued to expand, tangle, and unravel, with no central point of entry and mind-boggling rules at the federal, state, and local levels. Contemporaneously, the number of older people was increasing. Because long-term care management and chronic care management are not covered by Medicare, these types of care are considered discretionary purchases. In addition, many older people had large enough incomes and amounts of assets to be ineligible for publicly funded and community-based programs. The over-65 cohort is much more affluent than all the age groups under 45 years of age. Seventy percent of the wealth in the United States is controlled by people 50 years old and older. Households headed by persons older than 65 years have considerable purchasing power, controlling one-third of all the discretionary income in the country. Older people in this $800 billion market have at least $115 billion in discretionary income. Therefore, older people needed and could afford geriatric care management services.[6]

Two other factors contributed to the development of geriatric care management. First, more women began working out of the home. Although women remain the principal informal caregivers in the United States today—75% of all relatives who care for elders are women—they have accounted for a significant percentage of the work force since the 1950s. Women entered the work force partly because of societal change, including the women's movement, and families began to need two incomes to stay afloat. Fifty-five percent of all women today work, leaving not only children but older adults in need of care. Despite the crushing emotional, physical, and financial burdens, the US family has not abandoned its elders. A study done in the 1990s by the US House of Representatives showed that the average woman spends 17 years caring for her children and 18 years or more caring for her older parents. Piggybacked on this is another startling statistic: For the first time in US history, Americans today have more living parents than they have children.[8]

Second, most Americans tend to live far from their older family members. The United States is a mobile society. Individuals no longer stay where they grew up. They may work in many different locations while their parents stay in the hometown. According to a study by the American Association of Retired Persons, one third of all adult children in the United States live at least 30 minutes away from their aging parents.[9] Because the main system of support is still the family, this leaves older people vulnerable if they have a crisis. If the family lives far away, a crisis can turn into a megacrisis if there is no one to offer assistance.

All of these factors have led to the need for geriatric care management. Public and private case managers as well as nurses and social workers who chose to leave the system saw a wonderful niche to fill. They understood how to provide care professionally. Many understood case management. And they saw the frustration of many older people, who had the money to purchase services but were not sure which services to choose, and of families, usually adult daughters, who were overworked and lived far away. In addition, adult children realized they could do what they already did for housecleaning and other services: they could outsource help for their parents.

■ THE BIRTH OF GERIATRIC CARE MANAGEMENT ORGANIZATIONS

Geriatric care management became a profession gradually. Because the people who started the profession came from diverse fields, in the beginning there was no central meeting ground for them. Social workers belonged to the National Association of Social Workers, whereas nurses belonged to many different associations, including the American Nurses Association. To work on common goals and interests, the new GCMs started several organizations. The most important early ones were the National Association of Professional Geriatric Care Managers and the Case Management Society of America (CMSA).

GCM

The first 12 GCMs, who were scattered across the country, were originally drawn together through a 1984 article in the New York Times.[10] GCMs from different areas were surprised to learn that other people were doing what they were doing. Social workers who were interviewed in the article were asked to join a coalition. In January 1985, the first meeting of what would become the National Association of Professional Geriatric Care Managers was held in the home of Adele Elkind, a social worker who was the founding force of the organization.

Professionals who had expertise in this relatively new area began to share information to help each other run better businesses. They agreed that if they could help each other, they could help the public. They put together a brochure to describe their services and moved on to develop criteria to decide who could be a member of the group. They formalized their network into the Greater New York Network on Aging (GNYNA) and began to refer cases to each other. Sarah Cohen, a founding member, suggested the radical idea that the fledgling group have a national conference; in 1985, 100 human service professionals gathered in New York City to take part in the first National Conference of Private Geriatric Care Managers. The gathering was hosted by GNYNA, which was by then a growing group of social workers, psychologists, nurses, and clinical gerontologists. This group had the vision of forming a national association dedicated to private geriatric care management.[11]

In 1986, this vision became a reality when the same group had a conference in Philadelphia, adopted membership standards, and unanimously voted to found the National Association of Private Geriatric Care Managers. In 1992, the association changed its name to the National Association of Professional Geriatric Care Managers, reflecting the fact that members might be from public, private for-profit, or private nonprofit backgrounds.

The association began with 30 members; currently it has 2000. It has been able to bring unity and consistency to geriatric care management by configuring an information base for aspiring and practicing GCMs. In 22 years of meetings, its members have been able to

gather a body of research about the GCM field. This body of knowledge has been presented in yearly national and regional conferences and in the GCM Journal. The journal, in existence since 1990, publishes research and topical information about the field and addresses points of interest to GCMs, including business practice and clinical issues.

The association includes a resource on the website (www.caremanager.org) called "Find a Care Manager," where potential GCM clients can locate a GCM anywhere in the United States, and an e-mail list through which GCMs can communicate with other GCMs from all over the country. The association has committees that benefit individual members and the whole GCM field, including marketing and public relations committees that create national marketing and public relations tools to promote geriatric care management through the media and articles published across the country. A public policy committee monitors legislation on national and local levels to keep GCMs informed of any significant pending action.

The association has nine regional chapters that can provide members with peer support and supervision, business and professional development, educational opportunities, clinical information, leadership training, networking, and joint marketing opportunities. Each chapter has a website, and many can help members advertise GCM job opportunities.

In the association's store on its website, the National Association of Professional Geriatric Care Managers offers many products that are helpful to GCMs who are starting a geriatric care management business. Products can be ordered by contacting the association (see Appendix A).[12]

CMSA

The Case Management Society of America (CMSA) is another association that addresses the growth of GCMs. CMSA does not specifically focus on geriatric care management but addresses the entire field of case management, including geriatric care management. Many CMSA members work in settings involving geriatric care management. CMSA has workshops and products that meet the needs of GCMs.

CMSA was founded in 1990 to support and develop the profession of case management through education, networking, and public policy. CMSA first published its Standards of Practice for Case Managers in 1995, and in 2009 completed their second revision. CMSA supports over 11,500 members and 20,000 subscribers. It now has 75 affiliated chapters and is associated with CMS UK, CMSAustralia, and NCMN in Canada. The CMSA website (www.cmsa.org) offers tools and resources for all healthcare professionals, including their Standards of Practice in a PDF format at no charge. CMSA's mission is to provide professional collaboration across the healthcare continuum, to advocate for patients' well-being and improve healthcare outcomes through the following:

- Fostering case management growth and development
- Impacting healthcare policy
- Providing evidence-based tools

CMSA's strategic priorities are education, outcomes, public policy, and national partnerships.

Under the education priority, CMSA holds a large national annual conference and expo, fields more than 70 smaller training sessions nationwide, and holds a Public Policy Workshop in Washington, DC, supporting case and care managers in working with their public officials. The online educational library has an extensive offering of courses in basic, intermediate, and advanced work, plus courses to prepare for various industry certifications.

Under the outcomes priority, CMSA has developed the "Case Management Adherence Guidelines" (CMAG), now in its third phase, to address the issue of patient nonadherence to recommended medication use and treatment. CMSA has expanded the CMAG guidelines to include disease-specific adherence chapters such as diabetes, deep vein thrombosis, and depression.

CMSA's Public Policy Committee is active at both the federal and state levels addressing such issues as transitions of care and the need for nurse licensure portability from state to state. CMSA chairs the National Transitions of Care Coalition in partnership with sanofi-aventis, US, which brings together 32 national healthcare associations to create collaboration and consensus on the issues facing seniors and their family caregivers with transitions of care.

Benefits of Membership

For a new GCM, joining an association is a wise step. As with any new professional, new GCMs can learn from those with experience in their chosen field, and associations are a good place to find knowledgeable people who might even become mentors. A rich body of information exists in the field of geriatric care management. Because this profession is relatively new, information is still mainly available through workshops and journals, both of which are produced by associations. However, many courses that offer a certificate and degree in geriatric care management have become available in the past 10 years.

By spending time with other members of professional associations, newcomers to geriatric care management can learn the pitfalls to avoid as they enter the field. GCMs who have practiced for any length of time have opinions in many areas, including whether becoming a GCM is a good idea. They can also provide tips about billing, setting up an office, hiring staff members, conducting geriatric assessments, using prefabricated forms, dealing with the stress of running a small business, and developing a business despite these stresses and pressures.

■ ACADEMIC PROGRAMS IN GERIATRIC CARE MANAGEMENT

In the past few years, several academic courses, certificate programs, and one master's program have emerged in geriatric care management. These programs offer a career path for students heading into the geriatric care management field or for GCMs who want further education in the business.

San Francisco State University Gerontology Graduate Program (master of arts) offers comprehensive coursework on aging. GCM content is taught in a special graduate course on the continuum of care. In addition, students may undertake an internship experience of practice in GCM and complete a culminating experience that focuses upon the multidimensional aspects of GCM.

The University of Florida offers a graduate certificate and specialty master's degree in geriatric care management. The curriculum covers topics such as client assessment, advanced care planning, and developing a private practice. The program is entirely online and designed to meet the needs of today's working professionals. The website is http://gcm.dce.ufl.edu.

The Brookdale Center for Aging and Longevity of Hunter College/CUNY and Continuing Education at Hunter offers several certificate programs in aging, including a geriatric care management certificate program through which a certificate in professional geriatric care management can be achieved. The website is www.hunter.cuny .edu/ce/courses-and-registration/certificate-programs/copy_of_brookdale-careers-in-gerontology.

The University of Utah Gerontology Interdisciplinary Program offers a 15-hour, fully online certificate with an emphasis in geriatric care management. Graduates are awarded a gerontology graduate certificate. The certificate is completed over three contiguous semesters (1 year), with students completing 5 credits each semester. Fall courses include Introduction to Gerontology and Physiology, and Psychology of Aging. Spring courses are Best Practices in Geriatric Care, and Geriatric Care Management I: Clinical Issues. Summer courses are Geriatric Care Management II: Professional, Legal, Financial and Business Issues, and the Geriatric Care Management Practicum/Seminar.

Their website is http://nursing.utah.edu/ gerontology/index.html.

Kaplan University offers an online geriatric care management certificate program. The student receives a certificate of completion at the end of the program. The website is www.kaplanonlineprograms.com.

Virginia Commonwealth University offers a master of science in gerontology. Coursework includes both didactic classes including GCM texts and field experiences where students are placed with a GCM. Following this experience many of these students continue the GCM specialty as part of their final fieldwork (600 hours) required for the program. Contact the program at www.sahp.vcu.edu/ gerontology.

The University of Wisconsin has a Case Management Certificate Program. The program offers professional continuing education in the field of aging and long-term care. They also offer an introduction to case management and advanced case management. Both are held at the University of Wisconsin-Madison. More information is available at www.dcs.wisc.edu/ classes/aging.htm.

College Misericordia in Dallas, Pennsylvania, offers a professional geriatric care manager graduate certificate. This is a web-based distance education program offering 15 credits and designed to be completed over a 15-month period. The website is www. misericordia.edu/misericordia_pg_sub. cfm?sub_page_id=775&subcat_id=133&page _id=370.

■ CONCLUSION

The geriatric care management profession developed in response to a societal need: a wide array of fragmented senior services was available, but older people and their adult children were having trouble figuring out which senior services would be helpful. GCMs are caring problem solvers who match older people to the appropriate senior services and monitor their care. Professionals who provide this very personalized service have organized into associations to help define and advance the geriatric care management field.

■ REFERENCES

1. Parker M. Private care management: how families are served. *J Case Manage*. 1992;1:108–112.
2. Cress C. The business of for-profit case management. *J Case Manage*. 1992;1:113–116.
3. Secord L, Parker M. *Private Case Management for Older Persons and Their Families*. Excelsior, MN: Interstudy; 1987.
4. US Department of Health and Human Services. *A National Agenda for Geriatric Education*. Vol. 1. Rockville, MD: Interdisciplinary Geriatrics and Allied Health Branch, Division of Associated Dental and Public Health Professions, Bureau of Health Professions; 1998.
5. Mullahay CM. *The Case Manager's Handbook*. Gaithersburg, MD: Aspen Publishers; 1998.
6. Kaye LW. The evolution of private care management. *J Case Manage*. 1992;1:103–107.
7. Cress C. Care management news takes hold in long term care. *Aging Int*. September 1992;19.
8. Kilborn B. Eldercare: its impact on the workplace. *Update Aging*. 1990;16.
9. American Association of Retired Persons. *A Profile of Older Americans*. Washington, DC: AARP Fulfillment; 1998.
10. Collins G. Long distance care for the elderly. *New York Times*. January 1984.
11. Elkind A. Development and growth of a regional network. GNYNA: the first two years, joys and growing pains. *Geri Gazette*. 1986;1:1–4.
12. National Association of Professional Geriatric Care Managers. GCM *Directory of Members*. Tucson, AZ: National Association of Professional Geriatric Care Managers; 1999.

■ WEBSITES

- Brookdale Center for Aging and Longevity of Hunter College/CUNY—www.hunter.cuny.edu/ce/courses-and-registration/certificate-programs/copy_of_brookdale-careers-in-gerontology
- Kaplan University—www.kaplanonlineprograms.com
- Misericordia University—www.misericordia.edu
- San Francisco State University—http://socwork.sfsu.edu/pdfs/gero/program_overview.pdf
- University of Florida—http://gcm.dce.ufl.edu
- University of Utah—http://nursing.utah.edu/gerontology/index.html
- University of Wisconsin—www.dcs.wisc.edu/classes/aging.htm
- Virginia Commonwealth University—www.sahp.vcu.edu/gerontology

Chapter 2

Ethics and Geriatric Care Management

Cathy Jo Cress

What is ethics? Ethics is a process of studying ourselves and our behavior, according to Nancy Alexander, a geriatric care manager (GCM), social worker, and attorney who has written much on ethics and geriatric care management.[1] According to John Banja, a noted writer on ethics and case management, the word *ethics* derives from the Greek *ethikos*. Banja says that the word *ethikos* means character; for people like Plato and Aristotle, an ethical person had a good character and many virtues.[2]

This idea of virtues had a renaissance in William B. Bennett's best-selling book, *The Book of Virtues: A Treasury of Good Moral Stories*.[2] Banja notes that to the Greeks, being ethical was not difficult. The Greeks simply assumed that a person of good character would make ethical decisions because he or she knew right from wrong. When tough ethical decisions had to be made, Aristotle simply suggested that a group of reasonable and upstanding people decide together. Banja notes that Aristotle believed this process was as good as any decision-making process because deciding what is moral and traversing dilemmas along the way are so complex that there are no simple rules to follow.[2]

Aristotle and the Greeks did not make the process of discovering the ethical choice overly complex. There were no rigid formulas to give one the correct answer. In fact, even today, knowing the right behavior is relatively easy because this knowledge is so embedded in our societal understanding of the right path. We know the basics: we must pay our debts, be good parents, be honest, be respectful, and so forth. How do we know these basic truths? Some would hold, as Banja points out, that God or another creator imprinted these truths on our souls.[2] Banja then shows us another possible source.

Banja uses Edgar Schein's theories on organizational behavior to explain another way of learning basic truths.[2] Schein says that we first learn moral rules as young people because we are born into a system of ethics. We are taught this system by our parents and the institutions we are a part of (e.g., synagogues, churches, schools, communities). When we become a member of a group, we must then adapt to the external reality the group confronts. Groups then go through a second step, according to Schein's theory. That second step is to integrate their internal operations. This is done through role definition. In the family group, for example, one role is that of mother; in a university, professor; in geriatric care management, GCM.

Here is where morality or the right or wrong of an action comes in. Those who have a certain role within a group (e.g., a mother in the family group, a GCM in the field of geriatric care management) must act consistently in a manner that the group deems acceptable for a person in that role. Persons who have these roles must set aside their own beliefs and be socially responsible to the group and carry out their obligations to the group. Individuals who fail may be penalized by the group.

For instance, consider a young mother who gives in to her need to enjoy herself and leaves her children unattended while she goes out to a bar. She is reprimanded either by society or a group, perhaps by being arrested for child abandonment. She has exposed her children to harm and neglected her obligation as a mother to her family. Even though she has a desire for pleasure and happiness, which is natural and generally acceptable to most people, she does not act morally according to society's concept of harm and duty to the family. So, being a mother means that one has to act in a socially responsible way as defined by the group, setting one's other needs aside if they conflict with the group's expectations.

A GCM must be socially responsible to the group of GCMs and carry out the obligations of the GCM group as defined by the field's professional organizations, the Case Management Society of America (CMSA) and the National Association of Professional Geriatric Care Managers. For example, this means following the association's "Pledge of Ethics" (Exhibit 2–1).[3] The pledge states, among other things, that GCMs should always make referrals in the client's interest, not in the GCM's own interest. For example, if a GCM has a business relationship with a local physician, the GCM might be tempted to refer all clients to that physician to gain reciprocal business referrals from the physician, despite the facts that the physician may not offer appropriate services for every client and that clients should be offered multiple healthcare choices. In this situation, by referring all clients to this physician, the GCM has not set aside personal interests and has not put the client's interests first. This GCM also has ignored the obligation to be fair and do no harm to clients, an obligation codified by CMSA and the National Asso-

ciation of Professional Geriatric Care Managers. This GCM has violated the GCM Pledge of Ethics, which states:

> I will only refer you to services and organizations I believe to be appropriate and of good quality. I will fully explain to you any business relationship I have with any service I propose, and give you information on alternatives, if at all possible, so that you, or a person designated to act for you, can make an informed decision to accept or reject services recommended to you.[1]

Out of this theory of group ethics, we can see how ethical concepts such as goodness, harm, risk, and benefit emerge in a group. All groups develop an understanding of these ideas to help the group survive. We all have our own desires for pleasure or self-gain. However, to act morally in a group, we must go along with the group's understanding of the concepts of harm, benefit, duty, justice, and fairness. These become the rules of the group, and belonging to a group means complying with the group's rules or code of morality. The rules also involve policies, vocabulary, and a system of enforcement within the group. Rules are learned not only when a person joins a group, but also from the time of infancy during the normal socialization process.[2]

Banja points out that the case manager receives a code of moral concepts made up by his or her profession or group.[2] As part of the field of case management, GCMs also follow a professional moral code. For example, as mentioned earlier, GCMs must avoid conflicts of interest. If a conflict exists, the GCM must disclose the conflict to the interested party.[1] GCMs who refer clients to home health agencies in which the GCMs have financial interests violate the GCM code of ethics. The GCM must disclose that interest to the client.

A third step in Schein's theory of learning moral rules then comes up. Banja says that we learn moral rules through basic assumptions taught to us by a group. These basic assumptions both drive the system and explain its morality. He reasons that these assumptions

Exhibit 2–1   Pledge of Ethics for Members of the National Association of Professional Geriatric Care Managers

---

Provisions of Service

I will provide ongoing service to you only after I have assessed your needs and you, or a person designated to act for you, understand and agree to a plan of service, the results that may be expected from it, and the cost of service.

Self-Determination

I will base my plan of service on goals you, or a person designated to act for you, have defined, and which enhance the decisions you have made concerning your life.

Cooperation

I will strive to ensure cooperation between all of the individuals involved in providing service and care to you.

Referrals/Disclosure

I will refer you only to services and organizations I believe to be appropriate and of good quality. I will fully explain to you any business relationship I have with any service I propose, and give you information on alternatives, if at all possible, so that you, or a person designated to act for you, can make an informed decision to accept or reject the services I recommend to you.

Termination of Service

I will end service to you only after reasonable notice. I will recommend a plan for you to continue to receive the services as needed.

Confidentiality

I will hold in trust any confidence you give me, disclosing information to others only with your permission, or if I am compelled to do so by a belief that you will be seriously harmed by my silence, or if the laws of this state require me to do so.

Substitute Judgment

I will not substitute my judgment for yours unless I am acting in the role of your guardian, appointed by a Court of Law, or with your approval, or the approval of someone designated to act for you.

Loyalty

My first duty is loyalty to you. I will always provide services based on your best interest, even if this conflicts with my interests or the interests of others.

Qualifications

I am fully qualified in my profession to provide the services I undertake. I continue to improve my skills and knowledge by participating in professional development programs and maintaining certification and licensing in my profession.

Discrimination

I will not promote or sanction any form of discrimination.

Source: Reprinted with permission from: Pledge of ethics for members of the National Association of Professional Geriatric Care Managers. *GCM J.* 1999;9(4):4–5. ©1999, National Association of Geriatric Care Managers.

---

tell people when they have to do certain things in a group and what justifies that behavior. Basic assumptions begin to show us the group's policies, beliefs, and practices. These group tenets reveal the group's moral concepts. When we begin to look into this morality, we also look at whether the group's moral system is defensible or acceptable. We then enter the realm of ethics.[2]

Beauchamp and Childress, in their classic *Principles of Biomedical Ethics,* propose that there are four accepted guides to making ethical decisions: beneficence, nonmaleficence, justice, and autonomy (Exhibit 2–2).[4]

The four principles defined by Beauchamp and Childress are the moral principles accepted as guides in the medical field, and they can also be applied to geriatric care management. These are the basic assumptions referred to by Banja. These principles are in balance with each other, and no principle supersedes another. GCMs try to adhere to these principles. They sometimes have difficulty when they are unsure which principle applies or when one principle collides with another.[5] Here we are entering the world of ethical probing and ethical dilemmas.

■ WHAT IS AN ETHICAL DILEMMA?

Banja defines morality as a group's moral code—its policies and its understanding of right and wrong. Ethics, as Banja says, is a major step beyond morals.[2] Ethics considers whether a group's moral beliefs are defensible, coherent, factual, honorable, and fair.

If we are to accept Beauchamp and Childress's four tenets, how do we apply them to a society with limited resources?[2] For instance, if beneficence, or doing the greatest good for all older people, is a goal, why does Medicare not cover home care? We know that one answer given by the federal government is that having Medicare fund home care might damage the federal budget. This is an ethical dilemma. How does one choose between preserving government funds and helping older people?

Another example of an ethical dilemma might be the conflict between a legal mandate and a basic GCM assumption such as the autonomy of an older person. An older woman, for instance, might be having mem-

ory problems, forgetting to take her medications, and burning pots by forgetting to turn off the stove. Such behavior may lead her family members to believe that she can no longer care for herself and that a conservator may need to be appointed. Here an ethical dilemma concerning surrogate decision making might arise. GCMs believe in the basic assumption of autonomy, respecting a person's freedom. However, if the woman's safety or health is compromised by her poor decisions and unsafe actions, should her freedom be curtailed through conservatorship? Is she no longer legally competent—capable of making decisions, understanding, and acting reasonably? The GCM can take a step in solving this dilemma by obtaining the family's and the woman's permission to do a mental competency exam.

In a survey of 251 case managers in 10 states, Rosalie Kane and Arthur Caplan uncovered other ethical dilemmas case managers regularly encounter.[6] Case managers' dilemmas included the following:

- Case managers overwhelmingly agreed that case managers should ensure that clients receive all possible services. But at the same time, the case managers agreed almost as strongly that they should be responsible for seeing that taxpayers' money is well spent. This creates an ongoing ethical dilemma: it is difficult to both restrict costs and provide all the services necessary.
- Case managers believed that family members should care for their older relatives. Yet at the same time, case managers supported the idea that if older people want to keep family members out of their business, they have the right to do so.
- Case managers believed that a client should have the right to die at home. But at the same time, the case managers felt that if the agency could not arrange

Exhibit 2–2
Principles of Biomedical Ethics

- Autonomy: Respecting the client's worth
- Nonmaleficence: Refraining from harm
- Beneficence: Advancing an individual's benefit
- Justice: Acting in fairness and equitably giving clients the services they need

enough services for the client to be safe in the home, the agency should withdraw services altogether, perhaps resulting in the client being forced into an institution and not being able to die at home.

Other types of ethical dilemmas described by Kane and Caplan are discussed below.

Here is a more detailed account of one GCM's ethical dilemma. Mary, a GCM, contracts with a senior housing complex to do geriatric assessments. Her employer, Pleasant Gardens, wants her to do a geriatric assessment on a particular resident. Pleasant Gardens has a rule that if a resident scores a 7 or higher on the mental status quotient (MSQ) exam section of the geriatric assessment, the resident is deemed too confused to live independently and is asked to move. Mary knows this. Mary also knows that when the resident's unit is rented again to another client, Pleasant Gardens receives triple the current rent because housing for older people is in great demand.

Eighty-eight-year-old resident Becca Virden's neighbors state that they have seen her putting silverware in the clothes washing machine, that there is spoiled food in her refrigerator, and that she sometimes wears two dresses at the same time. Mary conducts the geriatric assessment. Becca scores higher than a 7 on the MSQ section. There is some spoiled food in the refrigerator, but Becca has limited vision and may not have been able to see the spoilage. She was not wearing two dresses during the assessment, but her clothes, although clean, are worn and shoddy compared to those of her neighbors, who are obviously more affluent than Becca is. Becca says that she does

not want to move out of her apartment where she has lived for 10 years, and she tells Mary that she is terrified to go into a nursing home. She also says that the neighbors who have moved into the complex in the last few years are "hoity-toity," or above her class, and don't like her because she uses common language and was never well-to-do or a "ladies luncheon" person.

Here an ethical dilemma arises. Should Mary tell the Pleasant Gardens staff that Becca has an MSQ score high enough for her to be evicted from her unit, which would almost surely cause her to end up in a nursing home? Mary has contracted with Pleasant Gardens as a consultant, so she is not obligated to report the MSQ score to the Pleasant Gardens staff. Is there anything wrong when a GCM's assessment causes an older person to be forced to move out of her residence, given that the move is certainly in the senior housing facility's fiscal interest? Does the fact that Mary is paid by Pleasant Gardens force her to disclose everything about a resident's assessment? If Pleasant Gardens finds out Mary did not reveal information, could the facility sue her? Before doing the assessment, should Mary have told Becca that she could not promise confidentiality of the results?

If Mary reveals information that results in Becca being moved, will Mary be violating her responsibility as a GCM to always safeguard the best interests of the client? Mary must ask herself who her client is, Becca or Pleasant Gardens? Is Mary inherently unethical if she does not disclose to Becca before the assessment that she works for Pleasant Gardens? Mary now faces the ultimate conundrum. She has been hired, as Banja says, to serve two masters—her employer and her client.[2]

A Collision of Moral Systems

Two different GCMs could easily make totally different decisions about Mary's ethical dilemma. Both individuals might believe that their analysis of the situation is objective and that they have found the ethical answer. Being ethical simply means considering a situation and deciding what response is correct.

This is why, Banja says, we run into ethical dilemmas. If a person's actions are called into question by multiple parties and the ethics of the person's decision is debated, each debating party can reach a different conclusion, with an excellent supporting argument. For example, in ethical dilemmas about such charged issues as physician-assisted suicide and abortion, each side can give fine reasons to justify its position. Each side believes that it has the "most right position," as Banja says.[2(p45)] Each side is calling on its own moral system, which it believes to be superior. These types of unresolved dilemmas usually involve the collision of two moral systems.

For example, a young woman who is unmarried and pregnant might see both a counselor at a women's health clinic and a counselor at a right-to-life clinic to help her decide whether to terminate the pregnancy. Both counselors will give the young woman advice according to their own moral principles. The right-to-life counselor might advise the young woman to carry out the pregnancy, advice based on the counselor's highest religious principles. The woman's health counselor might give the young woman the option of carrying out the pregnancy and the option of a legal abortion, based on the counselor's belief in a woman's freedom of choice. Both counselors would believe that their advice was justified and moral.

▪ ETHICAL CONFLICTS BETWEEN THE CLIENT'S NEEDS AND THE CLIENT'S WANTS

As this chapter has already made clear, GCMs encounter many ethical conflicts. Frequently, these revolve around the lack of harmony between what the client needs and what the client wants. In an analysis of the study done on the ethics of home care and case managers, Kane and Caplan refer to this tension.[6] In the study, case managers pointed out the ethical dilemma encountered when the client chooses to do something that the case manager does not feel is healthy, given the client's condition. An example of this is an older woman who is depressed and who is prescribed the drug Zoloft (sertraline), with the specific instruction not to drink alcohol. Despite the warning, the older woman drinks three glasses of wine a day, two before dinner and one with dinner. She never appears drunk or acts inappropriately. Her family hires a GCM to assess her for depression. The GCM knows that the excess alcohol intake might contribute to her depression. The GCM's assessment mentions the need to help the client stop consuming alcohol.

The woman is mentally competent and not under the legal authority of a conservator. She states that she enjoys the wine and is not going to stop drinking it every night. The GCM is then caught between the client's assessed need and the client's right to choose what to do. This kind of tension often frustrates GCMs.

CASE STUDIES

Here are two detailed examples of GCMs facing the conflict between client needs and client wants. John Powers is an 81-year-old colonel and a former aeronautical engineer who worked on many famous US missile systems before retiring because he had Parkinson's disease. He is an attractive, dignified, and mentally competent older man who enjoys the company of his female caregivers, who are there 24 hours a day. He has reached a stage in his Parkinson's where he has several falls a month. Although the private caregivers use transfer belts and do standby assistance at all times, they occasionally must leave him to go to the bathroom or do something else outside his room. When the caregivers are out of the room, John often gets up by himself. He refuses to wear headgear to protect his head from the falls that result from his Parkinson's. He says that he is still in charge of his life and does not want to be restrained in any way or wear anything as unattractive as a helmet.

He is visited weekly by a GCM (who is also a registered nurse [RN]), and she is quite frustrated. She has assessed his need to be protected from falls but is sympathetic to his refusal to wear the headgear. She understands his desire to preserve his dignity and be independent. He is mentally competent and has no appointed conservator, so he has the choice to refuse the restraints and helmet, and his family refuses to force the issue. The GCM is experiencing a dilemma because the client's desires conflict with her assessment of his physical needs.

Alice Manges is a 79-year-old woman who has a gastrointestinal tube inserted in her stomach. She had throat cancer and after the operation could not eat solid foods or drink liquids. She has 24-hour care, and the caregivers are monitored and supervised by both a GCM who is a social worker and a GCM who is an RN. Alice, the GCMs discover, is an alcoholic who had been very protected by her husband, a respected judge in the community. He recently died. The couple have no children, and her nephew is in charge of her care but lives far away. The RN GCM assesses Alice in the beginning of the case and creates a care plan that says to bring no alcohol into the home and to not let Alice drink. Alice is mentally competent, has no conservator and, when given an MSQ, scores perfectly. The care providers start to report

that Alice has a cleaning person bring wine into the house every week. In addition, they report that Alice is drinking the wine through her feeding tube. When the social worker GCM discovers this, she orders the care providers to discard the alcohol. Alice calls her attorney and her trust officer. The attorney reviews the situation and says that Alice is mentally clear, not in need of a conservator, and has the right to drink alcohol even if it may damage her health. The nephew reluctantly agrees, as does the trust officer. Both the RN GCM and the social worker GCM are caught between the client's choice of lifestyle and the client's health needs.

■ THE ETHICAL CONFLICT REGARDING CLIENT EXPLOITATION

Another dilemma mentioned in Kane and Caplan's study is the ethical conflict case managers experience if their clients are associating with individuals who could exploit the clients.[6] Older people who are lonely often end up in new relationships, frequently with members of the opposite sex, because many older people are widowed or divorced. However, these new relationships can alarm case managers and family members if it seems like the new companion might take advantage of the older person by getting cash or having their name added to the older person's will. If the older person is competent, how can the case manager address this dilemma?

CASE STUDY

Emily Jones is a 78-year-old woman who has been married to an alcoholic 82-year-old man for 20 years. This is her second marriage. She is a very attractive older woman who has retained her figure, loves to dress beautifully, and she always looks attractive. Harold Jones, her husband, was well-to-do when they first married, but Emily's extravagant lifestyle and Harold's alcoholism have severely diminished their finances. They have been friends with another couple, Tommy and Heidi Smith, for 15 years. Tommy always flirted with Emily, but it was socially acceptable among the couples and never led to anything more.

Heidi died after a long illness, and Tommy moved 50 miles away but always kept in touch with Emily and Harold because he was very lonely and distraught over the death of his wife of 44 years. Over a 5-year period, a relationship started between Emily and Tommy. They have lunch together frequently, at Emily's instigation and without Harold's knowledge, and are obviously increasingly attracted to each other. Harold's alcoholism causes him to act inappropriately in social situations. Emily has been thinking of leaving Harold for Tommy. One night at a party following a bar mitzvah, Harold acts very inappropriately after drinking. Angry, Emily moves out to a friend's house that evening. However, her real reason for leaving is her attraction to Tommy.

Eventually, Emily moves in with Tommy. She is impoverished because she and Harold had little money, and now she has only her meager Social Security income. Tommy pays all the bills, and his adult children are angry, viewing Emily as a "money grubber." Eventually, Emily talks Tommy into letting her live in his house if he should die, and then when she dies the house will go to his children. Tommy changes his will to this effect. Tommy's children are incensed and tell Tommy they do not approve. Tommy refuses to cooperate,

saying he loves Emily and wants her to have a place to live until she dies. The children believe that Tommy is being exploited and want to force him to make Emily move out and change his will again. They want to move him to the home of one of his children who lives 500 miles away to get him away from Emily. Because Tommy is in his eighties, they feel he will eventually give in to their wishes. They have also talked to Emily's children, who feel bad about the situation and are willing to take her in.

Tommy's children's attorney advises them to get an assessment from a GCM, and the children call in a local GCM. After assessing the situation, the GCM concludes that Emily has influenced Tommy to change his will. The GCM states in her assessment that Emily has been exploitive in this relationship and has influenced Tommy to change his will to her benefit. Tommy's loneliness after his wife's death made him more open to Emily's flirtations. However, the GCM assesses Tommy's mental status and finds him fully competent, with the right to make this choice, even if his children disapprove. The GCM advises the children not to move him at this time. She, however, encourages further assessment if his will is changed again. So, as Kane and Caplan's study points out, the GCM is left with an ethical dilemma between the client's wants and the client's needs.[6] The client is associating with an exploitive person but, in this case at least, has the right to continue the association.

■ CONFLICT BETWEEN THE CLIENT'S SAFETY AND THE CLIENT'S AUTONOMY

Another type of ethical dilemma discussed by Kane and Caplan involves case managers with clients who live a life that involves high risk.[5]

An example of this is older men or women who insist on driving even though they have compromised eyesight, limited response times, or confusion. Does a person's right to be independent supersede his or her safety or the public's safety? If the person has passed a driver's test, what can a case manager do?

■ CONFLICTS AROUND CONFIDENTIALITY AND DISCLOSURE

Kane and Caplan's study also found that case managers experienced ethical conflicts around the issues of confidentiality and disclosure. The largest group of respondents (22%) reported having conflicts over what to disclose to family members. The second-largest group (17%) reported having conflicts over what to disclose to agency providers. More than 50% of those GCMs who reported having conflicts over confidentiality stated that they used their judgment to resolve what to disclose and to whom.[6] The conflict that the GCM Mary experienced with regard to her client Becca, discussed earlier, was partly a conflict involving confidentiality and disclosure. Another example of this type of conflict follows.

CASE STUDY

The White family daughters hired a GCM to do a geriatric assessment of their mother, Blanche. Blanche lived with one son and his wife, whom the other family members suspected of physically abusing, overmedicating, and intimidating their mother. In doing the assessment, the GCM found evidence of potential physical and medication abuse, which warranted turning the situation in to Adult Protective Services (APS). However, the GCM knew that APS was so underfunded and understaffed that it might not do anything about the situation immediately, although by law it would make an investigative visit, which would tip off the son and his wife to the problems uncovered.

The geriatric assessment confirmed the children's fear that the son and his wife were physically abusing the mother and overmedicating her. The other children decided to send their mother to stay with her daughter in Atlanta. One daughter who lived near the son planned to take Blanche out for a supposed day trip and would actually put her on a plane to Atlanta to go live with the sister, who would implement all the GCM's suggestions. These suggestions included a medication review by a geriatric RN, a possible reduction of medication, and attendance at an adult day care program for additional socialization. The family members did not want to tell the brother with whom the mother lived because they feared he would stop them and might harm the mother.

The GCM was in a ethical dilemma. The family members did not want her to report the case to APS until they got their mother on the plane to Atlanta. The GCM worked for the family. However, by law the GCM was obligated to report the case to APS, even though she knew it might stop the plans to get the mother away from the abusive son. The GCM had a conflict about confidentiality involving what to disclose to an agency.

■ ANALYZING ETHICAL DILEMMAS

Patricia Burbank provides one framework for analyzing ethical problems (Exhibit 2–3). Burbank suggests many avenues to help in ethical decision making and states that analysis does not have to be done in isolation. Among her suggestions is using ethics review boards in institutions because they are there to help health professionals resolve ethical dilemmas. If this option is not possible, she suggests team conferences that include all the parties involved

Exhibit 2–3   Analyzing Ethical Problems

1. Review the situation.
   - What health problems exist?
   - What decisions need to be made?
   - Which components are ethical and which are based on scientific knowledge?
2. Gather additional information necessary to make a decision.
3. What are relevant ethical principles?
   - What are the historical, philosophical, and religious bases for each of the principles?
4. What are your values and beliefs?
   - From your family and other personal experience?
   - From your professional code of ethics?
5. What are the values and beliefs of others in the situation?

6. What are the value conflicts in the situation?
7. Who is the best person to make the decision?
8. What is the fullest range of possible decisions and actions?
   - What are the implications or consequences of possible decisions and actions?
   - Do the possible decisions and actions and your professional code of ethics agree?
9. Decide on a course of action and take steps to implement it.
10. Evaluate the outcomes of the decisions and use this information for future decision making.

Source: Reprinted with permission from: Legal and ethical issues in health care of older adults. *GCM J.* 1999;9(4):28. © 1999, National Association of Professional Geriatric Care Managers.

in the dilemma. She also suggests reaching out to other professionals, while always respecting the confidentiality of the client.[5] GCMs could also use the National Association of Professional Geriatric Care Managers, CMSA, the National Association of Social Workers, or any other professional association with a code of ethics and an ethics committee (see Appendix A for contact information).[5]

E. Haavi Morreim proposes another possible method of ethical dilemma analysis.[7] He suggests that the first step is fact-finding. The GCM should seek the primary sources of information, not rely on secondhand information. The GCM should not make unwarranted assumptions or depend on other people's assumptions. Objectively gathering facts to discover basic problems is the first step in routine geriatric assessment. Therefore, it should be familiar to GCMs.

Morreim's second step is to identify all those whose interests and wishes might be affected by the results (e.g., family members, friends, other agencies, other professionals). The client is the GCM's highest responsibility, but Morreim says GCMs must uncover all the other players and then uncover all the values that are at stake (e.g., autonomy, justice, freedom).

The third step involves creative problem solving. Like the other steps in the process, creative problem solving is part of a GCM's basic skill set in geriatric assessment and general geriatric care management. Morreim advises GCMs to respect the important moral values in the problem and not only consider obvious options but try to devise creative new options.[7]

■ HOW TO RESOLVE ETHICAL DILEMMAS

Resolving ethical dilemmas is difficult at best. The body of literature on ethics and case or care management—a body of literature that grew considerably in the late 1990s—suggests several different pathways.

In Kane and Caplan's study, case managers who had ethical dilemmas with other case managers or agencies tended to resolve the conflict in various ways. Negotiation and compromise were used by 31% of the case managers responding to the survey. Ten percent mentioned overriding their providers and colleagues. Another 10% said they occasionally appealed to a higher authority and went over the head of the individual who caused difficulty. A strategy of winning the confidence of their providers and colleagues was used by only 6%. Kane and Caplan state that case managers sometimes assisted the client in finding another agency or simply refused to refer again to an organization or professional that caused a conflict. However, Kane and Caplan state that most case managers had a difficult time with the concept of blackballing.[6]

Sixty-eight percent, the largest percentage of case managers in the study, used discussion with their supervisors to solve ethical dilemmas. Because many GCMs operate as entrepreneurs and have no supervisors, GCMs might consider the second most common approach to resolving ethical dilemmas found in Kane and Caplan's study: discussion with colleagues. This method was used by 39% of case managers. Seventeen percent said they used care and case conferences, where professional care managers meet to discuss client problems and resolve ethical dilemmas.[6] If a GCM works for an agency or has many other GCMs in his or her own agency, this is an excellent avenue to consider.

Banja says that the process of resolving ethical dilemmas may reveal not only what to do but also what not to do.[2] He makes another interesting point: When resolving an ethical dilemma, both sides can become very emotional. The average person gets defensive, making all kinds of excuses when there is an allegation of error. A prominent flaw in the majority of the poor reasons used to justify a type of conduct is that the poor reasons rarely address the problems at hand. Instead, these reasons avoid the real issue and involve justifications for disregarding the real issue, causing the ethical dilemma.

■ CONCLUSION

As geriatric care management and case management evolve as professions, GCMs have a great opportunity to learn how to think ethically. GCMs have the codes of ethics of both the National Association of Professional Geriatric Care Managers and CMSA to govern their ethics and help with ethical dilemmas. Both associations also offer ethics committees to help clarify and resolve problems. Both associations have rules, disciplinary procedures, and penalties for breaking these codes. Membership in an association also gives GCMs access to colleagues with whom they can discuss ethical problems—just as the Greeks would have done. As Kane and Caplan's survey shows, professionals find many ways to resolve these interesting but painful ethical dilemmas.

■ REFERENCES

1. Alexander N. An international code of ethics for care/case managers. *GCM J.* 1999;4:6.

2. Banja J. Ethical decision making: origins, process, and applications to case management. *Case Manager.* 1999;9:41–42.

3. Brostoff PM. A short history of drafting the GCM Pledge of Ethics. *GCM J.* 1999;10:6.

4. Beauchamp T, Childress J. *Principles of Biomedical Ethics.* 4th ed. New York: Oxford University Press; 1994.

5. Burbank PM. Legal and ethical issues in health care of older adults. *GCM J.* 1999;27.

6. Kane R, Caplan AL. *Ethical Conflicts in the Management of Home Care: The Case Manager's Dilemma.* New York: Springer; 1993.

7. Morreim E. Ethical issues in care management: case studies in moral problem solving. *GCM J.* 1999;9.

PART 2

Geriatric Assessment, Planning and Care Monitoring

Chapter 3

Psychosocial Assessment

Carmen L. Morano and Barbara Morano

Psychosocial assessment along with the functional assessment (discussed in Chapter 4) provides the foundation for all the care management that follows. Combined, the functional and the psychosocial assessments are not only critical to developing a relevant and appropriate care plan, but in fact they provide an in-depth perspective of the older adult's quality of life.[1] The goals of clinicians and researchers alike have moved from focusing on how long a particular intervention can extend an older adult's life to a more holistic approach that recognizes the importance of increasing the quality of the older adult's life.[1] (See Chapter 10 for a more complete discussion on quality of life.) Within the fields of social work and care management there has also been a shift from focusing on assessing client deficits (impairment or disease) to a broader perspective that focuses on the strengths of clients and their family systems.

The knowledge gained from a comprehensive psychosocial assessment provides objective measurable information about the cognitive, social, psychological, spiritual, financial, and legal dimensions of the client system, as well as important subjective information about the entire client system's coping mechanisms and relationships. There is no one model or approach to completing a psychosocial assessment or even a unified consensus on what specific dimensions (cognitive,

psychological, financial, social, etc.) make up a comprehensive psychosocial assessment. The care manager must develop a psychosocial assessment that best meets the needs of the clients served, and one that helps to inform, guide, or contribute to making professional judgments about an appropriate care plan.[2] This chapter primarily focuses on the cognitive, psychological, economic, and social dimensions, as well as assessing the potential for substance abuse and elder maltreatment. Spiritual assessment is covered in Chapter 8.

"Underlying good care management is good assessment."[3] Although the psychosocial aspects of an assessment can be labeled the heart and soul of the comprehensive geriatric assessment, it is important that they represent dimensions of the assessment that can only be understood within the context of all other dimensions of a comprehensive assessment. The GCM takes a historical perspective that encompasses the individual, familial, and systemic perspectives. This understanding of the client's behavior, strengths, coping mechanisms, motivations, and the nature of relationships provides the foundation of the care plan. Once the assessment is completed, the care manager is able to engage the client more successfully as well as engage the entire client system in a collaborative working relationship.

The psychosocial assessment begins when a call is made to inquire about care management services for an older adult. Frequently this is precipitated by an unexpected trauma or crises (e.g., hospitalization, sudden behavioral change, accident). Consequently, most practice models start with a family assessment to obtain reliable information about the family system and to understand the problem more fully from the family perspective. During this initial call the care manager is inquiring about the reason for the call at this particular time, rather than at some previous time, and the rationale for who actually is making this call, rather than other family members, or even the older adult. The information obtained during this initial call or visit is valuable for developing an approach for the initial engagement of the older adult, as well as other family members who may be involved with the older adult.

Care management is unique in that there are frequently multiple clients, most notably spouses or life partners, adult children or step-children, and their spouses, nieces, nephews, and grandchildren. Any member of the entire client system, most frequently the older adult, can be resistant to engaging a care manager, yet alone agreeing to an intervention. This resistance can be a function of a general denial of the problem, anger at family interference, fear of the unknown, inability to cope with the situation, or losing control of one's self, family, or situation. By initiating the assessment process with the family, the care manager can understand who this client is within a larger familial context and how to appropriately manage potential resistance from the initial engagement, through the assessment, and ultimately during the intervention.

This chapter delineates the essential elements of the psychosocial assessment. A comprehensive psychosocial assessment is time consuming and involves inquiring about sensitive and personal information that for some families and cultures can be intrusive. There-fore, it is not uncommon to defer certain areas for subsequent visits when the care manager has established a relationship with the client and family members and can better gauge their comfort with some of the questions that will ultimately have to be asked. Because every care manager must initially assess for safety and risk factors in the client's day-to-day living situation, it is imperative that the cognitive, psychological, and support systems are assessed at the time of the first visit.

The demographic information gathered during the initial family meeting is required to complete an assessment fully. Although a standardized tool does not exist, the following information about the older adult must be obtained:

- Birth date and place
- Nationality/history of immigration
- Religion/affiliation/importance
- Siblings/alive/deceased/relationships/health
- Childhood
- Education
- Military history
- Marital history/significant others
- Offspring/birth order/relationship to parent(s) and each other/current living arrangement/availability
- Occupation
- Hobbies/interests
- Retirement

As the information about each of the family members is gathered, it can be used to construct a genogram. The authors suggest the use of a genogram (see Figure 3–1) to illustrate graphically who is part of the family system and each person's relationship to the identified client. Information about the age, health status, and relationship (good, strained, distant, etc.) to the identified client can be included in the genogram. This enhances the basic genogram that depicts connections members have to each other by providing a richer description of each of the members included.

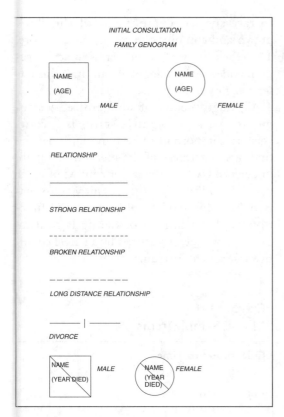

INITIAL CONSULTATION

FAMILY GENOGRAM

NAME
(AGE)

MALE

NAME
(AGE)

FEMALE

RELATIONSHIP

STRONG RELATIONSHIP

BROKEN RELATIONSHIP

LONG DISTANCE RELATIONSHIP

DIVORCE

NAME
(YEAR DIED)   MALE

NAME
(YEAR
DIED)   FEMALE

Figure 3–1   Genogram

■ COGNITIVE ASSESSMENT

Cognitive assessment is an integral part of detecting dementia.[4] Because the incidence and prevalence of dementing disorders increases in later life, it is necessary to assess the older adult's cognitive status to determine whether the current living arrangement is appropriate and safe. Research has shown the failure of physicians to perform mental status testing routinely on older patients;[5] therefore, it is wise not to assume a cognitive assessment has been done. In situations when cognitive assessment has reportedly been done by a primary physician, it is important to understand that many of those with cognitive impairment can behave in a socially appropriate manner, and they are therefore not recognized as having any impairment without for-

mal testing. Conversely, there are also situations where cognitive status has been accurately assessed with a diagnosis of mild to moderate dementia, yet the client can demonstrate the capacity to make appropriate decisions within their home or other familiar environment.

Assessment for mental capacity can be accomplished through both an unstructured and structured process using one or more screening tests. An unstructured form of cognitive assessment occurs throughout the entire evaluation process. Based on information provided by a family member, the care manager can ask the older adult many of the same questions initially asked of the family as a way to informally gauge memory and recall. Other informal ways to test memory include the following:

- Asking the older adult to perform a task that requires multiple and sequential steps (e.g., requesting a cold drink, necessitating sequential tasks of asking what drink is preferred, going to the kitchen, retrieving a glass)
- Asking the older adult to identify people in family photos
- Carrying on an informal conversation with the older adult using a few of the factual types of questions being asked at different times during the course of the interview and listening for inconsistencies in responses

Sometimes the most informative assessment could simply be to ask the older adult for an assessment of his or her own cognitive functioning. Regardless of the approach to the cognitive assessment, understanding the older adult's perception of his or her own functioning is especially informative to both the assessment and care plan. A lack of self-awareness or denial of a cognitive problem must be addressed when the care plan is developed and implementation strategies explored with the family.

Indirect assessment can also be completed by conversing with a family member or other close contact. Family members can provide useful information in this process because they have the historical context of change over time. "The caregiver is able to provide information regarding the mode of onset of cognitive dysfunction (abrupt vs. gradual), progression of symptoms (stepwise vs. continuous), and duration of symptoms."[4]

The most commonly used and most thoroughly researched formal screening test for dementia is the Mini Mental State Examination (MMSE) (Exhibit 3–1) developed by Folstein and colleagues.[6] Concentration, language, orientation, memory, and attention are tested in this short, usually 10-minute, 30-question test. A score of 23 or lower out of a possible 30 has been defined as indicating cognitive impairment. Shortcomings of the test include a wide variation of scoring and test administration styles, as well as inappropriateness for those with physical disability, sensory impairment, and poor command of the English language.

The Short Portable Mental Status Questionnaire (Exhibit 3–2) asks 10 questions with each error scored as 1 point.[7] Intact mental function is indicated by less than 2 errors, and severe mental impairment is indicated by 8 to 10 errors. The scoring is adjusted for educational level.

The Blessed Orientation-Memory-Concentration Test consists of all verbal questions, takes 3 to 6 minutes to administer, counts errors, and has a maximum score of 28, with a score of 10 indicating dementia.[8]

The Clock Drawing Test measures multiple cognitive and motor functions through a clock-drawing task.[9] The individual is given a piece of paper with a 4- to 6-inch circle drawn on it and is asked to write the numbers and draw the hands of the clock to show "10 past 11." Although many clinicians use a qualitative evaluation, there are scales to rank the drawing for completeness and correctness or to rate specific components of the clock drawn and combine the ratings into a score. The clock-drawing interpretation scale recommended by Mendez et al. falls into this latter category.

Although the use of standardized instruments to assess cognitive status is encouraged, it is important to keep in mind that the findings, regardless of the measure used, are understood within the larger context of older person's ability to process cognitive information. The ability of the older person to function safely within his or her daily routine cannot always be measured by a single cognitive assessment instrument.

Exhibit 3–1
MMSE Sample Items

Orientation to Time
"What is the date?"

Registration
"Listen carefully. I am going to say three words. You say them back after I stop.

Ready? Here they are . . .

APPLE (pause), PENNY (pause), TABLE (pause). Now repeat those words back to me." [Repeat up to 5 times, but score only the first trial.]

Naming
"What is this?" [Point to a pencil or pen.]

Reading
"Please read this and do what it says." [Show examinee the words on the stimulus form.]
CLOSE YOUR EYES

Source: Reproduced by special permission of the Publisher, Psychological Assessment Resources, Inc., 16204 North Florida Avenue, Lutz, Florida 33549, from the Mini Mental State Examination, by Marshal Folstein and Susan Folstein. Copyright 1975, 1998, 2001 by Mini Mental LLC, Inc. Published 2001 by Psychological Assessment Resources, Inc. Further reproduction is prohibited without permission of PAR, Inc. The MMSE can be purchased from PAR, Inc. by calling (813) 968-3003.

Exhibit 3–2 The Short Portable Mental Status Questionnaire (SPMSQ)

Scoring: Count the number of correct and incorrect responses.

Question	Correct Responses	Incorrect Responses
1. What are the date, month, and year?		
2. What is the day of the week?		
3. What is the name of this place?		
4. What is your phone number?		
5. How old are you?		
6. When were you born?		
7. Who is the current president?		
8. Who was the president before him?		
9. What was your mother's maiden name?		
10. Can you count backward from 20 by 3s?		

SCORING

0–2 errors: normal mental functioning
3–4 errors: mild cognitive impairment
5–7 errors: moderate cognitive impairment
8 or more errors: severe cognitive impairment

*One more error is allowed in the scoring if a patient has had a grade school education or less.
*One less error is allowed if the patient has had education beyond the high school level.

Source: Pfeiffer E. A short portable mental status questionnaire for the assessment of organic brain deficit in elderly patients. *J Am Geriatr Soc.* 1975;Oct. 23(10):433–441.

■ PSYCHOLOGICAL ASSESSMENT

Older adults are hesitant to discuss psychological problems because of a fear of being labeled as crazy, or because it may be perceived as a sign of weakness, or something to be ashamed of.[5] With numerous somatic or physical complaints, it is not uncommon for both the older adult and family to deny a diagnosis of depression. Frequently, sadness or anxiety is attributed to normal aging and/or illness. The care manager is in a good position to differentially assess psychological compromise from personality traits or cognitive decline.

Through the building of an ongoing and trusting relationship with the geriatric care manager, the older adult may become more comfortable discussing personal problems and fears. Additionally, over time the care manager can assess the older adult's psychological functioning by observing him or her in different circumstances, performing various tasks, and relating to family, friends, and other professionals. Although standardized measures are valuable screening tools, they are not the definitive assessment, but rather they are used in conjunction with direct observation and interviews with the older adult and support system.[10]

Depression

Depression is significantly underdiagnosed and undertreated in older adults.[11] Yet, of every 100,000 people ages 65 and older, 14.2 died by suicide, and 48 per 100,000 of white non-Hispanic men committed suicide. This is compared to only 10.9 per 100,000 in general population.[12] Given that older adults represent approximately 13% of the general population but account for 18% of deaths resulting from suicide, the underdiagnosing and underreporting are especially problematic.[13] It can affect performance on mental status tests and should be considered when cognitive impairment is suspected. As discussed by Gallo and Wittink:

> The person with the appearance of cognitive impairment secondary to depression remains oriented and with coaxing can perform cognitive tests. Clues that dementia may be secondary to depression include recent onset and rapid progression, a family history of depressive disorders, a personal history of affective disorders, and onset of the disorder after the age of 60 years.[12(p157)]

The Geriatric Depression Scale (GDS) designed by Yesavage[15] was the first depression assessment scale explicitly for older adults and remains widely used because of its simplicity. The GDS is a 30-question survey that includes yes-or-no questions. A point is given for each answer that matches the answer in parentheses. A score of 10 or more usually suggests depression.

The Beck Depression Inventory is a 21-item self-rating report that assesses symptoms of depression and includes a broad range of questions.[16] Individual questions are scored as 0, 1, 2, or 3. A total score of greater than 11 is indicative of depression. This scale relies heavily on physical symptoms, making it less useful for older adults with physical impairment. It is also difficult to use with those who have cognitive impairment and those with communication and hearing problems.

The PHQ-9 (Spitzer et al., 1999) is a nine-item instrument that is both brief and easy to use. Clients are asked a series of questions preceded by "How many days during the past 2 weeks...." Sample questions include: *Have you had little interest? Have you been down, depressed, or hopeless?* The scoring is; 0 = no days, 1 = several days, 2 = more than half the time, and 3 = nearly all the days. A response of "several days" or "more than half the time" in more than five questions is suggestive of needing treatment for depression. In addition to the brevity of this nine-item scale, the first two items can be used as a screen for suicidal ideation. This measure has also been used to objectively assess improvement or lack of improvement resulting from treatment. The complete instrument and scoring is available at www.depression-primarycare.org

Anxiety

With community-living older adults, generalized anxiety, more commonly stated as worry, is the most frequently encountered disorder—it is even more prevalent than depression.[17] Anxiety and depression coexist and can overlap in older adults with symptoms stated as sleeplessness or fatigue. Other symptoms of anxiety can include fear, nervousness, dread, shortness of breath, and rapid heartbeat. All of these symptoms can be misdiagnosed as various medical conditions, such as cardiovascular problems, Parkinson's disease, Alzheimer's disease, or hormonal imbalances. Anxiety is easily confused with worry, which is an emotional reaction to health and safety concerns rather than a pathological response. Assessing an older adult's concerns during the assessment process is necessary to make this distinction.

The Beck Anxiety Inventory is a 21-item self-report questionnaire of common anxiety symptoms.[18] Respondents rate the intensity of each symptom as 0, 1, 2, or 3, with a score of 22 to 35 indicating moderate anxiety, and a score of more than 36 as severe. It should be noted that there are other anxiety instruments, none of which appear to be used that frequently by care managers.

■ SOCIAL SUPPORT

Social support as presented in the context of this chapter and text refers to both the formal and informal sources of support. Formal supports such as home health care, custodial care, case management, and day care among others, are supportive services that are either purchased by the client or reimbursed through a third-party source (e.g., Medicare,

Medicaid) or other local, state, or federal program. Informal support is provided by family members, extended kin, friends, or neighbors. Although this section focuses primarily on informal social support, the eco-map (see Figure 3–2) is an excellent tool that can be used to display all forms of social support, both informal and formal.

As illustrated in Figure 3–2, the eco-map can be used to display all supports, both formal and informal in a single document. The eco-map can be used to display supports that are in place at the time of the assessment, as well as additional supports that might be indicated

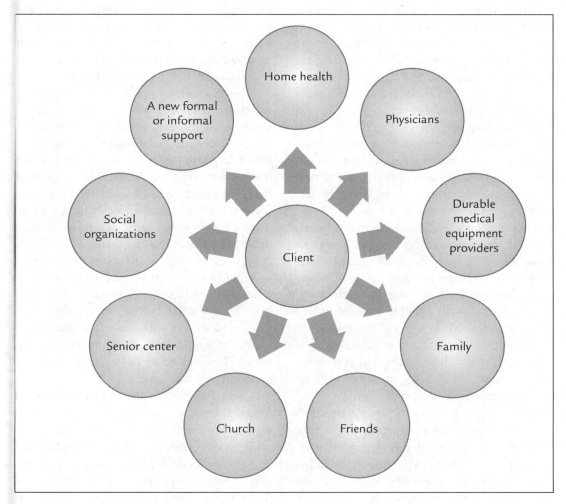

Figure 3–2   Eco-Map

as part of the care plan. Arrows can be unidirectional or bi-directional, as well as indicated if the interactions between the client and support is positive or negative. Together the genogram and eco-map provides tools that allow the care manager to illustrate important information about the members of the client's family system as well as current and future sources of formal and informal support. The process of conducting an assessment of formal and informal support provides important subjective and objective information that is critical to the development, and ultimately the success, of the care plan.

Approximately 80% of all support to older adults is provided on an informal basis by either an adult child or a spouse.[19] As previously discussed, assessing informal support begins with the very first call to the care manager. Most often, the initial call to the care manager comes from an adult child, frequently the older adult's daughter or daughter-in-law. Understanding why the call to the care manager is being made now as well why this particular person is making the call initiates the assessment of informal support. In addition to being concerned about a parent(s), this person is often already involved with providing informal support or coordinating formal support. In 2005, family members providing care to someone with a memory impairment provided on average 30 hours per week of care.[20] Many of the family systems working with a care manager will have both primary and secondary caregivers involved with providing varying levels of support. Thus, it is not surprising that those involved with providing support, especially to someone with cognitive impairment, can experience significant strain.[21,22]

Identifying all primary and secondary informal caregivers, perhaps starting with those represented in the genogram and then expanding to include other family, extended kin, friends, or neighbors who might be involved or have the potential to become involved, can be the starting point for assess-

ment of social support. As discussed previously, the genogram is a useful tool that depicts not only the relationship each family member has to the identified patient, but it can also be useful when assigning roles and responsibilities for the care plan.

Because the entire informal support system may not be present during the initial assessment, it is important to establish an accurate assessment of the motivation of both those present and involved as well as those who are not present but who might be involved. The assessment of social support should ultimately reflect an accurate picture of who makes up the informal support network, the nature of the relationships with the older person, and the capacity for serving as a source of support. Frequently, some of those who are most involved are also reported to have the most strained relationship with the older person.[23]

Some care managers use an informal, semistructured interviewing process to assess social support, whereas others, the authors included, use a combination of a semistructured interview along with one of the many standardized instruments that can measure informal support. The semistructured interview process can provide the care manager with valuable information about how individuals relate to each other as well as to the care manager, whereas a standardized instrument reports quantified information that can be used as an objective outcome to evaluate the effects of the intervention. Whatever format the care manager uses, the size of the network and the availability of assistance for the client, as well as the caregiver, should be assessed by the conclusion of the social support assessment.

A number of standardized instruments measure social support, but not in a uniform way. Some focus only on family members, some focus on both family and friends,[23] and still others focus only on the older person's perception of support.[21] The Lubben Social Support Scale uses a series of nine questions to assess the client's social support system, including family and friends.[24] This instrument can be used equally well with the client and the caregiver to provide a broad-based picture about the size of the support network and its availability to assist with care and decision making. Another formal assessment instrument is the Norbeck Social Support Questionnaire.[25] This scale has also been shown to have strong validity, and it has demonstrated its usefulness for measuring social support not only with caregivers but also for the clients themselves. The Norbeck subscales permit some determination of the areas in which a person perceives adequate social support and those areas in which the person perceives social support as lacking. As previously mentioned, in addition to assessing the availability of support, it is important to then measure the level of strain or burden that those involved with providing support might be experiencing.

Not all supportive relationships are positive relationships. In fact, overwhelming evidence shows that being a caregiver, especially a primary caregiver, can result in feelings of strain or burden,[26-28] and a growing body of evidence shows that some caregivers also report positive feelings or what is referred to as caregiver gain.[28,29] If there is evidence, or if the care manager has an intuitive feeling that a particular caregiver is at risk of becoming overwhelmed, it is advisable to assess the caregiver's level of burden. As with social support, a number of instruments can be used to assess the caregiver's burden and satisfaction. The Lawton Scale of Appraised Burden and Appraised Satisfaction,[30] the Caregiver Burden Inventory,[31] and the Caregiver Strain Index (CSI)[32] are just some of the multidimensional scales that can be used to measure strain. The CSI has 13 items that assess five dimensions or sources of strain (financial, physical, time, social, and employment). A positive response to more than seven indicates a need for a more focused assessment to determine the most appropriate intervention.

ELDER MISTREATMENT

The actual rate of elder mistreatment is probably much higher than is reported because secrecy and isolation, common in all forms of intimate abuse, prevent an accurate count. The National Elder Abuse Incidence Study calculated that for every case reported to Adult Protective Services (APS), five additional cases were known to community agencies.[33] Furthermore, less than one-half of reported cases are substantiated.[34] Elders are vulnerable to abuse and neglect because of a greater likelihood of suffering from physical and cognitive impairments and the resultant need to rely on caregivers and family members for basic physical care.[1]

For purposes of the psychosocial assessment, elder mistreatment is defined as physical, psychological or emotional, financial, or sexual abuse, as well as financial exploitation, use of undue influence, neglect, and self-neglect inflicted actively, passively, or unintentionally. All states have some form of protection and services for vulnerable older adults, yet at the time this chapter was being prepared, four states do not have mandatory reporting (Colorado, New Jersey, New York, and North Dakota).

As with other areas of psychosocial assessment, elder mistreatment can be assessed both formally and informally. The care manager is directly involved with the older adult and his or her caregiver and can assess mistreatment by direct observation, interview, or by report from others. An unexplainable sudden decline in the older adult's functional, cognitive, or psychological status can be an indicator of mistreatment. "The assessment of elder mistreatment begins when there is a suspicion that the elders' relationships are contributing to unnecessary suffering, or when elders hint at or directly report relationship problems."[33]

The instruments used to assess elder mistreatment are designed to assess the risk for abuse, cognitive ability, and functional status. The Elder Assessment Instrument developed by

Fulmer, Street, and Carr is a 46-item instrument that reviews signs, symptoms, and subjective complaints of elder abuse, neglect, exploitation, and abandonment.[35] There is no score, but this instrument is used as a guide for referral to APS if the following conditions exist:

1. If there is any evidence of mistreatment without sufficient clinical explanation
2. Whenever there is a subjective complaint by the elder of mistreatment
3. Whenever the clinician believes there is a high risk of or probable abuse, neglect, exploitation, or abandonment

■ ECONOMIC AND LEGAL ASSESSMENT

Developing an appropriate care plan requires an accurate picture of the older adult's economic status. If the care plan is not affordable, or a particular community-based service is not accessible or available, the plan is inappropriate. A thorough financial assessment helps to screen for risk of financial exploitation, the unintentional and perhaps inappropriate dissipation of assets, as well as to facilitate the access to future community-based or long-term-care services. Unfortunately, many older adults are uncomfortable or hesitant to disclose the particulars of their finances to their own children or to the care manager. It is not uncommon that the adult child or children will not have a clear picture of the older adult's financial status and are uncomfortable in broaching the subject.

A complete financial assessment needs to include an evaluation of income and assets, as well as health insurance and long-term care insurance. If the care manager senses any discomfort or resistance in this area, assessing the older adult's financial resources can be initiated by asking a few indirect questions to assess their openness to discussing this especially sensitive area. Questions such as, "Do you worry about your finances?" "Have you ever delayed getting a prescription filled?" "Do you have sufficient healthy foods?" can help initiate discussion about finances. Because many older adults are living on a fixed income, unexpected expenses, such as for additional medications, special nutritional supplements, or home care or day care, can be difficult to manage.

Although social security frequently represents a significant percentage of monthly income, income from retirement pensions, annuities, interest income, employment, and/or income from real estate must be accounted for. Information about the source of the income, as well as conditions attached to the income (taxable or tax free, time limited or for life, etc.), should also be obtained.

In addition to obtaining reliable information about income, it is important to include the older adult's assets as part of the financial assessment. Given the increased lifespan and years spent in retirement, what was once considered as adequate income and savings for retirement might turn out to be inadequate for meeting the older adult's future health and care needs. Additionally, most entitlement programs have specific income and asset qualifying limits. Therefore, just as with income, a complete and accurate assessment of assets must be obtained to determine the affordability of a care plan and also to determine eligibility for various entitlement programs. Accurate information about all assets (e.g., home, stocks, bonds, life insurance, property) must be accounted for. A referral to an elder law attorney or estate planner can be considered when there are considerable, or even reasonable, assets to plan for future care needs or to protect assets for a well spouse.

Many older adults, as well as their adult children, do not understand eligibility requirements for community-based entitlement programs and long-term care. False assumptions about what older adults are entitled to or not entitled to must be addressed. And although not every care management client will need to access an entitlement program, it is important that the care manager provides current and accurate information about any relevant entitlement programs and services. Care managers can use their knowledge of the various local programs and their expertise in navigating the bureaucracy to access these programs to increase the older adult's willingness to provide accurate information about finances.

In addition to income and assets, a comprehensive economic assessment should include an assessment of the older adult's insurance policies, including health, life, pharmaceutical, home, and long-term care insurance. It is especially important that the care manager confirm that all insurance policies are current and in effect, and that they represent adequate and practical coverage. For example, some long-term care policies have long waiting periods (elimination days), some as long as 90 days, before benefits can be accessed. Also, other restrictions can limit the policyholder's choice of provider, eligible diagnoses, or type of care.

A final dimension of the economic assessment includes an assessment of the older adult's legal affairs and advance directives (e.g., healthcare proxy, power of attorney, living will). This is another area in which the care manager is advised to confirm and verify the status of these documents. Although many older adults have some, or even all, of these documents, the documents may be outdated, not compliant with current law, executed in a state other than where the older adult is currently residing, or inappropriate as a result of the death or cognitive decline of the appointed agent. The care manager must be knowledgeable of the state's laws with respect to advance directives and must make an immediate referral to an appropriate elder law attorney to initiate or update these documents.

■ SUBSTANCE ABUSE

Substance abuse or dependence, including alcohol use, drug misuse, and nicotine use, can have severe negative physical, cognitive, and psychological consequences for the older adult. Screening for this is essential, not only

to detect the problem, but to identify potentially harmful interactions with other physical and mental conditions that could lead to high blood pressure, falls, or memory loss. Improper substance use can increase comorbidities and interfere in the treatment process, and therefore increase medical complexity.[36]

"Heavy drinking, even in the absence of abuse and dependence, can be detrimental to the care of older adults; however, moderate drinking may be associated with certain health benefits."[36(p176)] Having a clear definition of what constitutes problem drinking in the elderly is difficult, though. With younger adults, clear criteria are defined in the *Diagnostic and Statistical Manual of Mental Disorders,* including disruption of role function, financial instability, and decreasing social networks.[37] These criteria can be present in the older adult population at large without a substance abuse problem. Additionally, substance abuse problems are masked by other problems associated with aging, including falls, injury, confusion, self-neglect, depression, emotional liability, memory loss, sleep disturbance, and adverse drug interactions. Furthermore, an elder's tendency to use alcohol frequently or heavily is dismissed as "the only vice she has left" or "something to help him sleep."[1]

Even though the frequency of drinking and the amount consumed often declines with age, it is estimated that 49.4% of persons over the age of 65 drink alcohol at least on a semi-regular basis, compared to 73.1% of persons between the ages of 18 and 29 years. Approximately 10% of elders are defined as problem drinkers.[1] Of significance is the acceptance and casual attitude of alcohol consumption and drug use in the younger population, including the baby boomers, suggesting a dramatic increase in substance abuse in the elderly in coming decades.

Formally assessing alcohol abuse in older adults is difficult because most screening instruments are not age specific and rely on self-report. The Short Michigan Alcoholism Screening Test—Geriatric Version was developed as the first short-form screening instrument for the elderly.[38] A score of two or more "Yes" responses suggests an alcohol problem. The goal of the screening is to identify an at-risk population of older adults who use alcohol on a regular basis.

More commonly used is the following CAGE screening questionnaire, a simple-to-administer, four-question instrument.[39] A positive response to any question indicates the need for further evaluation. The major drawback to the validity of this instrument is the reliance on self-report. The older adult may deny any problem when confronted with these questions.

The CAGE Screening Questionnaire consists of these four questions:

1. Have you ever felt you should *cut down* on your drinking?
2. Have people *annoyed* you by criticizing your drinking?
3. Have you ever felt bad or *guilty* about your drinking?
4. Have you ever had a drink first thing in the morning to steady your nerves or get rid of a hangover (*eye-opener*)?

The care manager must also rely on observation to detect alcohol use or abuse. Such indicators as deteriorating hygiene, increased number of falls, slurred speech, the smell of alcohol, and moodiness may indicate a potential problem with alcohol. As mentioned earlier, other physical and cognitive impairments must be ruled out first.

Drug dependency and misuse in the elderly population entails both the use of illicit drugs and the misuse of prescription medications. Drug dependency develops faster in this population because of an older adult's slower metabolic process. The kidneys and liver are not as efficient in removing these substances from the bodies of older adults. Currently, a very small number of older adults have a life-long history of illegal drug use. However, this number will rise dramatically as a result of the longer life expectancies and the wide-spread acceptance of recreational drug use among more recent generations.[1]

The most common drug misuse among older adults is with psychoactive medications for the treatment of depression, anxiety, and pain. These medications can cause both physical and psychological dependency. Women are more at risk for drug dependency because they are more likely to seek treatment for somatic complaints and other emotional problems. The care manager must pay close attention to all medications currently prescribed by the older adult's physicians and must be aware of multiple pharmacies to prevent duplication that could potentially lead to lethal dosages.

■ CONCLUSION

Psychosocial assessment is important both for what it can accomplish and what can happen if it is not completed thoroughly and correctly. A comprehensive and accurate psychosocial assessment can better ensure the development of an appropriate intervention and successful care plan. The accurate and timely use of psychosocial assessment tools must be combined with good interviewing skills. The ability to develop and maintain relationships, knowledge of human behavior, understanding of family and caregiver dynamics, knowledge of the effects of aging and disability, and the awareness of community resources and services are critical to all that follows.[2] An assessment that either is incomplete or ignores good clinical and professional judgment can result in the failure to develop a healthy relationship between the care manager and older adult, which can only result in eventual failure of even the best care plan.

The National Association of Professional Geriatric Care Managers has developed a book of forms as a benefit for its members. Included in this comprehensive manual are many assessment forms a new care manager can use, as well as a number of the assessment tools mentioned in this chapter (e.g., MMSE, GDS). As stated earlier, the care manager must adapt the psychosocial assessment to the population served to ensure appropriate and relevant information is obtained to develop the care plan. Care must be taken to use only those forms, or those sections of forms, found in the manual that are reflective of the needs of the individual practice population.

■ REFERENCES

1. McInnis-Dittrich K. *Social Work with Elders: A Biopsychosocial Approach.* 2nd ed. Boston, MA: Allyn & Bacon; 2005.

2. Geron D. Guidelines for case management practice across the long-term care continuum. *Report of the National Advisory Committee on Long-Term Care Case Management.* Bristol, CT: Connecticut Community Care, Inc; 1994.

3. Aronson J. Assessment: the linchpin of geriatric care management. *Geriatr Care Manage.* 1998;8(1):11–14.

4. Langley LK. Cognitive assessment of older adults. In: Kane RLKRA, ed. *Assessing Older Persons.* New York: Oxford University Press; 2002.

5. Gallo JJ. Cognitive assessment. In: Gallo JJ, Fulmer T, Paveza GJ, eds. *Handbook of Geriatric Assessment.* 4th ed. Sudbury, MA: Jones and Bartlett Publishers; 2006:46.

6. Folstein MF, Folstein SE, McHugh PR. Mini-Mental State: a practical method for grading the cognitive state of patients for the clinician. *J Psychiat Res.* 1975;12(3):189–198.

7. Pfeiffer E. A short portable mental status questionnaire for the assessment of organic brain deficit in elder patients. *J Am Geriatr Soc.* 1975;23:433–441.

8. Katzman R, Brown T, Fuld P, Peck A, Schechter R, Schimmel H. Validation of a short Orientation-Memory-Concentration Test of cognitive impairment. *Am J Psychiatry.* 1983;140:734–739.

9. Mendez MF, Ala T, Underwood KL. Development of scoring criteria for the clock drawing task in Alzheimer's disease. *J Am Geriatr Soc.* 1992;40:1095–1099.

10. Berkman BJ, Maramaldi P, Breon EA, Howe JL. Social Work Gerontological Assessment revisited. *Gerontol So Work.* 2002;40(1/2).

11. Grann JD. Assessment of emotions in older adults: mood disorders, anxiety, psychological well-being, and hope. In: Kane RLKRA, ed. *Assessing Older Persons.* New York: Oxford University Press; 2000:129–169.

12. National Institute of Mental Health. Suicide in the U.S.: statistics and prevention. http://www.nimh.nih.gov/health/publications/suicide-in-the-us-statistics-and-prevention/index.shtml#adults. Accessed July 2, 2010.

13. Mitty E, Flores S. Suicide in late life. *J Geriatr Nurs.* 2008;29(3):160–165.

14. Gallo JW. Depression assessment. In: Gallo JJ, Fulmer T, Paveza GJ, eds. *Handbook of Geriatric Assessment.* Sudbury, MA: Jones and Bartlett Publishers; 2006: 20.

15. Yesavage TL. Development and validation of a geriatric depression scale: a preliminary report. *J Psychiatr Res.* 1983;17:37–49.

16. Beck AT, Ward CH, Mendelson M, Mock J, Erbaugh J. An inventory for measuring depression. *Arch Gen Psychiatry.* 1961;4:561–571.

17. Gellis Z. Older adults with mental and emotional problems. In: Berkman B, ed. *Handbook of Social Work and Health in Aging.* New York: Oxford University Press; 2006:10.

18. Beck AT, Epstein N, Brown G, Steer R. An inventory for measuring clinical anxiety: psychometric properties. *J Consult Clin Psychol.* 1988;56:893–897.

19. Albert S. *Public Health and Aging.* New York: Springer; 2004.

20. Albert SM, Sano M, Bell K, Merchant C, Small S, Stern Y. Hourly care received by people with Alzheimer's disease; results from an urban, community-based survey. *Gerontologist.* 1998;38(6):704–714.

21. Pearlin LI, Mullan JT, Semple SJ, Skaff MM. Caregiving and the stress process: an overview of concepts and their measures. *Gerontologist.* 1990;30:583–594.

22. Schulz R, O'Brien AT, Bookwala J, et al. Psychiatric and physical morbidity effects of dementia caregiving: prevalence, correlates, and causes. *Gerontologist.* 1995;35(6):771–791.

23. Antonucci TC, Sherman AM, Vanderwater EA. Measures of social support and caregiver burden. *Generations.* 1997;XXI(1):48–51.

24. Lubben J. Assessing social networks among elderly populations. *Fam Community Health.* 1988;11:42–52.

25. Norbeck JS, Lindsey AM, Carrieri VL. The development of an instrument to measure social support. *Nurs Res.* 1981;30:264–269.

26. Aneshensel CS, Pearlin LI, Schuler RH. Stress, role captivity, and the cessation of caregiving. *J Health Soc Behav*. 1993;34:54–70.

27. Schulz R. Caregiving as a risk factor for mortality: the caregiver health effects study. *JAMA*. 1999;282:2215–2219.

28. Morano C. Appraisal and coping: moderators or mediators of stress in Alzheimer's disease caregivers? *J Soc Work Res*. 2003;27:116–128.

29. Kramer BJ. Gain in the caregiving experience: where are we? What next? *Gerontologist*. 1997;37(2):218–232.

30. Lawton MP, Kleban MH, Moss M, Rovine M, Glicksman A. Measuring caregiving appraisal. *J Gerontol*. 1989;44(3):P61–P71.

31. Novak M, Guest C. Application of a Multidimensional Caregiver Burden Inventory. *Gerontologist*. 1989;29:798–803.

32. Robinson BC. Validation of a Caregiver Strain Index. *J Gerontol*. 1983;38(3):344–348.

33. Tomita S. Mistreated and neglected elders. In: Berkman IB, ed. *Handbook of Social Work and Health in Aging*. New York: Oxford University Press; 2006:219–230.

34. National Center on Elder Abuse. NCEA national incidence study—1998. http://www.elderabusecenter.org/. Accessed October 15, 2010.

35. Fulmer T, Street S, Carr K. Abuse of the elderly: screening and detection. *J Emerg Nurs*. 1984;10(3):131–140.

36. Zanjani D. Substance use and abuse assessment In: Gallo JJ, Fulmer T, Paveza GJ, eds. *Handbook of Geriatric Assessment*. Sudbury, MA: Jones and Bartlett Publishers; 2006:175–192.

37. American Psychiatric Association. *Diagnostic and Statistical Manual—Text Revision* (DSM-TR). Washington, DC: American Psychiatric Association; 2000.

38. Blow FC, Gillespie BW, Barry KL, et al. Brief screening for alcohol problems in elder populations using the Short Michigan Alcoholism Screening Test—Geriatric Version (SMAST-G). *Alcohol Clin Exp Res*. 1998;22:13A.

39. Ewing JA. Detecting alcoholism: the CAGE Questionnaire. *JAMA*. 1984;252:1905–1907.

■ STANDARDIZED INSTRUMENTS AVAILABLE ONLINE

Iowa Geriatric Education Center
   www.healthcare.uiowa.edu/igec/tools/Default.asp
- Clock drawing test
- Katz-ADL
- Tinetti-Fall
- Caregiver Burden Inventory
- SPMSQ

Internet Stroke Center, Washington University Medical Center
   www.strokecenter.org/trials/scales/bd_imct.html
- Blessed Memory Orientation

Louisiana State University—Health Sciences Center
   www.sh.lsuhsc.edu/fammed/OutpatientManual/Short%20MAST%2013.htm
- Short Michigan Alcoholism Screening Instrument—Geriatric Version

Carolinas Health Care System
   www.carolinashealthcare.org/services/behavioral/tests/cage.cfm
- CAGE

Family Practice Notebook
   www.fpnotebook.com/Psych/Exam/BckDprsnInvntry.htm
- Beck Depression Scale

Hartford Institute for Geriatric Nursing
www.hartfordign.org
- Geriatric Depression Scale
- Lawton Scale of Appraised Burden

Chapter 4

Functional Assessment

Deborah Newquist, Connie Rosenberg, and Carolyn Barber

■ INTRODUCTION

One maxim of geriatric care management is to promote the autonomy of older individuals to the greatest extent possible. A careful and competent functional assessment of the older person provides information that is critical to ascertaining how that person's autonomy can be maximized through medical, social, mechanical, and environmental manipulations.[1] For this reason the ability to function is a central focus of all geriatric care management evaluations. It is not enough to know about a person's diagnoses because this information alone is insufficient to predict the impact of health problems on a person's daily life. The ability to live as one chooses and to perform basic activities throughout the day is affected by a multitude of factors—health problems, attitude, environmental features, social roles, and resources, to name a few. Evaluation of an older person's functional status is fundamental to helping that person maintain his or her autonomy and quality of life because functional abilities are of paramount importance to overall health, well-being, and potential need for services.

The functional assessment should be done by a professional, certified geriatric care manager (GCM). Functional ability is assessed through the measurement of the basic skills of role function. This includes measurement of the performance of basic activities of daily liv-

ing (ADLs), such as bathing, grooming, dressing, eating, transferring, and toileting; and the more advanced instrumental activities of daily living (IADLs), including handling financial matters appropriately, finding one's way out of the home and back, and managing medication regimens. Evaluation of the older person's functional abilities is a critical component of the geriatric assessment. "One of the goals of a responsive healthcare system is to assist clients in maintaining their functional well-being. Functional status in the older person is characterized by the gradual decreases in organ function that accompany normal aging and the more rapid declines associated with acute and chronic illness."[2] A review of medical symptoms and diagnoses does not by itself predict an individual's functional impairments. These impairments may be the determining factor in decisions about the living situation that person will require. Together, the medical diagnosis and a description and appraisal of the client's function provide the most accurate assessment. Impairments in ADLs have been identified as risk factors for falls, injuries, and institutionalization.

As stated by Gallo, functional assessment helps set priorities around which the available medical, social, and economic resources can be rallied.[3] Changes in function signal a problem whose source should be addressed and whose solution may not be a medical response but a realignment of the social situation.[4] In older persons, functional assessment is critical for use with ongoing clients as well as at the time of initial assessment because functional assessment is a barometer of health status in this age group. Loss of functional ability is the most sensitive indicator for identifying new disease and monitoring the progress of treatment.[3] According to Fretwell, most older persons have one "most vulnerable function" (e.g., cognition, memory, continence, ability to walk).[5] Disorders such as pneumonia, urinary tract infection, myocardial infarction, and heart failure may present initially as confusion, incontinence, and other function-related symptoms in certain older adults. Having knowledge of a person's baseline functional status allows early detection of disease, and the subsequent improvement of that functional impairment is a sensitive indicator of recovery.

Some impairments can be identified by interview or observation of the older person performing common everyday functions. Others require the use of screening tools and methods to differentiate them from other impairments and conditions and to determine their severity. Functional impairment of ADLs and IADLs can often be identified by history taking and by demonstration and observation. When questioning the older person, it is more effective to ask about recent activities such as, "Did you drive here today?" rather than "Are you still driving?" and, "Did you dress yourself this morning?" rather than "Do you dress yourself?" Asking questions in this manner helps focus the older person on what is possible right now and minimizes the reporting of inaccurate information. If the older person is cognitively impaired, responses should be confirmed with a caregiver. Observation of the client's behavior and abilities at the time of the assessment meeting, such as ability to rise from a chair, ambulate, and respond appropriately when speaking, can provide much valuable information. It is also critical to note whether any activities performed are done slowly, with difficulty, unsafely, or only partially.[6]

In some cases it may be important to evaluate the client on more than one occasion to observe and note variations in functional ability throughout the day. For example, a client may be fatigued in the afternoon and function better in the morning. Knowing both the high and low functional points can help the care manager plan effectively. In addition, it is important that the care manager adjust the duration of the assessment meeting to accommodate the client's stamina and tolerance. A good rule of thumb is to not exceed 90 minutes (120 minutes at the most) at one assessment interval. Not all information needs to be gathered at one sitting. Also the care manager should guard against overassessment of the client. Identifying areas of concern is the first step and follow-up referrals to appropriate medical or mental health professionals for targeted assessments is an important care management function.

If deficits in ADLs are identified, it is important to try to determine the underlying cause of the loss of function and how long ago it occurred. This information will help the care manager determine whether the condition is permanent or is potentially reversible and perhaps just a symptom of an illness that can be treated, restoring function. Many factors affect the ability to perform ADLs safely and completely. No matter what the determination, it is usually wise to involve the client in treatment to alter the dysfunction because, with the proper treatment, many clients have the ability to regain at least partial function. Living with a growing loss of function has a major impact on the quality of life of older people and their caregivers.[6]

■ MEASURING ACTIVITIES OF DAILY LIVING

A variety of tools are available to assist the care manager in evaluating the needs of the client. Below are some of the commonly used tools.

The Tools[6]

The instrument most familiar to researchers and clinicians for performing functional assessments is the Katz Index of ADL (Exhibit 4-1). This instrument measures independence of function in bathing, dressing, toileting, transfers, continence, and feeding. It is widely used for assessing treatment outcomes of older persons and the chronically ill. It provides a standardized measure of biological and psychological function and a framework for assessing the ability to live independently. When deficiencies are found, it provides guidelines for care planning for correction of those deficiencies. The client is ideally witnessed by the GCM while performing the ADLs and rated either independent or dependent based on the definitions for performance of each ADL as established by Katz.[7] Caregiver report is often used in situations where it is not practical for the GCM to witness ADL activities. The need for assistance is further broken down into categories for supervision, direction, or personal assistance so that subjectivity of the clinician is minimized. A client refusing to perform any function is categorized as not performing the function even though it might be obvious to the tester that, based on the overall functional abilities, the client is capable of performing the particular ADL. A combined measure of the six ADL functions can be used to quantify changes over time. Although this instrument is easy to use in a home or facility environment, it is somewhat time consuming to administer and might be of more use to the GCM who is assessing the client on an ongoing basis rather than one performing a one-time assessment.

The Rapid Disability Rating Scale-2 (Exhibit 4-2) rates individuals' performance of ADLs and their degree of disability on a 4-point scale from "None" (needing no assistance) to "Total" (needing total assistance). It includes a selection of both ADL and IADL tasks and has sections for "degree of disability" and "degree of special problems." As with other scales, it is important to rate the client on what the client does, not what the client says he or she does. This scale is useful for monitoring changes in clients' conditions over time.[6]

Other comprehensive assessment tools that include the functional domain, along with other components identified as determining factors of ability to live independently, are useful in assessment and care planning. The most widely mentioned in the literature are the Barthel Index, which rates 10 different items[8]; the Older American Rehabilitation Services (OARS), which includes within its extensive format of many health parameters the same items as the Katz Index but relies on self-reports of clients[9]; and the PULSES (Physical, Upper Limbs, Lower Limbs, Sensory, and Social Factors) Profile, which measures wider dimensions of functions but includes ADLs.[10]

One instrument, mainly used in nursing homes, is the Minimum Data Set (MDS). The MDS is based on direct observations made by professionals and a review of clinical records.[11] The Minimum Data Set for Home Care is now a tool required by several states to assess the needs of persons living at home. It is a multidimensional assessment instrument similar to the long-term-care MDS and is used in combination with the Clinical Assessment Protocols (CAPs) to form the Resident Assessment Instrument—Home Care. CAPs provide guidelines for individualized care planning of triggered problems.[12]

Disease-related assessment scales are available for some conditions, such as gait and balance dysfunction. The Tinetti Balance and Gait Evaluation (Exhibit 4-3) is a 28-point assessment tool that is performed by a trained evaluator.[13]

A condensed version of the Tinetti is also available. This test, the Get Up and Go Test, is simple to administer, requires no special equipment, and can be conducted in a brief amount of time.[14] The test begins with the client sitting up straight in a high-seat chair,

Exhibit 4–1   Katz Index of ADL

Independence means without supervision, direction, or active personal assistance, except as specifically noted below. This is based on actual status and not ability. A patient who refuses to perform a function is considered as not performing the function, even though he or she is deemed able.

Bathing (Sponge, shower, or tub)

Independent: assistance only in bathing a single part (back or disabled extremity) or bathes self completely

Dependent: assistance in bathing more than one part of body; assistance in getting in or out of tub; does not bathe self

Dressing

Independent: gets clothes from closets and drawers; puts on clothes, outer garments, braces; manages fasteners; act of tying shoes is excluded

Dependent: does not dress self or remains partly undressed

Going to Toilet

Independent: gets to toilet; gets on and off toilet; arranges clothes; cleans organs of excretion (may manage own bedpan used at night only and may or may not be using mechanical supports)

Dependent: uses bedpan or commode or receives assistance in getting to and using toilet

Transfer

Independent: moves in and out of bed and in and out of chair independently (may or may not be using mechanical supports)

Dependent: assistance in moving in or out of bed and/or chair; does not perform one or more transfers

Continence

Independent: urination and defecation entirely self-controlled

Dependent: partial or total incontinence in urination or defecation; partial or total control by enemas, catheters, or regulated use of urinals and/or bedpans

Feeding

Independent: gets food from plate or its equivalent into mouth (precutting of meat and preparation of food, as buttering bread, are excluded from evaluation)

Dependent: assistance in act of feeding (see above); does not eat at all or parenteral feeding

Evaluation Form

Name _____

Date of Evaluation _____

For each area of functioning listed below, circle description that applies (the word "assistance" means supervision, direction, or personal assistance).

Bathing—either sponge bath, tub bath, or shower

Receives no assistance (gets in and out of tub by self if tub is usual means of bathing)
Receives assistance in bathing only one part of body (such as back or a leg)
Receives assistance in bathing more than one part of body (or does not bathe self)

Dressing—gets clothes from closets and drawers; puts on clothes, including underclothes, outer garments; manages fasteners (including braces, if worn)

Gets clothes and gets completely dressed without assistance
Gets clothes and gets dressed without assistance except for tying shoes
Receives assistance in getting clothes or in getting dressed or stays partly or
    completely undressed

continues

Exhibit 4–1   Katz Index of ADL (continued)

Toileting—going to the "toilet room" for bowel and urine elimination; cleaning self after elimination and arranging clothes

Goes to "toilet room," cleans self, and arranges clothes without assistance (may use object for support such as cane, walker, or wheelchair and may manage night bedpan or commode, emptying same in morning)

Receives assistance in going to "toilet room" or in cleansing self or in arranging clothes after elimination or in use of night bedpan or commode

Does not go to room termed "toilet" for the elimination process

Transfer

Moves in and out of bed and in and out of chair without assistance (may use object for support such as cane or walker)

Moves in or out of bed or chair with assistance

Does not get out of bed

Continence

Controls urination and bowel movement completely by self

Has occasional "accidents"

Supervision helps keep urine or bowel control; catheter is used or is incontinent

Feeding

Feeds self without assistance

Feeds self except for getting assistance in cutting meat or buttering bread

Receives assistance in feeding or is fed partly or completely by tubes or intravenous fluids

Source: Republished with permission of the Gerontological Society of America, 1030 15th Street, NW, Suite 250, Washington, DC 20005. *Progress in the Development of the Index of ADL* (Tool), S. Katz, T.D. Downs, H.R. Cash, et al., *Gerontologist*, 1970, Vol. 1. Reproduced by permission of the publisher via Copyright Clearance Center, Inc.

---

which allows the person to sit with hips at a 90-degree angle to knees. The client is then instructed to (1) get up (without using armrests if possible), (2) stand still, (3) walk forward 10 feet, (4) turn around and walk back to the chair, and (5) turn and be seated. The evaluator notes sitting balance; transfers from sitting to standing; pace and stability of walking; and ability to turn without staggering. Statistical verification of the test by the developers showed good correlation between test scores and other measures of gait, which in some cases involved more sophisticated laboratory-based measures of balance and gait.

The Activities of Daily Living

Below are the activities of daily living assessed by the care manager during an evaluation.

Bathing

Determining the exact amount of assistance that a person needs in each ADL is necessary to make the best recommendations in a plan of care. For example, in bathing, if we find that the person needs only standby assistance in getting into and out of the tub or shower, the person might need the assistance of a companion (or family member) who can provide this service rather than assistance by a certified home health aide. Each state has

Exhibit 4–2   Rapid Disability Rating Scale (RDRS-2)

Directions: Rate what the person does to reflect current behavior. Circle one of the four choices for each item. Consider rating with any aids or prostheses normally used. None = completely independent or normal behavior. Total = that person cannot, will not, or may not (because of medical restriction) perform a behavior or has the most severe form of disability or problem.

Assistance with Activities of Daily Living

Eating	None	A little	A lot	Spoon-fed; intravenous tube
Walking (with cane or walker if used)	None	A little	A lot	Does not walk
Mobility (going outside and getting about with wheelchair, etc., if used)	None	A little	A lot	Is housebound
Bathing (include getting supplies, supervising)	None	A little	A lot	Must be bathed
Dressing (include help in selecting clothes)	None	A little	A lot	Must be dressed
Toileting (include help with clothes, cleaning, or help with ostomy/catheter)	None	A little	A lot	Uses bedpan or unable to care for ostomy/catheter
Grooming (shaving for men, hairdressing for women, nails, teeth)	None	A little	A lot	Must be groomed
Adaptive tasks (managing money/ possessions; telephoning; buying newspaper, toilet articles, snacks)	None	A little	A lot	Cannot manage

Degree of Disability

Communication (expressing self)	None	A little	A lot	Does not communicate
Hearing (with aid, if used)	None	A little	A lot	Does not seem to hear
Sight (with glasses, if used)	None	A little	A lot	Does not see
Diet (deviation from normal)	None	A little	A lot	Fed by intravenous tube
In bed during day (ordered or self-initiated)	None	A little (< 3 hr)	A lot	Most/all of the time
Incontinence (urine/feces, with catheter or prosthesis, if used)	None	Some-times	Frequently (weekly +)	Does not control
Medication	None	Some-times	Daily, taken orally	Daily; injection (+oral if used)

Degree of Special Problems

Mental confusion	None	A little	A lot	Extreme
Uncooperativeness (combats efforts to help with care)	None	A little	A lot	Extreme
Depression	None	A little	A lot	Extreme

Source: Linn MW, Linn BS. The rapid disability rating scale-2. *J Am Geriatr Soc.* 1982;30(6):378–382. Reproduced by permission of Blackwell Publishing LTD.

Exhibit 4–3   Tinetti Balance and Gait Evaluation

Balance

Instructions: Subject is seated in hard, armless chair. The following maneuvers are tested.

1. Sitting balance

Leans or slides in chair	=	0
Steady, safe	=	1 _____

2. Arises

Unable without help	=	0
Able but uses arms to help	=	1
Able without use of arms	=	2 _____

3. Attempts to arise

Unable without help	=	0
Able but requires more than 1 attempt	=	1
Able to arise with 1 attempt	=	2 _____

4. Immediate standing balance (first 5 sec)

Unsteady (staggers, moves feet, marked trunk sway)	=	0
Steady but uses walker or cane or grabs other objects for support	=	1
Steady without walker or cane or other support	=	2 _____

5. Standing balance

Unsteady	=	0
Steady but wide stance (medial heels more than 4 in. apart) or uses cane, walker, or other support	=	1
Narrow stance without support	=	2 _____

6. Nudged (subject at maximum position with feet as close together as possible, examiner pushes lightly on subject's sternum with palm of hand 3 times)

Begins to fall	=	0
Staggers, grabs, but catches self	=	1
Steady	=	2 _____

7. Eyes closed (at maximum position No. 6)

Unsteady	=	0
Steady	=	1 _____

8. Turning 360°

Discontinuous steps	=	0
Continuous	=	1
Unsteady (grabs, staggers)	=	0
Steady	=	1 _____

9. Sitting down

Unsafe (misjudged distance, falls into chair)	=	0
Uses arms or not a smooth motion	=	1
Safe, smooth motion	=	2 _____

Balance score: _____/16

continues

Exhibit 4–3 Tinetti Balance and Gait Evaluation (continued)

Gait

Instructions: Subject stands with examiner; walks down hallway or across room, first at his "usual" pace, then back at "rapid, but safe" pace (using usual walking aid such as cane, walker).

10. Initiation of gait (immediately after told to "go")

Any hesitancy or multiple attempts to start	=	0
No hesitancy	=	1 ____

11. Step length and height

a. Right swing foot

Does not pass left stance foot with step	=	0
Passes left stance foot	=	1
Right foot does not clear floor completely with step	=	0
Right foot completely clears floor	=	1 ____

b. Left swing foot

Does not pass right stance foot with step	=	0
Passes right stance foot	=	1
Left foot does not clear floor completely with step	=	0
Left foot completely clears floor	=	1 ____

12. Step symmetry

Right and left step length not equal (estimate)	=	0
Right and left step appear equal	=	1 ____

13. Step continuity

Stopping or discontinuity between steps	=	0
Steps appear continuous	=	1 ____

14. Path (estimated in relation to floor tiles, 12-in. diameter; observe excursion of 1 foot over about 10 ft of the course)

Marked deviation	=	0
Mild/moderate deviation or uses walking aid	=	1
Straight without walking aid	=	2 ____

15. Trunk

Marked sway or uses walking aid	=	0
No sway but flexion of knees or back or spreads arms out while walking	=	1
No sway, no flexion, no use of arms, and no use of walking aid	=	2 ____

16. Walking stance

Heels apart	=	0
Heels almost touching while walking	=	1 ____

Gait score: ____/12

Total score: ____/28

Source: Tinetti ME. Performance-oriented assessment of mobility problems in elderly patients. *J Am Geriatr Soc.* 1986;34:119–126. Reproduced by permission Blackwell Publishing LTD.

its own laws regarding who can legally provide what service in a home care setting. If the person indicates that he or she isn't showering because of a fear of falling, the person might only need to have the security of a shower chair and handheld shower spray. If the person has dementia and the family reports that he or she is not bathing, the person might only need reminders to bathe.

More specific knowledge of joint function is also helpful in determining the amount and type of assistance that a person might need. For example, if the person has limited range of motion in one or both shoulders, will that person be able to bathe him- or herself? Will physical therapy improve shoulder function?

Grooming

Oftentimes, a care manager can make recommendations that will improve a person's grooming and allow for continued independence. For example, switching from a regular razor to an electric razor can make shaving easier and safer for a person who may have hand tremors or arthritis. Encouraging a woman to go to the assisted-living beauty salon for manicures and hair washes can provide her with the feeling of "treating" herself plus improve hygiene. Cueing for clients with dementia to brush their teeth or comb their hair can give them a continued sense of accomplishment and independence.

Dressing

Again, detailed questioning can assist the care manager in making the most appropriate recommendations. If the family reports that the client is wearing soiled clothes, it may be that the person has a visual impairment that is preventing him or her from seeing that the soiled clothes should be changed. However, it may also be that, if the person has dementia, he or she is forgetting to change clothes and might just need reminders or need to have a caregiver lay out the appropriate clothes to wear. If a person can get dressed unassisted

except for shoes and socks, recommending that the person use adaptive devices such as a long shoehorn will enable the person to continue to be independent. Persons who need hands-on assistance because they are unable to dress themselves because of physical problems, such as Parkinson's disease or cognitive loss, will need a referral to a home health aide if family members are not available.

Pain is an often-overlooked problem. Frequently, pain can be great enough to inhibit a person from functioning independently. Pain can definitely be a problem that affects a person's ability to dress him- or herself. The care manager needs to be aware of whether pain is decreasing a person's function and recommend a pain evaluation. In addition, a referral for physical therapy for range-of-motion exercises or other therapeutic interventions may assist with improving function in dressing as well as accomplishing other ADLs and IADLs.

Toileting

A person who needs assistance getting on and off the toilet because of physical problems may also need a referral for a home health aide. However, installing a raised toilet seat or adding a grab bar next to the toilet may help to keep this person independent. If a person has difficulty getting to the toilet, for example, at night, having a commode next to the bed may allow him or her to toilet safely alone without waking a caregiver. In addition, if in a review of medications the care manager notes that the person is taking a diuretic in the afternoon and getting up frequently to toilet at night, a change to a morning dosage can be suggested to the person's physician.

Transfers

Is the person having difficulty getting in or out of bed? The care manager can recommend that the bed be lowered so that it is closer to the floor or that the person rent a hospital bed so that he or she can use the side rails to assist with the transfer. Also, check to see whether a pillow-top mattress is making the bed too high.

Does the person have difficulty getting in or out of a chair? A chairlift can ease the transfer, or perhaps the person can even use a walker for added support. If physical assistance is needed, the care manager should always ask whether a person needs assistance from one or two people. This can make the difference between a person being able to stay at home with one caregiver or needing to be placed in a nursing home. In some instances, the care manager may recommend a Hoyer lift to be used at home so that a transfer is safe for the person and the caregiver.

Continence

Fifteen percent to 30% of adults living in the community and almost 50% of nursing home residents are affected by urinary incontinence.[15] The prevalence in older women is twice that of prevalence in older men. Despite the fact that incontinence is common in aging, it should never be considered a normal condition of aging. Various methods of managing and reducing incontinence have been developed, and many older persons have been assisted with incontinence so that the quality of their lives is not so greatly affected.

Because of embarrassment and worry about appearance and odor, clients may not report incontinence unless asked directly. It is isolating and has a major impact on quality of life. Incontinence also increases the risk of falls in older persons. The development of incontinence is often the final factor influencing family caregivers to institutionalize those they care for.

Few older people realize that incontinence can be treatable. Oftentimes, they will self-treat by decreasing fluid intake, which in turn can lead to dehydration, which in turn can lead to falls. The care manager should refer the person to the primary care physician or a urologist for a workup before assuming that the incontinence is untreatable. Many times,

this condition can be caused by an acute urinary tract infection.

Also, other strategies can be recommended to increase continence, such as frequent reminders to toilet or developing the habit of sitting on the toilet to have a bowel movement at the same time every day. Using disposable undergarments that pull up and down easily may also allow a person with incontinence to be more independent in managing his or her incontinence.

Eating

This is not to be confused with meal preparation. The functional ability to eat refers to a person's ability to get food from the plate into his or her mouth. A referral to an occupational therapist by the care manager may improve the person's independence in this area. For example, the therapist may suggest adaptive utensils for a person with arthritis who is unable to grasp a common fork. For persons who are blind, having a dish with a straight rim allows them to feel when they have touched the edge of the plate. Cups that have lids with spouts prevent spills for persons with tremors from Parkinson's, for example. Think adaptive to keep a person independent.

Also, for a person with dementia, providing finger foods or cueing to continue eating may improve nutrition and allow for more independence. Having the caregiver cut food into bite-size pieces and setting up drinks so they can be more easily reached are other useful strategies for persons with cognitive or physical impairments.

The care manager needs to be alert to the fact that problems in this area can seriously affect the client's nutritional status. Asking questions about weight loss will provide added information. If the client is in a nursing home setting, it is important to look at the monthly weight chart. If there is weight loss, the client may not be finishing meals as a result of dementia or the physical inability to continue feeding him- or herself. The nursing home physician may need to order nutritional supplements, and the staff may need to provide more oversight at mealtimes. Visiting a client at mealtime in a nursing home or assisted living facility can provide invaluable information for the care plan.

■ AMBULATION AND MOBILITY

One factor influencing ADL performance is mobility. Direct observation can identify problems in gait and balance. Early detection of deficits in mobility can identify those clients at risk of injury. Whenever possible, rehabilitation can then assist in restoring functional losses and reduce the risk of falls. For those deficits that cannot be rehabilitated, assistive equipment such as a cane or walker can be provided.

Immobility and inactivity can lead to the older person becoming chair- or bed-bound. These older persons often go on to develop edema, contractures, incontinence, or pressure sores. These complications place them at increased risk of falls and nursing home placement. It is important to inquire about recent falls and the circumstances under which they occurred and to test gait performance in all older adults. One tool, as noted earlier, is the Tinetti Balance and Gait Evaluation tool. Those at high risk can be identified so that preventive measures can be taken as part of care planning. Factors increasing risk include confusion, incontinence, impaired mobility, generalized weakness, use of sedating medications and alcohol, postural hypotension, and history of previous falls.[6 (p183)]

To note the character of the gait it is best for the care manager to observe the person ambulating. Is the gait slow and shuffling or too fast and without concern for the environment? Note the person's balance. Does the person need to grab onto furniture to prevent a fall? Can he or she walk up a flight of steps to get to the bedroom or even up the two steps from the living room to the kitchen? Would a stair lift provide improved safety? It is important to observe footwear. Is the stylish older woman still wearing a shoe with a raised heel? Is the stylish older man still wearing a slip-on shoe that does not provide proper support? Recommending proper footwear can be the first step in preventing falls. Asking the person for a tour of the home is an excellent way to observe how he or she gets around and to make observations regarding home safety.

What about ambulating outside? Does the person need adaptive equipment outside because of uneven surfaces even if he or she is fine when ambulating on a smooth floor inside? Is the person able to get up the outside stairs? Are there railings to keep the person safe? Does the person need a ramp? Is the person cognitively intact enough to use a scooter for longer distances traveled in the nursing home? Does the person need a prescription for a wheelchair because he or she is unable to walk the long distance to the doctor's office?

Falls

Every year, approximately 30% of older persons living at home fall. As stated earlier, getting more information about where falls occur is vital. A practical mnemonic for reviewing the actual fall is as follows[16]:

S   Symptoms experienced at the time of fall
P   Previous number of falls or near-falls
L   Location of falls
A   Activity engaged in or attempted at time of fall
T   Time (hour) of fall
T   Trauma (e.g., physical or psychological) associated with falls

Prevention of falls is of utmost importance because after a fall the fear of another fall can become a vicious cycle. Fear leads to inactivity that then results in decreased strength that then leads to increased risk of another fall.[17]

Many falls by older persons occur in the bathroom. Adaptations in the environment can decrease the risk. If your client is falling at night, ask about the use of sedating medications at bedtime. Or perhaps does the person fall because he or she ambulates slowly and needs to rush to answer the only phone in the home, which is located on the kitchen wall? Getting a portable telephone may decrease the risk of another fall. Was the person experiencing specific symptoms secondary to medical problems, for example, dizziness or postural hypotension? Reviewing these symptoms with the physician can result in treatment or change in medications that will reduce the risk of a repeat fall.[18]

Changes in the environment, attention to adaptations, and medical evaluation will make it safer for a person with impaired mobility to get around the home. In addition, with the goal of improved mobility and balance, the care manager should think about the possibility of physical therapy for strength training, personal trainers who can come to the home or the assisted living facility to do light exercise, or even a membership at a local senior-friendly gym that offers tai chi classes, which are known to improve balance. In addition, for clients in nursing homes the care manager needs to advocate for needed therapies and medical evaluations to improve mobility and decrease falls.

■ MEASURING INSTRUMENTAL ACTIVITIES OF DAILY LIVING

The wide range of abilities involved in IADLs (not only physical but mental and social variables) and the complexity and variation of interpretations of the test results mean that there are more problems with IADL instruments than there are with ADL instruments. IADL scales sometimes result in falsely low scores for men and women who have not performed certain food preparation or financial tasks during their lifetime, but who are perfectly capable of performing other IADL functions. The gold standard scale, most widely used and with well-documented reliability and validity in the older population, is the IADL Scale developed by Lawton and Brody (Exhibit 4–4).[19] The scale measures eight aspects of living that are critical to those living independently.[6]

The Lawton IADL Scale was the first tool to measure more complex activities related to a person's ability to adapt and function in the environment. It was designed for use as a guide

Exhibit 4–4   IADL Scale

Male Score		Female Score
	A. Ability to use telephone	
1	1. Operates telephone on own initiative; looks up and dials numbers, etc.	1
1	2. Dials a few well-known numbers	1
1	3. Answers telephone but does not dial	1
0	4. Does not use telephone at all	0
	B. Shopping	
1	1. Takes care of all shopping needs independently	1
0	2. Shops independently for small purchases	0
0	3. Needs to be accompanied on any shopping trip	0
0	4. Completely unable to shop	0

Exhibit 4–4   IADL Scale (continued)

Male Score		Female Score
	C. Food preparation	
	1. Plans, prepares, and serves adequate meals independently	1
	2. Prepares adequate meals if supplied with ingredients	0
	3. Heats and serves prepared meals, or prepares meals but does not maintain adequate diet	0
	4. Needs to have meals prepared and served	0
	D. Housekeeping	
	1. Maintains house alone or with occasional assistance (e.g., heavy-work domestic help)	1
	2. Performs light daily tasks such as dish washing and bed making	1
	3. Performs light daily tasks but cannot maintain acceptable level of cleanliness	1
	4. Needs help with all home maintenance tasks	1
	5. Does not participate in any housekeeping tasks	0
	E. Laundry	
	1. Does personal laundry completely	1
	2. Launders small items; rinses socks, stockings, etc.	1
	3. All laundry must be done by others	0
	F. Mode of transportation	
1	1. Travels independently on public transportation or drives own car	1
1	2. Arranges own travel via taxi, but does not otherwise use public transportation	1
0	3. Travels on public transportation when assisted or accompanied by another	1
0	4. Travel limited to taxi or automobile, with assistance of another	0
0	5. Does not travel at all	0
	G. Responsibility for own medication	
1	1. Is responsible for taking medication in correct dosages at correct time	1
0	2. Takes responsibility if medication is prepared in advance in separate dosages	0
0	3. Is not capable of dispensing own medication	0
	H. Ability to handle finances	
1	1. Manages financial matters independently (budgets, writes checks, pays rent and bills, goes to bank); collects and keeps track of income	1
1	2. Manages day-to-day purchases, but needs help with bank for managing purchases, etc.	1
0	3. Incapable of handling money	0

Source: Republished with permission of the Gerontological Society of America, 1030 15th Street, NW, Suite 250, Washington, DC 20005. *Assessment of Older People: Self-monitoring and Instrumental Activities of Daily Living* (Scale), M.P. Lawton and E.M. Brody, *Gerontologist*, 1969, Vol. 9. Reproduced by permission of the publisher via Copyright Clearance Center, Inc.

in determining appropriate living environments for older persons. It measures performance rather than ability and therefore is subject to sex role biases that need to be accounted for during use. Originally, it was intended that eight items would be used for women and five items for men, but common use has blurred this approach. The items are ordered in a Guttman scale form with the first item, ability to use a phone, being the lowest level, and handling finances the highest functional activity.

Another widely used tool for IADL assessment is the instrument called the Older Americans Resources and Services Multidimensional Functional Assessment Questionnaire (OARS-IADL).[20] The OARS questionnaire assesses five domains of functioning: social, economic, mental health, physical health, and self-care capacity and service utilization. The IADL component has been developed into a separate, seven-item tool that uses a self-reporting approach.[21] (See Exhibit 4–5.) Unlike the Lawton instrument, all items are to be used with both men and women. The tool is useful as a screen for determining the need for more in-depth evaluation and for service planning.

IADL tools generally are viewed as concentrating on activities necessary for independent living in the community. They incorporate an inherent emphasis on cognitive functioning with items such as financial and medication management. Cultural and sex role issues need to be considered in their use so as to avoid unreliable results.

Dementia and Function

Incipient or more pronounced dementia by definition impairs functional performance. Indeed, the diagnosis of dementia requires that a cognitive condition be severe enough to interfere with the performance of daily activities. It is through functional problems that dementia is often first noticed by patients and their families. IADL instruments, which measure higher-level functioning, are particularly helpful in detecting incipient dementias. Changes in habits indicating difficulty paying bills and managing finances or troubles with medication regimens are often telltale signs that cognitive changes are afoot. These, in fact, may be clues to care managers that other problems, less apparent superficially, are present.

Dementia can also pose challenges to the care manager in conducting an assessment of

Exhibit 4–5   OARS-IADL Scale

	Response Option		
	Without help (2)	With help (1)	Unable (0)
Question			
Can you use the telephone?			
Can you get to places out of walking distance?			
Can you go shopping (groceries/clothing)?			
Can you prepare your own meals?			
Can you do your own housework?			
Can you take your own medications?			
Can you handle your own money?			

Source: "Components of the Older American's Resources and Services Instrumental Activities of Daily Living" (Scale). From Fillenbaum GG. Screening the elderly: a brief instrumental activities of daily living measure. *J Am Geriatr Soc.* 1985;33(10):698-706. Reproduced by permission Blackwell Publishing LTD.

IADLs. This is because the reliability of self-reports may be eroded in dementia patients. It is important, therefore, that care managers probe to learn what the person is actually doing, not just what the person says he or she can do, and also for the care manager to gather information about past patterns to determine whether recent changes have occurred. Sorting out capacity from behavior—what the person can do but chooses not to do, versus what he or she can no longer do but makes the excuse of preferring not to do—takes experience and judgment on the part of the care manager.

Gathering information from various sources—the older persons themselves, their caregivers (ideally in private conversations), observation of the person in the environment, and keen observation of the environment itself—all provide clues about functioning. For example, are medication bottles or systems organized, or are bottles of current and past medications scattered throughout the house? Are random pills left on countertops or tables? Can the person show you which medications he or she takes and tell you his or her routines? Does the person evidence difficulty remembering which medications are taken and when, and if so, can the person problem solve to tell you the routine accurately?

If appropriate (i.e., if needed and with permission of the patient), count the medications in the bottle and calculate the number that should be there based on the prescription instructions and date the prescription was filled. Check the cupboards and refrigerator to see if they are well stocked and kept current. Are there numerous spoiled and/or expired foods in the refrigerator? Are there abundant numbers of the same item in the cupboard, which can indicate the person forgets what is in the cupboards and buys foods repeatedly out of habit, is not able to make a shopping list, or is unable to remember what supplies are needed. (Of course, everyone does these things to some extent, but the care man-ager must look at degrees of problems and whether any patterns are present.)

Are bills and papers organized, or is the house heavily cluttered with stacks of papers? Have there been reports that utilities or other services have been discontinued or threatened to be shut off because of nonpayment? Are there signs of mail "contests" and other solicitations for "charities" present and in abundance? If the person will let you see his or her checkbook, is it in order or does it show signs of frequent errors, double payments, transposed numbers, and the like?

Dementia interferes with many higher-level functions and, in its more advanced stages, with basic ADLs. Assessing the older person's functional performance can help guide the care manager's plan of care, direct communication with other professionals when further diagnostic tests might be needed, or tailor appropriate supports when independence is no longer possible.

IADL Tasks

Several core functional activities form the bases of IADL assessments. How an older person performs on these activities gives important information about that person's ability to live independently with safety and quality of life.

Telephone Use

Determining a person's ability to make and receive phone calls can help identify home safety issues. From higher-level activities, such as locating or remembering a phone number or looking up a number, to following through to place a call and completing a call all give clues to a person's ability to manage independently and safely at home. If there were a fire, could or would the person be able to call for help? Can the person call the doctor's office and make an appointment? If there were a water leak, could the older person locate and call a plumber, or would the person need to call a family member or friend to get that person to locate help?

Determining capacity in this regard can be tricky. First, determine whether the person has the physical capacity to use the phone: can the person reach the phone, hold it, and hear well enough to use it? Asking the person to place a call to the doctor to reconfirm an appointment is one method of evaluating behavior. Another is to ask what the person would do in an emergency. Then ask the person to give the numbers of the persons he or she would need to call. Document the person's responses. When conducting assessments for IADLs, there is the risk that people will give false-positive responses—stating they can perform a function when in fact they may have difficulty performing it. Observation and gathering information from several sources help the care manager pinpoint areas of strength and limitations.

Shopping

Is the older person able to assess needs for supplies and plan and execute shopping excursions independently? What type and level of help are needed if the older person cannot do these tasks alone? Asking the person questions about who does the shopping and having the person describe his or her last shopping trip can give information useful for care planning. Some persons may have difficulty carrying grocery bags but be able to make a shopping list and drive to the store. Others may have cognitive problems that interfere with the ability to survey needs, make a list, find the items in the store, and pay accurate amounts at the checkout counter. Other persons may have ambulation difficulties or low stamina as a result of a heart condition, for example, which precludes the person from walking up and down grocery aisles or going to the mall to buy clothing.

Food Preparation

This task is subject to classic sex role influences. The care manager needs to ascertain past and current role behaviors and inte-

grate that information into the assessment evaluation.

Food preparation involves cognitive functions, including memory, executive function, forecasting, sequencing, and visual-spatial abilities. In addition, physical abilities involving manual dexterity; stamina; ability to reach, stoop, lift, and carry; and balance and gait are involved as a person moves about the kitchen cooking. Deciding what to eat, obtaining the foods to eat, preparing the foods, and storing and cleaning up after meal preparation are all involved. The level of complexity of the meals and their nutritional value are important considerations for the care manager to note. Safety issues are also involved in remembering to turn off the stove or to regulate cooking temperatures, deciding whether a food is safe to eat or past its expiration date, and storing foods at appropriate temperatures.

It is helpful for the care manager both to ask questions and to observe for telltale signs of trouble. Is the refrigerator stocked with fresh, healthy foods? Is the cupboard or pantry bare, or are there adequate staples on hand? Are there any signs of burnt pans? Are there signs that the meal described was prepared? Are breakfast dishes in the sink? It is very helpful if a visit is close to a time when the care manager has been told the older person normally eats. It gives the care manager a chance to see whether meal preparations are underway. Asking for a tour of the home or for a drink of cold water is an easy way to observe the kitchen unobtrusively if an older person is not forthcoming with information in this area.

Housekeeping

Again, sex role differences can influence responses on this item, and the care manager needs to take account of these issues. Also, some people use the services of a housekeeper and may have for years, so their nonperformance in this area needs to reflect long-established patterns. Finally, individual standards of cleanliness vary, and these need to be acknowledged.

A tour of the house of the older person, in addition to asking direct questions about housekeeping habits, provides information for the care manager to consider. In addition, information about past practices helps the care manager to ascertain whether functioning has changed and when. The care manager should look for signs of neglect. Also signs of hoarding should be noted. Safety issues in the home are also important to record for future follow-up.

Laundry

Like housekeeping, laundry tasks are subject to sex role and support (housekeeping) staff practices. It is important to note actual behavior and health issues or disabilities that interfere with the behavior, if any. Any changes in habits should be followed to learn what triggered or caused the behavior change. Also note the person's general appearance. Is the person wearing soiled clothing? Is the person reported to wear the same clothes day in and day out? When touring the house, note whether there are signs of neglect, heavily soiled towels in the bathroom, for example. Where is the laundry room? Is it down a flight of stairs in the basement? Does that pose a risk or difficulty if the person must carry laundry baskets back and forth? Is the laundry in another building or outside in the garage? In the winter, are there environmental difficulties or risks involved in doing the laundry? For example, does a person with unsteady gait or arthritis in the knees need to go down snow- or ice-covered steps to get to the laundry facilities?

Mode of Transportation

In our automobile-oriented society, many people drive as their normal mode of transportation. Age-related changes can threaten driving ability, however. Health problems can interfere with functioning in this area in obvious and less obvious ways. Problems with vision, reaction time, information processing, concentration, and visual-spatial abilities all interplay to influence driving capacity. Motor skills and coordination also affect performance.

Determine through discussion the older person's usual mode of transportation. Then integrate that with information about the person's lifelong habits. Did the person ever drive? How much? It is also important to screen for any concerns about whether the person should be driving and to probe and gather information from various sources to ascertain whether the self-reported behavior can be corroborated. Observing the car itself can also be helpful to see whether there are dents or scratches present and, if so, to learn about their origin.

For many men and women, driving is both a symbolic and a functional basic necessity. It affords freedom to come and go when and where one chooses, even for persons who no longer venture far, and thus is the hallmark of independence and full personhood. The idea that one can go when, where, and whether one chooses is key to many people's sense of autonomy. It is not surprising, then, that many people hold fast to driving as a basic right. Not surprisingly, too, many people continue to drive even when age or infirmity, or even the removal of their driver's license, dictate that they should not.

It is not within the GCM scope of practice to evaluate a person's driving capacity. The care manager should, however, screen for problems and concerns in this area, note transportation modes being used, and note any need for intervention, evaluation, or assistance to afford the older client continued opportunities for freedom of movement.

Older drivers have a higher risk of traffic fatalities because they are involved in more accidents per mile driven than middle-aged drivers are and because they are more fragile and therefore more likely to suffer more serious injuries should an accident occur.[22] For their safety and the safety of others, it is important that concerns about driving ability be addressed. The American Medical Association (AMA) established the Older Drivers Project to educate physicians about the public health issues related to older driver safety. It has developed a *Physician's Guide to Assessing and Counseling Older Drivers* to aid in addressing issues surrounding fitness to drive. Driver rehabilitation and older driver safety training initiatives are available in many communities. Occupational therapists and driver evaluation programs at universities, state motor vehicle departments, or specialty clinics can aid older persons and their families with driving concerns as well.

Medication Management

The ability to procure, organize, and follow medication regimens is vitally important. Medication mismanagement is widely prevalent in the elderly population. Its consequences can be profound, leading to preventable health declines, hospitalization, and sometimes even death. Moreover, physicians are often unable to ascertain whether or not their patient is compliant with the prescribed medications. Hence, medical management can become misguided inadvertently as a result of noncompliance behaviors. The care manager can play a critical role in evaluating this vital component of functioning among older clients.

In assessing functioning in this area, it is important to combine information gathered from self-reports, reports of others close to the patient, and direct observation. Incipient dementia can interfere with abilities to manage medications, as noted earlier. This is compounded when a person's medication regimen is complicated, for example, take this pill 1 hour before meals, this one with meals, this one 2 hours after eating; sit up for 30 minutes after taking this medication, and so forth. Early-stage dementia patients may forget that they forget to take their medications and may give you false reports about their behavior. Or

they may try to cover their deficits and minimize or fail to reveal difficulties. It is therefore important to observe, count medications if possible, and gather information from others as well as the older person. Suggest the use of a pillbox if one is not present. Other more targeted pill organizers and reminders may also be needed and can be recommended as part of the care plan. Many new devices and technological supports are now available, as is discussed in Chapter 11.

Handling Financial Affairs

Can the older person plan, budget, manage investments, pay bills, balance a checkbook, and manage day-to-day purchases without assistance? Is the person at risk for scams, undue influence, credit problems, or other financial difficulties because of functional limitations? Does the person show good judgment in regard to finances? Has the person changed lifelong habits in how he or she manages money?

On first meeting someone, often it is difficult to gain enough trust to fully assess functioning in this area. As a first step, questions about who pays the bills and manages investments opens up the topic. Based on responses to earlier less threatening questions, the care manager may detect some clues that can shed light on functional capacity here. For example, if someone has difficulty shopping because Alzheimer's disease has affected his or her ability to make a shopping list and go through the market independently to shop, it is expected that this person will need assistance with bookkeeping and money matters. Because the Lawton scale is ordered, it is important to recall that the less demanding tasks are presented first and those requiring higher cognitive functioning are presented later. Thus, difficulties performing the easier tasks indicate the likelihood of difficulties performing the higher-order functions.

When the care manager tours the house, he or she can discreetly and with permission look for unpaid bills lying about or piles of mail that need attention. Stacks of solicitations for charities and/or contests should be noted. Enlisting information from key informants, such as adult children, is important to round out the evaluation of this area. Adult children may be able to review the older person's checkbook to make sure things are in order. They may be aware of utilities or insurances that have threatened termination for nonpayment. They may know whether the older adult participates in "contests" or gives more money than ever before to charities. Financial advisors for the older person may also be a source of information for assistance in evaluating functional performance. Because finances are a very private topic in many families, this subject needs to be handled with delicacy and discretion.

■ SENSORY LOSS

Hearing

Hearing loss affects significantly more persons as they age and the majority of persons over age 70.[24] Hearing loss affects one's ability to drive or use the telephone or perhaps hear a smoke alarm sound. This in turn affects the client's safety. It is important for the care manager to ask about the client's perception of his or her own hearing. If there is a question, just doing a simple test of whispering so that the lips cannot be read or asking the person whether he or she can hear a ticking watch can be a quick screening tool.

Oftentimes, clients just assume that experiencing a sensory loss is a normal part of aging, when in fact, their ears may be filled with wax. Thus, it is important for the care manager to recommend that the person first see the primary care physician if this has not already been done. Then a referral for an evaluation for treatable causes and for testing is appropriate. Many clients are very resistant to getting hearing aids that will correct their hearing problem. They don't always realize the extent of their loss and what they are not hearing until they

have the aids in place. Many are too embarrassed to ask people to repeat themselves and thus may simply nod and smile when they have not heard what has been said. Asking the client to repeat what you have just said is helpful in making sure that the person has heard you.

In addition to an evaluation for a hearing aid, other adaptations are useful. One example is a handheld assistive device that amplifies sound and can be used on an as-needed basis. Other adaptations include doorbells or telephones that trigger a light to go on when they ring. Telephones made especially to be used with hearing aids can make hearing on the phone easier. In addition, adapters for televisions are available that will enable a spouse without hearing loss to listen to the TV at normal sound and the person with the hearing impairment to wear headphones that amplify the volume.

Hearing loss can lead to social isolation and depression,[24] which can in turn lead to other complications that affect function. It is important for the care manager to recommend a plan of care that decreases the likelihood of this occurring and improves the person's quality of life, for example, eating out in restaurants that are not noisy or going in off-hours when it may be the most quiet. Informing others in the person's social circle that the person has hearing loss helps ensure that the person is included in conversations. The care manager can see whether area theaters and performing arts centers have devices available that amplify sound for those with hearing impairment. For clients in a nursing home or an assisted living facility, the staff needs to be alerted to the person's need to be wearing a hearing aid. It is important to keep the client with hearing impairment involved as a part of his or her community.

Vision

Visual impairment is very common in older persons and has a major impact on performance of daily activities. Data from the National Health Interview Survey show that approximately 12% of persons age 65 and older have difficulty seeing words and letters in ordinary newspapers even when wearing glasses or contact lenses.[23] Age-related illnesses resulting in progressive vision loss include macular degeneration, cataracts, glaucoma, and diabetic retinopathy. Acute vision loss can be caused by stroke or giant cell arteritis. Many older people are unaware of losses in peripheral vision and central acuity.

Visual acuity information pertaining to the ability to function in the environment can be gathered by observing the client walking, shaking hands, and completing forms. The client can be asked by the care manager to read a headline and a sentence from the newspaper. Ability to read both denotes normal visual acuity. Ability to read only the headline signifies moderate impairment, and inability to read either indicates severe impairment.[6 (p186)]

Vision loss can affect a person's ability to perform many ADLs and IADLs. Older persons with vision loss may experience the following:

- Problems with ambulation because they do not see obstacles in their path or changes in the ground surfaces outside
- Problems with dressing because they do not see that their clothes are soiled or do not match
- Problems with feeding because they do not see the food clearly on their plate
- Problems with the telephone because they don't see the numbers
- Problems with food preparation because they can't read directions
- Problems with transportation because of the inability to drive
- Problems with medication use because they can't identify the pills or see that they have dropped them on the floor
- Problems with finances because they can't see to write checks.

The list of potential problems can go on and on.

To begin, the care manager should ask whether the person wears glasses and ascertain that the glasses are being worn, especially in a nursing home or assisted living facility where the glasses may be kept in a drawer. Next, the care manager should know when the last ophthalmology exam was performed. Frequently, older persons forget to have their eyes examined, especially if they perceive that they are seeing well enough. However, checks for glaucoma and other eye disease should be done annually. Other clients may require a referral to a low-vision center that can offer adaptations, such as specialty magnifiers, to improve vision.[25] In addition, the care manager can recommend changes in the home to prevent falls such as applying brightly colored tape on the last step, using color contrast when the floor surface changes, or improving contrast in the environment such as not using a light-colored chair on a light-colored carpet. Improved lighting and removing clutter also reduce the risk of falls. In addition, large clocks, calendars, and telephone dials can improve independence in function. An excellent source for strategies on dealing with vision loss is The Lighthouse (1-800-829-0500), which also provides a website for purchasing products that improve independence.

■ SLEEP

Lack of sleep can have a definite impact on clients' quality of life and their ability to participate in their ADLs and IADLs. Thus, part of every care manager's assessment should include questions about the client's sleep pattern, such as, "What time do you fall asleep at night?" "Do you get up in the middle of the night?" "Do you fall back to sleep without problems?" "What time do you wake up in the morning?" If there are indications of problems with sleep, a follow-up question should be asked about whether the client naps during the day to see if this is why the person cannot sleep at night. Also the care manager should ask whether there have been recent changes in sleep patterns.

Oftentimes, a person with dementia can have marked sleep problems that include a reversal of sleeping and awake hours. This has a major effect on family caregivers and may result in placement into an assisted living or nursing home because the client may not have the funds to pay for a caregiver or home health aide who can be awake at night.

Inadequate amounts of sleep can affect the amount of energy the person has to dress in the morning, make breakfast, or go grocery shopping. It is important to attempt to find out the reasons for the poor sleep. Is arthritic pain keeping the person awake at night? Is the person drinking alcohol, which affects the ability to stay awake, or caffeinated soft drinks, which may impair sleep? Would increased exercise during the day improve sleep at night? Is the person depressed? Is the person getting up to toilet too frequently because of a urological problem that can be improved with medication? Is the person taking medications that have side effects that disturb sleep such as causing nightmares or leg movements? Have there been recent changes in medications, or are there possible new medical problems that might be contributing to the sleep disturbance? For clients in a facility, the problem may be staff checkups at night or early in the morning that may awaken them. Attempts to address the root of the problem are important before prescribing medications for sleep that may then have the added problematic effect of increasing the risk of falls or causing oversedation in the morning. The care manager may consider having an evaluation at a sleep center conducted, which can diagnose problems such as sleep apnea. Changes in bedtime routine such as taking a bath, drinking warm milk, having a snack, listening to soothing music, or removing the television from the bedroom may have a positive effect on the ability to fall and stay asleep.

■ HOME ENVIRONMENT ASSESSMENT[6(pp196–200)]

Over one fifth of all households in the United States have one or more persons aged 65 and older.[26] The overwhelming majority of people choose to remain in their current residence as they age. The living situations of this group are diverse. In addition, conventional housing is not easily adaptable to meet the changing needs of people over their lifetimes. Older persons are more vulnerable to the problems of inadequate, unsafe housing as a result. The three most common housing-related problems of older persons are adequacy of housing for the individual's needs, suitability of the neighborhood, and cost.[5] The homes of older persons are more likely to have physical defects because of age than homes lived in by younger persons. Some of these defects, such as inadequate insulation, may actually increase the costs of day-to-day living for older persons, who often live on fixed incomes.

Other vital components of the home (e.g., wiring, roofing) may need repairs and upgrades that the older person cannot afford. As a result of the factors listed earlier and the reluctance of some older persons to consider making any changes to accommodate physical disabilities, such as the installation of grab bars in bathrooms, relocation to a downstairs area for sleeping, and the addition of ramps for safe entry and exit, some older persons are living in unsafe conditions. This group is at increased risk for falls and fractures and the institutionalization that frequently follows such events.

It is very important and necessary to perform a home assessment as part of the geriatric assessment process. The assessment should include the evaluation of safety factors (e.g., functioning smoke alarms, adequate wiring) and how effectively the older person is able to function within the floor plan and room arrangement of his or her home. While the home might be safe for a person without disabilities or cognitive impairments, if there are features (e.g., a second story, sunken rooms or hallways, tiny bathrooms) that are obstacles or potential dangers to a person needing assistive devices or forgetful of steps, that home is not safe for that person. Observation of the client as he or she performs ADLs is invaluable for assessment of the client's home safety and environmental needs as well as functional abilities.

Using a checklist is a time-efficient and comprehensive method for ascertaining the safety of a home. The Home Safety Checklist (Exhibit 4–6) is one tool that can be used to identify fall hazards in the home.[27] Its detailed questions provide some education to the older person in practices that can be initiated to minimize the likelihood of falling. As part of the assessment, caregivers can be educated to be alert for haz-

ards and to evaluate the need for added safety features (e.g., alarms on outside doors, grab bars, raised toilet seats) that the older person may need as his or her condition progresses.

Once safety hazards have been identified and necessary changes have been listed and explained to the client, the care manager has to make sure that changes will be made by addressing hazards as problems in the care plan and writing an intervention for their solution. Often, older persons are unable or unwilling to make changes. Suggested changes should be addressed with the older person, and every attempt should be made to get the person to agree and plan for the prompt implementation needed. If the older person resists, family or other support persons should be notified of the risk to the older person in remaining in the unchanged environment. These persons often can influence the older person and assist with the practical matters of implementation of changes.

Exhibit 4–6   Consumer Product Safety Commission's "Safety for Older Consumers: Home Safety Checklist"

TOP TEN SAFETY CHECKLIST FOR OLDER CONSUMERS

☑ Install smoke and carbon monoxide alarms throughout your home.

☑ Have an emergency escape plan and pre-arrange for a family member or caregiver to help you escape, if needed.

☑ Keep a fire extinguisher handy in the kitchen in case of fire.

☑ Make sure there is good lighting inside and outside your home to help prevent falls.

☑ Make sure walking surfaces are flat, slip resistant, free of objects, and in good condition to avoid falls.

☑ Keep ashtrays, smoking materials, candles, hot plates, and other potential fire sources away from curtains, furniture, beds and bedding.

☑ Have fuel burning appliances including furnaces and chimneys inspected by a professional every year to make sure they are working properly and not leaking poisonous carbon monoxide.

☑ Install ground fault circuit interrupters, or GFCIs, in potentially damp locations such as the kitchen, bathroom, garage, near utility tubs or sinks, and on the exterior of the house to protect against electrocution.

☑ Make sure all medications are stored in child-resistant enclosures and are clearly marked to prevent children from accessing the medication and being poisoned.

☑ Set your hot water heater to no more than 120°F to help prevent burns.

Exhibit 4–6   Consumer Product Safety Commission's "Safety for Older Consumers: Home Safety Checklist" (continued)

PREPARE FOR AN EMERGENCY

☑ Install smoke and carbon monoxide alarms throughout your home.

☑ Have an emergency escape plan and pre-arrange for a family member or caregiver to help you escape the home in a fire, if needed.

Smoke and Carbon Monoxide (CO) Alarms

☐ *Smoke alarms are installed on every level of my home, outside sleeping areas and inside bedrooms. Carbon monoxide (CO) alarms are installed on every level of my home and outside sleeping areas.*

Smoke alarms are critical for the early detection of a fire and could mean the difference between life and death. About two-thirds of home fire deaths occur in homes without working smoke alarms.

All homes should also have carbon monoxide (CO) alarms installed. CO is an invisible and odorless gas that can kill you in minutes. Any fuel-burning appliance in your home is a potential CO source, but even all-electric homes could have sources of CO such as a car running in an attached garage or a portable generator operating outside. CO alarms should not be installed in basements, attics, or garages unless they contain sleeping areas.

☐ *I have tested my smoke and CO alarms within the last month, and they are working properly.*

Alarms that use voice warnings may help you to distinguish smoke alarms from CO alarms. If you are hearing-impaired and are unable to hear the sound from a smoke or CO alarm, install alarms with strobe lights to notify you during the day and use an assistive device that vibrates the bed and pillow to awaken you when the alarms sound at night.

☐ *I have replaced the batteries in all of my alarms within the last year.*

Emergency Escape Plan

☐ *I have an emergency escape plan.*

Once a fire starts, it spreads rapidly. An escape plan can reduce the amount of time required for you and your family to get out safely, and can improve your chances of surviving a fire or similar emergency. To the extent possible, identify two ways to escape from every room and avoid escape routes that require the use of escape ladders or similar items that could put you at risk of a fall. If there is a fire in your home, do not waste time trying to save property. Get out as fast as possible, and remember: ONCE OUT – STAY OUT!

☐ *I have practiced my fire escape plan with my family within the last 6 months, during both the day and night.*

Emergency Contact Information

☐ *Emergency numbers are posted on or near all telephones.*

Make certain that telephone numbers are readily available for the Police, Fire Department, and local Poison Control Center, along with numbers for your doctor(s) and a trusted neighbor or family member. If you have impaired vision or difficulty seeing the numbers on a regular telephone, choose a phone that has large, lighted number keys.

☐ *Telephones are positioned low enough so I can reach them if I have an accident that leaves me unable to stand.*

Keeping telephones at a low height is helpful in the event that you have an accident that leaves you unable to stand. As an alternative, consider obtaining a wearable medical alert device that provides a "Call for Help" pushbutton.

☐ *A telephone is located in my bedroom in case a fire traps me there.*

continues

Exhibit 4–6   Consumer Product Safety Commission's "Safety for Older Consumers: Home Safety Checklist" (continued)

CHECK THROUGHOUT THE HOME

☑ Make sure walking surfaces are flat, slip resistant, free of objects, and in good condition to avoid falls.

☑ Install ground fault circuit interrupters, or GFCIs, in potentially damp locations such as the kitchen, bathroom, garage, near utility tubs or sinks, and on the exterior of the house to protect against electrocution.

Walking Surfaces

☐ *All walking surfaces are free of electrical cords, boxes, furniture, appliances, and other objects that could pose a tripping hazard, especially in the event of an emergency or fire.*

Falls are associated with more than half of all product-related visits to the emergency room among adults aged 65 to 74, and with more than three-quarters of visits among adults 75 years and older. Tripping over loose carpets, cords, or other obstacles on the floor is a common fall scenario.

☐ *All flooring is in good condition, is flat and uniform, and is slip-resistant or is covered with slip-resistant carpeting, rugs, mats, or similar materials.*

Slip-resistant surfaces are especially important in potentially wet locations such as bathrooms, kitchens, and entryways. There should be no loose floorboards, missing tiles, or similar problems that could pose a tripping hazard. Carpeting should be low pile and free of tears, holes, or wear that could cause slips or trips.

Steps and Stairways

☐ *All steps are in good condition, have flat, even surfaces and are free of objects that could pose a tripping hazard.*

☐ *All stair treads are in good condition, and have slip-resistant surfaces such as dense, low-pile carpeting or slip-resistant strips that are securely attached to the steps.*

☐ *Light switches are located at both the top and bottom of the stairs.*

If no other light is available, keep an operating flashlight in a convenient location.

☐ *All stairs have solidly mounted handrails that run continuously along the full length of the stairs on both sides. Handrails are easily graspable.*

Lighting

☐ *Walkways and rooms in which I am likely to be reading—for example, the bedroom, bathrooms, and the kitchen—are especially well-lit or have additional lighting available.*

Lighting is an important factor in preventing falls since areas that are poorly lit or in shadow can hide slipping and tripping hazards. Indirect lighting or frosted bulbs can be used to reduce glare.

☐ *All light bulbs are of the appropriate wattage and type for the lamp or light fixture in which they are installed.*

For those fixtures that do not identify the correct wattage, installed bulbs should not exceed 60 watts, or 25 watts for bulbs with a miniature base (candelabra). Consider using compact-fluorescent or similar energy-efficient bulbs, which produce more light per watt than incandescent bulbs.

Exhibit 4–6   Consumer Product Safety Commission's "Safety for Older Consumers: Home Safety Checklist" (continued)

Electrical Outlets and Switches

☐ *All electrical outlets that are located in potentially damp locations, such as the kitchen, bathroom, garage, near the utility tub or sink, and on the exterior of the house, have ground-fault circuit interrupters, or GFCIs, installed to protect against electrical shock.*

☐ *I have tested all GFCI receptacles within the last month and have found them to be working properly.*

GFCI receptacles can provide power even when they are no longer providing shock protection. Test a GFCI receptacle monthly by plugging a night-light or lamp into the receptacle and switching it on. When you press the TEST button on the GFCI receptacle, the RESET button should pop forward and the light should go out. Pressing the RESET button should restore power to the outlet.

☐ *No electrical outlets or switches are unusually warm or hot to the touch.*

Hot or unusually warm electrical outlets or switches may indicate an unsafe wiring condition. Stop using these electrical outlets and have an electrician check them as soon as possible.

☐ *All electrical outlets and switches have cover plates installed so no wiring is exposed.*

☐ *Unused receptacles have safety covers installed to prevent access by young children.*

Electrical Cords

☐ *All electrical, extension, and telephone cords are out of the flow of foot traffic since they pose a tripping hazard.*

☐ *Electrical cords are not beneath furniture, rugs, or carpeting. Cords are not pinched against the wall by furniture and are not wrapped tightly around objects.*

☐ *All electrical cords are in good condition and are free of damage such as fraying, cracking, and staple or nail holes.*

☐ *Extension cords are not overloaded. In other words, the total wattage of all appliances plugged into an extension cord does not exceed the rated capacity of the extension cord.*

If the cord rating is exceeded, switch to a higher-rated cord or unplug some of the appliances. Standard 16-gauge extension cords can carry 1625 watts. Discard older extension cords that use small 18 gauge wires.

☐ *All extension cords have polarized-plug receptacles; that is, receptacles with one wide plug slot and one narrow plug slot.*

CHECK KITCHENS

☑ Keep a fire extinguisher handy in the kitchen in case of fire.

☐ *A fire extinguisher is in the kitchen in case of fire.*

☐ *Towels, curtains, potholders, and other objects that might catch fire are located away from the range.*

☐ *Kitchen ventilation systems or range exhausts are functioning properly.*

Indoor air pollutants and CO may accumulate to unhealthy levels in a kitchen with gas or kerosene-fired appliances. Use ventilation systems or open windows to clear the air of vapors and smoke. Never use your range or stove to heat your home.

continues

Exhibit 4–6   Consumer Product Safety Commission's "Safety for Older Consumers: Home Safety Checklist" (continued)

☐ *Electrical appliance and extension cords are away from the sink and other water sources and are away from hot surfaces such as the range.*

☐ *Electrical receptacles that supply countertop appliances, such as coffeemakers and toasters, are protected by ground-fault circuit interrupters, or GFCIs.*

Test all GFCI receptacles monthly to make sure they are working properly.

☐ *Kitchen lighting is bright and even, especially near the stove, sink and countertop work areas.*

☐ *A stable step stool with a handrail is easily accessible for reaching high items.*

Standing on chairs, boxes, or other makeshift items to reach high shelves can result in falls. Buy a step stool if you don't have one. Choose a sturdy one with a handrail that you can grasp while standing on the top step. Before climbing on any step stool, make sure it is fully opened and stable on a flat surface. Discard step stools that are not stable or have broken parts.

CHECK LIVING ROOMS AND FAMILY ROOMS

☑ Have fuel-burning appliances, including furnaces and chimneys, inspected by a professional every year to make sure they are working properly and not leaking poisonous carbon monoxide.

☐ *All chimneys have been professionally inspected and cleaned within the last year, and chimney openings are clear of leaves and other debris that could clog them.*

A clogged chimney can cause poisonous carbon monoxide (CO) to enter your home. Burning wood in a fireplace can cause creosote, a highly flammable substance, to build-up inside the chimney. This material can ignite and result in a serious chimney fire.

☐ *All portable space heaters and woodburning heating equipment are at least 3 feet from walls, furniture, curtains, rugs, newspapers, and other flammable or combustible materials.*

☐ *All portable space heaters are stable and located away from walkways.*

☐ *The surface of each fireplace is fireproof, and all wood-burning heating equipment is installed on fireproof flooring or on an approved non-combustible floor protector.*

Burning material can be ejected from an open fireplace. Fire resistant hearthrugs, made of wool, fiberglass, or other synthetics, are readily available to protect the area in front of a fireplace.

☐ *Candles, smoking materials, and other potential fire sources are located away from curtains, furniture, and other flammable or combustible objects and are never left out unattended.*

CHECK BATHROOMS

☑ Make sure all medications are stored in child-resistant enclosures and are clearly marked to prevent children from accessing the medications and being poisoned.

☐ *All medications are stored in child-resistant enclosures and are clearly marked.*

If grandchildren or other youngsters are visitors, purchase medicines in containers with child-resistant caps, and close the caps properly after each use. Store all medicines out of the reach of children. Many poisonings occur when children visiting grandparents go

Exhibit 4–6   Consumer Product Safety Commission's "Safety for Older Consumers: Home Safety Checklist" (continued)

through the medicine cabinet or their grandmother's purse. Only request non-child-resistant enclosures if you are physically unable to use child-resistant enclosures. Medications that are not clearly and accurately labeled can be easily mixed up, causing you to take the wrong medicine or to miss a required dosage of medicine. Be sure that all containers are clearly marked with the contents, doctor's instructions, expiration date, and patient's name. Dispose of outdated medicines properly. Because of their environmental impact, disposing expired medication in the toilet may not be an acceptable method. Your doctor or pharmacist can advise you on the best method of disposal.

☐ *All bathtubs and showers are equipped with non-skid mats, abrasive strips, or surfaces that are not slippery and have at least one secure and easily graspable grab bar.*

☐ *The bathroom floor is slip-resistant or is covered with secure slip-resistant materials.*

☐ *All hair dryers, shavers, curling irons, and other small electrical appliances not currently in use are unplugged.*

☐ *All small electrical appliances are away from sinks, tubs, and other sources of water.*
Never reach into water to retrieve a fallen appliance without being sure that the appliance is unplugged.

☐ *Electrical receptacles in the bathroom are protected by ground-fault circuit interrupters, or GFCIs.*
Test all GFCI receptacles monthly to make sure they are working properly.

CHECK BEDROOMS

☑ Keep ashtrays, smoking materials, candles, hot plates, and other potential fire sources away from curtains, furniture, beds, and bedding.

☐ *Ash trays, smoking materials, candles, hot plates, and other potential fire sources are located away from curtains, furniture, beds, and bedding.*
Burns associated with personal use products were the most frequently reported cause of accidental death among seniors. Smoking is one of the major contributors to this problem. Never smoke in bed. Remove sources of heat or flame from areas around beds, and do not leave the room or fall asleep while a candle is burning.

☐ *A flashlight is within reach of the bed in case of a power outage.*

☐ *A telephone is within reach of the bed in case of an emergency.*

☐ *My mattress meets the new federal flammability standard.*
Newer mattresses are more resistant to fires from open flames such as candles, lighters, and matches, and have tags indicating that they meet the federal standard.

☐ *Electrically heated blankets are not folded, covered by other objects, or "tucked in," when in use. The power cord is not pinched or crushed by the bed, between a wall or the floor.*
Objects that cover the blanket's heating elements or controls can cause overheating. Do not allow anything, including other blankets, comforters, and even sleeping pets, on top of the electric blanket while it is in use. "Tucking in" electric blankets also can cause excessive heat buildup and start a fire. The edges of your electric blanket should hang freely over the sides and end of the bed. Always turn off your heating pad before you go to sleep. It can cause serious burns even at relatively low settings.

continues

Exhibit 4–6 Consumer Product Safety Commission's "Safety for Older Consumers: Home Safety Checklist" (continued)

☐ *As recommended by the fire safety community, smoke alarms are placed inside and just outside bedrooms and they have been tested within the last month and are working. CO alarms are located outside sleeping areas, have been tested within the last month, and are working properly. The batteries have been replaced within the last year.*

CHECK BASEMENTS, GARAGES, WORKSHOPS, AND STORAGE AREAS

☑ Set your hot water heater to no more than 120 degrees Fahrenheit to help prevent burns.

☐ *The water heater is set to no more than 120 degrees Fahrenheit.*

Water above 120 degrees can burn your skin. Lower the setting to 120 degrees or "low." If you are unfamiliar with the setting, ask a qualified person to adjust it for you; if your hot water system is controlled by the landlord, ask the landlord to consider lowering the temperature.

☐ *Work areas, especially those where power tools are used, are well-lit.*

Basements, garages, and storage areas can contain many tripping hazards. Sharp or pointed tools can make a fall even more hazardous. Power tools and workshop equipment have been associated with many emergency room-treated injuries to people 65 and older.

☐ *For electrical panels with fuses, the fuses are the correct size (amperage) for the circuit.*

If you do not know the correct electrical rating, have an electrician label the fuse box with the sizes you should use or replace the fuse panel with a circuit breaker panel. Fuses rated 15 and 20 amperes are typical in homes. If you find that all or most of the fuses in your fuse box are rated higher than 20 amperes, there is a good chance that some of the fuses are rated too high for residential circuits and can present a serious fire hazard.

☐ *All power tools are either equipped with a 3-prong plug or marked to show that they are double-insulated. All space heaters with 3-prong plugs are plugged into 3-hole receptacles or are connected with a properly attached and certified adapter.*

Three-prong plugs and double insulation reduce the risk of an electric shock. Consider replacing old tools that lack a 3-prong plug and are not double-insulated. Improperly grounded tools and appliances can lead to electrical shock. Never defeat the grounding feature by removing the round grounding prong on the plug. Check with your service person or an electrician if you are in doubt.

☐ *Electrical receptacles in garages, unfinished basements, and workshops are protected by ground-fault circuit interrupters, or GFCIs.*

Test all GFCIs monthly to make sure they are working properly.

☐ *All fuel-burning appliances, including furnaces, boilers, fireplaces, wood stoves, and water heaters, as well as chimneys, flues, and vents have been inspected professionally within the last year.*

A heater operating without proper ventilation and air supply produces carbon monoxide (CO), and older consumers may be more susceptible to CO exposure. CO is an invisible killer. It's a colorless, odorless, poisonous gas. The first line of defense against CO poisoning is to have a qualified professional inspect all fuel-burning heating systems, including furnaces, boilers, fireplaces, wood stoves, water heaters, chimneys, flues and vents.

Exhibit 4–6   Consumer Product Safety Commission's "Safety for Older Consumers: Home Safety Checklist" (continued)

☐ *All kerosene, natural gas, and similar space-heating equipment has adequate ventilation.*

Always use the correct fuel, as recommended by the manufacturer. Never pour gasoline into a kerosene heater. Review the installation and operating instructions. Call the manufacturer or your local fire department if you have additional questions.

☐ *No containers of flammable and combustible liquids are stored inside the house.*

The vapors that can escape from damaged or loosely closed containers of flammable or combustible liquids may be toxic when inhaled and may cause fires. Do not store gasoline or other highly flammable liquids in the house, utility room, garage or near the water heater. Portable gasoline containers intended for use by consumers are required to have child-resistant closures effective January 2009.

☐ *Portable generators are not operating in the basement, garage, or anywhere near the house.*

People have been killed by operating a portable generator in their basement or garage. Generators quickly produce high levels of poisonous CO and should never be used indoors, including inside a home, basement, shed, or garage, even if doors or windows are open. CO from a generator used indoors can kill you and your family in minutes. Consumers should use portable generators outside only and far from windows, doors, and vents to their homes.

CHECK ENTRYWAYS AND THE HOME EXTERIOR

☑ Make sure there is good lighting inside and outside your home to help prevent falls.

☐ *The porch, entryway, and approach to the entryway are all well-illuminated.*

☐ *The light switch is located near the entryway.*

☐ *Outside steps, entryways, and approaches to the entryway are in good condition and are slip-resistant.*

☐ *Outside steps have handrails that are easily graspable.*

☐ *All outside electrical outlets are GFCI-protected and in weatherproof covers or enclosures.*

☐ *Portable generators are located far from windows, doors, and vents to the home.*

☐ *All outdoor electrical tools and equipment have 3-prong cords and have not been modified to plug into 2-prong outlets.*

Source: Consumer Product Safety Commission. *Safety for Older Consumers—Home Safety Checklist.* CPSC Document #701. Available at: http://www.cpsc.gov/cpscpub/pubs/701.pdf. Accessed October 21, 2010.

■ CONCLUSION

The evaluation of an older person's functional status is key to helping that person maintain his or her autonomy and quality of life. Functional abilities are of paramount importance to overall health, well-being, and potential need for services. The functional assessment helps set priorities around which the available medical, social, and economic resources can be rallied. Once the functional assessment, psychosocial assessment, and cognitive assessments (see Chapter 3) are completed, the care manager can develop a plan of care (see Chapter 5).

■ REFERENCES

1. Kane RL, Ouslander JG, Abrass IB. *Essentials of Clinical Geriatrics*. New York: McGraw-Hill, Health Professions Division; 1999.

2. Newcomer R, Harrington C, Kane R. Implications of managed care for older persons. In: Katz P, Kane R, Mezey M, eds. *Emerging Systems in Long-Term Care*. New York: Springer Publishers; 1999:118–148.

3. Gallo J. *Handbook of Geriatric Assessment*. 3rd ed. Gaithersburg, MD: Aspen Publishers; 1999.

4. American Geriatrics Society. Comprehensive Geriatric Assessment Position Statement. October 1996. Available at: http://www.american geriatrics.org. Accessed March 15, 1999.

5. Fretwell M. Comprehensive functional assessment. In: Abrams W, Berkow R, eds. *The Merck Manual of Geriatrics*. Rahway, NJ: Merck & Co.; 1990:170–174.

6. Barber C. Geriatric assessment. In: Cress C, ed. *Handbook of Geriatric Care Management*. Gaithersburg, MD: Aspen Publishers; 2001:187–194.

7. Katz S, Downs T, Cash H. Progress in the development of the index of ADL. *Gerontologist*. 1970;10:20–30.

8. Mahoney F, Barthel D. Functional evaluation: the Barthel Index. *Md State Med J*. 1965;14:61–65.

9. Fillenbaum G, Smyer M. The development, validity and reliability of the OARS multidimensional functional assessment questionnaire. *J Gerontol*. 1981;36:428–434.

10. Moskowitz E, McCann C. Classification of disability in the chronically ill and aging. *J Chronic Dis*. 1957;5:342–346.

11. Morris J, Harues C, Murphy K. Designing the National Resident Assessment Instrument for Nursing Homes. *Gerontologist*. 1990;30:293–307.

12. Heeren T, Lagaay A, vonBeck W, Rooymans H, Hijman W. Reference values for the Mini-Mental State Examination in octo- and nonagenarians. *J Am Geriatr Soc*. 1990;38:1093–1096.

13. Tinetti M. Performance oriented assessment of mobility: problems in elderly patients. *J Am Geriatr Soc*. 1986;34:119–126.

14. Mathias S, Nayak U, Issacs B. Balance in elderly patients: the Get Up and Go Test. *Arch Phys Med Rehab*. 1986;67:387–389.

15. Resnick N, Wells T. Maintaining and restoring continence. In: Funk S, Tornquist M, Champagne M, Weise R, eds. *Key Aspects of Elder Care*. New York: Springer Publishers; 1992:135–154.

16. Tideiksaar R. *Falls in Older Persons, Prevention and Management*. 2nd ed. Baltimore, MD: Health Professions Press; 1998.

17. Davies G, Scully F. *Fall Prevention: Stay on Your Own Two Feet*. West Conshohocken, PA: Infinity Publishing; 2006.

18. Castle S, Opava-Rutter D. Practical fall risk assessment in older adults with multiple medical problems and/or chronic disease. *Geriatric Care Manage J*. Summer–Fall 2003;13(2):17–23.

19. Lawton M, Brody E. Assessment of older people: self-maintaining and instrumental activities of daily living. *Gerontologist*. 1969;9:179–186.

20. Pearson VI. Assessment of function in older adults. In: Kane R, Kane R, eds. *Assessing Older Persons*. New York: Oxford University Press; 2000:17–48.

21. Fillenbaum GG. Screening the elderly. A brief instrumental activities of daily living measure. *J Am Geriatr Soc*. 1985;33(10):698–706.

22. American Medical Association. Safety and the older driver, physician's guide to assessing and counseling older drivers. 2010. http://www.ama-assn.org/ama/pub/physician-resources/public-health/promoting-healthy-lifestyles/geriatric-health/older-driver-safety/assessing-counseling-older-drivers.shtml. Accessed November 7, 2010.

23. Lighthouse International. National (US) Estimates, all ages, of prevalence of vision impairment. http://www.lighthouse.org/research/statistics-on-vision-impairment/prevalence-of-vision-impairment/#national. Accessed July 5, 2010.

24. Weinstein BE. Hearing loss and hearing aides. *Geriatric Care Manage J*. Summer 2002;12(2):7.

25. Strand CH. Vision loss—a focus on function. *Geriatric Care Manage J*. Summer 2002;12(2):3.

26. Pynoos J, Caraviello R, Cicero C. Lifelong housing: the anchor in aging-friendly communities. *Generations*. 2009;33(2):26.

27. U.S. Consumer Product Safety Commission, Safety for Older Consumers Home Safety Checklist. CPSC Document #701. Available at: http://www.cpsc.gov/cpscpub/pubs/701.html. Accessed August 21, 2006.

■ WEBSITES AND RESOURCES

- Driver Safety Program at AARP:
  www.aarp.org/home-garden/transportation/
  driver_safety

- Fall prevention resources from National
  Council on Aging:
  www.healthyagingprograms.org

- Hearing information:
  www.betterhearing.org

- Home safety for people with Alzheimer's:
  www.nia.nih.gov/Alzheimers/publications/
  homesafety.htm

- Sleep information:
  www.sleepfoundation.org

- Urinary incontinence:
  www.mayoclinic.com/health/urinary-
  incontinence/DS00404

- Visual impairment resources:
  www.lighthouse.org

Chapter 5

Care Planning and Geriatric Assessment

Cathy Jo Cress

■ INTRODUCTION

The process of geriatric assessment is like the method detectives use to solve a crime. Just as detectives meticulously sift through clues, leave no stone unturned, ensure all evidence is taken into account before reaching conclusions, so must geriatric care managers (GCMs). Like Sherlock Holmes, GCMs conducting a geriatric assessment must strive to make sure all facts have been gathered and examined, both individually and in combination with one another, before writing a report and developing a care plan. However, unlike Sherlock Holmes, GCMs often have to first meet a client because of an immediate crisis, and they sometimes have to begin to assist that client without being able to gather all of the information they might like.

Comprehensive geriatric assessment has been defined as a "multidisciplinary evaluation in which the multiple problems of older people are uncovered, described, and explained, if possible, and in which the resources and strengths of the person are catalogued, need for services assessed, and a coordinated care plan developed to focus on interventions of the person's problems."[1] Additionally, the resources and strengths of the older person must be ascertained and evaluated so that they can be part of the development of a care plan, in recognition of the uniqueness and individuality of that person. Assessment of the impact of illnesses and the aging process on an older person's physical, emotional, spiritual, and social functioning is a critical component of the provision of appropriate health care. Performing comprehensive geriatric assessments and care planning is a challenge for GCMs.

The Comprehensive Geriatric Assessment Position Statement of the American Geriatrics Society includes the following statements: "Comprehensive geriatric assessment has demonstrated usefulness in improving the health status of frail, older patients. Therefore, elements of Comprehensive Geriatric Assessment should be incorporated into the acute and long-term care provided to these elderly individuals," and "Medicare and other insurers should recognize as a reimbursable service or procedure: (1) periodic assessment of patients, and (2) the support services required for effective application on Comprehensive Geriatric Assessment."[2]

A comprehensive assessment is essential to provide the right services at the right time. Older people often have complex health problems with atypical presentations. Elders have cognitive and affective problems that make history taking difficult. They react strongly to medication, are frequently socially isolated, and can be economically compromised. If a comprehensive assessment is not done, older people may be at risk for premature or inappropriate institutionalization. Problems often involve more than one domain of the assessment. Treatment of a medical problem or living condition can sometimes affect cognitive or functional status. On the other hand, the client's cognitive and functional status and values must often be taken into account before deciding how aggressively medical problems should be approached.

The geriatric assessment should be carried out by an experienced GCM. This person is usually either a registered nurse (RN) or human services professional such as a gerontologist or social worker. As more classes, certificates, and concentrations in geriatric care management evolve throughout the United States, GCMs can actually have specific educational backgrounds in geriatric care management. Many have passed a certification exam in geriatric care management. A team approach involving an RN and a social worker can be very effective, but a non-RN GCM using a functional assessment tool can gather both the health and psychosocial information needed for a comprehensive assessment.

The assessment process begins with a case-finding approach and employs screening instruments and techniques, unless this information is already available from the client's medical record. Based on the initial interview, more detailed assessments may be recommended. This may mean referrals to a number of professional disciplines, such as audiology, psychology, nutrition, physical therapy, occupational therapy, pharmacy, and speech therapy. The assessment should take account of the older person's physical and emotional health. It should reflect his or her ethnic and spiritual background and quality-of-life preferences, finances, and support systems so realistic plans for long-term care can be made if necessary. The older person's own goals and wishes should be taken into account in the planning as much as possible.

The initial assessment is also the GCM's first contact with the client and family. First impressions are important, so the GCM should present him- or herself in a professional manner by being on time, well dressed, and thorough. The GCM must be the quality professional the client and family want to work with on an ongoing basis. This assessment is also the basis for getting paid a fee, so making an excellent initial impression is essential if you want to do further work with the client and family.

■ GOALS OF A WRITTEN GERIATRIC ASSESSMENT

The GCM does a geriatric assessment to create a care plan, which proposes recommendations to repair the holes in the older client's personal safety net using the family system and the continuum of care. The recommendations suggest services at the right time for the right amount of money.

The first GCM goal of a written geriatric assessment is to convey in an organized and thorough manner the information gathered and recorded with the assessment tools, interviews, and observations. These pieces of information are all the clues. The second goal is to draw conclusions from that information or clues and present them in a persuasive manner. The final goal is for the GCM to prepare recommendations based on the conclusions. These conclusions are presented to the client, family, or third party who requested the assessment. It is hoped they are convincing enough that the family or third party will agree with those needed solutions to the documented problems. By preparing a thorough, well-reasoned geriatric care assessment, the GCM has begun the process of developing an ongoing relationship with that client and family.

■ ELEMENTS OF THE ASSESSMENT

The first step the GCM takes in a basic geriatric assessment is looking at the client's physical and mental health and social, spiritual, economic, functional, and environmental status. Much like Sherlock Holmes or his new sleuthing wife, Mary Russell, you observe the clients through the lens of a magnifying glass, which is the GCM's assessment tools.

You measure change in an assessment—change in the client's present problems; change in the client's present functioning; change in the support system that might necessitate need for different solutions. As an example of this process, consider a client we will call Mamie Nixon, who lives in Santa Cruz, California. Her son calls you and asks you to assess his mother because she drove to the grocery store, got lost, and was picked up by the highway patrol, disoriented and confused. Mamie has actually had difficulty driving for 20 years, first ameliorated by eyeglasses and, then, 10 years later, she agreed not to drive at night. But now a new problem has developed. Her original visual issue is now complicated by mental confusion. So, a client could have a long-term change in functional ability. Twenty years later, she can't remember well enough to drive from home to the supermarket.

Mamie also experienced a change in appearance. She dressed appropriately a year ago, and now is always dressed in dirty, unmatched clothes. A year ago Mamie walked around unaided, and now she needs to use a cane. Twelve months ago she was mentally clear enough to execute a will, but now her mental status has declined to the point where she may not have the capacity to change her will. She could pay her bills a year ago, but now she can't. Twelve months ago she regularly attended the Live Oak Senior Center, but last month she stopped going to the classes in current affairs she has always loved. During the course of the geriatric care assessment, you discovered and reported all these changes in Mamie.

The next step is to recommend ways to repair the holes in Mamie's safety net: a secure way to shop, get to church, and attend to her activities of daily living (ADLs) such as bathing, grooming, and washing her clothes. In preparing your recommendations, you will consider her strengths and what resources she has to fill these holes. For example, Mamie's resources include her son Pete Nixon, the geriatric psychiatrist at Dominican Mental Health Center, the home care aides available through Senior Network Services, and adequate financial resources from Mamie's income and assets to pay for these services.

Physical Health

The first element of a geriatric assessment is a physical assessment that identifies specific diseases or symptoms for which curative, restorative, palliative, or preventive treatment may be available. Special attention is directed toward visual or hearing impairment, nutritional status, incontinence, and conditions that may contribute to falling or difficulty in ambulation. Of course, any actual physical examination should be done by a nurse practitioner or a physician. Gathering health information about the client and reporting it to the physician, through assessment tools, can be done by the GCM who has a background in gerontology, the health sciences, or social work or psychology.

Psychosocial Status

The GCM evaluates the cognitive, behavioral, and emotional status of a client. Identification of signs of dementia, delirium, and depression is particularly important. A range of assessment instruments is available for screening and differentiating among these conditions. Following screening, the care manager may refer clients for a thorough psychiatric or neurological consultation.

Caregiving and Ethnic, Social, Spiritual, and Economic Status

Identification of present and potential caregivers and assessment of their willingness, competence, and acceptability to the older person is determined through interviews with the client's family and the social network. Caregiver stress and the support network of the client are also evaluated. (See Chapter 17 on the family and Chapter 15 on caregivers.) Assessment of the older person's cultural, ethnic, and spiritual values should also be included in a geriatric assessment. The older person's concept of what constitutes quality of life should be assessed. End-of-life decisions and verification of written advance directives should be included as well, although this information may not be appropriate to gather in an initial interview. (See Chapter 6 on ethnic assessment, Chapter 14 on spiritual assessment, Chapter 17 on family assessment, Chapter 3 on psychosocial assessment, and Chapter 19 on quality of life.)

Economic resources also need to be evaluated because they are crucial for planning for the provision of personal care and the living arrangements of the client and can be a factor in compliance with medical treatment. (See Chapter 3 on psychosocial assessment.)

Functional Status

A functional assessment is a measure of the person's ability to adequately and safely perform basic ADLs, including bathing, dressing, toileting, transferring, and feeding. Instrumental activities of daily living (IADLs), such as meal preparation, shopping, housework, financial management, medication management, use of the telephone, and driving, are evaluated by direct observation in the home, interviews with the client and family, and administration of standardized questionnaires. (See Chapter 4 on functional assessment.)

Environment

Evaluation of the client's physical environment is essential. Home safety must be evaluated. Problem areas must be identified and corrected if the client is to remain in the home environment. (See Chapter 4 on functional assessment and Chapter 16 on late life relocation.) Evaluating the physical environment in combination with an understanding of the client's ability to perform the ADLs enables the care manager to understand the level of care the client needs. This is the basis for recommending when a client should consider a move to another setting.

Goals of Geriatric Assessment

In 1987, the Consensus Development Conference on Geriatric Assessment Methods for Clinical Decision Making established five goals of comprehensive geriatric assessment: (1) to improve diagnostic accuracy, (2) to guide the selection of interventions to restore or preserve health, (3) to recommend an optimal environment for care, (4) to predict outcomes, and (5) to monitor clinical change over time.[3] The effectiveness of geriatric assessment has been demonstrated most convincingly with clients in geriatric and rehabilitation units and inpatient geriatric units. Less evidence is available regarding home and ambulatory settings.[3] Outcomes demonstrated include improved diagnostic accuracy, prolonged survival, reduced medical care costs, reduced use of acute hospitals, and reduced use of nursing.

■ CARE PLAN

After the initial assessment information is gathered, a comprehensive list of the client's problems and interventions should be generated at a multidisciplinary team conference with other GCMs on staff. This list is called a care plan. If you practice alone, having an agreement with a more experienced GCM, mentor, or a consultant to review your care plans is an excellent idea.

A care plan is a strategy to repair the holes in your clients' web or safety net. Your client is experiencing problems because the web of support or his or her own functioning has deficits or holes. The care plan suggests a way to repair those holes by recommending the right services at the right time for the right amount of money. Again, you are Charlotte, the crafty spider from Charlotte's Web, using the large continuum of care in your community to recommend ways to repair holes in the older person's personal web.

The care plan is also like a prescribed remedy. The GCM identifies each problem the client is experiencing in the problem section and gives an intervention for each problem in the intervention section of the care plan. You, the GCM, are like a health practitioner. You examine your patient—using your psychosocial and functional assessment tools plus any other needed assessments (spiritual, dementia, etc.). You then make a diagnosis based on your assessments—the problem list in the care plan. Then, you prescribe the solution to the client's problems—the interventions or solution in the care plan. (See Exhibit 5–1.)

How do you create a care plan or your professional opinion of what the family ought to do to solve its problems? You begin by gathering all of the data with your assessment tools: your functional assessment data (see Chapter 4 on functional assessment) and your psychosocial assessment data (see Chapter 3 on psychosocial assessment). You then add additional data you have gleaned from any specialized assessment you have done, such as depression, spiritual, or quality of life.

The next step is to sort through these data, like Holmes.

This is where you sift through clues, leaving no stone unturned, to ensure that all evidence has been taken into account before reaching conclusions. You must examine the clues closely. Talk to each person in the formal or informal support system and make sure all evidence is taken into account. Everyone has a different version of what happened. Analyze the client's problems from all perspectives and then synthesize all the opinions into one truth, which will form your professional opinion. Collect all the data, and then look at each person's point of view to come up with your own professional GCM point of view.

As a GCM, you should start your care plan with the problem you were asked to solve initially. Why was your agency called in? For example, was the client very dirty and unable to shower alone when the out-of-town son visited? Start there. This becomes your first problem in your care plan. Always start with the initial presenting problem.

How do you find the remaining problems in the care plan? After addressing the first problem, continue by listing the client's functional problems. What are the deficits you discovered in your functional assessment? A few examples might be the following: unable to prepare meals, unable to walk without a cane, unable to bathe, in pain, or poor diet.

Next, list problems you found through the psychosocial assessments. Some examples are as follows: unable to handle finances, unable to drive to the store because driver's license was taken away, or unable to participate in activities as a result of depression.

Frequently, many older clients have similar deficits as they age. See Exhibit 5–2 for a sample problem list that presents problems older people often develop when they become more frail and vulnerable. Most care plans will include one or more of these problems, and it is good to incorporate this list into your assessment tools.

Exhibit 5–1   Care Plan

1. Examine the client = Assessment
2. Come up with a diagnosis = Problems list
3. Prescribe the solution to the problems = Intervention list

    2 + 3 = Care Plan

Exhibit 5–2   Sample Care Plan
Problem Checklist

Below is a list of the most frequent problems older people experience. If these
problems are not addressed by an assessment tool, keep this list handy to draw
from when you create a care plan.

- ❑   Self-care deficit
- ❑   Impaired home management
- ❑   Alternation in nutrition
- ❑   Impaired mobility
- ❑   Knowledge deficit
- ❑   Alteration in bowel elimination
- ❑   Alteration in urinary elimination
- ❑   Impaired skin integrity
- ❑   Loneliness
- ❑   Depression
- ❑   Pain
- ❑   Caregiver burnout

■ INTERVENTIONS IN THE CARE PLAN

Where do you get the interventions or solutions for the problems listed in your care
plan? In part, you take them from the continuum of care. In Chapter 17 on the family,
GCM Anne Rosenthall wisely states, "Just as
no man is an island—no GCM stands alone."

Every GCM must know a staggering array
of other experts who make up the web of senior services in the community. These experts
practice in areas where GCM skills do not
reach (attorneys, trust officers, moving companies, plumbers). It is the care manager's
expert knowledge of the continuum of care in
the community that is the heart of the care
management role. As stated in Chapter 1, a
GCM is like Charlotte, the friendly spider.
The GCM runs across the web of senior services (continuum of care), linking services,
repairing gaps, spinning new solutions, and
coordinating answers. You need to know how
to locate all these services to implement your

care plan and find interventions to the problems you have uncovered.

Finding Interventions for the Care Plan

How do you find this continuum? As a GCM,
you should already have significant experience in this continuum before you open your
GCM door for business. In Chapter 7, this is
what is meant by your core competence to
open a geriatric care management business.
You need to know your community's continuum of care from day one.

However, because the web billows, expands,
compresses, and changes constantly, you need
the World Wide Web to help you keep up. You
can access most areas of the continuum of
care and all its changes (new businesses, new
senior services offered) through the Internet.
You can access your county's or Area Agency
on Aging website, which will usually list all the
current senior services available in your town.
You can review your business plan and find all
the sources you listed there such as the
National Association of Elder Law Attorneys
website for elder law attorneys. In 2010, most
organizations serving seniors maintained a
website. Of course, you should only recommend services that you know to be competent
and able to solve the particular problem you
are seeking to ameliorate. For example, if you
recommend a local conservator or guardian,
there should be an organization in your
county of guardians with a website.

You can expand your knowledge beyond
your local continuum of care nationally by
using the Eldercare Locator, which is available
at www.eldercare.gov.

Crafting Interventions

Interventions in a care plan to be placed in
the older person's residence followed by care
providers are less complex at times than interventions in a written geriatric assessment sent
to a judge. The judge and attorneys are not

healthcare providers and may need less jargon-free interventions.

Once you know where to find the interventions for your care plan, tailor these interventions to the client. For example, consider another of Mamie Nixon's problems in her care plan—her self-care deficit, namely, that she is apparently unable to bathe without supervision. The intervention to this problem might be hiring a paid care provider to come for 2 hours, 3 days a week to bathe Mamie. Each intervention must have a clear plan. You must state in your intervention who will carry out the intervention, how it will be carried out, the number of times it will be carried out, and how you will measure that it was carried out.

Make Interventions Doable

In the example of recommending an aide to bathe Mamie 3 days a week, you could suggest that the family call a home care agency in the community that provides bonded care providers for 2-hour blocks of time. Also, someone has to carry out the intervention or you risk that it will not be done. Who will carry it out? Your intervention could specify that the family will locate care providers by calling three home care agencies as recommended by the GCM. But before you recommend this, check with the family and confirm they will do this. It may be that the family wants you to interview the care providers and recommend which one they should hire. So, remember to create a solution based on facts. This makes the solution doable.

Make Interventions Measurable

Your recommended interventions should be measurable. This means you should specify the number of times an intervention will be carried out. For example, the agency will send an aide 3 times a week, for 2 hours each time. You need to show the family exactly how to measure whether the intervention was com-

pleted. For example the care provider might fill out and sign a charting page for his shift. This also provides the GCM monitoring the care of the older person a basis to review both the status of the older person and whether the care provider was present. If the care provider has come only once a week, you know you need to follow up. If the family wants to monitor the care, this approach also tells them how to measure the care.

Make Interventions Understandable

Each intervention must be written in straightforward and objective language so that the person carrying out the plan can understand it. It is important to communicate clearly to families, who need jargon-free language. Unskilled caregivers, who may think in another language, need you to use simple, straightforward sentences. The care providers should read the care plan and understand it completely because they are the people who will carry it out in many cases.

Make Interventions with a Timeline

Your intervention should have measurable goals based on a timeline. For example, the problem of loneliness: Mrs. Virden recently lost her husband of 50 years, and she is not socializing and resists outside help. Intervention: The GCM will visit weekly for 1 month to help Mrs. Virden accept community services to relieve some of her loneliness and ongoing grief.

■ MULTIPLE INTERVENTIONS

The GCM can recommend more than one intervention to solve a single problem. For example, an additional intervention to assist Mrs. Virden could be as follows:

> Intervention: GCM will arrange a friendly visitor to visit Mrs. Virden weekly for 6 months.

Intervention: GCM to call the Blessed Christian Church to ask whether a minister could visit Mrs. Virden weekly for 1 month and offer spiritual comfort and encouragement to attend church on Sundays after that month.

Intervention: GCM to encourage Mrs. Virden to attend weekly adult exercise class at local senior center within 1 month.

Because older clients often have chronic disease, the absence of disease, a cure for the problem, or a return to normal is rarely a goal. Mrs. Virden may not fully recover from the death of her husband, but the GCM can fashion interventions that will help her better accept his death over time, and these interventions can be written in a way that you, the client, and her family can measure.

Care Plan Is Subject to Change

Everyone who follows the care plan must understand that it is subject to change. Mrs. Virden may start to attend her church on Sundays, make a male friend at the Blessed Christian Church, and decide to remarry, or she may refuse to accept the friendly visitor you have arranged.

Care Plan Needs to Be Acceptable: Dealing with Rejected Interventions

Sometimes the family or third party may not accept your intervention. For example, you discover that Mrs. C is pouring wine brought in by the cleaning lady down her gastrointestinal tube. The intervention you advise: The trust officer is to replace the cleaning lady within 24 hours, and all alcohol is to be removed from the home by the GCM.

However, the GCM may find that a planned intervention cannot be carried out. For example, Mrs. C may call her attorney, who may insist that a geriatrician hired by the court has tested Mrs. C's competency and

concluded that she is competent and has the right to drink alcohol if she wishes. In this case, the GCM has developed an intervention that the client rejects and will not carry out. When care plans are rejected, the GCM may have to wait until the client or the family will accept the solution. If they do not, the GCM will have to accept the wishes of the legally competent client and family. If the GCM feels that not carrying out the solution will seriously endanger the client's health and safety, the GCM can report the situation to Adult Protective Services. The GCM should consult with Adult Protective Services and an attorney about mandatory reporting state laws.

Care Plan Needs to Be Affordable

The care plan must be something that the older person's assets and income can afford or that the family is willing to pay for. If your client has a self-care deficit, cannot bathe or groom without assistance, and requires ongoing oversight to remain safely in her home, you may recommend 24-hour care. However, if the client cannot afford 24-hour care, you must offer other, cost-effective solutions, such as having the client move in with a family member or be cared for by the informal support system. This is why a financial assessment is needed before you can prepare your care plan. Financial resources should be investigated on the psychosocial intake form.

Consider this example: Mrs. Scott is unable to get to Happy Trails assisted living dining room every night. A solution would be for the daughter to hire a care provider from a home health agency to take Mrs. Scott to the dining room 7 nights a week. However, the family says they cannot afford a care provider. You may have to ask the assisted living facility if it provides a free service to transport clients, or you may have to ask a neighbor in the assisted living facility (part of her informal support system), to escort Mrs. Scott to the dining room. Finding an affordable solution is one of the challenges to the creativity of the GCM in preparing the care plan.

Care Plan Needs Consensus: Getting Family, Client, and Third Party Buy-In

The GCM always needs to remember that the care plan is about solving the problems and meeting the goals of the client and/or family. Listening to family members, fiduciaries, and legal representatives during the assessment process can help the GCM understand how to craft a care plan that is most likely to be accepted. The greater number of interested individuals who support the plan, the better chance the plan has of being implemented. However, the GCM must seek primary approval from the party who requested the care plan initially and who is paying for the assessment. If the assessment and plan were ordered in a court case by the court, the GCM must provide the answers to the questions the court has asked and should have an attorney review the geriatric assessment before it is submitted to the court. Ask an attorney what to do in this type of situation.

If you have the permission of the client or the client's power of attorney or guardian, and if the client does not make a decision, a way to get support for your care plan from all involved parties may be presenting your care plan at a family meeting or having a conference call with all parties. If not, you may call all parties and present your care plan or fax it to all parties with a follow-up phone call. If you can gain consensus for your care plan by these steps, you have a much better chance of having the family members help the older person accept it, and you have a lesser chance of family members sabotaging the care plan.

Care Plan Needs to Be Impartial Yet Creative

Given the same set of problems, several GCMs may come up with different care plans. It is important that the care plan be suitable to the particular client. Because most clients come to care managers because they or their families have been unable to solve their problems themselves, care plans often involve creative problem solving. A creative care plan is crafted by thinking about the client's identified problems imaginatively and using your experience with and knowledge of community resources to suggest a unique solution. However much creativity it involves, the care plan must begin with standardized assessment tools that have been developed with multiple-choice answers that result in objective information with which to develop the care plan. Refer to the assessment tools discussed in various chapters. Also, the National Association of Professional Geriatric Care Managers offers standardized assessment tools through its GCM Forms Book and CD.

For example, you are asked to consult with a couple. The wife has had Parkinson's disease for a number of years, and the couple lives in a house that they retrofitted for her care with a wheel-in shower, lower counters in the kitchen, no steps, and everything, including the laundry, on one floor. The husband is now confronted with having an operation that will require 6 to 8 weeks of rehabilitation. They are trying to figure out if they should hire a live-in worker, try to get their current help to commit to 24/7 care for a month, or hire a new agency to fill in the extra hours. You use standardized functional and psychosocial assessment tools to assess their problem. Then, in discussing their options, you suggest the creative solution that both of them move to a facility for 6 weeks because they do not seem very eager to have a live-in.

Why Add a Budget to a Geriatric Assessment and Care Plan?

It is a good idea to send a projected budget out along with your geriatric assessment. Many families will need to budget for care management expenses, the majority of which are not reimbursed by insurance (private or Medicare). These families will likely ask during the initial consultation about the expenses they can expect to incur for care management, so you will need a process to estimate the amount of time and fees the client will be billed. We suggest you complete this task for each new client, whether you share the estimate with the family or not. The overall process involves translating the care plan into a monthly breakdown of hours across the primary category of tasks recommended in the care plan.

The care plan is your strategy to repair the holes in your client's safety net. In this sense you are like a mechanic working on a car. The car has problems, like your client's life and safety net. Your time, skills, and GCM tools as a human services mechanic will, it is hoped, fix the older person's problems. Like the person who brought the older model auto in to be repaired, the family of the older person hiring you as a GCM, needs an estimate of the number of hours you predict it will take to repair the older person's safety net. They also need to know how much money they will spend to fix the issues or concerns in the older person's life.

Creating a Monthly Budget

What are the steps you take? First you will have the client sign a service agreement with the understanding that you will complete a geriatric assessment and care plan, in which you will make recommendations for next steps and provide an estimate of the time and fees over the next 2–3 months it will take to implement your solutions.

You then do your geriatric assessment, and create your care plan including specific recommendations and next steps. Then, for each following month, you will group the activities into 4 to 6 categories. For instance, the recommendations from the care plan for the

first month may include home visits, medical advocacy in helping obtain a diagnosis, lining up home care, and communicating with the adult children regarding the issues, recommendations, and outcomes. Based on the activities in this example, you now have four categories for Month 1: home visits, doctor visits, communication, and home care. You will then estimate the amount of time you'll spend on activities in each category.

Don't forget to address travel—either include it within the estimates for each category or make travel its own category if you bill separately for travel time. Then, add all the estimated time up for month 1 and multiply it by your hourly rate to provide the estimated fees for month 1. Repeat this process for Months 2 and 3.

What if there is a change in health status that requires a higher level of commitment, time, coordination, and communication? You are giving the family a general idea of what you think it will cost to fix the problems at hand. There can always be a crisis between the time you do your initial assessment, care plan, and budget. You can't predict that, and you will set the expectation up front with the family that you will notify them if circumstances change requiring additional GCM resources. In others words, your budget is not set in stone. Say if you went to a garage to have your transmission fixed. The mechanic would give you an estimate of his time. But what if the brakes went after the car was repaired? The mechanic could not predict that. The key is not in being able to predict, but instead providing frequent updates to families if circumstances and assumptions about recommended care change.

Once you've provided the family an estimate, you'll then want to manage your time against this estimate. You may want to create a calendar for each client by adding appointments and estimated activities (see Table 5–1). You will also need to check your progress against your estimate periodically throughout

Table 5-1 Care Management Monthly Fee—Estimate			
Budget (hours per month)	Month 1	Month 2	Month 3
GGCM home visits	4	3	3
GCM doctor visits	10	4	4
GCM establishing home care	6	2	2
GCM communication/reports	3	3	3
Other	0	0	0
Total hours/total fees	23 hours/ $2300	12 hours/ $1200	12 hours/ $1200

Note: Estimate assumes no significant change in health status.

the month; you can do this by running a quick report in your time-tracking software to determine the number of hours spent. To do this, you'll need to ensure your tracking software contains the latest activities for your clients. Finally, if you find that you're exceeding the estimate, contact the family members as quickly as possible to communicate the cause for the overage (e.g., more complex medical issues than anticipated) and a revised breakdown. This will help prevent any unpleasant surprises for the clients once you send an invoice; it will also help you ensure you collect on all amounts you invoice.

■ CARE MONITORING: UPDATING YOUR CARE PLAN

Care monitoring is measuring whether your care plan is really working. As an example, consider again Mrs. Virden, who was widowed after 50 years of marriage. The problem you identified in your care plan is Mrs. Virden's social isolation and loneliness. Your solution or intervention is to make a weekly monitoring visit and to have a neighbor drive Mrs. Virden to the senior center twice a week. During your first monitoring visit, you find out that the neighbor forgot to take her to the senior center, so you change your care plan to arrange for senior transportation to pick up

Mrs. Virden two times a week to take her to the senior center. When you then check with the client to make sure that senior transportation is arriving at the correct time and that she feels comfortable in the van, you are able to state that your plan has succeeded.

Monitor Your Client to Measure Change

GCMs monitor the services they have recommended to find out whether the client's needs have changed, whether the services originally arranged are still appropriate, and whether the client needs new services or needs to stop receiving services. You monitor to find any holes in the care plan, and then rewrite the care plan and follow up to create new interventions.

Monitoring visits are usually done by appointment with the client. However, it may be appropriate to drop in to visit the client or make unannounced visits if your purpose is to oversee the quality of care being provided. For example, you can drop in to observe the care in an assisted living facility outside of regular office hours. When you make a home visit, use a form to record your monitoring visit (see Exhibit 5-3).

The purpose of a monitoring visit is to observe how the client is doing and to see whether the care plan is being implemented. After you have met with the client, you should also speak to any care provider in the

Exhibit 5–3   GCM Field Evaluation/Care Management Service

Date: 11/18/04   **Client Name:** Zeke Zeigler
SW Name: Miss Full Charge

		(1-excellent 5-poor)		

General Home Environment: 1   **2**   3   4   5
Facility was pleasant. Zeke Zeigler was seated in his wheelchair across from the nurses' station next to the lounge. The lounge was busy yet felt organized.

General Home Cleanliness: 1   **2**   3   4   5
The facility was generally clean and free of odor.

Supplies: **1**   2   3   4   5
(food, cleaning supplies, attends, expense $, Ensure, etc.)
Provided by the facility

Client's Physical Condition: 1   **2**   3   4   5
(personal grooming, overall condition, behavior, etc.)

Zeke Zeigler was seated on his chair dressed and ready for his doctor's appt. He was neat and well groomed. Overall he was relaxed.

Client's Mental Condition: 1   2   **3**   4   5
(oriented, moderately confused, very confused)

Zeke Zeigler was alert although he was not oriented to time, place, and person. When Zeke Zeigler entered The Stroke Institute, he read the sign and clearly said "Stroke Institute." While waiting for Dr. Feelgood, Zeke Zeigler read a few words accurately from a magazine, but could not connect words together. During the doctor's visit, he responded clearly when Dr. Feelgood asked his name but started singing when asked about his age, family, or symptoms.

New Psychosocial Problems:
Julia Nimble, social worker at Agility Skilled Nursing Facility, reported that his humming, singing, and general agitation bothered Mr. Zeigler's roommate. However, this behavior did not impact Zeke Zeigler and his relation to the outside world. No other psychosocial problems were apparent. He was pleasant and interacted with the GCM, the nurse, and Dr. Feelgood.

List of Medications:
(include quantity and expiration date)
During this visit, Dr. Feelgood prescribed Seroquel 25mg, 1/2 to 1 tab daily at bedtime to decrease the agitation and allow him to sleep better.

Specific Concerns:
Dr. Feelgood noted that Mr. Zeigler's right hand was contracted and stiff. He suggested botox treatment on his forearm to paralyze the stiffened muscles and decrease the contractures. This will ease the movement of his right hand and also make it easier for a caregiver to dress him. Dr. Feelgood will do the botox treatment at Mr. Zeigler's next appointment.

continues

Exhibit 5-3   GCM Field Evaluation/Care Management Service (continued)

Actions:

GCM rode with Zeke Zeigler in Medical Transport vehicle from Agility Skilled Nursing Facility Care to The Stroke Institute.

GCM sat with Zeke Zeigler during his visit with Dr. Feelgood. Dr. Feelgood took over from Dr. Baseline and spent this visit reviewing symptoms, current therapy, and getting to know Mr. Zeigler.

GCM waited with Zeke Zeigler until Medical Transport came to pick them up. Due to the time of day, we had to wait for over an hour for transport back to Agility Skilled Nursing Facility Care.

Plan:

Return visit was set for Thursday, February 10, 2005 @ 9:45 a.m. During that visit, Dr. Feelgood plans a botox treatment to decrease the contracture of Mr. Zeigler's hand.

Summary of Visit:

Miss Full Charge, GCM accompanied Zeke Zeigler to a doctor's appointment at The Stroke Institute scheduled for 4:30 p.m. Pick-up was scheduled for an hour before the appointment. Zeke Zeigler was seated on his chair dressed and ready for his doctor's appt. He was neat and well groomed. Overall he was relaxed. Zeke Zeigler was alert although he was not oriented to time, place, and person. When Zeke Zeigler entered The Stroke Institute, he read the sign and clearly said "Stroke Institute." While waiting for Dr. Feelgood, Zeke Zeigler read a few words accurately from a magazine, but could not connect words together. During the doctor's visit, he responded clearly when Dr. Feelgood asked his name but started singing when asked about his age, family, or symptoms.

Source: Cresscare, Case Management for Elders, Cathy Cress, Director, 2006.

home, paid or unpaid. If the client lives in a residential care setting, you could speak to the residential care provider, and if the client lives in a skilled nursing facility (SNF), you could speak to either the director of nursing or the social worker and/or the direct service worker if possible. In addition, in a facility setting, you can review the written record.

In all of these conversations, discuss the previous time period between visits by reviewing historical problems in the care plan. For example, if the older person was wandering but has not wandered for months, ask whether there has been a reoccurrence of wandering. Discuss ongoing psychosocial and functional problems included in the care plan, and probe for any new psychosocial or functional problems, any problems with

patient care, any problems with care staff, and any household problems.

During a monitoring visit, check the condition of the environment, cleanliness of the home, and whether there are enough supplies (adult diapers, food, etc.). Check the client's physical condition, mental condition, new medications, and compliance with the current medication regimen. Chart the medications each time you visit. You should then record on the care monitoring form any specific concerns and actions you plan to take. If you find any changes in the client's situation, update the care plan and make sure the new version is given to the care provider responsible for implementing the plan or to the residence (SNF, board and care, etc.). If you create an updated care plan and no one is aware of the changes, it will, of course, fail to be implemented, and your care monitoring will flounder.

New recommendations are integrated into a plan of care as interventions. The goal is to achieve the outcomes that the team has determined are desired despite any changes that might occur in a client's situation. Recommendations must then be communicated to the appropriate care providers and to the client if possible. Periodic reassessment and modification of the care plan are critical to the success of the plan.

■ WRITING A GERIATRIC ASSESSMENT AND DESIGNING THE CARE PLAN

The GCM creates the care plan after the intake and then begins service. At times families, trust officers, attorneys, or other third parties ask the GCM to integrate the care plan into a more in-depth written report called a geriatric assessment and recommendations.

What triggers a written geriatric assessment? A problem does. As a GCM, you are a problem solver, and you solve an older person's problems through a geriatric assessment. You take the same steps to discover the client's problems and solutions as you use during assessment.

The purpose of a written assessment is to impart to families the information you gathered using the assessment tools to help the family know what the next step in care of the client may be. Occasionally, a written assessment is used by attorneys and judges as an outside professional opinion about how to solve the client's problem: should the person be conserved, should the person move from the home, or which adult child would serve best as a guardian.

A written assessment also transmits information from other sources, such as court records, facility records, medical records, and conversations with family members or others that you documented in service notes. Most important, the written assessment communicates all this information in an organized and convincing manner. Here, you are much like an attorney: you are making a case to convince the family, physician, court, and so forth (jury) that the older client has X problems and they can be solved by Y solutions. Last, the purpose of the geriatric assessment is to complete the first significant task the client asked you to do.

Consider Mrs. Hurricane. Her daughter, Miss Tornado, hires you to write a geriatric assessment because Mrs. Hurricane has had several falls. You begin your written geriatric assessment stating that GCM Care Solvers was hired by Miss Tina Tornado to do a geriatric assessment on her mother Hannah Hurricane because the mother has fallen five times at home in the past 2 weeks and refuses to accept care or move to a different level of care.

To begin the written assessment, you take the steps as outlined in this chapter to gather data. You perform the assessments. Gathering the information to write the geriatric assessment is done as outlined in Chapter 4, functional assessment, and Chapter 3, psychosocial assessment. Once you have gathered all the information, you must analyze it in a systematic, logical manner. Written assessment questionnaires assist in the categorization of data. Data can be classified according to a number of different parameters, including identified problems, functional deficits, chronic or acute illnesses, and coping mechanisms and deficits. The sorting and classification of data lead to the identification of areas of intervention. Intervention strategies must be individualized in a geriatric assessment. Included in Exhibit 5–4 is an outline of Phyllis Brostoff's assessment and care plan recommendations, which was presented in her report "How to Write a Professional Assessment and Recommendations" at the Geriatric Care Management National Conference in 2004. This can be helpful in categorizing your data into problem types and areas of intervention before you write your geriatric assessment.[3]

Exhibit 5–4   Assessment, Care Plan, and Recommendations Outline

1. Date assessment and care plan and recommendations were prepared: _____

2. Client demographic information:
   a. Name
   b. Address
   c. Phone number
   d. Current living arrangement
   e. DOB
   f. Marital status or primary relationship
   g. Gender
   h. Primary language if not English

3. Information on individual who requested assessment:
   a. Name
   b. Address
   c. Phone number
   d. Relationship to client

4. Informants other than client who provided information, relationship to client, and dates of contact

5. Presenting problem (the problem that precipitated the referral for this assessment)

6. Social network status (include current activities and interests, occupational background, spiritual life, living arrangements, nature and frequency of significant social relationships; describe a typical week in the life of the client such as outings, contacts with others)

7. Physical and mental health/medical status (include current medical diagnoses; medications; name of primary care physician, other specialists, dentist, podiatrist; any problems with sleeping, vision, hearing, elimination, speech, respiration, nutritional status, and diet). When listing current conditions, observe whether they are stable, worsening, or improving.

8. Activities of daily living status (include assessment of ability to ambulate, bathe, dress, communicate, eat, maintain continence, shave, maintain oral health, toilet, transfer alone or with assistance; if assisted, indicate by whom or with what equipment)

9. Instrumental activities of daily living status (include ability to shop, prepare meals, do housekeeping and laundry, use telephone, manage medication, do own finances alone or with assistance; if assisted, indicate by whom or with what equipment)

10. Legal status (include whether there are signed Health Care and Financial Powers of Attorney and who the agents are in these documents, whether there is guardianship, whether a living will is signed, whether a current will is in place)

11. Financial status (include current income and assets to determine eligibility for state/federal programs or Veterans Administration programs; include how the client is managing daily money matters and whether there is a trust administrator)

12. Insurance coverage (include information on primary and secondary insurance, long-term-care insurance, VA benefits)

13. Summary of concerns and identification of risk factors (specify concerns uncovered in the assessment under the following areas and identify any potential problems you are aware of regarding possible solutions to these problems, such as client resistance, limited financial resources, or family conflict)
    a. Safety concerns (include risks identified in the home setting such as hazards on stairs, in kitchen, in bedroom, in bathroom, in living room)

continues

Exhibit 5–4   Assessment, Care Plan, and Recommendations Outline (continued)

b. Mental health, behavioral, or cognitive concerns (include outcome of mental status assessments such as depression screens, mini-mental screens, suicide potential, relevant psychiatric history)

c. Driving safety concerns (include whether there is evidence that the client may be driving unsafely)

d. Nutrition concerns (include information on change in weight, unhealthy/unbalanced diet, difficulty preparing food)

e. Fall risks (include information on fear, clutter, medications, balance, strength, specific conditions)

f. Abuse risks (include information on physical, emotional, financial, psychological, neglect, or self-neglect issues)

g. Medications/substance abuse/smoking risks (note any compliance issues, polypharmacy issues, obstacles to attaining medications or taking them appropriately, alcohol or over-the-counter medication abuse)

14. Care plan and recommendations (identify each problem/concern uncovered in the assessment. Explain your rationale for each recommendation, and provide at least two alternatives and the cost associated with each alternative). Include referrals needed to any medical or other specialists.

Source: "How to Write a Professional Assessment and Recommendations." Phyllis Brostoff at GCM National Conference in 2004.

Presenting Problem Section

The report always begins with a statement describing the presenting problem. Why did someone ask you to write the assessment? Take the example of Mrs. Hurricane again. Following is a sample Presenting Problem section.

> Tina Tornado contacted GCM Care concerning her mother, Hannah Hurricane, and asked that we complete a geriatric assessment. Ms. Tornado is concerned because her mother has fallen five times during the 2-week period from October 15 to October 31. She states Mrs. Hurricane refuses to have help at home and refuses to move from her home to a higher level of care.

Writing the History Section

The History section follows the Presenting Problem section. It should include a brief history of the client from birth until the time of this current problem. Use the psychosocial assessment form to gather these data. The data should include birth date, where the client grew up, education, job held through most of life, and marriage date. The important part here is to describe this elder as a person who had a life before this major problem or crisis. You do this to give him or her three dimensions. It also gives the attorney and/or family members reading the written assessment a quick history of this person. The history must be brief, succinct, clear, and no more than three paragraphs but contain all relevant information. Following is an example History section.

> Hannah Hurricane was born on September 12, 1918, and grew up in Monterey, California. After Hannah graduated from high school, she attended San Jose State Teachers College. After graduation she worked as an English teacher in the Mon-

terey school system for 10 years. She married Mr. Harold Hurricane in 1942, began to raise her family, and gave up her teaching career to become a homemaker for more than 50 years.

Mrs. Hurricane has three children: Tina Tornado, James and Steve Hurricane. Steve and James live in Washington, D.C., and Tina lives nearby in Santa Cruz, California. Hannah was widowed when her husband died 13 years ago.

Mrs. Hurricane moved to Park Lane, a residence for seniors in Monterey, after her husband died. Approximately seven years ago, she moved to a condominium in Carmel, where she presently resides. Until recently, she tutored students in English as a Second Language. Mrs. Hurricane also attended social activities and lunches at the Carmel Foundation, a senior center in downtown Carmel. Mrs. Hurricane is a Christian Scientist.

Writing the Functional Assessment Section

Write the chronological history of functional problems that led to the main problem. Describe the health history, including the diagnosis, physician's evaluation, and information from the functional assessment tool. Include present medications and assessment of ADLs and IADLs and home safety. Describe your observations on gait, environment, and so forth as recorded in service notes or a functional assessment form. Following is an example Functional Assessment section.

Carolyn Hellsapoppen GCM from Care Solvers GCM made a home visit to the client on November 27, 2010 because Mrs. Hurricane had a recent history of five falls. The GCM observed Mrs. Hurricane ambulate. She watched the client arise from the couch and walk to the kitchen with difficulty, assisted by her cane. The Get Up and Go Test was administered by asking Mrs. Hurricane to get up from a kitchen chair, stand still, walk forward 10 feet, turn around, walk back to the chair, and then turn and be seated. The GCM noted Mrs. Hurricane's sitting balance, transfers from sitting to standing, pace, and stability of walking. Mrs. Hurricane scored a 3 on this test, indicating she needs to be further evaluated by a primary physician.

Mrs. Hurricane's daughter, Tina, reported to Carolyn Hellsapoppen in a phone conversation on November 26, 2003, that her mother had fallen on the dates October 15, 20, 21, 26, and 31. The first two falls happened while she was putting her laundry in the washer, which is located down the stairs on the lower level of the house. The last three falls were reported to have happened in the kitchen, as Mrs. Hurricane rushed to get to a boiling teapot. Ms. Tornado stated that there were no apparent injuries from these falls, but that her mother did lie on the ground for 3 to 4 hours after the first fall. However, in all instances, Mrs. Hurricane was not able to summon help.

Mrs. Hurricane is slightly hard of hearing. The GCM had to repeat some questions before she understood them. She has no hearing aid.

On the home visit of November 27, Mrs. Hurricane told the GCM she was depressed. She identified depression as the cause of her symptoms of a burning sensation in her upper back, neck, and both arms. Mrs. Hurricane stated these feelings come upon her at night and are quite uncomfortable. Mrs. Hurricane also stated to Carolyn Hellsapoppen that she had not seen a physician since these symptoms began.

Mrs. Hurricane was administered a Katz ADL by the GCM, which identified that she needs assistance with bathing because of her balance problems and should be watched on transfers. She is independent in dressing, continence, and feeding. She was administered an IADL test by the GCM.

Mrs. Hurricane is independent in telephone use, managing medication, and financial management. Mrs. Hurricane needs assistance with food preparation, housekeeping, driving at night, doing laundry, and shopping because of ambulation difficulties and recent falls. A physician's report, received on December 7, 2002, was completed by Mrs. Hurricane's physician, Dr. Feelbetter. The report stated Mrs. Hurricane has diabetes, high blood pressure, a history of interstitial cystitis, and is noncompliant with doctor's appointments and orders. Mrs. Hurricane was also reported by her doctor to be mentally clear.

Carolyn Hellsapoppen, GCM, reported that Mrs. Hurricane is a non-insulin-dependent diabetic and, according to Mrs. Hurricane, her blood sugar values are "quite high" despite her avoidance of sweets and the use of the prescription drug Glucophage (metformin). She feels this drug has caused a 2- to 3-week bout of diarrhea, which she says is now resolved. She stated to Ms. Hellsapoppen that she has discontinued taking this drug.

As reported to Carolyn Hellsapoppen of GCM Care by Mrs. Hurricane, Mrs. Hurricane had one of her kidneys removed in 1994 and had a urostomy performed in 1990, following several years of interstitial cystitis. Dr. Olsen's physician's report stated this as well. Mrs. Hurricane stated to Ms. Hellsapoppen on her visit of November 27, 2002, that she can usually manage her urostomy well but has had some episodes of skin irritation of the stoma and the surrounding tissue to the point of bleeding. In March 2002, Mrs. Hurricane was admitted to Community Hospital Emergency Room in Santa Cruz. She had an irritation of her urostomy. After treatment, she was released and sent home. There have been no other hospitalizations before this or after this incident, according to Tina Tornado. These periodic irritations of her urostomy prompted Tina Tornado to request a home health aide, who Mrs. Hurricane discharged after two months. Mrs. Hurricane reported to Carolyn Hellsapoppen that she is now using a moisture barrier before applying the urostomy bag and has had good results with it.

As examined by GCM Carolyn Hellsapoppen, RN, on her visit of November 27, 2002, Mrs. Hurricane's lungs were clear; abdomen was soft; ankles were without swelling. Her blood pressure was elevated by 160/100; pulse was 88 and regular; respirations were 20 per minute. She stated that she feels she needs to lose weight. Her daughter Ms. Tornado reported to Amber Helpall, Social Worker for GCM Care, that her mother has lost approximately 20 pounds and weighs approximately 180 pounds. This weight was confirmed on the physician's report. Mrs. Hurricane also stated to Carolyn Hellsapoppen that she is not eating as much as she used to and is losing weight.

As was also reported to Carolyn Hellsapoppen, Mrs. Hurricane's doctor, Mabel Olsen, discharged Mrs. Hurricane as a patient approximately 3 months ago for missing three medical appointments. According to Mrs. Hurricane and her daughter, Dr. Ted Tittlemouse, endocrinologist, has also discontinued his services as her physician for noncompliance. The doctor recommended she either have 24-hour care or move to a board and care. Carolyn Hellsapoppen of GCM Care recommends that Mrs. Hurricane be evaluated as soon as possible by a new physician because of her elevated blood pressure and the recent falls. The fact that she is a diabetic also puts her at high risk of heart disease, according to Carolyn Hellsapoppen.

On a home safety check the GCM found the following: there is no handheld showerhead installed nor shower chair for safety in the bath. Smoke alarms are not working throughout the house. There are outside obstructions, such as tools and planter boxes, in the pathway that would make it easy to trip and fall. There is no cordless phone, which would prevent the client from rushing to answer phones. Teapot on stove needs to be replaced by an electric teapot so she does not have to hurry to turn it off.

Writing the Psychosocial Assessment Section

Write the chronological history of psychosocial and psychological events that led to the main problem. This could include mental status. If dementia is a part of the problem, break this out as its own section. The Psychosocial Assessment section should include information about moving from one level of care to another, death of a spouse, substance abuse, economic and legal issues including conservatorships, financial assets, insurance, both informal and formal support systems, activities, spiritual beliefs, recent life changes and life satisfaction, and ethnic background including preferences and needs. Following is a sample Psychosocial Assessment section.

Mrs. Hurricane has a history of noncompliance with doctors' orders and safety issues. She is a Christian Scientist and, because of her religious beliefs, she prefers to handle her medical problems by prayer first and medical care second. Mrs. Hurricane and her daughter asked for Carolyn Hellsapoppen's recommendation for physicians in the Monterey area. Carolyn was able to provide them with three names, one being Carl Handsome, MD, an internist in Carmel. Mrs. Hurricane has an appointment with Dr. Handsome on December 13, in 1 week.

Mrs. Hurricane was administered a short portable mental status questionnaire by the GCM, and her score of 1 error indicated she does not seem to need additional evaluation for memory loss. This was confirmed by Dr. Olsen's physician's report. There is no former or present substance abuse.

Upon discussion with Carolyn Hellsapoppen, Mrs. Hurricane stated that she is feeling depressed. The GCM observed she had a flat affect and appeared lethargic, and Mrs. Hurricane stated that she has felt depressed for days. She stated she did not want to go out of the house, hardly wanted to watch her favorite show Jeopardy anymore, and does not feel like going to the Carmel Foundation. GCM Carolyn Hellsapoppen interviewed Miss Service, a social worker at the Carmel Foundation. Miss Service stated Mrs. Hurricane attended until 1 month ago and repeated calls and follow-up home visits were made to find out what prevented Mrs. Hurricane from attending the foundation. Miss Service said she will work with the family and the GCM to reengage the client in foundation activities. Amber Helpall, social worker, discussed the possibility of Mrs. Hurricane having a pet. Mrs. Hurricane stated she would like one but is unable to have a dog or cat because of restrictions in the condominium complex where she lives.

Ms. Tornado, the adult child who lives closest to her mother, is the primary family care provider. Although Mrs. Hurricane's sons James and Steve live on the East Coast, they have both agreed to offer their mother whatever support is required, which might include taking her as respite, helping financially, or whatever is suggested by the GCM. Mrs. Hurricane's other social support is her 92-year-old neighbor, Mrs. Charlotte Murphy, who encourages Mrs. Hurricane to go to the Carmel Foundation and visits her most days for tea and conversation. Ms. Hellsapoppen interviewed Mrs. Murphy and Mrs. Murphy stated that Mrs. Hurricane seemed more "down in the dumps lately" and was staying in bed some days instead of watching Jeopardy. The two women have watched Jeopardy together for several years. Additional social supports were from the Carmel Foundation, where Mrs. Hurricane attended a women's support group, tutored English as a Second Language, and had daily lunches.

Daughter Ms. Tornado has the durable power of attorney for health care as well as the durable power of attorney for finances for her mother. These two documents were established in 2002 to prepare for her mother's future, according to Ms. Tornado. Mrs. Hurricane continues to handle her own finances, but Ms. Tornado "checks everything over" for her mother, according to Ms. Tornado. Mrs. Hurricane has adequate finances (about $1 million in assets) to pay for care. She has long-term care insurance through PERS because she was a teacher, plus Medicare and a Medicare supplement.

Mrs. Hurricane asserts that she does her own housekeeping and laundry, and that she needs a cleaning lady only once a week. Mrs. Hurricane's home was very neat and clean, according to the observation of Carolyn Hellsapoppen. However, because of her balance problems, it is recommended that a care provider do the daily light housework for the client. Mrs. Hurricane drives, but she does not drive at night, according to her daughter.

Writing the Medications Section

List all current medications in this section, including dosage. You should get this information from the physician report you send to the client's doctor. You can also find out about all medications by asking the client or client representative if you can look at each bottle of medication in the client's possession. By doing this, you can make a list of current medications and also find medications that are out of date and discover any polypharmacy issues.

Writing the Level of Care Section

In the Level of Care section, you recommend a level of care. You might recommend the same level of care as currently provided with no supports or the same level of care but including additional support systems such as care providers. You might have to recommend the client move to a higher level of care such as moving to an assisted living facility.

Your job as GCM is to be an expert in level of care. After you complete all your assessment tools, you should be able to state exactly what level of care your client needs. Again, evaluating the physical environment in combination with an understanding of the client's ability to perform the ADLs enables a care manager to understand the level of care the client needs. Following is a sample Level of Care section.

Ms. Tornado is concerned because her mother has fallen five times during the 2-week period of October 15 to October 31. She states Mrs. Hurricane refuses to have help at home and further declines to move from her home to a higher level of care. She would like the GCM's opinion on how to proceed in keeping her mother safe at her present level of care or on a plan to move to a higher level of care.

The GCM recommends that Mrs. Hurricane remain at home where she is in familiar surroundings, has a good neighbor, and is comfortable. If all home safety deficits are followed through and the client is provided assistance with her ADLs of food preparation, housekeeping, driving at night, doing her laundry, and shopping, Mrs. Hurricane can remain in her home with a live-in care provider. However, the GCM recommends that the daughter hire a live-in. Because Mrs. Hurricane is adverse to this level of care, the GCM suggests that she be allowed to counsel Mrs. Hurricane over a period of time to accept this assistance.

Writing the Care Plan Section

The care plan comes next. This care plan should include more details than the care plan you place in the home for care providers and update on an ongoing basis. The care plan in the geriatric assessment must paint a clear picture of the client's needs for a judge, attorney, family member, or third party, and others who are not GCMs. The care plan should be written in clear English, without jargon, and should be concise and readable. Start as stated earlier with the problem you were hired to assess in the first place. Following is a Care Plan example that would be included in a geriatric assessment.

Narrative Explanation of Care Plan

After the actual care plan, include a narrative explaining the care plan. For example, if the care plan states that Mrs. Hurricane is depressed and needs to see a mental health provider to be evaluated for depression and possible medications, you can insert the additional information that Mrs. Hurricane has only one friend in her informal support system and that a care provider should be hired. You can explain some of the things the care provider can do to allay the client's depression, such as taking Mrs. Hurricane on visits to the Monterey County SPCA because Mrs. Hurricane likes animals but cannot have one and taking Mrs. Hurricane to plays at the local theaters.

Problem	Intervention
1. Ms. Tornado is concerned because her mother has fallen five times during the 2-week period of October 15 to October 31. She states Mrs. Hurricane refuses to have help at home and further refuses to move from her home to a higher level of care. Ms. Tornado would like GCM Care's opinion about how to proceed with her mother's safety issues.	1. a. Within 1 week, daughter Ms. Tornado to hire live-in care providers for Monday through Friday and Saturday and Sunday who can drive, through a list of home care agencies given to her. b. GCM to visit weekly and as needed to help Mrs. Hurricane to accept care and problem solve with Mrs. Hurricane and care provider. c. Care provider to do standby assist at all times. d. Within 1 week, daughter to arrange for Lifeline alerts through Community Hospital of Mt. Peninsula or other source. e. Daughter to ask physician Dr. Handsome to evaluate reason for falls at next appointment on December 13th.
2. Washer and dryer are located down the stairs and outdoors and are one reason for recent falls.	2. Daughter to have care provider do laundry 1 time a week in basement on an ongoing basis.
3. Mrs. Hurricane presently has no primary physician because she has been noncompliant with doctor's appointments in the past.	3. a. Daughter to take Mrs. Hurricane to appointment with Dr. Handsome on December 13th and confirm that he will be Mrs. Hurricane's primary physician.

continues

Problem	Intervention
	b. If Dr. Handsome declines to follow up with Mrs. Hurricane on December 13 appointment, daughter to obtain a primary physician from list given by GCM within 1 week after December 13.
	c. After first appointment on December 13, care provider to keep track of all doctor's appointments and drive Mrs. Hurricane to each doctor's appointment.
4. Alteration in nutrition: recent loss of appetite. Mrs. Hurricane has lost approximately 20 pounds and weighs approximately 180 pounds.	4. a. Daughter to have Dr. Handsome evaluate Mrs. Hurricane's weight loss at December 13 appointment.
	b. Care provider to prepare breakfast and dinner and drive Mrs. Hurricane to the Carmel Foundation for daily lunch on an ongoing basis.
5. Alteration in urinary elimination: client has a urostomy.	5. Daughter to ask Dr. Handsome to evaluate Mrs. Hurricane's urostomy and urinary problems at December 13 appointment.
6. Alteration in bowel elimination: medication side effects of diarrhea.	6. Daughter to ask physician to evaluate urinary medication side effects at December 13 appointment.
7. Mrs. Hurricane has elevated blood pressure.	7. a. Daughter to ask Dr. Handsome to evaluate elevated blood pressure and monitor blood pressure at December 13 appointment.
	b. Care provider to prepare low-salt meals on an ongoing basis.
8. Pain: Mrs. Hurricane complains of burning sensation and pain in back and neck.	8. Daughter to ask Dr. Handsome to evaluate present pain and burning sensation at December 13 appointment.
9. Mrs. Hurricane is a non-insulin-dependent diabetic, and her blood sugar values are self-reported as "quite high" despite her avoidance of sweets and the use of the prescription drug Glucophage (metformin), which she has discontinued using.	9. a. Daughter to ask Dr. Handsome to evaluate diabetes and present diabetic medications for side effects at December 13 appointment.
	b. Care provider to prepare diabetic meals on an ongoing basis.
	c. Care provider to monitor sweet intake and chart on an ongoing basis.
	d. Daughter to call Carmel Foundation and order diabetic meals week before client returns to Carmel Foundation.

Problem	Intervention
	e. Daughter to investigate a diabetic support group for Mrs. Hurricane at Dominican Rehab Services held one Tuesday a month.
10. Mrs. Hurricane is hard of hearing and has no hearing aid.	10. GCM to take client to an audiologist to have hearing evaluated and to get possible prescription for hearing aid within 1 month.
11. Depression: Mrs. Hurricane expressed being depressed to the GCM, and she is no longer engaged in social activity that enhances her quality of life.	11. a. Daughter to arrange for mother to see mental health provider Martin Skirt at Community Hospital within 2 weeks to evaluate level of depression and assess for possible medications.
	b. Daughter to instruct care provider to drive Mrs. Hurricane to Carmel Foundation daily for lunch and socialization as soon as care provider is hired.
	c. GCM to contact social worker Miss Service at Carmel Foundation to find new activities that would benefit client or a continuation of old activities such as women's support group 1 week before client begins attending.
	d. GCM to work with Carmel Foundation social worker to make sure Mrs. Hurricane is engaged in activities and to work with any barriers the client may have in attending activities on an ongoing basis.
	e. Within 1 month, GCM to call Monterey School District to find out whether client could continue to tutor English as a second language if care provider accompanied her to site.
	f. Care provider to take Mrs. Hurricane to plays at Forrest Theater, to SPCA to visit animals, and to other activities suggested by GCM to engage Mrs. Hurricane in activities that improve her quality of life and increase her social engagement.
	g. Care provider to drive Mrs. Hurricane to have lunch with daughter 1 day a month, preferably on day the client attends the diabetic support group in Santa Cruz.

continues

Problem	Intervention
12. Home safety issues that may lead to more falls include shower lacks safety bars, shower lacks handheld showerhead, smoke alarms are not working, and outside obstructions are in pathway of client. Client does not have cordless phone and may rush to answer phone. Client fell rushing to take teapot off stove.	12. a. Daughter to arrange for shower bars to be installed in bathroom outside of shower on both sides, within 1 week. b. Daughter to arrange to have handheld showerhead installed within 1 week. c. Daughter to get a shower chair for mother at medical supply store or Carmel Foundation within 1 week. d. Daughter to arrange for repair person to hook up smoke alarms within 1 week. e. Daughter to have handyman remove outside obstructions in pathways, such as tools and planter boxes, within 1 week. f. Daughter to order cordless phone so mother does not have to rush to answer phone, within 2 weeks. g. Daughter to buy electric teapot that automatically turns off, within 2 weeks.
13. Mrs. Hurricane states that she cannot drive at night.	13. a. Daughter to take mother to have a thorough eye exam at an ophthalmologist within 1 month. b. Care provider to drive Mrs. Hurricane to all night events on an ongoing basis.
14. Mrs. Hurricane is opposed to medical treatment and thus is noncompliant because of her Christian Science beliefs.	14. a. GCM to contact the local Christian Science foundation in Monterey and make arrangements for a church member who specializes in working with elders to help problem solve so Mrs. Hurricane's health, safety, and spiritual issues can all be met. b. Care provider to drive Mrs. Hurricane to Christian Science services once a week.
15. Daughter is stressed by caregiver burden.	15. Daughter to consider attending on first and third Fridays caregiver support group through Del Mar Caregiver Resources in Santa Cruz, where she lives.
16. Mrs. Hurricane's care plan needs to be monitored on an ongoing basis.	16. a. To monitor care plan, care provider, activities, health issues, spiritual issues, and compliance issues GCM will visit Mrs. Hurricane every week for the first 2 months and then every other week after that if Mrs. Hurricane is stable. b. GCM to reevaluate weekly whether daughter is able to do all tasks and to take over tasks daughter wishes to delegate.

■ EVALUATING THE GERIATRIC ASSESSMENT

Proofread the first draft of the geriatric assessment to make sure you have all the correct information and that the information is well written, grammatically correct, and spelled correctly. The following sections describe some tools to help you accomplish this.

What Makes You a Good Detective?

When you complete the first draft of your geriatric assessment, go back and check that all elements are in place. In other words, did you gather all the clues? Did you talk to every person who could give you a point of view about the crisis? In Mrs. Hurricane's case, the daughter, the two other adult children, the friend, the Carmel Foundation social worker, and Mrs. Hurricane's former primary physician were involved.

Check that every line of your assessment tool was completely and accurately filled out. This is where you keep track of your clues. Too many GCMs are messy, leaving lines in assessment forms unfilled or skipping over lines or writing in haste. Don't miss any clues. As stated earlier, look at your assessment tools to make sure you slowly and meticulously sift through clues, leaving no stone unturned in your efforts to ensure that all evidence has been taken into account before reaching conclusions and announcing them. Following that, ask yourself these questions: Did you distill the sifted information into your care plan? Does your care plan have complete and well-written problems? Does it have complete and well-written solutions? Is your care plan measurable? Does your care plan tell the reader who will accomplish the solutions?

What Makes a Good Written Assessment?

In a workshop titled "How to Write a Professional Assessment and Recommendations," Phyllis Brostoff discussed the 4 Cs of writing a geriatric assessment that are invaluable in checking your document.[3] The first is clarity—make sure your facts are presented clearly. In Mrs. Hurricane's geriatric assessment, you would not say, "Mrs. Hurricane looked depressed." You would state, "When visiting Mrs. Hurricane on November 1, 2002, Mrs. Hurricane stated to the GCM that she was feeling depressed."

The second C is cohesiveness. This means organization. For example, don't put information about the client's depression in the Home Management section of your geriatric assessment. Follow the guidelines in Exhibit 5–5. Do not commingle sections. Write a tight outline, follow it, and make your written assessment cohesive.

The third C is completeness. You have conducted multiple assessments, but have you filled in every line like a good detective? Have you answered every question fully? With Mrs. Hurricane, did you answer the question of why she was having falls? The answers were many: having no care providers, having to walk down a flight of steps to the laundry, having no portable phone, having a teapot that could not turn itself off, not attending the Carmel Foundation where she had supervision, and so forth.

The fourth C is coherence. Your geriatric assessment must lead to logical conclusions. In the beginning of Mrs. Hurricane's geriatric assessment, her daughter Ms. Tornado wanted you to find out why her mother had multiple falls, and what level of care her mother belonged in. You need to offer a solution to these beginning problems in your conclusion section—why is Mrs. Hurricane falling, and where should she live?

Next, determine whether the items included in the geriatric assessment are actionable. When editing the first draft of your geriatric assessment, use Phyllis Brostoff's criteria to help you create an actionable care plan.[3] The solutions in your geriatric assessment must be actionable, which means they should be affordable, acceptable, and doable.

Exhibit 5–5   Elements of a Geriatric Assessment

Problem

- Brief client history from birth to crisis that prompted GCM to intervene
- Written summation of functional assessment
- Written summation of cognitive assessment
- List of all medications
- Written summation of psychosocial assessment
- Written summation of home environment assessment
- Written summary of any other pertinent assessment
- Care plan
- Written explanation of the care plan
- Summary of recommendations

- Are solutions affordable? In your geriatric assessment, you discovered that Mrs. Hurricane has about $1 million in assets and Ms. Tornado, who has durable power of attorney for finances, is open to spending the money on care and services for her mother. So it seems you have an affordable care plan.
- Are solutions acceptable? Will Ms. Tornado pay for a 7-day live-in? Ask her. Will the daughter carry through with all the interventions you are recommending to her? Did you discuss these recommendations with her? Will Mrs. Hurricane be noncompliant with another doctor? Will she accept a care provider? You can check whether some of these interventions are acceptable just by asking the client and family members. Whether interventions like the ones created for Mrs. Hurricane are acceptable will depend on whether the GCM can work with the client during care monitoring visits, as well as the quality of the care provider. Some of these interventions take time to become acceptable to the client.

- Is your plan doable? Can Ms. Tornado get Mrs. Hurricane to the mental health assessment at the community hospital? Will Ms. Tornado follow through, or is her relationship with her mother so strained that Mrs. Hurricane might not go with her? Would it be better to have the GCM take Mrs. Hurricane?

Did You Sell Your Services Well?

Your written geriatric assessment is your geriatric care management product. If you were selling a car, you would never put a vehicle on the car lot with smashed windows, torn seats, and an empty tank. If you sold a car to someone, you would not deliver the car late. So in your geriatric care management work, do not be sloppy. Check to see that you have gathered enough information to evaluate and solve the problems you were hired to solve without making errors. Don't present questionable or unfounded information in your written assessments. If you cannot check the facts, don't include them in the document. Make clear the source of the information and how reliable that source is. Do not include poor spelling, bad grammar, and awkward sentence structure. Have someone who knows how to write and edit review your document, even if you are a good writer. Organize your information by following the outline presented in this chapter. Base your conclusions on facts, not assumptions.

Also, make sure there is coherence between problems you have identified and interventions you are recommending. For example, if you are dealing with the problem that Mrs. Hurricane is depressed, don't simply recommend she go to a women's support group. Although that might help, a more complete recommendation would be for Mrs. Hurricane to be assessed by a mental health professional. Include the name of the professional, his or her phone number and address, and a recommended time frame for the appointment as part of your recommendation.

Do not be subjective. Always be objective. "I thought she appeared depressed" should be reworded as "On the GCM's visit of 6/6/10, GCM observed Mrs. Hurricane had a flat affect, appeared lethargic, and stated that she has felt depressed for days. She stated she did not want to go out of the house and hardly wanted to watch her favorite show Jeopardy anymore." Also, do not be vague—present measurable statements: "She should be evaluated for symptoms of depression by Martin Skirt, LCSW, within 2 weeks," not "She should see a mental health professional."

■ CONCLUSION

Once the assessment is completed, mailed out to the party who requested it with copies sent to the other relevant individuals, and discussed with all concerned parties, the job of the GCM may be finished or just begun, depending upon whether the GCM is asked to carry out the care plan. In this chapter's example, Ms. Tornado may say she will move forward with all the GCM's suggestions, or she may say she will wait on some. At times, the client or family may resist the changes recommended in the plan and decide that their connection with the GCM is finished. If and when a crisis arises in the life of the client, the GCM may be called upon again to become involved, adjust the plan to fit the needs of the current situation, and implement and manage the care plan. If this occurs, because the GCM has already acquired so much information about the client, the GCM is usually able to provide relatively quick assistance. In either case, the GCM has provided the client and family with a comprehensive blueprint of how to proceed and, it is hoped, has assisted them in seeing the value of using professionals for consultation and assistance.

■ REFERENCES

1. National Institutes of Health. Consensus Conference on Geriatric Assessment Methods for Clinical Decision-Making. October 19, 1987. Available at: http://www.nlm.nih.gov. Accessed April 4, 1999.

2. American Geriatrics Society. Comprehensive Geriatric Assessment Position Statement. October 1996. Available at: http://www.americangeriatrics.org. Accessed March 15, 1999.

3. Brostoff P. *How to Write a Professional Assessment and Recommendations*. Presented at: Geriatric Care Management National Conference. October 2004; Austin, TX.

Chapter 6

Ethnic and Cultural Considerations in Geriatric Care Management

Nancy Hikoyeda and Christina E. Miyawaki

■ INTRODUCTION

The United States has one of the world's most ethnically and culturally diverse populations. This diversity has important implications for the provision of high-quality, appropriate social, health, and long-term care services, including geriatric care management. This chapter focuses on older adults from different ethnic and cultural backgrounds and the needs and preferences that the professional geriatric care manager (GCM) should consider in assessments, care plans, recommendations, and monitoring to enhance the quality of life of his or her clientele. This chapter is designed to provide only a brief introduction to the health and long-term care complexities faced by an immigrant or ethnic elder. The intent is to increase awareness of the challenges a GCM can face and to serve as a starting point for available resources.

■ THE DEMOGRAPHIC IMPERATIVE

Population Growth

The U.S. population is rapidly growing older and increasingly more diverse. Nearly 39 million people are currently 65 years and older, and 19.6% are considered ethnic minorities. Of this number, census data from 2008 by race and Hispanic origin reported roughly 80% of the older population were white non-Hispanic; 8.3% were black; < 1% American Indian/Alaska Native; 3.4% Asian/Pacific Islander; 6.8% Hispanic; and 0.6% reported two or more races.[1] By 2020, the minority population is expected to grow to 12.9 million or 23.6% of those 65+. Based on the 2000 census, about 10% of those older than age 65 are foreign born with the majority (62%) entering the United States prior to 1970.[2] Roughly 13% of the foreign-born elders speak a language other than English at home: 38% Spanish, 44% Indo-European languages, and 14% Asian and Pacific Island languages.[2]

Although these four federally designated racial/ethnic categories are helpful in referring to the various population groups overall, the picture is incomplete because the numbers ignore numerous variations within and between groups. Levinson and Ember have identified 161 immigrant groups excluding indigenous populations such as American Indians.[3] To illustrate these distinctions, Asian/Pacific Islander elders include more than 60 subgroups (e.g., Chinese, Filipino, Asian Indian, Vietnamese, Fijians, and others) who speak more than 100 different languages and dialects.[4] Further distinctions exist because Chinese elders may come from mainland China, Hong Kong, Shanghai, Singapore, Taiwan, Malaysia, or other Asian countries. Even terms such as *Southeast Asian* may refer to Vietnamese, Cambodians, or Laotian (Hmong or Mien) populations. The country of origin for Hispanic elders may be Mexico, Cuba, Puerto Rico, Spain, or Latin or South America, and although they may theoretically have the Spanish language in common, there are numerous differences in dialect and colloquialisms. Black elders may be descendants of slaves or may have come from any one of the many African (e.g., Kenya, Tanzania, Ethiopia, Sudan), South American, or Caribbean nations (e.g., Jamaica, Haiti). American Indian/Alaska Natives include more than 550 indigenous tribal groups, each with distinct languages and customs. Even elders labeled as white may have immigrated from any number of European or other countries throughout the world. Thus, the GCM must consider the unique differences of each of these subgroups to provide culturally appropriate assistance.

Socioeconomic Status

Ethnic elders have also been characterized as "bimodal" in terms of income, education, and social status.[4] That is, some groups of ethnic elders enjoy very high income and education levels while others may live in poverty with little or no formal education. Most ethnic elders exist between the two extremes. For example, the highest incomes among immigrant descendants are earned by Japanese Americans, who are the most acculturated and assimilated. Currently, some of the poorest and least educated are Hmong elders who are relatively recent arrivals from the agrarian Laotian region. Elders who have lived in the United States a longer time tend to be better off than more recent immigrants and refugees.

There are also gender differences in socioeconomic status (SES) in ethnic communities. Older women, in general, tend to face societal inequities as they age—living alone, suffering from multiple chronic health conditions, lower incomes, or living at or near poverty. Women of color tend to be at even greater disadvantage as a result of their employment history of jobs with low pay and no benefits (e.g.,

domestic or janitorial work). The 2008 data reveal that the highest poverty rates were experienced among Hispanic (43.1%) and black (34.7%) older women living alone. These inequities and injustices continue to plague this segment of our population.

■ ACCULTURATION AND ASSIMILATION

The Acculturation Continuum

It is important to know how acculturated an immigrant client may be because it has implications for adjustment, SES, living arrangements, physical and mental health, and service utilization. Acculturation refers to the degree to which an outsider adopts the culture, values, and norms of the dominant population.[6] Hence, the longer an immigrant elder has resided in a particular country, the more it is assumed that he or she will begin to adopt the beliefs and behaviors of the majority. Assimilation refers to the abandonment of one's native culture, beliefs, norms, and traditions and the replacement of them with those of the dominant group.[7] Japanese Americans, for example, are considered to be the most assimilated of the immigrant groups because of their length of time in the United States (the first pioneers arrived in the 1860s) and the decreasing numbers of recent immigrants from Japan.[8] Furthermore, Japanese Americans marry outside their culture at a rate of more than 50%, which has further diluted traditional Japanese practices and beliefs.

In the past, it has been assumed that the foreign-born are either acculturated or not acculturated. However, it is more likely that people fluctuate from one extreme to the other and, on occasion, may occupy a position somewhere in between. For example, a third-generation Japanese American may be considered very acculturated, particularly in the workplace or in the company of other non-Japanese people—certainly this person is more "Americanized" than his or her grandparents or parents. However, during the New Year's holidays (a traditional observance for people of Japanese descent), that same individual may relish traditional Japanese foods, attend a Buddhist temple, and observe other rituals such as cleaning the house or completing old business to welcome the new year. Thus, at a particular point in time, the Japanese American may be more "Japanese" than at others. Other ways to assess the degree of acculturation are discussed in the following sections.

Length of Time Since Immigration and Circumstances of Relocation

The length of time the elder or family has been living in the United States and the circumstances of immigration are important in assessing acculturation status. How long has the elder been in the United States (1 year or decades)? Why did he or she come? For example, Vietnamese immigrants arrived in essentially two "waves" to escape communist oppression and economic hardship. Did the elder arrive with the first group of relatively well-educated, well-to-do Vietnamese Catholic immigrants who worked with the U.S. forces in the mid-1970s? Or did the person arrive with the second wave of essentially mixed, less-educated refugees (e.g., boat people)? Was the elder imprisoned in a reeducation camp, or did he or she spend time in a refugee camp in Malaysia, Thailand, or Indonesia? Have the family members been reunited, or are they still separated? Are the elders "followers of children" who entered the United States for educational or employment opportunities?[9]

Personal Preferences

Other indicators of acculturation include personal preferences for native language usage, ethnic food, media, service providers, and socialization. The GCM can ask which language is preferred and used primarily in the client's home. Food preference is important particularly when long-term care residential options are being considered. Does the elder prefer ethnic food on a daily basis (e.g., rice with every meal) or a variety of food choices? Ethnic media is also an indicator of degree of acculturation. Does the client prefer an ethnic newspaper or television/radio station? Does the elder prefer a provider from the same ethnic group? It should not be assumed that the elder prefers a service provider from the same ethnicity—but for those who are less acculturated or monolingual non-English-speaking, this is frequently the case. Finally, does the ethnic elder prefer to socialize exclusively with others from the same ethnic group, or does it matter? The most effective way to obtain this information is to ask the client. Although family members may be helpful in ascertaining this information, even close family members frequently make assumptions about an elder's personal preferences that are not entirely accurate.[10]

Ideally, every effort should be made to locate providers who can communicate with the elder in the person's language of choice. However, if this is not possible, trained interpreters should be available. Because of the sensitive nature of many medical/social service encounters, young children or family members should not be used as interpreters. Additionally, a "cultural guide," a knowledgeable person from the elder's particular ethnic community who is familiar with the culture and beliefs of the traditional society, could also be consulted.

■ COHORT HISTORY

A cohort is a group of people born around the same time, generally within a 5-year time span. A cohort analysis considers the historical experiences, both positive and negative, that have influenced the members of the cohort at the present time. The GCM should consider the ethnic elder's background when doing an assessment to gain insights about the client's values, beliefs, behaviors, and preferences.[9]

Specific examples follow; however, each individual is unique and may not have experienced these events in the same way.

Many Mexican American elders have experienced the long-term effects of discriminatory immigration policies that have exploited Mexican laborers for decades. For example, the *Bracero* program was started to ease the U.S. labor shortage during World War II by welcoming short-term contract laborers and promising them U.S. citizenship and other benefits. However, depending on the U.S. economy, this program fluctuated over time, and the informal immigration policies resulted in *Braceros* sometimes being confused with "illegals," culminating in raids and mass deportations. Because of fear, confusion, and broken promises, many *Braceros* did not apply for citizenship even if they were eligible.[9] Despite these inequities, Mexican American elders have contributed substantially to U.S. society economically, socially, and culturally.

The majority of today's U.S.-born black elders faced institutionalized racial discrimination when they were young in the form of the Ku Klux Klan attacks, Jim Crow laws, segregated schools, antimiscegenation laws, and the Tuskegee Alabama Syphilis Experiment. As a result, black elders may distrust the system that supported such injustices. Despite the discrimination, black elders have the legacy of the civil rights movement; the one million plus men and women who served in segregated units during World War II and the Korean and Vietnam Wars; Harlem Jazz and gospel music as well as the humanitarian contributions of such leaders as the Rev. Dr. Martin Luther King and others.

Similarly, other immigrants have also experienced discrimination and hardships. Older Japanese Americans remember World War II when 120,000 individuals of Japanese descent, most of them U.S. citizens, were incarcerated by the U.S. government in wartime relocation centers. Filipino World War II veterans were recruited to serve in the U.S. Army and Navy in exchange for U.S. citizenship; however, this promise was revoked in 1945. It was not until the 1990s that the Veterans Equity Bill was passed, which granted the aging Filipino veterans immediate citizenship but only upon resettlement on the U.S. mainland.

Many Jewish elders are survivors of the Holocaust. American Indian elders faced decades of abuse, including relocation of the young to reservations and boarding schools, the termination of 100 tribes from federal responsibility, and subsequent forced urbanization.[9] In the 1970s and 1980s, Muslim refugees from Afghanistan fled the war with Russia and are now aging in the United States.[11] These are just a few examples of significant events that ethnic elders carry in their memories.

Despite the injustices, ethnic elders have contributed enormously to the American way of life.

Cohort history also considers migration patterns and resettlement within the United States. Decades ago, black elders moved from the Deep South to work in the industrial plants of the North where there was greater economic security. The largest populations of Hmong elders in the United States reside in California and Minnesota where the earliest refugees were assigned. The greater San Francisco Bay Area in California is home to the largest populations of Portuguese from the Azores (Portugal); Afghanis from Afghanistan; Sikhs and other South Asians from India; South Vietnamese; Chinese from Taiwan; and Filipinos from the Philippines. The location of resettlement communities was largely due to ethnic enclaves where lay referral networks and ethnic service providers helped immigrant families adapt to the foreign way of life.

It is impossible for a GCM to know all the historical events that influenced all the different groups living in the United States today. However, knowing where to look for information and what resources are available is a necessary and important skill. (See the section titled "Resources" at the end of this chapter.)

■ FAMILY VALUE SYSTEMS IN ETHNIC COMMUNITIES

Ethnic/Cultural Group Norms

Ethnic elders and families may exhibit value orientations that differ from mainstream U.S. society. In the United States, the focus is placed on individualism—Americans are socialized to be independent, autonomous, aggressive, opportunistic, and in control of various aspects of their lives from birth to death. Assertiveness in communication is encouraged along with the mandate to question authority and demand individual rights. However, many cultures promote values and behaviors diametrically opposed to these highly regarded American norms.

In other cultures, the focus may not be on the individual but on the immediate or extended family, the tribe, or the entire village.[12] The benefits and burdens, the good and bad, are experienced by, and reflect upon, the family unit rather than individual family members—children are warned not to bring shame upon the family. Additionally, some cultures emphasize nonconfrontational behaviors, whereas others teach deference to authority. An understanding of these differences helps to enhance communication between clients and providers.

Communication Styles

The GCM must learn to establish trust and rapport with the ethnic elder. Early on, respect must be shown in an appropriate manner and the elder made to feel as comfortable as possible. This can be done by addressing the elder as *Mr.* or *Mrs.*, taking time to chat before starting to discuss serious matters, and listening carefully when the elder is speaking. Methods of communication may also vary by ethnic or cultural group. For example, many older Asians perceive that asking questions of a

health professional is insulting to the provider and implies that the information has not been explained clearly or adequately. Other elders were taught deference to authority and unquestioning compliance because of the provider's expertise. Asking a question may also make the elder feel "stupid" or embarrassed. Hence, the Asian elder may shake his or her head in the affirmative; however, the nod means "Yes, I hear you" and not "I understand" or "I agree." In some cultures, direct eye contact may be perceived as threatening. In others, standing or sitting too close may be uncomfortable and inappropriate.[13]

End-of-Life Decisions

There may be cultural differences in end-of-life decision making as a result of underlying cultural values regarding disclosure of a terminal illness and use of life-sustaining medical treatment. With the widespread availability of advanced medical technology in the United States, people are encouraged to do everything possible to seek a cure for a life-threatening medical condition or sustain a life. However, there are others for whom quality of life is more important than length of life. Providers must realize that quality of life differs for each individual.

There are some societies, such as Japan, where a terminal illness may not be disclosed to a patient and it is culturally inappropriate to discuss impending or imminent death.[14] For instance, among some Chinese, it is considered bad luck to discuss death because such talk may cause death to occur. Sometimes the ethnic elder is not expected to make healthcare decisions and the responsibility may be based on a traditional family hierarchy. For instance, in many Filipino families there may be a designated decision maker who is not the patient (e.g., the oldest son or a daughter or son who is a health professional) and who articulates the wishes of the elder or family. Other end-of-life decisions are based on religious tenets. In many Catholic immigrant communities, there may be strong resistance to an advance directive because the document would signify a "loss of hope" or be interpreted as suicide, which is against church doctrine. These beliefs may also influence the use of hospice services.

Many providers are not aware that alternative clauses for advance directives are available from various religious traditions that convey religious intent and attitudes toward end-of-life issues (e.g., Christian Science, Jewish, Roman Catholic documents). Additionally, if a provider cannot discuss end-of-life preferences directly with a patient or client, other types of documentation (e.g., personal values charts) may be helpful if collected over time.

■ ETHNICITY, AGING, AND HEALTH

Health Disparities

Significant racial and ethnic disparities in the health status of older adults have been documented in the United States. A panel convened by the National Academies on race, ethnicity, and health in later life attempted to explain some of the differences.[15] In the past, most research focused on black–white comparisons, which revealed that even though life expectancy is increasing and overall health status is improving among older adults, blacks continually experience lower life expectancy than whites.[15] In general, blacks and American Indian/Alaska Natives are less healthy than older whites, and some Hispanics and Asians tend to be healthier than older whites.[15] There are many groups for which there is little to no information available, particularly the recent foreign-born immigrants from Southeast Asia, Eastern Europe, and Latin America.

The underlying determinants of these differences have remained elusive because of the many complex factors that influence health outcomes. Furthermore, relatively little research has focused on older adults.[15] Health status in ethnic communities is influenced by macrosocial factors (e.g., socioeconomic status, discrimination, politics, residence, fam-

ily); behavioral risk factors (e.g., smoking, exercise, alcohol use); cumulative prejudice and discrimination; stress (both personal and environmental); health care access and quality (e.g., cost, insurance, availability); lack of culturally competent services; adaptive health behaviors (e.g., coping, social supports); health care behaviors (e.g., utilization, help seeking, self-care); and genetics. Furthermore, these factors must be considered across the life course because early behaviors influence health in later years.

Health Risks and Health Status

Providing detailed information regarding the health status and risks among ethnic elders is not possible in this limited space; however, a brief discussion of major health risks is necessary. This material is based on the four federally designated racial/ethnic categories; therefore, caution must be taken to avoid generalization to specific subpopulations. To begin, Hummer et al. summarized overall differences in mortality:[16(p14)]

> Blacks generally have worse health than other groups. American Indians and Alaska Natives, especially those on reservations, are also less healthy than other groups except blacks. Whites are usually taken as the standard against which other groups are compared, but they are not necessarily in the best health. Hispanics appear to be healthier than whites on a number of measures, though not all. Asians are generally in better health than any other group.

It is noteworthy that among the oldest-old (those 85 years and older), there appears to be a mortality crossover in some populations—black elders live longer than whites, and there is some evidence that American Indian/Alaska Native mortality falls below that of Hispanics and Asian/Pacific Islanders.[15]

In general, the six leading causes of death among ethnic elders is similar to whites—heart disease, neoplasms (cancers), cerebrovascular disease, lower respiratory conditions, influenza and pneumonia, and diabetes.[15] When compared to data on the health of whites, self-report of the most common diseases and health conditions by ethnic elders reveals that older blacks have more hypertension, diabetes, strokes, kidney disease, and dementia/Alzheimer's disease.[17] Among Hispanic elders, non-insulin-dependent diabetes mellitus is a significant problem particularly among Mexicans and Puerto Ricans, as are hypertension and cardiovascular disease, cognitive impairment, and affective disorders.[18,19] The major health problems of elderly American Indian/Alaska Natives include type 2 diabetes mellitus, high blood pressure, tuberculosis, heart disease, cancer, and liver/kidney disease. Additionally, when compared to the general U.S. population, American Indian/Alaska Natives have high death rates from alcoholism, tuberculosis, and accidents.[20]

Overall, Asian/Pacific Islanders have a lower prevalence than whites of heart disease, cancer, and cardiovascular disease, but again this depends on the subgroup of interest.[4] Asian Indians, Chinese, Filipinos, and Japanese tend to have better health status than whites do,[21] whereas Native Hawaiians and Samoans tend to have worse health.[22] However, distinct differences exist within groups—for instance, breast cancer incidence is twice as high among Japanese American as among Vietnamese American women, whereas cervical cancer is seven times as high among Vietnamese as among Japanese American women.[23] These differences are a reflection of health statistics that tend to lump data for various subpopulations into a single category (e.g., African American, Hispanic, Asian) rather than the distinct ethnic subgroups. This aggregation of relevant data distorts the true picture of minority health status.

Health Beliefs

Some cultures see illness and healing from a different perspective than mainstream elders. Given the diverse number of cultures in the United States, numerous explanations exist for various medical conditions. The patient or client's perception of the source or cause of an illness carries broad implications for the acceptance of prescribed therapies and adherence to treatments as well as the use of medical and social services.

Western vs. Traditional Systems of Health Beliefs

The Stanford Geriatric Education Center has categorized culturally based health belief systems from documented information. Health belief system origins and some of their major characteristics are shown here:

- Biomedical model (Western, allopathic)—Practiced in the United States, founded upon evidence-based medical research studies
- American Indian—Mind–body–spirit integration, spiritual healing, use of native plants, respect for nature and environment
- African, African American—Integration of American Indian, Christian, other European traditions, occult/spiritual illness, religious healing
- Asian—Combination of Chinese medicine, Japanese Kampo, Korean Hanbang, and Southeast Asian medicine; balance of yin/yang, vital energy (chi); Taoist and Buddhist influence; Indian Ayurvedic medicine shaped by Hinduism and mind–body–spirit integration; Hmong beliefs involve healers, spirits, loss of soul
- Latin American—Biomedical model blended with Native American, European, African beliefs
- Other European American—Folk and religious healing practices, herbs, osteopathy, homeopathy

Caution must be taken because medical pluralism is common in self-care. The Stanford Geriatric Education Center has identified three overlapping sectors in health care: the professional sector (organized Western or other healing traditions), the popular sector (self-treatment, family care), and the folk sector (non-Western practitioners and healers).[24] In ethnic families, these sectors frequently overlap, and the patient may or may not inform the provider.

Meaning of Health and Illness

In ethnic communities, the source of an illness or medical condition may be attributed to biomedical causes or reflect an alternative belief system. For example, in some cultures, illness is believed to be caused by evil spirits or demons rather than disease pathology. The best way to obtain information is to ask the individual. Kleinman recommends these eight questions[25]:

1. What do you think caused your problem?
2. Why do you think it started when it did?
3. How does your sickness work on your body?
4. How severe is your sickness?
5. How long do you think it will last?
6. What are the problems your illness has caused you?
7. Do you know others who have had this problem? What did they do to treat it?
8. Do you think there is any way to prevent this problem in the future?

The answers to these questions serve as a basis for adherence to treatment interventions. For example, the health professional should also be aware that some medical terms to identify a medical condition may not exist in another language. This is particularly true of mental health problems because of the associated stigma. For example, a study of Vietnamese family caregivers of elders with Alzheimer's disease revealed there was no word in Vietnamese for *dementia* and the symptoms were considered a normal part of aging.[26] Similar findings were noted among Hispanic family caregivers.[27]

Ethnic Family Caregiving

Caregiving among ethnic families has not been well studied. However, ethnic family caregivers describe a cultural mandate toward eldercare at home, regardless of the circumstances, as a result of values such as filial piety (duty or obligation for parental care). Thus, placing an elder in a nursing home may be perceived as abandonment, an act that brings shame upon the family unit.

The degree of stress/burden experienced by a family caregiver depends on a number of factors. These mitigating factors include the family relationships such as the strength of the bond between the caregiver and care recipient and the express needs of the elder such as type of care, intensity, duration, and prognosis. Caregiver needs are also important such as willingness to provide care, available time, other family/work commitments, financial means, skill level, social and other support, personality, and acculturation. In general, although ethnic families desire to care for their elders at home, the demands of modern society may discourage eldercare.[10]

Depending on the ethnic group, there may even be a reluctance to use available services. Support groups may be perceived as discussing private family matters in public. Respite care may be linked to shirking responsibility. Other caregivers may feel guilty for seeking assistance.

Elder Abuse

There is a paucity of information on elder abuse (EA) in ethnic communities. Overall, incidence of mistreatment is underreported, particularly if the perpetrators are family members.[28] Other reporting problems are systemic, such as the absence of a consistent definition for EA across states.

In the mainstream US population, the primary forms of EA are physical, psychological, emotional, financial, verbal, neglect, and self-neglect with physical abuse being the most common. Elder mistreatment is caused by a web of factors such as lack of information about EA, caregiver stress/burden, dysfunctional family relationships (retaliation, unresolved conflicts, lack of close bonds), exploitation caused by economics, mental illness (substance abuse), and vulnerability.[29] There is a belief that EA does not exist in ethnic communities because of the respect for elders taught early in life. This is not true because elder mistreatment can occur in any family, but the type of abuse may vary.

Generally speaking, ethnic elders live with family members because of cultural values such as filial piety, love, and respect; economic necessity; and poor health. The expectations for family care make it difficult for an elder to believe that a relative would take advantage of his or her dependence and vulnerability.[28] Ethnic elders are reluctant to report mistreatment and tend to consider the intent, circumstances, and nature of the harm and ultimately condone abusive behaviors to avoid bringing shame upon the family. Elders may also have different perceptions of abuse.[28] For example, in a study using hypothetical vignettes, a Korean adult child could spend a parent's money without permission, which is considered financial abuse in the United States. However, the parent may condone the act because (1) the child must have needed the money badly or for a very good reason, and (2) the adult child will inherit the money anyway.[30] There is also evidence that psychological and emotional abuse is more common in some ethnic families. Tomita found that persistent extreme silence was used by one Japanese daughter-in-law, which literally stripped her mother-in-law of personhood within the family.[31]

There is a need for outreach and education about EA among ethnic families and providers and improvements in the service delivery system.[28] Because of the complexity involved in such EA cases, creative and culturally appropriate interventions must be developed and used. Furthermore, cultural and family values and relationships must be considered and incorporated into EA interventions such as ways to overcome the stigma of having private family matters addressed by outsiders.

Spirituality

Spirituality is discussed at length in Chapter 14. Similar to mainstream populations, ethnic elders come from a wide array of religious traditions and belief systems. In assessing an ethnic elder, a GCM must use a holistic approach that considers the mind, body, and spirit; this necessitates some assessment of spiritual practices and beliefs.[32]

Spirituality is most important to quality of life because it defines a meaningful life and gives an individual's existence value and purpose.[32] Many ethnic families rely on spirituality when faced with adversity, and it can serve as a coping mechanism and provide support, hope, comfort, and guidance. Some healthcare providers believe that spiritual support assists in the healing process.

The role of spirituality appears to be similar across cultures. As mentioned previously, the best way to assess spirituality is to ask the client. What is important in life? What about the future? How is quality of life defined? This interaction can enhance the quality of an ethnic elder's existence.

Health Literacy

Another area of growing concern in ethnic communities is *health literacy*—the skills to access, read, process, understand, communicate, and act upon basic health information to make informed health and long-term-care decisions.[33] An increasing body of research exists on this topic; however, very little attention has been paid to older immigrant populations. The GCM must have some indication of the health literacy skills of the ethnic client, particularly if recommendations to healthcare providers and other services are to be made.

The goals of health literacy extend beyond simply having educational materials translated into other languages. Monolingual, non-English-speaking clients may be unable to make medical appointments, use public transportation, understand insurance benefits and billings, comprehend directions, read instructions for a treatment regimen, and/or to report back on progress.[34] Some ethnic elders are functionally illiterate in their native countries, unable to read or write in any language—some languages have no written form. Particularly troublesome are cases involving informed consent because the medical terminology and concepts are daunting to older adults.

Current efforts to improve health literacy in foreign-born populations include increasing practical health literacy topics in English as a Second Language (ESL) courses, providing tutors to assist in teaching health communication, and developing materials using different media (e.g., videos, audiotapes) to accommodate varied learning styles. Immigrant elders also require assistance navigating the complex US healthcare system. One frustration is the insufficient number of trained, linguistically and culturally competent medical interpreters even though federal law requires an interpreter be available in all settings that accept federal funds. Although telephone language banks are increasingly available, they may lack regional familiarity and personal attention required in medical encounters.[35] This is particularly important when body language and other indirect forms of communication are necessary for accurate diagnosis and treatment. The GCM can advocate for professional interpreters on behalf of ethnic clients and their families.

■ BARRIERS TO SERVICES AND PROGRAMS

Ethnic elders frequently encounter structural or conceptual barriers to services and programs.[4] Structural barriers are built into the bureaucracy and include affordability and the high costs of health and social services; the availability of services in ethnic communities; access issues such as inconvenient hours; inferior-quality services; the lack of information and outreach; and service providers that disregard diversity. Conceptual barriers are the personally unacceptable and inappropriate aspects of the service delivery system. Conceptual barriers include sociocultural factors (e.g., personal preferences); ethnic and racial discrimination or prejudice experienced in the past; lack of knowledge about available options such as health screenings to prevent illness; attitudes toward the use of various services; and the unfamiliar culture of the health and social services systems. All of these barriers can prevent ethnic elders from accessing needed services.

■ RECOMMENDATIONS

The following recommendations for the GCM can enhance the quality and appropriateness of geriatric care management services.

- Ask questions about the personal preferences and specific needs of ethnic elders; listen closely to their responses.
- Be aware of your own values, biases, and gaps in knowledge about ethnic aging.
- Learn as much as possible about the backgrounds of the ethnic clients.
- Be sensitive and accepting of differences in values, beliefs, and behaviors.
- Use trained language interpreters and cultural guides if necessary.
- Modify assessment instruments to incorporate personal experiences, beliefs, and needs of ethnic families.
- Refer clients to culturally competent service providers.
- Advocate for education, outreach, and referral in ethnic communities.

CASE STUDY

Objectives

1. The first objective of this case study is to illustrate the sensitivity to cultural differences that the GCM must have when working with an ethnic client. The GCM must be sensitive to traditional cultural practices such as the Japanese way of showing gratitude to those who provide assistance or services.
2. The second objective is to show that the GCM working with an ethnically diverse client may maximize the use of community resources (both mainstream and ethnic-specific) to accommodate the client's needs and preferences.

In October 2004, a discharge planner from the ABC Hospital called the professional GCM at the Japanese American Senior Agency (JASA), a Japanese-specific culturally sensitive social service agency for older adults, to ask for assistance in finding a caregiver for Mr. Ken Takaki. The hospital had received a call from a Dr. Bob Edward, Mr. Takaki's friend, reporting that the caregivers from the local home care agencies were not meeting Mr. Takaki's needs. Mr. Takaki did not feel comfortable with the caregivers (ethnic/racial issues), and he was not used to eating the food that the caregivers prepared for him (food preference issues). Mr. Takaki typically prepared only Japanese food for himself and was not fond of American food.

Mr. Takaki was an 84-year-old Nisei, a second-generation Japanese American. His Issei (first-generation) parents immigrated to Hawaii, where Mr. Takaki was born. He was bilingual and spoke Japanese with his parents and English among his friends. After his father's death when he was 15, Mr. Takaki left Honolulu and moved to California with his mother in search of a better-paying job. World War II broke out in 1942 and all people of Japanese descent living on the West Coast were incarcerated in War Relocation Authority camps. Mr. Takaki and his mother were no exception and were evacuated to Topaz, Utah.

In 1946, after returning to San Francisco from the camp, his mother became very frail and needed constant care at home. Mr. Takaki took a job as a janitor cleaning a dental office near his home at night for Dr. Edward, which enabled Mr. Takaki to care for his mother during the day. Mr. Takaki never married and lived with his mother until she passed away peacefully at the age of 74. He worked for Dr. Edward until the doctor retired in 2000. Although Mr. Takaki had a heart attack in 1987 at the age of 65, he continued working. He had very little social life, and his only enjoyment was an annual week-long trip to Reno. In September 2003, he found blood in his urine and in December 2003, he had a prostatectomy. Mr. Takaki stayed at a local board and care facility, RN Home, for 6 months and was discharged on July 1, 2004.

The JASA GCM referred Mr. Takaki and Dr. Edward to several Japanese caregivers, who were bilingual in Japanese and English and could cook Japanese food. Dr. Edward contacted the first caregiver, Ms. Chieko Saito, and they both interviewed her at Mr. Takaki's residence. Both liked her and hired her, 4 hours a day, twice a week starting right away. She was to do the housekeeping and laundry, shopping, food preparation, medication reminders, assist with walking, and so forth.

Mr. Takaki was very pleased with Ms. Saito's services. However, after a couple of weeks, Ms. Saito called JASA and reported that Mr. Takaki bought food for her every time they went grocery shopping, spending twice the amount of money he should. She did not feel comfortable taking groceries from him. If she refused the food, he did not buy his own groceries. Ms. Saito was aware that Mr. Takaki was on a fixed income; however, he used his ATM card. Mr. Takaki's attitude reflected the traditional Japanese custom of showing gratitude to those who provide services even though Ms. Saito was paid to provide care.

After discussion with Dr. Edward, who had Mr. Takaki's power of attorney for finances and health care, a care plan was developed that used both mainstream and Japanese community services. Meals-on-Wheels and JASA's home-delivered Asian meals fulfilled Mr. Takaki's dietary needs, thereby eliminating Ms. Saito's cooking responsibilities. She did not have to take him grocery shopping, which eliminated his excess spending. Ms. Saito no longer felt guilty and Mr. Takaki's independence remained intact. Mr. Takaki continued to be ambulatory and exercised by walking four long blocks four times alone. He was engaged in the community, read the Japanese newspaper, watched Japanese TV programs, and rented Japanese videos.

In January 2006, JASA received a call from Dr. Edward that Mr. Takaki was rushed to ABC Hospital because he became disoriented while at a nearby restaurant. His cognition appeared to be declining and he required 24-hour care. Dr. Edward asked JASA if there were any Japanese care homes for Mr. Takaki. A few facilities were Japanese-owned; however, there were no vacancies at that time. Dr. Edward and the JASA GCM visited a board and care facility, Grace's Care Home, and arranged for Mr. Takaki's care. While there, the home tried to accommodate his personal preferences—he continued to receive the Japanese newspaper, watched Japanese TV, and the Filipino caregiver cooked Asian, but not Japanese, food at least three times a week.

For about a month, there was no problem and Mr. Takaki seemed happy with his new home. The Filipino caregiver took him out three times a week for a walk. However, Mr. Takaki became bored with the suburban environment where his care home was located. He was used to walking around his house daily, which was in the center of the city. He also missed his favorite Japanese foods and videos.

To further accommodate Mr. Takaki's needs, a new care plan was established whereby the JASA GCM located some nearby Japanese/Asian grocery stores, listed his favorite Japanese foods in both Japanese and English, and asked the caregiver to buy and prepare some of the food for him. The JASA GCM arranged with a Japanese video store to mail a list of available Japanese videos to Mr. Takaki, so he could order the ones of interest. The JASA GCM also contacted the local county library to mail a list of its Japanese books. Mr. Takaki could call the library for a monthly bookmobile delivery to his care home. Mr. Takaki was occupied watching Japanese videos, reading Japanese books, and enjoying a taste of Japanese food.

The next step was to motivate Mr. Takaki to do some activities outside the care home to maintain his ambulatory abilities and avoid further decline.

Conclusion

1. The JASA GCM working with this ethnic client was sensitive to traditional cultural practices. Traditionally, Japanese people express their gratitude to service providers and others. In Mr. Takaki's case, buying groceries for Ms. Saito was probably the only way he could express his appreciation even though he paid for her services. To avoid Mr. Takaki's overspending, the JASA GCM changed Ms. Saito's responsibilities for meal planning and cooking by substituting community programs (mainstream and ethnic home-delivered meals).

2. The GCM working with an ethnic client must use community resources (both mainstream and ethnic). To meet the needs of a homebound elder is always a challenge. However, if the elder is from a different ethnic or cultural group, it can be a daunting task depending on the barriers faced by the client and the providers. Although Mr. Takaki did not have any language barrier, he still preferred Japanese foods and activities, which the GCM considered in the assessment. To satisfy and fulfill Mr. Takaki's needs, the GCM hired a Japanese-speaking caregiver; requested both mainstream and ethnic home-delivered meals; arranged for a subscription to an ethnic newspaper; used a Japanese video mail service; arranged for a bookmobile delivery from the local library; and gave instructions to the Filipino caregiver about purchasing and preparing the client's favorite Japanese foods.

CARE MONITORING

Objectives

1. The first objective of this case is to illustrate that, ideally, a GCM working with an ethnic client should speak the client's language and have an understanding of the client's cultural background and preferences.

2. The second objective is to show that the GCM should be aware of available agencies and resources that serve various ethnic communities.

Ms. Debbie Martin, discharge planner at Richmond Hospital, called the JASA about Mr. Jiro Ikeda. Mr. Ikeda was hospitalized after a neighbor found him disoriented in his truck in front of his home. He was diagnosed with dehydration caused by heat exhaustion and fatigue. Mr. Ikeda was a 74-year-old Japanese *Shin-Issei* (newcomer) who came to the United States as a typhoon refugee after the Immigration and Naturalization Services Act of 1965, which increased Asian immigrant quotas. He graduated from a Japanese high school. Although he had been living in the United States for more than 40 years, he could not understand, speak, or write in English because of his limited social network of Japanese-speaking associates. He worked as a gardener all his life, never married, lived alone in a small rented house, and had no social life. Mr. Ikeda had no relatives in the United States.

According to Ms. Martin, Mr. Ikeda was very cooperative at the hospital, followed doctors' directions, and was well-liked. His only support system appeared to be his employee, Mr. Jorge Martinez, who worked for Mr. Ikeda for seven years. While Mr. Ikeda was in the hospital, Mr. Martinez took care of Mr.

Ikeda's business and house, along with a friend, Ms. Elena Sanchez. Mr. Martinez was from Mexico and Ms. Sanchez came from Honduras. Mr. Martinez could not read or write in either Spanish or English and Ms. Sanchez had limited English language capability, and most of the time, they communicated in Spanish. Mr. Martinez and Ms. Sanchez had purchased a three-bedroom house and were willing to take Mr. Ikeda in as soon as the house was available. They were not planning to charge Mr. Ikeda any rent because he had given Mr. Martinez all his customers.

The JASA GCM, who was bilingual in Japanese and English, met with Ms. Martin, Mr. Ikeda, Mr. Martinez, and Ms. Sanchez at the hospital. Mr. Ikeda had had a thorough psychosocial assessment, and the GCM also did a functional assessment. Ms. Martin explained Mr. Ikeda's physical and psychological status in English and limited Spanish. Mr. Ikeda's physical condition was good and he was ambulatory. His cognition was fair, although he sometimes became confused and had mild dementia. He also needed assistance with some instrumental activities of daily living (IADLs). They concluded that Mr. Ikeda was ready to be discharged as long as he had 24-hour care. After thorough discussion, agreement was made on the following care options:

1. The GCM would do a home assessment and, if it was acceptable and safe to return home, the GCM would recommend a Japanese-speaking caregiver from JASA's caregiver directory two times a week, four hours a day until Mr. Ikeda's condition improved. The other three days, Mr. Martinez would have Mr.

Ikeda accompany him on his job, so that Mr. Ikeda could give advice. On weekends, both Mr. Martinez and Ms. Sanchez would watch over Mr. Ikeda. Payment would be discussed at a later time.
2. If his home was not safe enough for Mr. Ikeda to live by himself, the GCM would search for a board and care facility to aid in Mr. Ikeda's recovery.

Mr. Ikeda did not remember how much money he had in the bank. The JASA GCM contacted Ms. Maria Lopez, at Kyoto Bank, to get Mr. Ikeda's account information. Ms. Lopez, who spoke Spanish, also agreed to be a translator for Mr. Martinez and Ms. Sanchez to help Mr. Ikeda.

The GCM made a care monitoring and assessment visit. The condition of the house was totally uninhabitable, and the house was located between several busy streets, which posed a health hazard. Windows were broken and walls were damaged. None of the utilities were functioning. Therefore, the first plan was not an option.

The GCM informed Mr. Ikeda that he could not go back to his old home and that he needed to move out of the house. The GCM located a facility, Sierra Home, that accepted tenants for respite care on a monthly basis at a fixed rate ($2000). Mr. Ikeda agreed to move into the care home when he was discharged from the hospital.

As soon as Mr. Ikeda moved, the GCM received several calls from the owner, Mr. Ray Chang, complaining that Mr. Ikeda did not sleep at night and moved furniture around. He was also incontinent and needed to wear pads. This information was all new to the

GCM because the discharge planner had not mentioned these problems.

The GCM made a care monitoring visit to Mr. Ikeda the next day. Mr. Ikeda explained it would take a month to get used to the new place. He did not know why he could not get to the bathroom on time. He liked the food and had no problems. Mr. Chang said he would take Mr. Ikeda to his doctor and have him prescribe medication to help him sleep through the night.

A few days later, the GCM received another call from Mr. Chang reporting that Mr. Ikeda was taken to the doctor, but that he was still wandering and incontinent. Mr. Chang said that Mr. Ikeda wore a diaper, only to tear it off during the night and urinate on the floor. The GCM visited Mr. Ikeda again only to find out that because of his Japanese cultural background, he was not honest in his initial response. In Japan, information that might hurt someone else's feelings should be withheld, particularly if the person is trying to help (enryo). However, Mr. Ikeda's behavior revealed his true feelings. He actually did not want to stay in the home because he was uncomfortable with the Asian caregiver.

Mr. Ikeda stated that he wanted to move out of Sierra Home and move in with Mr. Martinez. To make sure that Mr. Martinez and Ms. Sanchez were responsible individuals, the GCM contacted Ms. Lopez from Kyoto Bank to act as a translator. Ms. Lopez, Mr. Martinez, Ms. Sanchez, and the GCM had a meeting. Mr. Martinez left Mr. Ikeda's checkbook with Ms. Lopez. Mr. Martinez explained their intent to care for Mr. Ikeda in their new house, but he did not want to assume the responsibility

for Mr. Ikeda's financial matters. The following care plan was developed:

1. Mr. Ikeda would move in with Mr. Martinez. Ms. Sanchez was to care for Mr. Ikeda on Mondays, Tuesdays, and Thursdays, and Mr. Martinez would watch over him on Wednesdays and Fridays. Both would share the responsibilities on weekends.
2. Ms. Lopez was to keep Mr. Ikeda's checkbook, and the JASA GCM was to help with check writing until other options could be investigated.

A couple of days after Mr. Ikeda moved, the GCM made a care monitoring visit. Mr. Ikeda looked happier and was cleaner. The house was spacious, clean, and orderly. However, Mr. Martinez reported that Mr. Ikeda did not sleep well and was incontinent at night. The GCM made an appointment with Mr. Ikeda's primary care physician and accompanied him to the doctor.

Subsequently, the GCM proposed that JASA become Mr. Ikeda's representative payee and also became Mr. Ikeda's agent for his durable power of attorney for finances and health care.

■ INTRODUCTION TO ASSESSMENT AND PLAN OF CARE FORMS

The following initial assessment and plan of care forms (Exhibits 6–1 and 6–2) are based on several existing geriatric care management tools currently used by both mainstream and ethnic-specific social service agencies and geriatric care management providers. These instruments were created for use with ethnic elders, including recent immigrants. The forms are comprehensive, but not all inclusive, because it is impossible to include all the different ethnic and cultural groups in one template. The purpose of these samples is to stimulate awareness of the diversity found in the elderly population and increase sensitivity to differences that exist.

The following websites can help the GCM to reflect upon his or her own cultural competence:

http://www.aafp.org/fpm/20001000/58cult.html
http://www.nccccurricula.info/assessment/index.html

■ CONCLUSION

The objective of this chapter is to increase awareness of the complexity of issues, concerns, and barriers that confront ethnic elders and their families today. Immigrant elders and their families are unique additions to the tapestry of life in the United States, and this cultural pluralism has contributed much to our society. To render appropriate assistance to this diverse population the GCM must have knowledge about the backgrounds, beliefs, and preferences of ethnic clients, as well as highly developed skills to guide clients in the right direction.

Exhibit 6–1   Initial Assessment Form

Date: _____

Client Name: First: _____   Middle: _____   Last: _____

How to Address Client: _____

How Client's Family Members Address Client: _____

DOB: _____   Sex: ❏ Male ❏ Female

Ethnicity/Race: _____

Street Address: _____

City: _____   State: _____   Zip: _____

Phone Numbers: Home: ( ) _____   Cell: ( ) _____

Live Alone: ❏ Yes ❏ No   Marital Status: _____

Client needs assistance in: ADL ❏ Eating   IADL ❏ Preparing meals
                                   ❏ Dressing   ❏ Shopping
                                   ❏ Bathing   ❏ Managing medications
                                   ❏ Toileting   ❏ Managing money
                                   ❏ Getting in/out of bed ❏ Using telephone
                                   ❏ Walking   ❏ Doing heavy housework
                                                           ❏ Doing light housework
                                                           ❏ Transportation ability

Primary Language: _____   Secondary Language: _____

Language Proficiency:

    English: ❏ Good ❏ Fair ❏ Not good
    Primary Language: ❏ Good ❏ Fair ❏ Not good
    Secondary Language: ❏ Good ❏ Fair ❏ Not good

Exhibit 6–1   Initial Assessment Form (continued)

Educational Level: Home Country: _____ Years   In the U.S.: _____ Years

Interpreter Need: ❏ Yes ❏ No

Interpreter Availability: ❏ Yes   If yes, who would it be? _____
                              ❏ No

Place (Country) of Birth: ❏ U.S.A.   ❏ Other   If other, which country? _____
                          Year when client moved to the U.S.: _____
                          Age when client immigrated to the U.S.: _____ years old
                          Reasons of immigration: _____

Cultural Needs: _____

Food Preferences (including Ethnic Food): _____

Dietary Needs: _____

Religious Preferences: _____

Emergency Contact Name: _____   Relationship: _____

Address: _____   Phone: ( ) _____

City: _____ State: _____   Zip: _____

Emergency Contact Name: _____   Relationship: _____

Address: _____   Phone: ( ) _____

City: _____ State: _____   Zip: _____

Caregiver Name: _____   Relationship: _____

Address: _____   Phone: ( ) _____

City: _____ State: _____   Zip: _____

Financial Resources: ❏ Social security   ❏ Supplementary security income (SSI)
                          ❏ Pension   ❏ Help from family members
                          ❏ Other

Insurance: ❏ Medicare   Policy #: _____
                          ❏ Private Health Insurance   Policy #: _____
                          ❏ Private Dental Insurance   Policy #: _____
                          ❏ Long-term Care Insurance   Policy #: _____
                          ❏ Other   Policy #: _____

Hobbies: Currently enjoy doing: _____
                          Used to enjoy doing: _____
                          Family activities: _____

Reasons for the initial contact:

_____
_____
_____
_____
_____
_____

Exhibit 6–2   Plan of Care Form

Date: _____

Name of Client: _____

Name of Care Manager: _____

Name of Agency: _____

Address: _____

Phone Number: (   ) _____   Cell Number: (   ) _____

Fax Number: (   ) _____   E-mail: _____

Ethnicity/Race of Care Manager: _____

Linguistic competency besides English: _____
(Name of Language)
❑ Speak   ❑ Read   ❑ Write

Name of Social Worker: _____

Name of Agency: _____

Address: _____

Phone Number: (   ) _____   Cell Number: (   ) _____

Fax Number: (   ) _____   E-mail: _____

Ethnicity/Race of Social Worker: _____

Linguistic competency besides English: _____
(Name of Language)
❑ Speak   ❑ Read   ❑ Write

Client - Personal Information

Client Name: First: _____   Middle: _____   Last: _____

How does the client prefer to be addressed? _____

How does the client's family address him/her? _____

DOB: _____   Sex: ❑ Male ❑ Female

Ethnicity/Race: _____

Street Address: _____

City: _____   State: _____   Zip: _____

Phone Numbers: Home: (   ) _____   Cell: (   ) _____

Former Occupation: U.S.A. _____   Other than U.S.A. _____

Live Alone: ❑ Yes ❑ No   Marital Status: _____

Other Living Arrangement: _____

_____
_____
_____

Exhibit 6–2   Plan of Care Form (continued)

Has the client had any change in residence in the past year?   ❑ Yes   ❑ No

If yes, how and why? _____

_____

Does the client wish to remain at home?   ❑ Yes   ❑ No

Has the client had any life event or traumatic experience
in the past year (hospitalization, move, etc.)?   ❑ Yes   ❑ No

If yes, what, when and why? _____

_____

Names, Addresses, and Phone Numbers of Children:

Name: _____   Relationship: _____
Address: _____   Phone: (   ) _____
City: _____ State: _____   Zip: _____

Name: _____   Relationship: _____
Address: _____   Phone: (   ) _____
City: _____ State: _____   Zip: _____

Name: _____   Relationship: _____
Address: _____   Phone: (   ) _____
City: _____ State: _____   Zip: _____

Current Care Arrangements among Family Members: _____

_____
_____
_____

Preferable Language: _____
Interpreter needed: ❑ Yes   ❑ No
Names of Interpreters: _____
Cultural Needs: _____
Food Preferences (including Ethnic Food): _____
Dietary Needs: _____
Religious Preferences: _____

Emergency Contact Name: _____   Relationship: _____
Address: _____   Phone: (   ) _____
City: _____ State: _____   Zip: _____

Emergency Contact Name: _____   Relationship: _____
Address: _____   Phone: (   ) _____
City: _____ State: _____   Zip: _____

Caregiver Name: _____   Relationship: _____
Address: _____   Phone: (   ) _____
City: _____ State: _____   Zip: _____

continues

Exhibit 6–2   Plan of Care Form (continued)

Medical Information

Primary Physician: _____   Phone: ( ) _____

Hospital: _____   Phone: ( ) _____

Interpreter Available: ❏ Yes ❏ No

Dentist: _____   Phone: ( ) _____

Interpreter Available: ❏ Yes ❏ No

Pharmacy: _____   Phone: ( ) _____

Interpreter Available: ❏ Yes ❏ No

Name of Health Insurance: _____
Address: _____
Phone Number: ( ) _____   Fax Number: ( ) _____
Policy #: _____

Name of Dental Insurance: _____
Address: _____
Phone Number: ( ) _____   Fax Number: ( ) _____
Policy #: _____

Name of Long-term Care Insurance: _____
Address: _____
Phone Number: ( ) _____   Fax Number: ( ) _____
Policy #: _____

Physical Health Symptoms: _____
_____
_____

Mental/Cognitive Symptoms: _____
_____
_____

Scheduled Medication

Name of Medication	Dosage	Time of Day	Instruction

Exhibit 6–2   Plan of Care Form (continued)

Does the client have a Durable Power of Attorney for Health Care? ❑ Yes ❑ No

    Name of the person/agent: _____ Relationship: _____

    Address: _____

    Phone Number: ( ) _____ Fax Number: ( ) _____

If no, who will make the client's healthcare decisions?

    Name of the person: _____ Relationship: _____

    Address: _____

    Phone Number: ( ) _____

    Name of the person: _____ Relationship: _____

    Address: _____

    Phone Number: ( ) _____

Does the client have a Do-Not-Resuscitate Order (DNR)? ❑ Yes ❑ No

If no, who will make decisions on behalf of the client?

    Name of the person: _____ Relationship: _____

    Address: _____

    Phone Number: ( ) _____

    Name of the person: _____ Relationship: _____

    Address: _____

    Phone Number: ( ) _____

Personal Care

	Needs Assist	Devices
Ambulation		
Bathing		
Dressing		
Feeding		
Foot Care		
Grooming		
Medication		
Oral Care		
Skin Care		
Toileting		
Transfers		
Vision Care		
Other Care		

continues

Exhibit 6–2   Plan of Care Form (continued)

Meal Preparation

Food Preferences (including ethnic food): _____

_____

Dietary Needs: _____

_____

Breakfast: _____
     Time: _____
     Eating Arrangements: _____

Lunch: _____
     Time: _____
     Eating Arrangements: _____

Dinner: _____
     Time: _____
     Eating Arrangements: _____

Snacks: _____
     Time: _____
     Eating Arrangements: _____

Meals-on-Wheels (MOW) requested?   ❑ Yes   ❑ No

     MOW: ❑ Yes   ❑ No   Which days? _____

     Ethnic MOW: ❑ Yes   ❑ No   Which days? _____

Is the client able to receive MOW without assistance?   ❑ Yes   ❑ No

Time of MOW delivery: MOW: _____   Ethnic MOW: _____

Additional Meal Instructions:_____

Housework

	Need Assist	Frequency/Instructions
Dishwashing		
Dusting		
Kitchen cleaning		
Bathroom cleaning		
Floor cleaning		
Laundry		
Vacuuming		
Other Housework		
Other Housework		

Exhibit 6–2   Plan of Care Form (continued)

Schedule of Activities

Daily Activities:

      Morning: _____

      Afternoon: _____

Hobbies: _____

_____

Outside Group Activities: _____

_____

Religious Activities: _____

_____

Exercises: _____

_____

Additional Arrangements (such as ethnic video, mobile book programs, etc.):

_____

_____

_____

Finances

Is the client able to manage his/her finances without assistance?   ❑ Yes   ❑ No

Does the client have agents (representative payee, conservator, power of attorney for finances, etc.)

     Finances?   ❑ Yes   ❑ No

     Name of the person/agent: _____   Relationship: _____

     Address: _____

     Phone Number: (   ) _____   Fax Number: (   ) _____

If no, who makes financial decisions for the client?

     Name of the person: _____   Relationship: _____

     Address: _____

     Phone Number: (   ) _____

     Name of the person: _____   Relationship: _____

     Address: _____

     Phone Number: (   ) _____

■ REFERENCES

1. US Census Bureau. *National Center on Health Statistics and the Bureau of Labor Statistics. A Profile of Older Americans: 2009.* Washington, DC: Administration on Aging.

2. US Census Bureau. *We the People: Aging in the United States. Census 2000 Special Reports.* Washington, DC: US Census Bureau; 2004.

3. Levinson D, Ember M. *American Immigrant Cultures: Builders of a Nation.* New York: Simon and Schuster Macmillan; 1997.

4. Kagawa-Singer M, Hikoyeda N, Tanjasiri SP. Aging, chronic conditions, and physical disabilities in Asian Pacific Islander Americans. In: Markides KS, Miranda MR, eds. *Minorities, Aging, and Health.* Thousand Oaks, CA: Sage Publications; 1997:149–180.

5. Mutran E, Sudha S. Ethnic and racial groups, similar or different, and how do we measure? *Res Aging.* 2000;22(6):589–598.

6. Spector RE. *Cultural Diversity in Health and Illness.* 5th ed. Upper Saddle River, NJ: Prentice Hall Health; 2000.

7. Barresi CM, Stull DE. *Ethnic Elderly and Long-Term Care.* New York: Springer Publishing; 1993.

8. Kitano HHL. *Generations and Identity: The Japanese American.* Needham Heights, MA: Ginn Press; 1993.

9. Yeo G, Hikoyeda N, McBride M, Chin S-Y, Edmonds M, Hendrix L. *Cohort Analysis as a Tool in Ethnogeriatrics: Historical Profiles of Elders from Eight Ethnic Populations in the United States.* Palo Alto, CA: Stanford Geriatric Education Center; 1998.

10. Hikoyeda N, Wallace SP. Do ethnic-specific long term care facilities improve resident quality of life? In: Choi NG, ed. *Social Work Practice with the Asian American Elderly.* New York: Haworth Press; 2001:63–82.

11. Morioka-Douglas N, Sacks T, Yeo G. Issues in caring for Afghan American elders: insights from literature and a focus group. *J Cross-Cultural Gerontol.* 2004;19:27–40.

12. Fugita SS, O'Brien DJ. *Japanese American Ethnicity: The Persistence of Community.* Seattle, WA: University of Washington Press; 1991.

13. McBride MR, Morioka-Douglas N, Yeo G. *Aging and Health: Asian and Pacific Islander American Elders.* Palo Alto, CA: Stanford Geriatric Education Center; 1996.

14. Braun KL, Pietsch JH, Blanchette PL. *Cultural Issues in End-of-Life Decision Making.* Thousand Oaks, CA: Sage Publications; 2000.

15. Bulatao RA, Anderson NA. Racial and ethnic disparities in health and mortality among the US elderly population. In: Anderson NA, Bulatao RA, Cohen B, eds. *Critical Perspectives on Racial and Ethnic Differences in Health in Later Life.* Washington, DC: National Academies Press; 2004.

16. Hummer R, Benjamin MR, Rogers RG. Racial and ethnic disparities in health and mortality among the US elderly population. In: Anderson NA, Bulatao RA, Cohen B, eds. *Critical Perspectives on Racial and Ethnic Differences in Health in Later Life.* Washington, DC: National Academies Press; 2004.

17. Hayward MD, Crimmins EM, Miles TP, Yang Y. The significance of socioeconomic status in explaining the racial gap in chronic health conditions. *Am Sociol Rev.* 2000;65:910–930.

18. Pleis JR, Coles R. Summary health statistics for US adults: National Health Interview Survey, 1998. *Vital Health Stat.* 2002;10:209.

19. Manly JJ, Mayeux R. Ethnic differences in dementia and Alzheimer's disease. In: Anderson NA, Bulatao RA, Cohen B, eds. *Critical Perspectives on Racial and Ethnic Differences in Health in Later Life.* Washington, DC: National Academies Press; 2004.

20. McCabe M, Cuellar J. *Aging and Health: American Indian/Alaska Native Elders.* 2nd ed. Palo Alto, CA: Stanford Geriatric Education Center; 1994.

21. Kuo WH, Porter K. Health status of Asian Americans: United States, 1992–04. *Advance Data from Vital Health Statistics,* No. 298. Hyattsville, MD: National Center for Health Statistics; 1998.

22. Hoyert DL, Kung H. Asian or Pacific Islander mortality, selected states, 1992. *Mon Vital Stat Rep.* 1997;45(suppl 1): 1–64.

23. Miller B, Kolonel L, Bernstein L, Young Jr JL, Swanson G, West D, et al. *Racial/Ethnic Patterns of Cancer in the United States, 1988–1992.* NIH Pub. No. 96-4101. Bethesda, MD: National Cancer Institute; 1996.

24. Levkoff S, Chee YK, Reynoloso-Vallejo H, Mendez J. Culturally appropriate geriatric care:

fund of knowledge. In: Yeo G, ed. *Core Curriculum in Ethnogeriatrics.* 2nd ed. Palo Alto, CA: Stanford Geriatric Education Center; 2000.

25. Kleinman A. *Patients and Healers in the Context of Culture.* Berkeley, CA: University of California Press; 1980.

26. Yeo G, Tran JNU, Hikoyeda N, Hinton L. Conceptions of dementia among Vietnamese American caregivers. In: Choi NG, ed. *Social Work Practice with the Asian American Elderly.* New York: Haworth Press; 2001:131–154.

27. Villa ML, Cuellar J, Gamel N, Yeo G. *Aging and Health: Hispanic American Elders.* 2nd ed. Palo Alto, CA: Stanford Geriatric Education Center; 1993.

28. Tatara T. *Understanding Elder Abuse in Minority Populations.* Philadelphia: Brunner/Mazel; 1999.

29. Rittman M, Kuzmeskus LB, Flum MA. A synthesis of current knowledge on minority elder abuse. In: Tatara T, ed. *Understanding Elder Abuse in Minority Populations.* Philadelphia: Brunner/Mazel; 1999:221–238.

30. Moon A. Elder abuse and neglect among the Korean elderly in the United States. In: Tatara T, ed. *Understanding Elder Abuse in Minority Populations.* Philadelphia: Brunner/Mazel; 1999: 109–118.

31. Tomita SK. Exploration of elder mistreatment among the Japanese. In: Tatara T, ed. *Understanding Elder Abuse in Minority Populations.* Philadelphia: Brunner/Mazel; 1999:119–142.

32. Barton J, Grudzen M, Zielske R. *Vital Connections in Long-Term Care: Spiritual Resources for Staff and Residents.* Baltimore, MD: Health Professions Press; 2003.

33. Ratzan SC, Parker RM. Introduction. In: Selden CR, Zorn M, Ratzan SC, Parker RM, eds. *Natural Library of Medicine Current Bibliographies in Medicine: Health Literacy.* NLM Pub. No. CBM 2000-1. Bethesda, MD: National Institutes of Health; 2000.

34. Williams MV, Parker RM, Baker DW, et al. Inadequate functional health literacy among patients at two public hospitals. *JAMA.* 1995;274(21):1677–1682.

35. Gordon D, Yoshida H, Hikoyeda N, David D. *Patient Listening: Health Communication Needs of Older Immigrants.* Philadelphia: Temple University Center for Intergenerational Learning; 2006.

■ SUGGESTED READINGS

Adler RN, Kamel HK, eds. *Doorway Thoughts: Cross-Cultural Health Care for Older Adults.* Sudbury, MA: Jones and Bartlett Publishers; 2004.

Cress C. *Handbook of Geriatric Care Management.* Gaithersburg, MD: Aspen Publishers; 2001.

Gallo JJ. The content of geriatric care. In: Fulmer T, Gallo JJ, Paveza GJ, eds. *Handbook of Geriatric Assessment.* 3rd ed. Gaithersburg, MD: Aspen Publishers; 2000:1–12.

Goode TD. *Promoting Cultural and Linguistic Competency Self-Assessment Checklist for Personnel Providing Primary Health Care.* Adapted from: *Promoting Cultural Competence and Cultural Diversity for Personnel Providing Services and Supports to Children with Special Health Care Needs and Their Families.* Washington, DC: Georgetown University Center for Child and Human Development; 2004.

Kane RJ, Kane RA, eds. *Assessing Older Persons: Measures, Meaning, and Practical Applications.* New York: Oxford University Press; 2000.

Mouton CP, Esparza YB. Ethnicity and geriatric assessment. In: Fulmer T, Gallo JJ, Paveza GJ et al, eds. *Handbook of Geriatric Assessment.* 3rd ed. Gaithersburg, MD: Aspen Publishers; 2000.

■ RESOURCES

The following are resources for further information about ethnicity, aging, and health. However, this is not a comprehensive listing of all that is available.

Stanford Geriatric Education Center
1215 Welch Road, Modular B,
Stanford, CA 94304-5403
Phone (650) 721-1023; fax (650) 721-1026
http://sgec.stanford.edu

Materials available:
- Ethnogeriatric curriculum materials and monographs on aging, ethnicity, and health in specific disciplines (nutrition, social work, medicine, spirituality, and many other fields)
- Mental Health Aspects of Diabetes in Elders from Diverse Ethnic Backgrounds
- Online training modules on various aspects of ethnogeriatrics and ethnogerontology: (1) Test Your Ethnogeriatric IQ; (2) Improving Communication with Elders

of Different Cultures; (3) Diversity, Healing, and Healthcare; (4) Other Ethnogeriatric Educational Resources.

Cross Cultural Health Care Program (cross-cultural health care and training programs for medical interpreters)
   http://www.xculture.org

Culture Clues (tip sheets designed for clinicians)
   http://depts.washington.edu/pfes/
   cultureclues.htm

Diversity Rx (promotes language and cultural competence to improve quality of health care)
   http://www.diversityrx.org

Ethnomed
   http://www.ethnomed.org

California Health Literacy Initiative (health literacy information and training)
   http://www.cahealthliteracy.org/resource_
   center.html

Office of Minority Health Resource Center;
800-444-6472
   http://www.omhrc.gov

Chapter 7

Integrating Late-Life Relocation: The Role of the GCM

Cathie Ramey and Cathy Jo Cress

■ THE PSYCHOLOGY OF MOVING AN OLDER PERSON

Whether you're young or old; whether you live in a tiny apartment or a grandiose estate; for a multitude of reasons the familiar saying, "there's no place like home" resonates with all of us. When we ask an older person to leave their home we are stripping them of more than the four walls that hold their belongings, and it's not just "memories" that are being threatened.

What we often fail to recognize when considering the move of a senior are the important intangibles that make a house truly a home. These intangibles include the meaning of home, the meaning of personal belongings, the delicate balance between expectations and reality, and the need to have control over our lives. For a multitude of reasons, many of which we are not familiar with, most older people do not want to move and prefer to remain in their own home. The ability to age in place—growing older without having to move—becomes an increasingly important housing issue for older Americans. The goal of this chapter is to explore the meaning of home, why seniors relocate, and what the professional geriatric care manager should be aware of when helping an older adult with this transition.

A recent survey found that 83% of people between the ages of 65 and 74 years and 86% of those age 75 years and older want to remain in their own homes as they age.[1] In 2001, 80% of the 21.8 million households headed by seniors were owner occupied, and 20% were renters.[2,3]

Most older people are more likely to be homeowners and less likely to be renters. The majority of elders have a high level of attachment to their own homes, and if older people move, they tend to move locally. The census data from 2002 to 2003 shows that approximately 4% of adults age 65 and older moved during that 1-year period as compared to 14% of the population as a whole.[4] So, the decision to leave the home is not to be taken lightly nor treated as a mere change of location that takes place on moving day. Home is where the family memories are, where the familiar paths are, and where a lifetime of history has taken place. When considering late-life relocation, when both familiar objects and familiar routines of daily life are threatened and disrupted, it's important to develop a relocation strategy that calls for awareness and planning on the part of the geriatric care manager, older adult, family, and the support network involved in the relocation process.

■ THE MEANING OF HOME

What *home* means to the individual, how we endow our living environment with objects that become an extension of ourselves, our keen awareness of our environment, the way in which we become physically attuned to it and the sensory stimulation that we receive from it are all integral to our ability to endow our physical environment with feelings of attachment and significance.

When looking at the meaning of home, it's important to know that research has found three basic functions of the home environment for the individual: (1) maintenance, (2) stimulation, and (3) support.[4]

Maintenance refers to the process of executing our daily lives in the home environment. Ask yourself, how much attention do you pay each day to activities such as going to the bathroom, bathing, making your breakfast, or brushing your teeth? The answer is probably "not much" because we do these activities on autopilot, and because we do them on autopilot we are free to pursue other challenges and opportunities during the day.

Have you ever wondered why people often return from their vacations exhausted? Could it possibly be that by "living out of your suitcase" and in a new environment (one that may change daily depending on your itinerary) you have lost the maintenance function of your surroundings? Not only are you trying to do your activities of daily living in a new, unfamiliar space, you're eager to take on the new and exciting experiences and challenges that come with your vacation plan.

Let's look at how we often take steps to lessen the impact of living in a new environment and the subsequent loss of the maintenance function of our new, temporary home.

When we arrive in our hotel room or condo, we'll check out the floor plan; look for the ice machine; find the fire exit; locate the gym and the swimming pool; call the front desk to ask about room service or the hours of a complimentary breakfast. Often, we'll ask for recommendations for restaurants and local activities. In the room we'll open closets and drawers; check out the refrigerator and coffee maker; unpack our suitcases, hang up our clothes and move our toiletries into the bathroom. We call this getting settled and comfortable in our new "home."

When moving an older adult to a permanent, not temporary, new home, the process of getting settled and comfortable is even more important. While on vacation, if there's something in our new environment we don't like or find uncomfortable, we know that we're going to leave our temporary home behind and return to the comfortable, consistent, and convenient routines we've established in our permanent home. When seniors relocate, the new must become the permanent—there's no going back.

It is critical that a plan to relocate an older adult address the need to familiarize them with their new community and environment and reestablish the maintenance function of their new home. This allows them to move on to the business of reestablishing their lifestyle through making new friends, finding new activities, and taking on new challenges.

The second function of our home environment is stimulation. Stimulation occurs whenever an individual brings their environment into his or her conscious awareness. When we experience the challenge of decorating, cleaning, rearranging the furniture, or simply dealing with something that's out of place, our environment is stimulating us.[17] For someone moving out of his or her independent living environment and into another independent or assisted living environment there may be an overwhelming amount of stimulation to deal with. On the other hand, for someone who has gone from living in his or her own home to living in a nursing home, the lack of stimulation may be considerable.

Last but not least, is the function of support. The supportive role of your environment refers to the consistency of that environment and how, by virtue of that consistency, you are able to function more easily. After all, when you go to bed at night your bathroom is located at the end of your hallway and when you wake up in the morning you expect it to be where you left it. Imagine its location changing during the night, and you're not sure where to find it when you need to use it? Fortunately we don't have to go in search of our rooms and our furniture with each new day because of its unchanging nature.

By the same token, it's the unchanging nature of our environment that requires greater attention as we age.[17] Our home will not sprout grab bars in the bathroom, additional lighting in the hallways, or level entryways from the street as our need for these changes grows. Nor will we suddenly find ourselves closer to social activities, public transportation, or the grocery store should we lose our ability to drive or our personal mobility declines.

The unchanging nature of our environment may eventually lead to a decline in its supportive role in our lives due to our changing needs, with a relocation to a more supportive environment being the necessary outcome.

In addition to the important functions of maintenance, stimulation, and support that a home plays in our lives, the home is given meaning by the individual in three other critical ways: (1) the sociocultural order or the social-centered process, (2) the life course or the person-centered process, and (3) the body or the body-centered process.[18]

The social-centered process represents the way in which we order our home and interpret rules and behaviors. We develop expectations and standards for the way we live with family and others. When we live in our own home we concern ourselves with our own rules, behaviors, and expectations.

The significance of the social-centered process lies in understanding that for a relocating older adult, leaving the family home and moving into another environment may present a new set of rules, behaviors, and expectations that the older adult may no longer have control over yet be required to conform to. Relocation also then requires the creation of a whole new set of rules, behaviors, and expectations that are required for the new environment.

The person-centered process refers to the way in which our environment reflects our life course and our knowledge of the features within our home. A senior gives meaning to their current environment when it reflects specific events or features of his or her life.[18]

For example, a piano may have been a childhood gift from a family member and may represent a lifetime full of musical accomplishments and experiences for the older adult. To leave that piano behind may represent leaving the significance of its acquisition and its role in the life course of the older person behind as well. In this case, a piano is much more than a large piece of furniture to be disposed of.

The body-centered process refers to the way the older adult physically functions within the home and the ease in which he or she navigates the environment. The familiar placement of light switches, the distance from the sink to the refrigerator, and the arrangement of the furniture are examples of the way in which we adapt to their placement. In addition, research has found that subtle factors such as "space, light, color, visual imagery, activity, rhythm, content, pace, ambiance, and sound"[18] contribute to the body-centered process through sensory stimulation.

When moving an adult to a new environment, be sure to observe, compare, and evaluate the factors of sensory stimulation in the existing environment as well as the new environment under consideration.

■ PUSH TO MOVE

There is a "push-pull" effect in play when older people and their families are considering the possibility of a move in later life.[5] The "push" is usually a crisis or triggering event surrounding the older person, forcing the elder or the family to consider relocating the elder to a more supportive living environment. Examples of push effects are loss of social support, declining health, deferred home maintenance, decreasing finances, and questionable home safety. All of these factors contribute to a lessening ability to maintain an elder's existing level of function or independence in the current environment. It's important to note that by 2040, 21.4% of the US population 65 years of age and older is projected to have limitations in their activities of daily living (ADLs).[19]

A common push to relocate is often related to health challenges from chronic or sudden changes in health status. An example of a health "push" is a decrease in visual acuity. Perhaps the older person's vision declines to the point that he or she can no longer prepare meals safely. In this case, if other nutrition options are not readily available, relocation may be the ultimate outcome. Another health push arises when the lack of fit between the older adult and his or her environment begins to limit independence. A fall is a classic example of a triggering event that may force a relocation. A broken hip or the fear of negotiating steps will often lead seniors to living environments that are friendlier and more compatible with their new physical limitations. Stairs, the lack of a bathroom on the main floor, or multiple steps from the street to the entry can suddenly turn the family home into an environment of concern. Home modification has emerged as a vital resource to enable children, adults, and older adults who have mobility problems to remain in their homes.[6] Without such modifications, these individuals face the difficult choice of moving to a facility or remaining in unsafe, unsupportive environments, which do not facilitate independence or an active and participatory lifestyle.[7]

Both declining vision and limited mobility are health exigencies that may prompt thoughts of moving. The desire to feel safe and the ability to navigate the environment safely often play critical roles in the decision to leave the current home.

Another circumstance that pushes toward the need to move is the loss of social supports. Social support can be as simple as a neighbor making a daily reassurance phone call or picking up an occasional prescription at the pharmacy or as complicated as a network of formal and informal caregivers providing transportation, meal preparation, home maintenance, and social opportunities to an older adult. A spouse dying and close friends or relatives moving away are common events that result in loss of social support. The rug can be pulled out from under an older person who is depending on a friend for companionship or transportation if that person dies or moves away. Not only does the older person lose a friend, but the loss of a primary source of transportation may in turn limit present and future social opportunities, access to medical care, and the ability to shop for food, clothing, and other necessities, all of which are integral to aging in place.

Declining physical safety due to the declining physical condition of the home often creates an urgency to move. Home safety concerns and deferred home maintenance often share a symbiotic relationship. Loose stair railings, leaky roofs, old furnaces, and seeping gas appliances all result from deferred home maintenance and create an unsafe living environment. If the older adult lacks the ability to access qualified home maintenance and repair services, the push to move will surface once again, and a change in living environment may be considered. Decrements in vision and hearing, a lack of a strong support network, or financial limitations can make the ability to identify and contract with reputable home repair services nearly impossible. When the home environment is deemed no longer able to support the needs of the older adult, relocation may ensue.

This calls into question the availability of sufficient financial resources to pay for much-needed assistance in the face of declining health or support networks. Aside from structural changes to the home, an older person's lack of ambulation or ability to execute ADLs or instrumental ADLs (IADLs) may require paid caregivers. If the older person has insufficient financial resources to afford care or modify the house, this financial crisis may push an older person to consider moving.

To summarize, social support, health and functional abilities, home environment, safety, and finances are all factors affecting the degree of push an older adult or an elder's family may experience leading to the need for late-life relocation.

■ PULL TO MOVE

There is also a "pull" to move. The pull is usually not prompted by a crisis or decline but by the anticipation of an enhanced lifestyle in retirement resulting from the availability of desired social, recreational, or health opportunities. When the move occurs early in late adulthood, coinciding with retirement, it is called the "amenity move."[5] This move occurs when relocation offers an improved lifestyle or home environment for the older adult. Whether it's the pull of the vacation-style retirement community, warm weather, or reduced house payments, the amenity move pulls the older adult out of his or her existing home and into a new environment. An example of this is a 65-year-old Wyoming native who wants nicer winter weather or year-round, warm-weather recreational opportunities that a city such as Phoenix, Arizona has to offer.

Beyond the amenity move, another type of relocation is called the "kinship or assistance move."[5,8] This move is precipitated by the desire to live closer to family or to services to meet present or future needs. It may be similar to the situation of the elderly Stanford University alumnus who discovers the newly built senior living community adjacent to the university on the Stanford campus. By selecting this senior housing option, this elder can access the medical expertise of a world-respected hospital, enjoy the stimulating academic environment of his alma mater, and return to a setting with familiar, pleasant memories.

Another comparable example is the pull for an older person who anticipates gradual disability in aging and thus moves into a long-term care community that offers three levels of support. These three levels include (1) independent living in a private apartment, (2) assisted living, where help with many ADLs and IADLs is available, and (3) skilled nursing, where, in addition to assistance with ADLs and IADLs, the older adult receives care for any health condition that requires skilled nursing care.

Family is often a pull factor for older adults. A senior may want to move closer to family for two fundamental reasons: (1) to be near children and grandchildren, and (2) in anticipation of future disability coupled with an increased sense of vulnerability. This sense of vulnerability creates a desire to be near adult children for hands-on as well as psychological support.

■ FAMILIES MAKE THE DECISION TO MOVE THE ELDERLY PERSON

When a geriatric care manager (GCM) works with an older person, it is important for the GCM to remember that most times the client entity is twofold, consisting of both the older person and the family. The family may be fragmented, dysfunctional, long distance, or around the corner; however, families and the older person usually make the decision to move together, unless totally estranged from each other or the elder is conserved.

Family is involved in the decision to relocate because the triggering event has, to a greater degree than previously experienced, drawn them into the support system of the older adult. The trigger to begin a move might be prompted by the failure of a planned support system that has kept the older person at home. This may mean that Meals on Wheels was ordered, but the older person does not like the food and is no longer eating well. If the only other perceived choice for providing support to the older adult requires home care or the adult child bringing food by, this choice may tip the balance and prompt the family to consider placement.

If caregiving for the older person has increased to a level no longer able to be met by the formal and informal support systems, relocation may be considered. For example, consider the family member who cannot cope with the need to change his incontinent mother's diapers and the only other option available is hiring paid care to cover this caregiving task. If the paid care is too expensive, placement may be the only alternative.

Another family-related trigger for placement is the lack of consistent, stable services. When the elderly parent needs increased home care and dependable paid caregivers cannot be found, the family may be left feeling heavily burdened and over the edge. Finally, there is another circumstance that results in the family's decision to relocate the older person: caregiver burnout. Making care arrangements, flying long distances on a regular basis to supervise care, covering shifts if they live nearby, and receiving call after call at night are all experiences that may lead directly to caregiver burnout. Like a proverbial sandwich, the family members are situated between meeting their personal and family needs and attending to the care needs of their elderly parents. (See Chapter 9 on caregiving, and Chapter 20 on the normal aging family.)

■ WHEN A GCM PREVENTS A MOVE

In many cases, good geriatric care management can prevent a move. However, it may require the availability of alternative solutions to a variety of challenges, including meal preparation, home care, and ADL deficits. For example, if Meals on Wheels is rejected by the older adult who cannot prepare his or her own meals, you as the GCM might make arrangements for the older person to go to a senior center for a nutritious hot lunch each day. Additionally, if the older person is capable, you could ask a family member or a neighbor to buy a microwave and healthy microwaveable meals so the older person could prepare meals at home.

If the senior requires home care staffing and the paid caregiver staffing is not stable, you could find a new staffing agency. If the older person is incontinent and an adult day care health center is available, the older person might be placed there during the day and additional care can be arranged for nighttime.

Accommodations like these may tip the balance toward keeping the person at home because you make new arrangements and take away the burden of sorting through the vast continuum of care from the burned-out adult child.

It is important to remember, however, that in the event an alternative plan of care is not enough, and either (1) the person is ready to move or (2) the family's needs cannot be filled by a GCM, then a move must be considered. Evaluating the physical environment in combination with an understanding of the client's ability to perform the ADLs enables you to understand the level of care the client needs. This is the basis for recommending when a client should consider a move to another setting. (See Chapter 5, Care Planning and Geriatric Assessment.)

■ THE GCM's ROLE IN MAKING A MOVE

If you as a GCM want to add moving to your product list of services, it is important to plan ahead and develop a database of moving resources in your community. The database could include the names of moving companies, professional organizers, lists of all good antique dealers, second-hand furniture stores, estate sale and consignment companies, as well as charities that accept donated items. Remember, a successful move consists of the completion of a series of multiple steps prior to the move, and you will need resources for all of them.

An additional resource for you is the National Association of Senior Move Managers. This service provider can be of assistance with the physical task of relocation. Senior move managers offer a range of services that may include organizing, downsizing, and planning as well as packing, floor plan design, coordination of estate and consignment sales, unpacking, and setting up the new residence. For a complete list of services and senior move managers in your area, visit the association's website at www.nasmm.com.

Your role before, during, and after the move of an older adult is multifaceted. Not only might you provide move management services as well as postmove support and advocacy, but you might also assist the family and the older person through any difficulty or crisis that occurs before the move.

You are there to assess the needs of the older person and the family, to determine to what level of care the client should move in relationship to the budget, and to develop a clear understanding of the specific needs or wants of the relocating older person. You will also provide opportunities to enhance perceived control by the client as well as ensure, as much as possible, that perceived expectations for the move match the reality of the outcome. Examples of activities that support perceived control are (1) allowing the client to select which personal items he or she will take to the new living environment, and (2) encouraging him or her to participate as much as possible in the selection of that new environment. In addition, choices in food selection, social activities, and clothing for the day enhance perceived control. You can also guide

the client and family in the establishment of expectations equal to the reality of the new environment. Arranging for the client to make premove visits to the new living environment to meet staff and fellow residents, to sample the meals, and to familiarize him- or herself with the physical property can help achieve this goal. If a client is unable to visit his or her new residence beforehand, showing the person pictures of the administrative staff, the grounds, and common rooms, as well as of the apartments or rooms, can be helpful.

You can use assessment results to help the family find the level of care the older adult requires. Once the level of care is determined and a residence is selected, you can then actually assist with the many components of the physical move: packing, storing, mailing, and helping the elder and the family decide what furniture and personal belongings to bring. Also, you should be prepared to help the older person, and sometimes the family, mourn the loss of the family home. Once moving day arrives, either the family can actually move the older person or you can make all the transportation arrangements for the transition. Finally, you can help the older person adjust to the move, monitor the transition for the family, and help the family and the older person adjust to the new setting and loss of their old nest.

■ ASSESSING AN ELDER TO FIND THE RIGHT LEVEL AND PLACE TO MOVE

Although the elder and family may decide to move, often they need assistance in determining to which level of care to move and finding that level of care within their budget and that meets their preferences. Your first task in transitioning an older adult is to determine the level of care and appropriate living environment the client requires.

For example, Ms. Greenberg might ask you to arrange a move for her mom, Mrs. Jacobson, who is presently in an assisted living facility in Miami. The daughter wants her mother to move to an assisted living facility or an appropriate level of care in Philadelphia. The daughter wants her mother to be nearer to her home in Philadelphia because she needs to provide increased care and is burnt out from making constant trips to Miami. The daughter is currently juggling a full-time job and the responsibility of relocating her mother. She may need to outsource this process to you, a GCM, because of her limited time, her lack of comfort in selecting the level of care her mother requires, and her feeling that you, the GCM, are the expert in such matters.

The Moving Assessment Tool (Exhibit 7–1) can assist you in assessing not only the basic needs of the older person facing relocation, but the needs of his or her family as well.

The Moving Assessment Tool provides the means to determine the needs and preferences of the client and the family for important factors, including time frame, geographic location, budget, and level of care. The first area addressed is the timetable: when does the family want the move to occur? The second area addressed is geographic—where do they want the older person to move? If it is within a city, how far do they want the older person away from critical contacts, such as family? In the earlier example, if Mrs. Jacobson is to move to the Philadelphia area, how far from her daughter's home does her daughter want Mrs. Jacobson's new residence to be? Is public transportation nearby? What about stores and medical services? The next assessment area addressed is the budget. The family or older person will usually have a range within which they can afford to rent or buy. This is critical to planning a move. Additionally, if the older adult is restricted to low-income housing or skilled nursing that accepts Medicaid, you need to determine the availability of those options in the city or county to which he or she is moving.

The next step prior to moving the client is to determine the required level of care. GCMs can use psychosocial assessment and func-

tional assessment tools to evaluate the older client's ability to perform ADLs and IADLs in relationship to the person's present physical environment (see Chapter 3, Psychosocial Assessment, and Chapter 4, Functional Assessment). This enables you to establish a baseline for the level of care. Evaluating the older person's present physical environment in combination with an understanding of the client's ability to perform the ADLs enables the care manager to understand the level of care the client needs. From this baseline, you can determine which living environment options offer the required level of care. These assessments should be done with each client, in all cases, for each move. It may be more costly to the client to pay for the geriatric care management assessments, but there is no sense in spending unnecessary time and money finding a skilled nursing facility (SNF) when all the person really needs is an assisted living facility.

Once the required level of care is determined, you can assess the specific housing needs and preferences of the older person and/or the family and correlate that to the budget constraints. Once you have completed your initial moving assessment and psychosocial and functional assessments, you should be able to identify, based on your assessment results, what level of care your client requires in a living environment. The moving assessment enables you to determine geographic preferences and budget constraints. The intersections of these assessments enable you to narrow your housing choices for the client. If, after you have completed your assessments, you have an older person who functionally and psychosocially must (1) reside in an assisted living facility, (2) in Philadelphia, (3) within the $5,000-dollar-a-month range, and the facility must (4) be within 20 minutes of the daughter's home, (5) provide weekly transportation to temple services and physicians' offices, (6) observe holidays, (7) offer a Kosher diet, and (8) allow pets, then your choices are narrowed for the search.

Exhibit 7–1   Moving Assessment Tool

Date _____

Completed by: _____

Client Name _____

Address _____

City _____ State _____ Zip _____

Time Frame: _____ Week(s) / Month(s) (circle one)

Actual Moving Date: _____

GEOGRAPHIC LOCATION:

1st Choice: City _____ County _____ State _____

2nd Choice: City _____ County _____ State _____

3rd Choice: City _____ County _____ State _____

FINANCES

Monthly Housing Budget: $_____

Revenue Sources

❑ Medicare   ❑ MediCal   ❑ Pension   ❑ Social Security   ❑ Retirement Income

Notes: _____

_____

REQUIRED LIVING ENVIRONMENT:

Independent

❑ Gated Active Adult Community   ❑ Senior Independent   ❑ CCRC   ❑ Life Care

❑ Apartment (Senior)   ❑ Apartment (Community at Large)   ❑ With Family

❑ Townhouse / Condo / Duet   ❑ Purchase   ❑ Lease/Rental

❑ Detached Single Family Home   ❑ Purchase   ❑ Lease/Rental

Comments: _____

_____

_____

_____

Assisted Living

❑ Dementia Care

❑ Assisted Living Facility   ❑ Residential Board and Care   ❑ Foster Home

Comments: _____

_____

Skilled Nursing

Medical Spend-Down Accepted   ❑ Yes   ❑ No   _____ Projected Date

❑ Rehabilitation   ❑ Long Term   ❑ Dementia Care   ❑ Medicaid/MediCal Beds
❑ Feeding Services

Comments: _____

_____

_____ *continues*

Exhibit 7–1   Moving Assessment Tool (continued)

PROXIMITY TO:

Family
- ❑ Walking ❑ Driving ❑ Home ❑ Work
- ❑ 5–20 min ❑ 30 min ❑ 1 hour ❑ 2 hours

Notes: _____

Grocery and Drugstore
- ❑ Walking ❑ Driving ❑ Home ❑ Work
- ❑ 5–20 min ❑ 30 min ❑ 1 hour ❑ 2 hours

Shopping, Restaurants, and Entertainment
- ❑ Walking ❑ Driving ❑ Home ❑ Work
- ❑ 5–20 min ❑ 30 min ❑ 1 hour ❑ 2 hours

Church
- ❑ Walking ❑ Driving ❑ Home ❑ Work
- ❑ 5–20 min ❑ 30 min ❑ 1 hour ❑ 2 hours

Senior Center
- ❑ Walking ❑ Driving ❑ Home ❑ Work
- ❑ 5–20 min ❑ 30 min ❑ 1 hour ❑ 2 hours

Doctors' Offices
- ❑ Walking ❑ Driving ❑ Home ❑ Work
- ❑ 5–20 min ❑ 30 min ❑ 1 hour ❑ 2 hours

Hospital
- ❑ Walking ❑ Driving ❑ Home ❑ Work
- ❑ 5–20 min ❑ 30 min ❑ 1 hour ❑ 2 hours

Alternate/Public Transportation:
- ❑ 1 block ❑ 2 blocks ❑ 3–6 blocks ❑ Door to Door

SPECIFIC NEEDS
- ❑ Transportation ❑ Religious Services ❑ Pets ❑ Music ❑ Crafts
- ❑ Entertainment ❑ Special Events ❑ Holiday Observations
- ❑ Guest Visits (overnight) ❑ Private Dining Room

Diet and Nutrition
- ❑ Diabetic ❑ Low Cholesterol ❑ Low Sodium ❑ Vegetarian
- ❑ Kosher ❑ Halaal ❑ Other ❑ Food Allergies

Notes: _____

ADDITIONAL SERVICES: PRE-MOVE
- ❑ Medical ❑ Legal ❑ CPA ❑ Real Estate ❑ Interior Design
- ❑ Professional Organizer ❑ Estate/Consignment Sales ❑ Move Management

Other: _____

ADDITIONAL SERVICES: POST-MOVE
- ❑ GCM ❑ Medical ❑ Legal ❑ CPA ❑ Real Estate
- ❑ Interior Design ❑ Orientation ❑ Move Management (unpacking and setup)

Other: _____

■ ADDITIONAL CONSIDERATIONS: HOUSING NEEDS AND PREFERENCES

If the client is moving to an apartment by himself or herself, what amenities does the person want in that apartment? How large, how small? Does the person require privacy? A view? What will the budget allow? Is the person eligible for moderate or low-cost senior housing? Is there a waiting list for these apartments? Does the community have an on-site services coordinator? If the senior is going to rent a market rate apartment or senior housing, you can contact the Area Agency on Aging (AAA) in the county or the local senior center for a list of senior housing and apartments for review.

You also need to assess transportation, terrain, and social services requirements. Does the client need to be in close proximity to accessible public transportation? What about the distance to stores and medical services? Is there a grocery store or drugstore close by? What about terrain? Is the housing choice on a hill or on flat land? What is the policy and procedure for maintenance repair? How quickly does the management respond to requests for repairs? Are smoke detectors and carbon monoxide detectors installed? If not, can the person have them installed?

What about social amenities? Should you find an apartment that allows pets because the client's dog is a treasured companion? Should the apartment be near the religious or spiritual services practiced by the older person? Religious involvement is a way to engage the older person in a new community if the person includes that practice in the lifestyle. Does the person like to play bingo, mahjong, or bridge? If so, a new assisted living or senior housing facility should have those activities. If not, could you find a senior center nearby that offers them? No matter our age, we all desire to recreate our lifestyle in our new living environment.

■ EVALUATING SENIOR HOUSING, CONGREGATE HOUSING, SHARED HOUSING, AND CONTINUING CARE RETIREMENT COMMUNITIES

When you consider alternative living environments, you will find there are many types of senior living environments and many levels of care below an SNF from which to choose. One idea to keep in mind is that not all older adults want to be among seniors, so the community-at-large housing market can also be considered. All choices in your community should be reflected in your database and be updated constantly. You can get this information from your AAA, information and referral services in your community, or Elder Locator. You can also use a real estate agent with a Senior Real Estate Specialist designation to locate properties for the older person to rent, lease, or purchase in the community of choice.

Senior Housing

The Housing for Older Adults Act of 1995 describes senior housing as follows:

> Dwelling specifically designed for and occupied by elderly; or is occupied solely by persons who are 62 or older; or houses at least one person who is 55 or older in at least 80 percent of the occupied units, and adheres to a policy that demonstrates intent to house persons who are 55 or older. Therefore, housing that satisfies the legal definition of senior housing or housing for older persons described above can legally exclude families with children.[9]

To find a variety of descriptions for the various senior housing options from which you and your client can select, do a Web search using the keywords types of senior housing. Helpguide, a resource created by the Rotary Club and the Center for Healthy Aging in Santa Monica, California, can be found at www.helpguide.org/elder/senior_housing_residential_care_types.htm and offers consumer information as well as the following in-depth descriptions of senior housing:

- **Independent living for seniors:** A retirement community of peers, for healthy seniors who are self-sufficient and want the freedom and privacy of their own separate, easy-to-maintain apartment or house, along with the security, comfort, and social activities of a senior community.

- **Assisted living facilities for seniors:** Assisted living facilities for seniors: For people who do not have severe medical problems but who need help with personal care such as bathing, dressing, grooming, and eating. There is a great deal of variety both in the types of housing and the range of services provided, and not much government regulation at this time.

- **Board and care homes for seniors:** Board and care homes for seniors: A residence for people who need minimal help with personal care such as bathing, dressing, grooming, and eating, but who need or want communal meals and easy access to social contact with peers. Facilities are licensed by the state and may specialize in care for seniors, psychiatric patients, or those with Alzheimer's disease.

- **Nursing homes (SNFs):** Nursing homes (SNFs): Facilities with 24-hour medical care available, including short-term rehabilitation (physical therapy) as well as long-term care for people with chronic ailments or disabilities that require daily attention of registered nurses in addition to help with personal care such as bathing or dressing or getting around.

- **Congregate housing for seniors:** Congregate housing for seniors: Previously considered a unique combination of private living quarters combined with shared activities, including communal meals and other social activities, but now considered a type of assisted living.

- **Continuing-care retirement communities (CCRCs):** Continuing-care retirement communities (CCRCs): A complex of residences that include independent living, assisted living, and nursing home care, so seniors can stay in the same general location as their housing needs change over time, beginning when they are still healthy and active.[10]

Additional information regarding the variety of assisted living options for seniors can be found on the Assisted Living Federation of America website at www.alfa.org/files/public/ ALFAchecklist.pdf.

In addition to the previously mentioned living environments, two others should be included: life care facilities and active adult communities:

1. **Life care facilities:** The Episcopal Homes Foundation website describes life care as the following: "Life care is an arrangement by which persons pay an initial accommodation fee and monthly maintenance fees in exchange for living accommodations and services. All levels of care are provided, including acute care, physicians' and surgeons' services, skilled nursing care, and personal care on premises of the retirement community, with no change in fees based on level of care."[11] Other life care facilities may vary their services included or their financial arrangements.

2. **Active adult or planned adult communities:** Planned adult, active adult, and gated golfing communities for active adults over the age of 55 offer homes for purchase as well as a variety of social and athletic activities for residents. Golf courses, tennis courts, swimming pools, theaters, special interest groups and clubs, social events, and travel opportunities create a vacation environment for the over-55 adult who selects this type of housing. Monthly homeowner fees may cover maintenance and/or housekeeping services. Meals are usually not included.[12]

When conducting evaluations of various living environments, you are making evaluations of the same factors you would rate in an SNF: overall environment, health and safety features, resident environment and comfort, food service (if applicable), staff, and programming. AARP provides a checklist for evaluating an assisted living facility on its website at www.aarp.org/families/housing_choices/assisted_living/a2004-02-27-assistedlivingchecklist.html.

For additional checklists to assist you in the evaluation of all types of senior housing, you can access the resources available at www.helpguide.org/elder/senior_housing_residential_care_types.htm.

■ LIVING IN THE COMMUNITY AT LARGE

If the senior is buying a condo or townhouse, it is important he or she is connected with an appropriate real estate services provider. There are now real estate agents called Senior Real Estate Specialists (SRES) (see www.seniorrealestate.com).

Real estate agents are able to acquire an SRES designation by enrolling in a course provided by the Senior Advantage Real Estate Council (SAREC). To view the requirements for the SRES designation, visit www.seniorsrealestate. com/sarec/servlet/perspective/requirements.

Make sure you interview the real estate agent in depth before referring the client or the client's family to this person. The real estate agent used by a GCM should be someone who has experience with seniors, is a good listener, has a genuine concern for the senior's welfare, is patient with the needs of the GCM and the senior, and is available to see a senior through the stressful process of selling or buying a home.

Additionally, the real estate agent should have a history of executing contracts diligently and completing all paperwork in a timely and orderly fashion. His or her license should be in good standing and free of any disciplinary action by the state department of real estate or local board of real estate agents. The SRES designation is a good place to start in the process of finding a real estate agent for a client; it is one of several criteria that should be used when selecting a real estate agent to work with the client or client's family. Because relocation is a process, not an event, the people involved determine how smoothly the process takes place.

If the senior is downsizing and renting a home, townhouse, or condo in the new community, many real estate agents manage and lease properties for homeowners and could act as a resource for finding available housing. However, a home or apartment that is leased requires a signed contract. Any contract that's required to live in any housing choice, whether in the community at large or in a senior living community such as a CCRC, life care community, senior independent facility, assisted living, board and care, or SNF, should be reviewed by a family member and an attorney before it is signed. Housing available in the community at large on a month-to-month rental basis is another option to explore.

■ RELOCATING TO A SKILLED NURSING FACILITY

When relocating an older person to an SNF, you must evaluate many of the same living requirements you looked at for independent apartment living and assisted living. In terms of finances and budget, it is important to anticipate the need for Medicaid assistance. A critical budget question is this: Is Medicaid a factor now or in the future if a spend-down, spending an elder's financial assets down to the Medicaid level, is anticipated? If Medicaid is not a factor now but could be in the future, it is important to know if the SNF has Medicaid beds for Medicaid-eligible residents. Verifying eligible Medicaid beds today could prevent an involuntary move of the client tomorrow.

As in other living environments, services and amenities play an important role. If the client is at an SNF level, do religious services need to be on site? Does the person need special services for feeding, bathing, and toileting? Does the person desire animal therapy services? Does the facility need to be within driving distance or public transportation reach of family? Is bingo a must for this particular client? All these needs and preferences must be determined through your assessment before the move is planned.

■ CREATING AN IDEAL MODEL

After you have done the psychosocial assessment and the moving assessment, develop for the client an ideal model of the ideal residence where the senior will move. This model should include the following information:

1. Level of care
2. Budget
3. Geographic area
4. Specific services or amenities that must be available (e.g., a Catholic mass, pets allowed, near enough for the wife to visit, and a great view)

Following are a few examples of ideal plans.

CASE STUDY

Example 1: Mr. Remer
Mr. Remer ideally will be moved to an SNF in St. Joseph, Missouri, within a mile of his daughter Katherine, within a budget range of $3,000–$4,000 a month, where the facility allows spend-down to Medicaid eligibility. The facility will ideally allow pets (he would like to bring his 15-year-old dog), will have Lutheran services or general religious programs, and will have a recreation program that offers art therapy because he was a commercial artist when he worked.

The preceding describes Mr. Remer's ideal model, and your job is to find the living environment that approximates this ideal to as great a degree as possible.

CASE STUDY

Example 2: Mrs. Murphy's Father
Mrs. Murphy has a father in Kansas City and wants you, a GCM in Los Angeles, California, to find a placement for her dad in the Redondo Beach, California, area, where Mrs. Murphy lives. You contact a GCM in Kansas City and arrange for him to do the psychosocial and functional assessments and the moving assessment. You then, through phone conversations and e-mail, determine with the family members (1) the budget, (2) kind of space that would work best (Mrs. Murphy requests a view of the ocean and a single room), and (3) the kinds of services that must be in place. Next, you develop a model from that information and then find an appropriate facility using the model as your guide.

■ NARROWING DOWN SENIOR HOUSING TO PREVIEW

The selection of the type of senior housing the older person will move to should be made by the family and the older person based on (1) the results of your psychosocial and functional assessment, (2) your premove assessment, (3) their preferences, (4) budget, and (5) housing availability in the community. Other factors to include when selecting a living environment that offers services below the level of skilled nursing are (1) the size of the facility that would work best for the older person, (2) apartment size (small and cozy, or large and spacious), (3) privacy, (4) physical floor plan, and (5) amenities (does the person want to cook and need a kitchen?).

After the client and family have selected the level of care and type of senior housing, you should review the client profile and narrow down the choices to 10 possibilities or fewer. If the community offers few choices, you might not need to narrow down the list and might need to call all facilities that fit the profile on paper. For example, finding an assisted living facility with an ocean view in the Redondo Beach, California, area may be difficult. Therefore, it is imperative that the facility be evaluated by more than an "on-paper profile" to ensure the best environment with the finest fit for the client is selected.

Once you have made evaluation phone calls to each potential housing option and have confirmed the specific features that match the ideal profile, the family and older adult are brought into the process once again. They may be given the list of properties to visit on their own, or they may prefer that you visit and evaluate the choices with them or by yourself and report back to them. Because you are working for the client, remember to visit only properties that match your client's profile. If further research of other properties is required, you must secure permission to do research beforehand.

■ RESOURCES FOR RESEARCHING SENIOR LIVING: ASSISTED LIVING AND SKILLED NURSING FACILITIES

If the client and family have hired you to search for that ideal living environment for the elder person, numerous state and local governing bodies and resources can help you in your search.

If you are searching for an SNF, contact the local Area Agency on Aging (AAA) for a listing of all senior housing, a list of licensed facilities in the appropriate city, and licensing regulations in the corresponding state. Your state's licensing body is also a valuable resource and should be able to provide a list of facilities and information on specific facilities such as any

citations, the number of beds, as well as information on the availability of special units such as an Alzheimer's unit. To find the appropriate agency in your state, access the website of your state's department on aging.

For California, the California Advocates for Nursing Home Reform (CANHR) can provide valuable information. Otherwise, ask the local AAA if a group such as CANHR exists in the geographic area you are searching.

You can contact the Long-Term Care Ombudsman for help in choosing facilities as well. Beyond a list of facilities and whether they accept Medicaid, determine the number of citations each facility has received, which is a critical piece of information as well. You must recommend a facility with the fewest, preferably zero, citations; this is critical to giving weight to the best and safest facilities.

Once you have assembled this information in your database, it is essential that you update it regularly because the information is constantly changing. As the expert, you must know the continuum of care in your community to help you stay abreast of this information. For example, some facilities go out of business or change their acceptance criteria, and citations can happen at any time.

Once you have contacted all the housing resources and created your skilled nursing or assisted living list, narrow down the list of potentially ideal facilities to only facilities with minimal, preferably zero, citations. It is important to remember that quality of care and safety in an SNF or assisted living facility are the highest priority factors you are evaluating for. If the ideal model is not available with zero or minimal citations, consult the ombudsman for other suggestions. You may have to alter your model rather than recommend an unsafe facility.

If you are searching for senior apartment complexes or homes to buy, narrow down your list to only the complexes or the homes that match the ideal model (say, the ones with an ocean view, tennis courts, and bingo). You

should also add to your database of relocation information the contact information for
202 Housing (i.e., government-subsidized
housing for the elderly in your community). If
the older person's budget requires a housing
subsidy, and the person's level of care is
appropriate for an apartment in your ideal
model, you should readily be able to identify
the appropriate site.

After you have established your pared-
down priority list, you can, with the client's
approval, accompany the client to preview
these properties or preview them on the
client's behalf.

■ VISITING AND EVALUATING YOUR LIST OF SKILLED NURSING FACILITIES

The next step is to physically evaluate the facilities on your list by making a site visit. This, of
course, must be done with the client's or family's permission. The family may want to do
this themselves to cut costs. But if they wish
you to do the job, then you can use the Facility
Evaluation form shown in Exhibit 7–2.

Because there are so many factors to weigh
when selecting an SNF, it is recommended
that you review and incorporate where appropriate these additional supplementary facility
evaluations, which can be found online at the
following websites:

> www.medicare.gov/Nursing/Checklist.pdf
> www.carepathways.com/checklist-nh.cfm
> nursinghomeguide.org/pub/
>   eval_checklist.pdf

You should have already determined the
basic fees of each SNF and are visiting only
those in the client's budget range.

Next, make an on-site visit to the facilities
that fit the client's profile. Make an appointment on a busy day at the facility; ask to go to
lunch and for a meeting with the activity
director. Request to meet with the facility
director, not a subordinate staff member.

Prior to entering the facility, survey the surrounding neighborhood, the condition of the
street and surrounding buildings, and note
whether the building is in good repair.

When entering the front door, your initial
screening tools are sensory: how the facility
feels, smells, and tastes are things you cannot
evaluate on the phone or from a list. When
you walk into the facility, how does it feel?
Does it feel welcoming, like a pleasant new
home for your client? Use your intuition
here—the same intuition you would use for
yourself if you were picking a new apartment
or buying a home. On all facility evaluation
checklists there is a general environment
question; this is where you put your answer to
the question "How does it feel?"

Next, use your sense of smell. Most graphically, do you smell urine? What do you smell
in the facility—urine, strong disinfectant, lack
of cleanliness? Any GCM who has worked
with disadvantaged clients knows this smell.
Again, use your intuition, and use the same
guide that would assist you in choosing your
own new home.

Is the temperature comfortable? What's the
noise level? Peek in the corners. Go down hallways—are they free of clutter, and is the lighting good? Look up and see if there are smoke
detectors and sprinklers. Enter bathrooms—
are they clean and uncluttered? Check out the
toilet seats. Is the bathroom safety-adapted?
Walk through the dining room and check out
the kitchen. Note what the general condition
of all these areas is and evaluate what the
facility feels like, smells like, and looks like.
Try thinking "Would my mother like this?"

Next, use your sense of taste. Have lunch in
the dining room. Does the food smell and
look palatable? Does it taste good? Is the environment in the dining room relaxing, and
does it encourage residents to relax and enjoy
their food? Are residents rushed through
their meal? Are residents given some dietary
control by being offered a choice of foods on
the menu? If residents need help with eating

Exhibit 7–2   Facility Evaluation

Evaluator: _____   Date: _____

General Information:

Name of Facility: _____

Address: _____

Phone #: _____

FAX: _____

E-mail: _____

Facility type: ❑ Profit ❑ Nonprofit ❑ Private ❑ Government
                     ❑ Religious Affiliate ❑ Other: _____

Contact Information (Include Position, Phone #, Fax, E-mail):

Name: _____ Administrator / License # _____

Name: _____ Director of Nursing _____

Name: _____ Social Worker _____

_____

_____

Fees:

Basic Fees:
   Single Room _____
   Double _____
   Triple _____

Deposit: _____

Included in Fees:
   Medications: ❑ Yes   ❑ No
   Telephone: ❑ Yes   ❑ No   If no, how much? _____
   Cable TV: ❑ Yes   ❑ No   If no, how much? _____
   Laundry: ❑ Yes   ❑ No   If no, how much? _____

Other Amenities: _____

Immediate Availability: ❑ Yes   ❑ No

Payment:

Medicare: ❑ Yes   ❑ No
Medi-Cal: ❑ Yes   ❑ No
Long-term Care Insurance: ❑ Yes   ❑ No   If yes, will facility bill LTC insurance
                                              company directly? ❑ Yes   ❑ No

Other: _____

Recreational and Social Activities:

Daily Recreational Activities: _____

Weekly Recreational Activities: _____

Seasonal / Holiday
   Recreational Activities: _____   *continues*

Exhibit 7–2   Facility Evaluation (continued)

Religious Services and
   Chaplain Visits: ❑ Yes ❑ No
     If yes, denomination: _____
       Describe services: _____
     If no, is transportation available to and from
       religious services?   ❑ Yes ❑ No

Other social support: _____

Addressing Grievances:

Resident Council: ❑ Yes ❑ No
Family Council: ❑ Yes ❑ No

Other formal / informal avenues
   to address complaints: _____

Number of citations: _____

Type of citations: _____

Medical and Other Health-Related Services:

Availability of:
   Dementia Care: ❑ Yes ❑ No   If yes, describe service(s): _____
   Dental Services: ❑ Yes ❑ No   If yes, describe service(s): _____
   Optometry/Ophthalmology: ❑ Yes ❑ No   If yes, describe service(s): _____
   Podiatry: ❑ Yes ❑ No   If yes, describe service(s): _____
   Respiratory Therapy: ❑ Yes ❑ No   If yes, describe service(s): _____
   Physical Therapy: ❑ Yes ❑ No   If yes, describe service(s): _____
   Occupational Therapy: ❑ Yes ❑ No   If yes, describe service(s): _____
   Speech Therapy: ❑ Yes ❑ No   If yes, describe service(s): _____

Closest Hospital: _____

Other Hospitals: _____

Specialty Clinics: _____

Transportation:

Medical appointments: ❑ Yes ❑ No   Describe service(s): _____

Social and recreational activities: ❑ Yes ❑ No   Describe service(s): _____

Capacity:

Total # of beds: _____
# of private beds: _____
# of semiprivate beds: _____
# of triple beds: _____
# of current residents: _____

Staffing Ratios:

Shift 1   Shift structure: _____   Ratio: _____
Shift 2   Shift structure: _____   Ratio: _____
Shift 3   Shift structure: _____   Ratio: _____

Private care allowed?   ❑ Yes ❑ No

Exhibit 7–2   Facility Evaluation (continued)

Private care encouraged?	❑ Yes ❑ No
Type of Staff:	
In-house:	❑ Yes ❑ No
Registry:	❑ Yes ❑ No
Staff interaction with residents (describe):	_____
Is there enough staff to feed the residents?	❑ Yes ❑ No

General Environment:

Presentation: _____

Common Areas: _____

Odors: _____

Hallways: _____

Doors: _____

Bathrooms: _____

Window(s) / Doors to the outside: _____

Access to outside: _____

Dining Rooms: _____

   Feeding tables?   ❑ Yes   ❑ No

Other Considerations:

Types of residents accepted: _____

Types of residents not considered: _____

Alternative diets: ❑ Yes   ❑ No

Visitation Policy: _____

Evaluator's signature: _____

how is this help offered? Can the facility provide special health-compliant diets?

Go into a resident's room similar to the one the elder you represent will use. Look at the condition of the doorknobs and the phone. Does the resident's room have personal furniture? Are the doors marked with memory boxes or do they display the resident's name and picture? Are there water glasses and pitchers in the rooms?

Visit the recreational areas and talk to the activity director. What are the activity choices, by day, week, and season? Does the facility observe rituals such as birthdays, holidays, and culturally appropriate events? Is art or music therapy available? How often? Does the facility offer religious services or chaplain visits?

Go to the public areas. Is the furniture comfortable and nice looking? Look at the residents. Are they clean and well dressed? Try to talk to three residents or visiting family members. Ask how residents like living here. Ask important questions such as: Do staff members respond when you need help? What is the best thing about living here?

Observe the staff interaction with the residents. Do they seem to enjoy their exchanges with residents? Are they attentive to residents' needs? Are they friendly?

Finally, meet with the facility director. Ask these questions: What is the waiting period for admission? Is the administrator licensed? Is there a deposit, and what is included in the fee (medications, telephone, cable, laundry)? Does the facility do background checks on staff? What is the ratio of staff to patients? Remember, the lower the resident-to-staff ratio, the better. What is staff turnover? What is staff training? Are snacks available during the day and evening? What is the facility's emergency plan? Can you see it? Remember the horrible events in SNFs in New Orleans, post Katrina in 2006. (See Chapter 19, Preparing for Emergencies.)

Are citations posted? Try to bring the last inspection results with you. Has the SNF corrected these? Ask for a copy of the resident agreement or contract and marketing literature about the facility.

■ NARROW DOWN TO THREE CHOICES

Finally, the time has come to make the final decision. The family and the older person should make this decision. If you can, create an electronic spreadsheet that lists all factors in your patient profile and any others you might add and then rank each category for each facility. If the client and/or family have previewed the locations, then you can do this task with them. You or your client can double-check your evaluations by making one more unannounced visit to three facilities and asking any unanswered questions you or the client might have. If you are doing the

evaluations alone, be sure to obtain permission from the client and family prior to these additional visits because they must pay for the hours you spend. Once you or you and the client/family complete the spreadsheet, send the spreadsheet or a general facility description along with marketing literature that you received from the facility to the family. It is now the family's and older person's time to make the final selection of where to move.

■ GETTING THE OLDER PERSON AND FAMILY PSYCHOLOGICALLY AND SOCIALLY READY FOR THE MOVE

Usually, older persons experience the emotions of very traumatic loss when they move. They lose their familiar surroundings, familiar faces, and sometimes their independence. They lose personal items that orient them to their past and present, such as pictures of family, furniture that may link them to their life experiences, and the garden where familiar plants came up every year giving them joy and a sense of sameness every spring. If a long-time pet cannot be taken with them, they may also lose one of their trusted companions. Coping with this momentous loss is often like coping with death because, in a real way, this move can trigger a grief response.[13,14] Such a response was noted in one older woman, Mrs. Butler, who looked around when first placed in a nursing home and said, shaking her head, "I guess I'm at the end of the road."

Your role in muting this potentially devastating loss can be to offer emotional support and counseling. As a GCM, you can arrange help to lessen the pain of this loss by listening to the older person's grief and accepting it as real. You can make sure that familiar and treasured items move with the senior to make a bridge from the past to the present, orient the moved elder, and create a familiar living environment.[14]

Included in the familiar and treasured is the older adult's pet. If there is a pet involved, your search should be for a facility that accepts pets. The beloved pet companion provides an even more important bridge to the present than furniture can.

If someone is being moved to a different city and has not seen the facility or met the staff, ask the GCM or family in the area to send pictures of the facility and staff members and create an album for your client. Place all pictures in an album and identify them by name or site, especially the client's new room or apartment. Another option is to consider making a video of the facility, showing the client's new living environment and surrounding areas such as the dining room, the grounds, the lobby, or recreation room. Additionally, if possible, have staff members introduce themselves to the client individually by name and identify their role in the new living environment. With the use of a laptop computer, the client can view this video in advance of the move and have a better idea of what to expect. Hopefully, some personal belongings can be sent ahead so that the room or apartment looks and feels familiar when the senior arrives.

Meeting the Psychosocial Needs of the Adult Child Before the Move

Adult children have their own trials and tribulations before a parent's move. Often, they have a very difficult time coping with the slow pace with which the older person accepts the traumatic loss of moving. This is something you can warn adult children about as the process begins. Also, offer encouragement by reassuring the adult child that the move will take place and that you are there to help. That knowledge can often slow down their demands for a speedy process.

Adult children are harried at times because they are taking care of younger family members while arranging the move of their elderly parent. You can take the burden off the adult child by finding others in the continuum of care to complete the move or by providing agreed-upon services for a fee.

If the adult child has to find time to tour facilities, make the process easier by offering several time choices so that the task can be squeezed into an already busy schedule.

Counseling the adult child about this life transition is often as important as counseling the elder making the move and is a good fit for a GCM's skills. Adult children are often coping with their parent's mortality, a specter that hovers over the parent and the child, "Is this the end of the line?"

Once the place to move has been determined by the older person and the family, you can fill many roles in a move. Packing and organizing are areas you can cover, or you can find a moving specialist to do this. If you choose to offer this service, managing the move can include premoving preparations and activities. A major theme in premoving is to keep the older person involved constantly and have the person take part in all decisions. That way, the person will feel more in control, and this may minimize relocation stress syndrome.

■ WORKING WITH THE PHYSICAL PART OF THE MOVE

Once you have chosen a place and level of care to move to, make arrangements with another GCM or family member or someone very reliable to carry out the receiving end of the move, especially if this is in another geographic location. This should be done well in advance of the move.

Premove activities should include helping the client decide what to take to the new home, completing a checklist of what needs to be done before the move, assisting the older person in going through possessions, and arranging the donation, sale, or family distributions of the older person's belongings. More of your job is creating an inventory of all items to be moved, organizing items before the move, arranging for the mover, ordering boxes, and then packing. Packing responsibilities may be outsourced to a reliable senior moving company in your area. You can add disconnecting all utilities and stopping all present support services (cleaning, caregiving, Meals on Wheels, etc.) currently in place.

Assisting the older person to sort through possessions is an excellent GCM task. If the move location is far away from the area you serve, connect with a family member living nearby or another GCM to have them take the measurements of the final move site. This will enable you to select furniture and belongings that will fit in the space available in the new home.

There is potential for experiencing great loss through the disposition of personal belongings, furniture, pictures, even clothes, because they represent the older person's whole past, present safety, and family history. Although you might want an aide to do an inventory here, the crux of the sorting is not just what will be moved and what will be discarded but helping the older person through the trauma of leaving his or her past. Understand that the person is also discarding the present safe space by determining what items go and what items stay.

A general rule of thumb when sorting belongings: when in doubt, take the comfortable old friend. Help the client choose the chair he or she sits in every day, perhaps the recliner that is slightly tattered but like a cozy home to sink into. If there is a huge collection of an item, discuss taking a few to display in the new home and storing, selling, or distributing the rest. If the client has accumulated several craft items or sewing materials, for instance, suggest donating them to the local senior center craft group. (This is also good advice for those who have to sort and donate the hobby items of a spouse who has passed away. This age group likes to know that a "perfectly good" item is being used, not wasted.)

Even if the person will not cook, if there is a small dining or kitchen area, take a place setting for two or four in case the person has guests over. Unless your older client is moving to a single-family home or private home in a senior community, label all furniture and personal belongings with the older person's name. This is a good task to delegate.

After you know how many belongings the senior would like to move, you can execute two sorting events. The first sorting is to determine what will actually fit into the new space. The second sorting is for those items that mean the most to the senior and will provide a basis for creating a familiar environment in the new home. With these two filters you can begin to pare down the inventory of what goes with the older person and what must be put in storage, given away, or sold.

If your client is moving to a facility and space is limited, consider buying juvenile furniture for any pieces that are needed. It is sized smaller and fits more easily in smaller living quarters. You also may be able to get juvenile furniture at second-hand stores. Most assisted living facilities have a move-in coordinator. Check if one is available, and work with that staff member to make the move.

■ DISBURSEMENT AND DISPOSITION OF PERSONAL BELONGINGS

The family meeting to discuss the disbursement of family belongings is another opportunity for you to smooth the way. You can participate in a minimal way by suggesting family members visit the website, Who Gets Grandma's Yellow Pie Plate? (www.yellow-pieplate.umn.edu) and by suggesting the adult children have a family meeting with their parent or parents to discuss what family items go to whom after the move. Have a list of all items in the home ready for the family meeting. If this will be a contentious meeting, consider a licensed marriage and family therapist, or licensed clinical social worker who specializes in mediation. In the presence of strong words such as, "You got the Lenox dishes because Mom loved you best," you can facilitate this highly charged meeting. Sometimes the family prefers to do this in private. The elder who is moving must have a strong voice because, through the disposition of their belongings, he or she is passing history on.

Sometimes just knowing that a treasured item is passed on as a legacy helps the older person turn the loss into a gain and helps the adult children feel both nurtured and better prepared for the next stage of their parent's life. The family meeting can be a time whereby an agreement is made delineating which personal and household items go to which child. Keep this list handy for the actual physical moving stage. Once again, late-life relocation is a time that may include a role reversal or dependence by the parent on the adult child (see Chapter 20, Geriatric Care Management: Working with Nearly Normal Aging Families).

PERSONAL BELONGINGS: MOVING TO A SKILLED NURSING FACILITY OR ASSISTED LIVING FACILITY

If the older person is moving to a SNF or congregate facility, put the person's name on all furniture and bedding, consider laser printing all old family photos that cannot be replaced, and give the originals to family. Take familiar bedding, buy a bright inviting new comforter, and take the person's pillow. Ask whether the client wants flannel sheets, which are comforting. Bring along items that bring contentment. Take a radio, glasses, a watch, and a calendar. Make sure you take chocolate, knitting or hobby items, the person's TV, beloved books, and pen and paper. If the person is religious, bring religious objects.

If the person is moving to an SNF, bring bedclothes that are easy to get on and off and warm socks. If you have a local source of easy-to-get-on-and-off clothing for people with disabilities, order from there. All clothing, furniture, and personal belongings should have the new resident's name written on them (for clothing, use washable laundry markers). Check whether the facility will allow you to put a picture of the older person and, if allowed in the facility, a photo of the person's pet, on the door of the residence. Also ask family members to write a short biography of the older person and post this on the door so aides see your client not just as another older resident but someone with a history who made a difference in life. With client and/or family approval, you may be asked to write this personal biography. Use the Moving to a Skilled Nursing Facility Checklist (Exhibit 7–3) to help you assemble everything the client will need for the move.

MOVING DAY

Being on hand on moving day is a good idea if the family or client agrees to this arrangement. You can supervise where items are placed, offer support to the older person, and act as a traffic director. It is your job to make the move happen. Your role is to see that everything transpires as planned and everything arrives as expected. Remember, life offers the unexpected, and there is no perfect move. It will not always be smooth sailing. If the antique dresser is left behind, make new arrangements. If the antique dresser arrives but is in the wrong place or won't fit, find a solution. Just like a care plan, what you plan often requires reevaluation. Use the creative skills in your GCM repertoire and find new solutions.

To make moving day as simple as possible for your client, do as much as possible to prepare for the physical relocation that day. Pack a special bag just for moving day that contains any medications and instructions, special belongings, a change of clothes, toiletries, and special personal items the client might need (should there be a delay) or simply want to keep close. Preferably, the new living

Exhibit 7–3   Moving to a Skilled Nursing Facility Checklist

Date _____

Completed by: _____

Client Name _____

Address _____   Phone (   ) _____

City _____   State _____   Zip _____

Facility Name _____   Room Number ____

Address _____   Phone (   ) _____

City _____   State _____   Zip _____

Medical Supplies

Prescription Medications

1. _____   2. _____   3. _____   4. _____
5. _____   6. _____   7. _____   8. _____
9. _____   10. _____   11. _____   12. _____

Other _____

Over-the-Counter Medications

1. _____   2. _____   3. _____   4. _____

Medical Equipment

❏ Wheelchair   ❏ Walker   ❏ Cane   ❏ Transfer Board   ❏ Other
1. _____
2. _____
3. _____
4. _____

Personal Grooming Supplies

❏ Electric razor   ❏ Toothpaste
❏ Toothbrush   ❏ Soap
❏ Deodorant   ❏ Perfume
❏ Hand lotion   ❏ Incontinence supplies
❏ Hair brush   ❏ Other _____
❏ Hair spray
❏ Preferred shampoos   _____

Clothing

❏ Sleepwear (button up the front)   ❏ Sweat/fleece jackets (front closing)
❏ Warm socks   ❏ Sturdy shoes and socks
❏ Sweats/warm-up sets (several)   ❏ Underwear

Bedding

❏ Pillow   ❏ Sheets (hospital beds require single sheets)
❏ Blanket   ❏ Bright, colorful bedspread

Exhibit 7–3   Moving to a Skilled Nursing Facility Checklist (continued)

Furniture
- ❏ Favorite chair or recliner
- ❏ Favorite afghan or quilt
- ❏ Armoire (for TV/DVD/CD player or personal belongings)

Electronics
- ❏ Radio (the person can see without glasses)
- ❏ DVD player
- ❏ Remote controls
- ❏ CD player and favorite music CDs
- ❏ TV

Stationery
- ❏ Pencil
- ❏ Pen and paper
- ❏ Monthly calendar
- ❏ Greeting cards (variety)
- ❏ Stamps

Religious Objects
- ❏ Bible
- ❏ Other significant religious items

Jewelry
- ❏ A watch
- ❏ Inexpensive costume jewelry

Miscellaneous
- ❏ Books
- ❏ Snacks (chocolate, etc.)
- ❏ Pictures (home and family)
- ❏ Knitting/crocheting
- ❏ Cards
- ❏ All items are labeled
- ❏ Pet Supplies
  - ❏ Food
  - ❏ Food and water dishes
  - ❏ Leash
  - ❏ Grooming supplies
  - ❏ Bed or kennel

environment can be set up and readied for occupancy before the client arrives. If not, check whether you can arrange for a temporary "guest" room for the client to use until everything is set up.

■ AFTER THE MOVE: POSTMOVE SUPPORT

Family is an integral part of the successful relocation outcome for the older family member. Arrange in advance a visit from the adult child after the move. If appropriate, you or a family member can stay with the client on the first day to assist him or her with learning the physical layout of the new environment. This is especially important if the client is anxious or not looking forward to the move. After learning about and then mastering the new environment, the client is more free to work on social activities and tasks of adjusting to the transition.[15]

If family members cannot provide postmove support, and if the move is local, arrange to visit or to have church members, friends, or former social or interest group members such as those from a book club or craft group to visit. If the move is to a new city with a church or synagogue of your client's denomination, arrange for the institution's representative to visit your client as soon as possible. If the client was in a book club in the former city or town, check whether a similar group exists in the new town and investigate the possibility of a member visit for your client. Familiar people and activities can offer sameness even when the physical environment changes.

Your role does not always end after the move. It's important that the client's expectations match the reality of the outcome. If the client lives in your town, monitoring the effects of the move include making sure what you said would get there got there, and what the facility said it would provide is provided. If the client is moved to a different town, if the family wishes, make arrangements for another GCM to do the important follow-up process.

Older people who move can experience difficulty in coping with the relocation. They may resist being in the facility or new domicile. There is a greater possibility for a positive relocation outcome if the transition is smooth. You as the GCM are there to ensure a smooth move.

The facility itself can present problems such as not offering activities, staff, or the type of meals it said it would. If you move a pet, there can be pet problems.

As the older person adjusts to the move, you can add more activities from the continuum of care. For instance, if family members are not visiting or friends can't find the time to stop by, try to arrange for a friendly visitor, paid care provider, or new book club member to visit your client. If the meals are not satisfactory, talk to the facility director to have the food adjusted until the resident is satisfied. If the older person is not going to meals or sits at a table where he or she is not accepted, work with the facility to make adjustments.

You will wear many hats throughout the relocation process for each client. At certain points in the process, you will be a logistical coordinator, at other times, an information specialist. Additionally, and possibly most impor-

tant, you will be the advocate for, supportive advisor of, and confidant of the older adult client in search of a new place to call home.

■ MOVING A PERSON WITH MEMORY LOSS

The process of relocation for a senior experiencing memory loss has a unique set of challenges that older adults and their families often encounter. It is imperative, therefore, that the GCM take great care when assisting families and clients with this transition.

As the GCM works with families through this often difficult and emotional process, you will need to be aware of family dynamics, the medical, cognitive, and emotional needs of your client, and available community resources when creating a transition plan. Your role may also include locating appropriate living environments for the family to choose from, facilitating the actual move, and providing postrelocation support to the older adult and his or her family members.

To assist you with this challenge are the client's family and doctors, the staff of the new living facility, and community agencies such as your Area Agency on Aging. These are all valuable resources that you can consult with when creating a transition plan for a senior with memory loss.[16]

Relocation is not a one-size-fits-all experience for seniors with memory loss or their families. Your role is to transition your client (as well as his or her family) with the least amount of trauma possible through the use of a relocation plan custom tailored to his or her unique circumstances.

■ CONCLUSION

Relocation of an older adult is a multifaceted process involving the older adult, the family, numerous professionals, and select service providers. Relocation is accomplished over a variable amount of time and is unique to each individual. This transition requires the GCM to focus on the relocation of the social and psychological facets of the individual a well as their physical relocation, and the physical relocation of their personal belongings. The GCM supports the older adult through the process of relocation by providing insight, assistance, and support through each stage of the journey. Initially, this is done by offering the senior opportunities to participate in the decision-to-move process and by providing information to facilitate the selection of the new living environment. The GCM provides coordination and assistance with management of personal belongings and their physical relocation to the new home. And finally, the GCM is the trusted professional who provides follow-up assistance to the senior and the family, once the move has been completed. Friend, advisor, confidant, coordinator, facilitator, educator, resource expert; the role the GCM plays in relocation is invaluable and sets the stage for the older adult to achieve an optimal relocation outcome.

■ REFERENCES

1. Gaddy K. Special care environments: an overview of state laws for care of persons with Alzheimer's disease. *Bifocal: Newsletter of the ABA Commission on Legal Problems of the Elderly* (Washington, DC), 2000;21(2).

2. U.S. Census Bureau. Housing vacancies and homeownership (CPS/HVS). Available at: http://www.census.gov/hhes/www/housing/hvs/movingtoamerica2002/tab6.html. Accessed December 6, 2010.

3. U.S. Department of Commerce and U.S. Department of Housing and Urban Development. American housing survey for the United States in 2001, current housing reports (H150/01). Available at: http://www.census.gov/prod/2002pubs/h150-01.pdf. Accessed December 6, 2010.

4. U.S. Census Bureau. Geographic mobility: 2002 to 2003. March 2004. Available at: http://www.census.gov/prod/2004pubs/p20-549.pdf. Accessed December 10, 2010.

5. Wiseman RF. Why older people move. *Res Aging.* 1980;2(2):141–154.

6. Pynoos J, Overton J, De Meire M. *Home Modification Resource Guide.* Los Angeles, CA: University of Southern California; 1996.

7. Peterson K. *Home Modification.* Los Angeles: Andrus Gerontology Center, University of Southern California; 2005.

8. Wiseman RF, Roseman CC. A typology of elderly migration based on the decision making process. *Economic Geography.* 1979;55(4):324–337.

9. U.S. Department of Housing and Urban Development. Senior housing—what you should know. Homes and Communities. Available at: http://www.hud.gov/offices/fheo/seniors/index.cfm. Accessed December 6, 2010.

10. The Rotary Club of Santa Monica and Center for Healthy Aging. Choosing senior housing and residential care. Available at: http://www.helpguide.org/elder/senior_housing_residential_care_types.htm. Accessed December 6, 2010.

11. Episcopal Homes Foundation. Retirement communities with life care. 2006. Available at: http://www.ehf.org/cw/cwlifecare.html. Accessed September 20, 2006.

12. New Lifestyles. Types of senior housing. 2004. Available at: http://www.newlifestyles.com/resources/articles/Types_of_Senior_Housing.aspx. Accessed December 6, 2010.

13. Dimond M, McCance K, King K. Forced residential relocation: its impact on the well-being of older adults. *West J Nurs Res.* 1987;9(4):445–465.

14. Young H. Moving to congregate housing: the last chosen home. *J Aging Stud.* 1998;12(2).

15. Lawton MP. Three functions of the residential environment. *J Housing Elderly.* 1983;5(1):35–50.

16. Spencer B, White L. *Moving a relative with memory loss: a family caregiver's guide.* Santa Rosa, CA: Whisp Publications; 2000.

17. Lawton MP. Three functions of the residential environment. *J Housing Elderly.* 1983;5(1):35–50.

18. Rubenstein RL. The home environments of older people: a description of the psychosocial processes linking person to place. *J Gerontol* 1989; 44(2):S45–S53.

19. Administration on Aging. Aging into the 21st century. Available at: http://www.aoa.gov/AoARoot/Aging_Statistics/future_growth/aging21/preface.aspx. Accessed December 6, 2010.

Chapter 8

Incorporating a Spiritual Perspective into Geriatric Care Management

Leonie Nowitz

In the last decade, there has been a growing interest in spirituality in US society and an increasing appreciation for spirituality's valuable contribution to health and well-being.[1] In the healthcare literature, there is evidence that prayer and a belief in a higher power contribute to healing and a general sense of well-being. There is also growing interest in the search and creation of meaning in the second half of life as evidenced by the numerous conferences, courses, and books that address these issues under the title of "conscious aging."

The search for meaning and purpose in life often begins at times of illness, crisis, and suffering. A geriatric care manager (GCM) helps older persons and their families, friends, and paid caregivers find meaning and strength in coping with changes in function, increased caregiving, and reduced resources. A spiritual perspective offers the GCM an opportunity to broaden his or her vision of meaning and values and to be open to clients' viewpoints, struggles, and ways of finding meaning in life.

In 1975, the National Interfaith Coalition on Aging defined spiritual well-being as "the affirmation of life in a relationship with God, self, community and environment that nurtures and celebrates wholeness."[2] It is that which unites all aspects of ourselves and brings together concurrent paths of spiritual and psychological well-being. If GCMs can

view more positively the frailty and finiteness of life, they can help older persons and their families find meaning and value in their situations, helping them care for each other, accept life's realities, and transmit the value of caring to future generations.

A spiritual view challenges the negative attitudes about aging in a society that celebrates youth, achievement, financial success, and power. This perspective enables GCMs to help their clients find meaning when productivity fails and they become dependent on others.

This chapter addresses the meaning of spirituality for older persons and their families and considers the purpose and spiritual tasks of life's last stages. Assessment and intervention tools for the practitioner are offered. Qualities with which GCMs need to address clients' struggles are also discussed. The final section discusses the facilitation of spiritual connections with persons who have dementia and their families.

■ THE PURPOSE OF LIFE'S LAST STAGES

According to Carl Jung, "We cannot live the afternoon of life according to the program of life's morning, for what was great in the morning will be little in the evening and what in the morning was true will in the evening have become a lie."[3] To help clients evaluate their lives, GCMs need to ask several questions. What is the purpose of life after age 65? What are clients' values, wishes, and dreams? How can clients stay true to their values and accomplish their dreams?

After age 65, there may be a transition from professional work to volunteer work and from ability to disability. Social networks may diminish as friends move away or die, which leads to an increased focus on family. Changes in family roles may ensue as a result of changes in health and dwindling resources. Everyone in the family needs to make a shift. As some members increasingly need care, others may need to assume caregiving responsibilities in addition to their current work and family roles. Though painful, transition and loss provide the opportunity to reevaluate one's life goals. Who am I without my work role, when I am disabled and need to depend on others? Why am I here? What is it I still want to do and be? These important questions were inspired by the work of Schachter-Shalomi and Miller.[4]

By reflecting on these questions and attending to clients' thoughts and values, GCMs can help clients redefine themselves. GCMs can help their clients find meaning in loss by offering a loving presence and allowing a trusting relationship to develop. This process may involve listening to clients mourn and find meaning in their losses as they reflect on their lives, struggles, and strengths, and acknowledging the gifts clients have given and continue to give to others. The GCM needs to transcend the dominant culture's status- and youth-driven values and respect each client's feelings regardless of age, function, and status. When the GCM takes this approach, it can help clients shake off the culture's focus on autonomy and independence and instead see themselves as who they are based on a lifetime of experience.

It is important that GCMs acknowledge and respect a client's values. If a GCM notices a client's kindness, wisdom, dignity, depth, joy, integrity, wholeness, confidence, or peacefulness, the GCM should tell the client. This respect will help clients reestablish a connection within themselves, with other people, and with God, if they so choose.

Kenyon notes:

> Advanced human aging may also be a time for the possibility of a transition from having to being. Something new may now be taking place that goes beyond loss. Inner activity may increase. Silence provides an opportunity for simply being with oneself which can be peaceful or anxiety provoking through confrontation with new aspects of ourselves. The experience of inner silence and being can result in an increased ability to be present to others, involving the ability to be more open to others and less preoccupied with self.[5(pp4-5)]

To provide a broader framework, it is helpful to consider traditions that offer another perspective. The Hindu tradition embraces loss as a natural part of the life cycle and thinks of the third stage of life as one in which one frees oneself from daily roles and moves to the performing of rituals and the reciting of sacred texts with all energies directed toward union with Brahman, the divine ground of the universe. Losses are considered "modes of liberation contributing to spiritual growth."[6(pp17-21)]

The Western counterpart to the Hindu journey would look upon late life as a natural monastic period.

> The aging process often strips the person of the distracting pleasures of the world by shrinking both actual life space and even the physical ability to participate in the adventures of life. It's as if God offers a new kind of intimacy and says to the frail elderly person, "You have lived a long life enjoying the pleasures of my creation. Sometimes you have enjoyed creation more than you have ME, but I understand because creation is so won-

derful. Now that you are housebound and can no longer enjoy the physical and mental pleasures of your past, we have an opportunity to really get to know one another before we meet face to face at your death!"[7(p9)]

Accepting brokenness in a positive light is a part of many spiritual traditions. Most religious traditions view frailty and loss as meaningful, valuable parts of life. The Jewish rabbinical traditions speak of the value of brokenness. The Kotsker rabbi recognizes that nothing is as whole as a broken heart and that the brokenness and deficits create an opening up to possibilities of humility and seeking union with God.[8] Rav Kook noted that a broken heart was beloved before God, and Reb Nachman said that in the brokenness itself is the yearning for God.[8] Similarly, Ralph Waldo Emerson said, "There is a crack in everything God has made."[9] It has been said that as we age, the cracks begin to show. Are they just about darkness and brokenness? Or are they also a place for the light of spirit to stream through?

Spirituality has many faces and takes many forms. It is important to recognize the unique essence of clients, their families, and caregivers and to be open and available to the form of spirituality favored by individual clients and the people around them. There are four ways persons commonly experience their spirituality:

- As a connection to something beyond themselves that comforts and guides them
- As a connection to all living things, earth, and the universe
- As a part of a faith tradition or having a close personal relationship with God or both
- As a process of finding answers to life's difficult questions

Some older persons tend to turn inward. Others move from the inward view toward more meaningful relationships with others.

And others experience spiritual awareness through religious traditions that sustained them in the past.[10] Moberg describes "spiritual" as referring to the very essence of each human being that relates everything consciously or unconsciously and either positively or negatively to God and that makes everyone valuable.[11]

■ SPIRITUAL TASKS IN OLD AGE

Genevay and Richards question the nature of growth in old age. Is spiritual growth separate from psychological growth, or is there one concurrent path that leads to mental, emotional, and spiritual growth in the last stage of life?[12]

Many believe that there are spiritual tasks to be accomplished in late life. The following tasks were suggested by Father Richard Sweeney at the 1991 American Society on Aging Forum and church and mental health workers at the 1997 American Society on Aging annual meeting:

1. Making a conscious effort to know oneself and clarify one's personal values
2. Establishing a sense of self-worth apart from life's externals
3. Letting go of dimensions of life where there is no longer ability
4. Seeking and sharing wisdom and love
5. Mentoring others
6. Viewing life as imperfect and facing issues of death and the afterlife

Many writers have shared their viewpoints on making meaning. Victor Frankl, a concentration camp survivor, writes about the search for meaning and how one's attitude toward one's experience creates meaning.[13] His works focus on how to turn suffering into human triumph and the importance of self-discovery, responsibility, and self-transcendence. Zalman Schachter-Shalomi and R. S. Miller, in the book *From Age-ing to Sage-ing*, talk about the concept of generativity, harvesting gifts of a lifetime and giving them back to family, friends, and society: "The archetype of the Inner Elder is a divine image representing the wisdom of the ages. This image of the Inner Elder calls forth the wisdom of older people at a time when our culture desperately needs it."[4(p139)] Allan Chinen's work offers much richness in noting the tasks of the elder: "learning to heed the dictates of the soul, being generative in inspiring the younger generations with practical counsel and noble inspiration, seeking self-confrontation and transformation through painful insight and authentic reformation."[14]

Carter Catlett Williams talks about the wonderful opportunity for self-discovery in later years. Paying attention to one's inner life, a person can make later life a time for growth, self-reflection, rediscovery, and self-exploration.[15] Finding meaning through suffering is the focus of Polly Young-Eisendrath, a Jungian psychotherapist who shares stories of people who have sustained major losses to their health and of family members.[16] She describes how they transcended these losses to develop, through their pain, compassion for and understanding of others. Through this process, they learned to accept the impermanence of life and allowed the formation of a new identity.

If GCMs view frailty and brokenness as valuable, meaningful parts of life, they can witness and be present to the suffering of clients. Often GCMs will witness great wisdom, understanding, and courage of their clients and families.

■ WAYS TO FACILITATE THE SPIRITUAL PROCESS IN GERIATRIC CARE MANAGEMENT

Psychological and spiritual growth can be nurtured by introspection and a search for meaning in life. Some ways the GCM can foster spiritual connection and growth in clients are discussed in this section.

Life Review

In reviewing their lives with an empathetic listener, clients can find meaning. Clients can review the struggles and the wisdom gained, the values lived and acquired, the mistakes made, and the opportunities missed. Healing can come from the process of facing hurtful experiences and letting go. Telling one's story in the presence of an empathetic listener allows a reworking of it.

Chinen notes that "in remembering the past, older adults transform it. The reflective individual comes to terms with mistakes and opportunities missed, learning to forgive himself and others. The elder embraces the past, not to regress, but to illuminate all of life."[14]

This process can be facilitated by the GCM (who may be a social worker or a nurse), paid caregivers, and family members (to whom the shared stories can transmit history and legacy). GCMs can help get their clients involved in senior center and day care programs. Participating in storytelling and the creative arts can enrich older people's lives and cultivate a sense of community. "When elders hear others reveal dimensions of their lives, they notice similarities and differences with their own experiences. They can be empowered to claim and reclaim the wisdom of their own lives."[17]

The GCM needs to be sensitive to each client's willingness to engage in this process and should engage with clients at their own pace.

Ethical Wills

The tradition of bequeathing a spiritual legacy in a conventional will, a codicil, or a separate document has its roots in the Bible. The desire was to pass on an instructive account of ideas and values close to the older person's heart—an ethical will.[18]

An ethical will can be used to pass values and a sense of what is important in life to future generations. If clients have no family members, the GCM can listen to clients' account of their values, a process that will strengthen the connection between the GCM and the clients. If clients are unable to articulate their values, GCMs can tell clients what they know of them based on stories the GCMs have heard that reflect the clients' values and character. This process will help clients feel that they are being understood and valued. Additionally, it helps clients recall old memories and gives them an opportunity to receive positive feedback and be seen for their deeper values.

For instance, Mr. K, a 96-year-old widower with a moderate degree of dementia, was working with a GCM. The GCM acknowledged Mr. K's generosity to his family and political causes as well as the extensive care he gave to his wife before she died. Although he did not initially remember some of these actions, he began to remember his wife, how he loved her, and how important it was for him to make her life comfortable when she was ill. As this example illustrates, when the GCM shares his or her view of the older person's values as exemplified by his or her life story, the older person is validated. This can stimulate memories in an environment of trust.

Prayer and Meditation

Prayer and meditation are common in all religious and spiritual traditions. Eighty-one percent of caregivers for people with Alzheimer's disease say they use prayer in coping with the demands of caregiving.[19] GCMs might consider praying with their clients. They might want to check with family members whether the older person has prayed in the past. GCMs would ask family members whether opportunities for prayer should be provided to the older person. If a GCM is uncomfortable praying with a client or comes from a tradition different from the client's, the GCM could find another professional on the care team (e.g., a nurse, a social worker) who is familiar with the client's religious tradition.

Many home care workers are comfortable with prayer and are willing to read from the scriptures and pray with clients, which can give clients a sense of peace and well-being.

Sacred and Secular Rituals

Performing sacred and secular rituals can help clients experience familiar memories and reconnect them with their faith and communal traditions. The GCM can find out what traditions and practices are familiar to clients and help re-create them. For instance, a traditional Christmas or Passover meal could be made. The GCM can ask clients and caregivers to help with planning (e.g., what foods they would like, what readings they would like to have) and can be present at a Passover Seder or Christmas meal. In addition, the GCM can help clients attend services by contacting places of worship to find out about wheelchair accessibility. The GCM can arrange for a friend to accompany the client and/or a caregiver to create more of a feeling of family and community.

Grief Counseling

Grief counseling to resolve the current and multiple losses of a lifetime is important to help clients heal their pain in the presence of a caring and empathic listener. The GCM can provide this counseling or can refer the client to another professional.

Focusing

In focusing, a GCM helps a client clarify and resolve all kinds of issues (e.g., unresolved relationship issues) and make all kinds of decisions (e.g., decisions about health care).

For example, Ms. F's aunt was not able to swallow food after surgery. Her physicians felt that the insertion of a peg tube was necessary to ensure adequate nutrition and hydration. Ms. F was ambivalent about this procedure. She questioned the quality of life of her aunt, who had recently experienced the onset of dementia. Ms. F thought her aunt would not tolerate being mentally and physically dependent. The GCM helped Ms. F explore her feelings about other relatives who had lived in a seriously vegetative state for several years. The GCM encouraged Ms. F to think about her aunt's life and what interests and people had sustained her. The GCM shared with the niece the possibility that the peg tube might not always be needed if her aunt's condition improved. She encouraged Ms. F to talk with other relatives and explore what Ms. F's aunt would want for herself. Her aunt had not expressed any negative feelings about being ill and dependent. After discussion with family members and review of her aunt's life and her own reactions to others who were disabled, the niece recognized that she needed to come to terms with her aunt's changed functioning. She also realized that her aunt was not as debilitated as her other relatives. The GCM listened to Ms. F's fears about the quality of her aunt's life and helped Ms. F clarify her decision regarding surgery. Ms. F's aunt got the peg tube and after several weeks regained her capacity to swallow.

Broadening Clients' View of Themselves to Include Deeper Values

Many older persons who have suffered losses of family and friends and changes in health tend to view themselves in a negative light. It is helpful to appreciate the deeper values that have sustained and enriched the client.

For example, Mrs. D, a widow who suffered from dementia, had no friends and only a distant relative. She reminisced with the GCM about her life with her husband, a famous physician, and how she enjoyed traveling. "Those were the good days, and they are no more," she said. She described her present existence as one in which God was punishing her by squeezing the life out of her little by little. She focused on her past life, talking about how she was valued for being the beautiful

wife of a famous physician. "Then I was something; now I'm nothing," she said. The GCM said, "Mrs. D, I see how valuable your past was to you in terms of your beauty and your sense of adventure. But in addition, I see a woman who has an inner beauty, who loved her husband and took care of him. You were hospitable to his friends and later you volunteered at a hospital and brought much caring to sick people. You visited them and gave so much of yourself." Mrs. D listened but did not respond. The GCM repeated her viewpoint many times because Mrs. D continued to think negatively about herself. The GCM talked to her about the wholeness of life and that if persons defined themselves by only one time in their lives they were bound to feel unworthy at other times that were different. The GCM continued to listen compassionately to Mrs. D's pain and sadness about the losses in her life. She shared what she valued about Mrs. D: "I value your courage and ability to endure the pain of so many losses, your warmth, your kindness, and your wisdom and ability to laugh at life." By reflecting on Mrs. D's lifelong values, the GCM attempted to help Mrs. D appreciate her many positive attributes and acknowledge her inner resources. The GCM brought small problems to Mrs. D from time to time, and Mrs. D reveled in the opportunity to share her wisdom by providing practical solutions. Mrs. D continued to view herself in a diminished capacity but also showed more comfort in being valued and grew more trusting in her relationship with the GCM and her caregivers.

Hearing the Spirit Beneath the Words

GCMs working with clients, especially those with dementia, need to listen to the meaning behind the spoken words. Older persons may not always be able to say precisely what they mean, but an attentive and sensitive listener will hear what an older person is really saying.

For example, Mrs. T was frightened of "men" in her bedroom. Her caregivers would check her room each evening to assure her it was empty. She was a religious woman and the GCM asked her pastor to visit her. On his visits he prayed with Mrs. T for God to protect her and keep her safe. He dealt with her feelings without specifically talking about the "men." By praying with her, the pastor acknowledged Mrs. T's fears and offered comfort and a sense of safety.[20]

Awareness of Countertransference

"Countertransference describes the personal feelings that a professional experiences in relation to a client that can affect his or her professional interventions."[21]

In facilitating the spiritual process, GCMs need to be aware of their own values. They can ask, "How can we facilitate resolution of past issues and letting go of emotional baggage that hinders at the end of life? Can we listen to older people and allow them to come to their own recognition of what they need?"[12(pp4-5)] To be effective, the GCM needs to be in touch with his or her own concerns and how he or she resolves them. The client may have a different perspective that needs to be respected, particularly when it conflicts with the GCM's view.

The next section discusses how GCMs can go about examining their own values, spiritual beliefs, and family history.

■ GCMs LOOK AT THEIR OWN VALUES, SPIRITUAL BELIEFS, AND FAMILY HISTORY

In helping clients deal with the multiple losses in their lives, GCMs are offered the opportunity to examine their own feelings about aging and dying and consider their own values. GCMs should ask themselves these questions: How do I view my own aging? What models of care do I embrace for myself? What makes me anxious and reactive to clients? With what family systems am I most comfortable and uncomfort-

able? GCMs need to consider values that are acquired from three sources:

- Their family
- Their culture
- Their professional training

GCMs need to be aware of the values they transmit to their clients and the impact of their values on their clients. The following exercise can help GCMs consider their own values at different stages of the life cycle and understand their clients' evolving values and beliefs. By answering the questions for themselves and considering how their clients might answer them, GCMs will broaden their perspective and learn to not impose their values on their clients. The questions were inspired by the work of Schachter-Shalomi and Miller.[4]

- How have you valued yourself at different times of your life?
- What were your beliefs about aging, interdependence, and family connections as a child, as an adolescent, as an adult, and as a person with an illness or a disability?
- Have your values been similar at different stages, or have they changed as you have aged?
- How has your belief system served you throughout your life?
- How does it serve you at a time of loss and diminishment?
- What is the meaning of your life now, despite losses that have taken place?

■ ASSESSMENT OF CLIENTS' VALUES AND SOURCES OF MEANING

In *Assessing Spiritual Needs: A Guide for Caregivers*, George Fitchett includes a spiritual assessment tool that can help GCMs evaluate their clients' spiritual life and struggles (Exhibit 8–1).[22] The tool contains a number of categories that GCMs need to consider.

Exhibit 8–1
Spiritual Assessment Tool

1. Beliefs of the client that give meaning and purpose to the client's life
2. Vocation and obligation: beliefs that create a sense of duty or moral obligation.
3. Experience and emotion that may be related to the sacred, the divine, or the demonic
4. Courage and growth
5. Ritual and practice
6. Community
7. Authority and guidance

Source: Copyright © George Fitchett.

This spiritual assessment is part of a holistic assessment that includes the medical, psychological, family systems, psychosocial, ethnic, racial, cultural, and social dimensions that affect older persons. This tool provides a comprehensive picture of a client. The following text considers each of the seven dimensions listed in Exhibit 8–1 in turn, with illustrative cases discussed for each dimension.

Beliefs That Give Meaning and Purpose

GCMs should ask what beliefs a person has that give meaning and purpose to his or her life. These can be religious beliefs and practices of the past. There are also other sources from which persons derive meaning and purpose.

CASE STUDY

Mrs. N
Mrs. N, a 75-year-old African American woman who was divorced and living alone and was a very feisty and strong-spirited person, lost one of her daughters a few years ago. She had another daughter who lived out of town, as did several siblings. Diagnosed with Alzheimer's disease, she gradually accepted a few hours of home care over a long period of time and sporadically visited a day care center. A woman who was very autonomous, she found it difficult to receive help. During one visit the GCM asked her what gave her the strength to deal with her memory loss and life situation. She said she had been raised as a Catholic and went to church all her life. She talked about God in personal terms, "I feel God is close to me—whatever happens during the day I talk to him at night and he listens. I couldn't be this age and in the world without God. He gives me strength in difficult times." The GCM asked Mrs. N about the times things did not work out the way she had hoped. She said, "I accept God's will. My mother died; she might have suffered more if she had lived. God does what is best." Mrs. N's faith and personal relationship with God gave her courage and strength to face her deteriorating health and the losses in her life. The GCM's interest in what gave Mrs. N strength encouraged Mrs. N to talk about her strong belief in and relationship with God.

CASE STUDY

Mrs. B
Mrs. B, who had a moderate dementia, talked about her very strong connection to nature by reflecting on the woods outside her apartment and how comforting it was to have the trees there. "I have always loved nature; my family found it a source of nourishment and strength," she said. Some of Mrs. B's frightening dreams found resolution in the woods. Mrs. B's source of healing and support was her lifetime connection with nature. Nature was a nurturing and

reassuring presence in times of difficulty. The GCM acknowledged and helped Mrs. B remember her connection with and comfort in nature.

CASE STUDY

Mr. J

Mr. J was a 95-year-old widower with severe sensory losses who walked minimally and suffered from moderate to severe dementia. Prior to his illness, he was an engineer who traveled extensively with his wife. Although his interests were wide-ranging prior to his illness, once he was ill Mr. J was confined to his apartment, where he watched ball-games and nature shows and enjoyed going to the nearby park to feed the squirrels and watch the boats sail by. These activities were the central focus of his day. Mr. J drew pleasure and a sense of connection from the park (he always loved nature) and from ball-games; these were activities he enjoyed in the past and could continue to enjoy. The GCM shared Mr. J's enthusiasm for ballgames. She also discussed with him the pleasure he got from feeding the squirrels and watching activities in the park.

CASE STUDY

Mrs. C

Mrs. C's health was deteriorating rapidly due to her congestive heart failure and multiple health problems. Her daughter hired a GCM to assess her mother's situation and to provide counseling to her mother as her health declined. She also had the GCM arrange home care and access other resources. The daughter was very stressed but continued to coordinate her mother's medical care and call her daily. The GCM noted the stress the daughter experienced because of the time associated with Mrs. C's care and the emotional drain of her mother's illness and decline. The GCM listened to her concerns about her mother and the emotional drain of caregiving. The GCM offered to help her with some tasks, but the daughter refused, feeling obliged to continue her role as primary caregiver. In ongoing discussions, she talked about the stress and drain of caregiving. After several months of the daughter refusing to accept any help, the GCM asked the daughter why she continued to do as much as she did. She said it helped her feel connected to her mother. This helped the GCM understand the meaning of her sense of obligation and to continue to be respectful of her wishes. In time the daughter was able to let go of the daily coordination of care and continued her daily calls to her mother, which gave her that continued sense of connection.

Vocation and Obligation

It is important to consider the client's or their caregivers' beliefs and whether they create a sense of duty or moral obligation. Are clients or their caregivers able to fulfill these obligations, or are clients and caregivers frustrated and guilty about not being able to fulfill them? Both the older client's and the family member's sense of obligation may provide stress, but there may be positive experiences such as a strengthened relationship.

It is important for a GCM to understand the meaning of the caregiver's caregiving experiences and to be respectful of the caregiver while acknowledging the stress of caregiving. The GCM needs to respect the caregiver's timetable and wait until he or she is willing to relinquish tasks to the GCM or to others in the system.

Experience and Emotion

The GCM needs to ask what direct contact with the sacred, divine, or demonic the older person has had. What emotions or moods are associated with these contacts and with the person's beliefs and sense of meaning in life? What past illnesses or crises in life were connected with spiritual experiences? How does spirituality affect the current situation? What sources or rituals provide comfort?

CASE STUDY

Mrs. G

Mrs. G was a 91-year-old widow, a musician who lived with her caregivers and who was visited by her two sons regularly. Her sons hired the GCM to oversee Mrs. G's care, because they were frequently out of town. Mrs. G had strong mood swings, which may have been caused by a long-standing personality disorder or dementia. A strong-willed woman who was not able to walk, she viewed herself as capable and was often frustrated in her efforts to care for herself. Her sense of self fluctuated depending on her mood. During visits, the GCM listened to her fears and frustration and encouraged her to tell stories about herself and her accomplishments and to reminisce about things that came to mind. Although Mrs. G's family was Jewish, they observed no rituals. Mrs. G told the GCM many times that she did not believe in God and did not like her caregivers reading the Bible or praying. In one of the conversations, she talked about preparing for death. "I keep wondering at night how I continue to survive. Perhaps with the help of the Lord."

"Do you believe in God?" the GCM asked.

Mrs. G answered, "I talk a lot to God when anything goes wrong. I blame God with great pleasure and affection, but then I think what a hell of a job he has." She went on to say that she felt God was somewhere around but that she had told him to go away. The GCM asked if Mrs. G was concerned about seeing God. She said she was. "If he comes close, I will die." The GCM asked if Mrs. G believed God comes for persons when they die. Mrs. G said yes.

"So you're not ready to die now?" the GCM asked.

"Not at all; there is time." The GCM asked Mrs. G about whether she believed in connecting with God after death, as the soul rises to take its place with God—which is part of the Jewish tradition. Mrs. G thought that would be a great thing but thought God was too busy for her. After reflection, she said, "There is a mysterious thing that guides us. If I try to go too far I get lost. Something in us guides us; it's not a person, it's a mystery. We just have to follow it." The GCM asked her if she was talking about her soul or God. She said, "I would rather not put a finger on it." Mrs. G is not involved in any rituals or practice, but she has strong spiritual connections.

It is important for the GCM to be aware of spiritual resources that give clients meaning and strength and to be open to the conversation about such resources even if clients deny them. The GCM's interest and openness give the client the opportunity to share his or her beliefs and fears. The GCM should be guided by the client's expression and support the beliefs of the client. If the client's beliefs create fear, the GCM can listen to these fears and offer additional opportunities to resolve these fears by encouraging familiar clergy or family members to comfort the client.

Courage and Growth

Must new experiences, including problems, always be explained by a person's preexisting beliefs, or can a person let go of existing beliefs to allow new ones to emerge? When do persons' new life experiences challenge their existing beliefs in God? Do crises of faith or self-doubt result? It requires courage to enter the dark night of the soul, come to terms with a new set of circumstances, and accept changes in oneself. How can GCMs help their clients accept changes?

CASE STUDY

Ms. H

Ms. H was a 77-year-old single woman who had had a stroke, was able to walk with assistance, and had a moderate degree of dementia, which affected her memory and made it difficult for her to articulate her thoughts. Ms. H's sister, who lived several thousand miles away, was her only living relative. The sister hired a GCM to oversee Ms. H's care and be accountable to the sister.

Ms. H was initially an opera singer and later worked in an administrative capacity for a major corporation. She was very knowledgeable about music and art and went to many concerts and museums. Her sense of self was diminished by her strong negative attitude toward being old and a societally induced emphasis on youth and beauty. It was difficult for her to say anything positive about herself.

The GCM tried to expand Ms. H's sense of self, encouraging her to modify her lifelong beliefs about youth and beauty. She tried to help Ms. H value her experience, wisdom, and knowledge and the fact that she was witty, caring, and loving. At times Ms. H was able to take this in. The GCM encouraged the caregivers to acknowledge Ms. H's strengths, points of view, and kindness, and Ms. H was receptive at times. At other times she stuck to her old negative beliefs about herself. The challenge of the GCM's work with Ms. H and her caregivers was to acknowledge her losses and traumas and help her view herself in a positive framework by mirroring positive views of her, to stretch her beyond her old beliefs.

Many clients have negative beliefs about aging and disability. To help clients accept their situations, GCMs can help clients explore their feelings toward God, if they express any feelings toward God at all. If clients do not have a religious connection, helping clients like Ms. H view themselves in more affirming ways can help them let go of entrenched beliefs that cause them to suffer.

Ritual and Practice

It is important for the GCM to know what the client's rituals and practices are and what they were in the past. This would include traditional religious practices, services, prayers, and holiday celebrations. It would also include nonreligious rituals such as family gatherings for celebrations or birthdays. If the GCM's clients do not have family or do not participate in any rituals, the GCM needs to find out what events were celebrated in clients' lives that had meaning to them. The GCM might ask what the clients would like to do (e.g., go to church or synagogue, receive communion at home, or have their priest or rabbi visit). Would clients like to say prayers with caregivers or have scriptures or other spiritual material read aloud? What holidays would they like to celebrate and how? The GCM can work with caregivers to provide holiday foods and organize or participate in holiday celebrations. Providing a service for older persons in their homes generates a sense of community for clients and caregivers. When clients have forgotten rituals of their past, the GCM can find out about these rituals by trial and error, by saying a familiar prayer, lighting candles, or singing familiar songs or hymns from the person's religious tradition. These rituals can engender a sense of deep connection to clients' past and tradition. The GCM needs to respect clients' wishes and move in a sensitive manner.

CASE STUDY

Mr. G

Mr. G was Jewish but did not remember the rituals of his childhood in an orthodox home. During Chanukah, the GCM asked him if she could say a prayer when he lit the menorah candle. At first he declined and said he was agnostic. The GCM accepted his wishes, but he was curious and encouraged her to do so. She read the prayer slowly in Hebrew and English while Mr. G watched attentively. He later told her he appreciated her saying the prayer. Mr. G insisted on lighting the candles on all future Jewish holidays, including lighting the menorah on Passover.

Clients can be responsive to music from their tradition. Responses to the singing of melodies can range from joyful participation to the more subtle response of a smile or tapping finger. It is important to follow the older person's lead in this. It is helpful to involve pastoral connections and staff familiar with the rituals to say prayers and sing religious songs. In these ways, the GCM will help clients build a sense of connection to the past and create a sense of well-being.

Community

Is the person part of one or more formal or informal communities of shared beliefs, ritu-als, or practices? What is the person's participation in these communities? The GCM may ask what it means to the client to be part of the community and how active the client is in the community. The GCM should consider both spiritual and other communities of family, friends, organizations, neighbors, and caregivers. The GCM may have to educate the clergy or lay volunteer if the client has dementia or is aphasic as to how to respond appropriately to the client. It is important to stress to the spiritual leader how valuable his or her visit would be to the client, as would other types of connection with the community of faith.

Past versus Current Communities

Frail, homebound clients tend to have small communities. Families may live far away, and the clients may have lost touch with friends who have moved or are too ill to visit. Other friends and family members may have died. Because of illness, clients may not currently be connected to religious organizations. If a client is not part of any faith community, the GCM should assess past involvement in and current willingness to be part of a faith community. Would clients want to participate in services outside their home, or would they like the members of their former community to visit? It is important to talk with clients about their current community as well as their emotional connections to organizations or communities that had meaning to them in the past. The GCM can help access important people from the client's past by asking the client and his or her family for names. The GCM can encourage clients to contact whoever they were close to or offer to make the calls on behalf of clients. In addition, the GCM can arrange for new opportunities to widen clients' circles, such as attending day care programs or respite programs, having friendly visitor volunteers, and participating in activities the client likes.

Mr. R

Mr. R was a 95-year-old client who was a successful artist and was cognitively impaired. The GCM encouraged Mr. R's caregivers to take him to art shows where his work was represented. He was significantly affected by his dementia, but he loved to see familiar faces at these shows and receive acknowledgment for his work. The connection to the art community affirmed his self-worth. It is important for a GCM to involve a client with those who have had meaning in the client's life (e.g., former associates, neighbors, friends).

Home Care Community

The community of home care providers often becomes the surrogate family, providing great meaning for and connection with the client. It is important to support the home care staff so that they maintain good relationships with clients and care for clients' well-being. Many home care workers are spiritual people and view their work as the work of God, so they take naturally to caring for and loving their clients.

Mr. H

Mr. H suffered from dementia and physical incapacity. He was often agitated. His care workers were religious and had a daily ritual of saying prayers at the morning shift. At times he told them to stop. At other times, he joined the workers in their prayers. GCMs need to be vigilant that the caregivers are not imposing their viewpoints on clients, making clients uncomfortable.

Authority and Guidance

The GCM should consider where clients look for guidance when faced with doubt, confusion, tragedy, or conflict. To what extent do clients look within or outside themselves for guidance?

Mrs. L

Mrs. L's family lived out of town and hired a GCM to oversee her care. Mrs. L was visually impaired and at home in bed after a fall in which her arm and leg were injured. She could hardly move. She talked to the GCM about the difficult hospital experience. She hated not being in control and was glad to be at home in her bed. "I'm just lying here wondering what purpose I have. I don't know, but I know I've been through a lot of difficult struggles. I'm a tough egg. I've gone through difficult times but met people who had substance—that's what made the difference."

"So you valued the connections with people?" the GCM asked.

"Yes, that is right—I really liked them a lot."

"Do you wonder about the meaning of your life now?" continued the GCM.

"Yes, I don't know what I'm needed for, but that's all right, I am here and observing."

"So instead of thinking of what to do, you're just living in the present moment."

"Yes, that is what I am doing," said Mrs. L. She was quiet for a few moments. "I love listening to the music and to the voice that is coming from you."

"I appreciate that," the GCM responded. "I know you have meaning to your family."

"For a time I didn't think so, but they seem interested in me now."

"How do you feel about that?" the GCM asked.

"Oh, I love them visiting and talking with them; I really enjoy that." The GCM asked Mrs. L about her grandson. "That's right, I am a grandmother," said Mrs. L. "I remember Steve's visits a long time ago." The GCM reassured her that the caregivers and the GCM cared and loved her and that she meant a lot to them. Mrs. L said she was glad to hear that. The GCM's goal was to follow up on Mrs. L's statement about the purpose of her life and encourage her to reflect on the meaning of her life. GCMs need to listen to the thoughts and feelings that guide clients and to follow the clients' lead as they reflect on their lives.

CASE STUDY

Mrs. N

A GCM worked with an adult daughter who had difficulty caring for her autocratic, independent mother, Mrs. N, who had a significant dementia, was visually impaired, smoked incessantly, and lived alone in a tiny apartment. Mrs. N, a refugee who worked and brought her family to the United States, where she fought for the rights of workers in a union, was a proud woman who was writing about her martyred father who was killed in Eastern Europe.

For 2 years, the GCM provided consultation to her daughter concerning providing care to her mother, who often refused it, and helped the daughter in her efforts to balance caring for her mother with caring for her own family. In the process the daughter discussed her unresolved relationship issues with her mother. She admired her mother but was saddened by her mother's limited emotional nurturing. The daughter found students to read to her mother and introduced home care in a sensitive manner, using the GCM's services intermittently when problems arose.

The daughter brought her mother to her home for holidays, despite the difficulty in providing care. Mrs. N had another stroke, and the daughter honored her wishes in not taking her to the hospital. Mrs. N's daughter moved into her mother's apartment and took care of her. The GCM talked with the daughter about her mother's condition. A hospice program began to provide care to her mother; the hospice program did not provide workers on a few shifts, but the daughter stoically filled in the gaps in physical and emotional care.

A week after the stroke took place, the daughter called to tell the GCM that her mother had died the previous night. The daughter said the experience had been perfect; it was beautiful to be alone with her mother. She had gone out with friends for dinner and came home relaxed. She sat on the floor and spoke to her mother.

> I told her gently that she was dying— that she had been sick since Monday and now it was Friday. I talked about all her accomplishments, how everyone admired her, including her home care workers. I told her I loved her and that I knew how much she loved me. It was an exquisite moment. I went on to say that I knew that she didn't believe in heaven but suggested that if it were possible that there is a heaven, then perhaps mother could meet and continue her discussions with Roger [a family friend] in heaven.

Mrs. N was very deaf, very ill, and cognitively impaired and her daughter was not sure she had heard her. But Mrs. N smiled, took a few breaths, and then stopped breathing. The GCM said it was wonderful that the daughter could be so present to her mother. The daughter said that she did not feel guilty but perfectly at peace.

Initially, Mrs. N's daughter had great difficulty providing care for her mother because her mother resisted it. Over time, with the support and encouragement of the GCM, she was able to help her mother come to accept the help she needed, while the daughter did what she found possible. Despite her sadness at her mother's earlier emotional unavailability, the daughter was able to care for her mother consistently or use the GCM when she was not able to do so. She was able to help her mother die by being present to her both physically and emotionally, acknowledging her life's gifts and enabling her mother to leave her life with good feelings about herself and her daughter, and with hope for the future. The GCM's support, acknowledgment of the daughter's feelings throughout the difficult caretaking period, and help in providing the daughter with home care assistance and the GCM's presence when needed were all important to the daughter. The daughter was able to rise above her ambivalent feelings and provide care and nurturing to her mother in a loving manner. The GCM witnessed the daughter's inner resources and strength as her mother died and supported all the daughter did for her mother. By being present to their clients' struggles and providing emotional support and concrete assistance, GCMs can help people solidify their own authority to care for their parents.

Ways to Affirm Clients' Spiritual Needs

There are seven ways that GCMs can affirm clients' spiritual needs.

- GCMs can develop a trusting relationship with clients and help them feel safe to express their suffering. Being present to their pain helps clients feel cared for, valued, and respected.
- GCMs can be open to the meaning of illness and loss and to their clients' view of the world.
- GCMs can help clients view themselves beyond just their roles (e.g., father, wife).
- GCMs can talk with clients about clients' beliefs and what has brought meaning to their lives.
- GCMs can appreciate clients' life stories and acknowledge their strengths, struggles, triumphs, and losses.
- GCMs can respect clients' agenda, words, and ways of doing things.[23]
- GCMs can be open to learning from clients and interactions with them, being open-minded and nonjudgmental.[23]

■ FACILITATING SPIRITUAL CONNECTIONS WITH PEOPLE WHO HAVE DEMENTIA AND THEIR FAMILIES

How do GCMs overcome society's negative attitudes toward people with dementia and treat impaired clients with dignity and value, maintaining a person-centered approach? One way is to empathize with the frustrations of clients, whose symptoms will vary over the course of the illness. They will experience changes in their ability to do everyday tasks and will have to abandon work and familiar activities. They may have difficulty communicating and expressing their wishes clearly, have changes in personality and mood, and lack initiative. All these changes can lead to feelings of anger, frustration, fearfulness, anxiety, and sadness. "Living with Alzheimer's means living in a world of fragments. There is a lack of connection. How did I get here? What am I supposed to do next?"[24]

To preserve the humanity of persons who have lost what this culture considers the defining quality of human beings—the ability to think and reason—GCMs need to move to an ethos of care based upon the emotional and relational qualities of human life.[25] GCMs are able to experience the person with dementia without having the emotions of the family, who have witnessed the changes in functioning of the person. In addition to listening to caregivers discuss their difficulties, the GCM should find out what the person's past interests, activities, and roles were and what has changed. What are the person's remaining cognitive abilities, and what does he or she like to do now? Listen to music? Take walks? The caregivers and friends can provide information on the client's values, such as working hard or caring for family members, as well as his or her life story. This helps the GCM better understand the person and be sensitive to the client's values and traditions.

It is important to understand each client's needs and to help the client feel respected, appreciated, loved, known, and understood. Persons with dementia need a sense of belonging—to feel part of a community, to share and give love, and to be productive, helpful, and useful. Because those with dementia lose their ability to fulfill these needs, they may feel frustrated, confused, isolated, and embarrassed.[26]

GCMs need to help clients experience positive connections with caregivers and the GCM. It is important for the GCM to be patient, sensitive, responsive, caring, encouraging, enabling, and empowering in his or her work and to serve as a model for both family and professional caregivers.

Being loved, responded to empathetically, and cared for can help the person with dementia feel more whole and provide a sense of security and peace. Bell and Troxel elucidate a positive and interpersonal approach in working with people with dementia and their families.[26]

Improving Spiritual Connections

In helping persons with dementia experience spiritual connections, it is important to have an idea about their traditions and bring familiar rituals to them to broaden their connections and sense of well-being. For persons with Alzheimer's, familiar symbols of faith connect with the heart rather than the intellect. The emotional or sensory aspects of spirituality take on a greater significance. "Music, hymns, prayers, familiar bible passages and rituals learned early in childhood can reach people with dementia and become a way to express themselves and receive comfort."[27(p2)] GCMs should ask clients and families what these familiar aspects of spirituality might be. "Touch, pictures, poetry, music and faith symbols can be used to communicate in individual contacts and in communal worship."[27(p2)] Clients may respond by joining in or showing nonverbal responses such as nodding, tapping a finger, or moving their body. Rituals of faith are usually learned early in life and can be part of a lifetime of religious practice. "Because they do not completely depend on the intellect they reach emotional levels and tap earlier memory which can connect the client to his past."[27(p2)]

If the client is religious, going to a church or synagogue or otherwise participating in a religious community can help the client feel God's presence as a reassuring haven of stability. It can also provide spiritual assurance that the client is worth more than just his or her cognitive capacity and offer hope to overcome fears about diminished capacity and the uncontrollable. For those without a specific faith tradition or belief system, spiritual needs may be addressed in other ways, such as sharing a sunset, listening to music, holding hands, praying together, or watching services on television.

Improving Family Connections

There are practical, emotional, and spiritual components to working with families whose relatives have dementia. In the following example, a GCM helps some adult children through the various stages of their father's illness and an adult daughter is able to experience her father in a holistic frame, beyond just his illness.

CASE STUDY

Mr. K

A GCM was contacted by the daughter of a 93-year-old man who had dementia, Mr. K. She lived out of town and needed assistance in providing care for her father. Her stepsister lived near her father. The GCM's relationship with the K family spanned 5 years. During this period, the GCM met regularly with the daughters on a schedule that fit into their visits with the father. She focused on understanding how the experience of dementia affected them and helped them listen to each other's perspectives. The GCM encouraged discussion about Mr. K's changed functioning, his forgetfulness, and his intermittent confusion. She encouraged them to reflect on the changes in his behavior, to share their feelings, to empathize with each other, and to work together. The GCM shared information about dementia with the daughters, acknowledging the changes they experienced and recommending books, tapes, and educational meetings to them. She encouraged the daughters to seek support from their partners and friends.

The GCM helped the daughters grieve over losses in their father's functioning while remaining receptive to Mr. K's remaining ability to share his love, his

point of view, and his sense of humor. His daughters shared their good experiences in taking him to the ballet, watching him enjoy art shows, and helping with his care. They continued to share a warm and loving relationship with him.

The GCM engaged the daughters in discussions along the continuum of care from 8 hours a day to two 12-hour shifts of care. The daughters thought a day care program would be helpful for their father. The GCM helped Mr. K get accepted into a day care program that he enjoyed and that provided stimulation for him and oversight of his home attendants. The GCM helped the daughters plan in small steps care for the future, arranging visits to facilities and helping them decide to have the father remain in his home unless it was medically necessary to transfer him to a nursing home. The GCM visited Mr. K and his caregivers and oversaw his care. She provided feedback to his daughters on a regular basis.

Mr. K died peacefully in his home at the age of 98. The tribute that his daughter wrote to him after his death speaks of her love, care, and spiritual growth and the importance of her connection to her father. In this poem she recognizes the contribution her father made as an artist and as a communist: his struggle to make art accessible to the people and for a living wage for artists.

Were you kidding around with me or was this for real?
I found this both disturbing and amusing
I struggled to make sense of what was happening
You didn't know who I was?

I began to feel like I was your memory
you were 93 years old, the main man in my life

*we were kindred spirits, though we were
    separated by 59 years
and you were always there when I got home
    from school*

*Your loss of memory coincided with the
    collapse of the Soviet Union.
I was careful to protect you from knowing that
    your cherished system was crumbling*

*I wondered if you lost your cognitive
    memory to spare yourself the
pain of watching the capitalist class
    toot its triumphant horn
I remind myself that you were 23 when the
    Russian revolution shook
the world up, and you with it.*

*Your loss of memory coming as it does in
    the middle of these celebrations
makes me feel like the context of my youth
    is slipping away
I rush to remember the historic moments
    that became family mantras
the Spanish civil war, the state murder of
    Ethel and Julius Rosenberg
the FBI's witchhunt against communists,
    gay people and labor unions*

*Have I now become a messenger of this
    history that you no longer remember?*

*As you aged, body connection became our
    major communicator.
It was difficult to watch you lose your memory
one of my mirrors was gone
but like you I am learning to be in the moment
not lacking history but assuming it
At some point I stopped reminding you that
    I was your daughter
Our relationship had been transformed by
    your loss of memory
we just were
Because of you I now understand that
    memory is most importantly
about our bodies and our hearts.
without these we cannot do justice to
    our histories*

*Your memory of the struggle was
    embedded in your body and in
    your heart
but the details were gone*

*You had a physical and emotional memory
    of justice and fundamental truth
You had an emotional essence
You were an essence in your stillness
You are the essence of Harry. That's what
    I get:
little fleeting moments of the essence of Harry.
It is a different way of seeing the world and
I take it as a gift.[28]*

This daughter's experience of her father throughout her life as a wonderful caregiver helped her value the positive connections between them that continued despite his dementia.

GCMs' work with families whose relatives have dementia challenges GCMs to help families go beyond grief to find the positive in the situation. The GCM can help the family shift their expectations of their relative, see their relative beyond the dementia, accept the situation, and live in the present. The family member can try to appreciate the relative's deeper values and the values of mutuality and caring throughout the life cycle. GCMs can encourage family members to draw on their inner strength and spiritual resources. Family members can think about how their parent cared for them or how they wish they were cared for. In being fully present to family members, GCMs can help them shift to being present to their relative, as they resolve their grief. Dementia offers persons the opportunity to treasure the moments they share together and live more fully in the present.

■ CONCLUSION

By incorporating a spiritual perspective, GCMs can be a resource in building compassionate communities of care. This perspective broadens the GCM's scope in working with chronically ill and elderly clients and their families in an attempt to help them find meaning and value in their lives.

By viewing the client's frailty as a potentially meaningful part of life, the GCM can share with the client the contributions he or she has made and continues to make. In reviewing his or her own values and spiritual beliefs, the GCM can discern the differences between personal values and client values and be open to and interested in the diverse ways clients find meaning in their lives.

As delineated in this chapter, the spiritual process can be facilitated in many different ways. It is important to enable family members and caregivers to experience the client's spirit beyond his or her illness, and encourage the client to share personal spiritual resources by valuing him or her, carrying out rituals, and being present to the client. In this way, the client's sense of connection to himself or herself, the community, and God can be enhanced.

■ REFERENCES

1. Atchley B. Atchley on aging and spiritual growth. In: Seeber J, ed. *American Society on Aging, Forum on Religion and Spirituality.* 1998;10:6.

2. National Interfaith Coalition on Aging. Spiritual well being: a definition. Presented at: National Interfaith Coalition on Aging; 1975; Athens, GA.

3. Jung C. *Modern Man in Search of Soul.* New York: Harcourt Brace; 1933.

4. Schachter-Shalomi Z, Miller R, eds. *From Ageing to Sage-ing: A Profound New Vision of Growing Older.* New York: Time Warner; 1995.

5. Kenyon GM. Aging and possibilities for being. *Aging and the Human Spirit.* 1992;2:4–5.

6. Leder D. *Spiritual Passages: Embracing Life's Sacred Journey.* New York: Tarcher/Putnam; 1997.

7. Thibault JM. Review of spiritual passages: embracing life's sacred journey. *Aging and the Human Spirit.* 1997;7:9.

8. Magid S. Wrestling with despair: a Jewish response to worry and depression. Presented by the Drisha Institute and the National Center for Jewish Healing; June 14, 1998; New York.

9. Emerson RW. *Essays: First Series.* 1841. New York: Thomas Y Crowell Company; 1926.

10. Atchley RC. The continuity of the spiritual self. In: Kimble MA, McFadden SH, Ellor JW, Seeber J, eds. *Aging, Spirituality and Religion.* Minneapolis, MN: Fortress Press; 1995:68–73.

11. Moberg DO. Spiritual well-being defined. In: Ellor JW, ed. *American Society on Aging, Forum on Religion and Spirituality.*1997:2–3.

12. Genevay B, Richards M. Spiritual growth and psychological development: a concurrent path as we age. *Aging and Spirituality.* 1997;9:4–5.

13. Frankl VD. *Man's Search for Meaning.* Boston, MA: Beacon Press; 1959.

14. Chinen AB. *In the Ever After: Fairy Tales and the Second Half of Life.* Wilmette, IL: Chiron Publications; 1989.

15. Williams CC. Explorers without a map: charting a course to value and meaning. Presented at: American Society on Aging Annual Conference; 1998; San Francisco, CA.

16. Young-Eisendrath P. *The Resilient Spirit: Transforming Suffering into Insight and Renewal.* Reading, MA: Addison Wesley; 1996.

17. Snorton TE. From struggles, dilemmas, and events in ages past. *Aging and Spirituality.* 1995;7:3.

18. Riemer J. *So That Your Values Live On: Ethical Wills and How to Prepare Them.* Woodstock, VT: Jewish Lights Publishing; 1991.

19. Alzheimer's Association, National Alliance for Caregiving. *Who Cares? Families Caring for Persons with Alzheimer's Disease.* Washington, DC: Alzheimer's Association, National Alliance for Caregiving; 1999.

20. Personal communication with Marty Richards, 1999.

21. Genevay B, Katz RS. *Countertransference and Older Clients.* Newburg Park, CA: Sage Publications; 1990.

22. Fitchett G. *Assessing Spiritual Needs. A Guide for Caregivers.* MN: Augsburg Fortress; 1992.

23. Simon D. Healing and the spirit: tapping spiritual resources to facilitate a more positive experience of life's final stage. Presented at: American Society on Aging, Summer Series; July 1998; New York.

24. Gwyther L. Helping congregations maintain a connection to spirit in the Alzheimer's disease experience. Presented at: Annual Meeting of the American Society on Aging; March 1999; Orlando, FL.

25. Post SG. *The Moral Challenge of Alzheimer Disease.* Baltimore, MD: Johns Hopkins University Press; 1995.

26. Bell V, Troxel D. *The Best Friends Approach to Alzheimer's Care.* Baltimore, MD: Health Professionals Press; 1997.

27. Richards M. Meeting the spiritual needs of the cognitively impaired. *Aging and Spirituality.* 1994;7:2.

28. Gottlieb A. In Living Memory [videotape]. Toronto, Ontario: VTape; 1997.

Chapter 9

Assessing and Supporting the Family Caregiver

Cathy Jo Cress

■ BACKGROUND

Family caregiving is the snapping spine of America's long-term care system. Today, it is estimated that approximately 65 million adults provide unpaid assistance as well as physical and emotional support to their relatives and friends, with an attributed economic value of $275 billion annually. This staggering figure exceeds the combined costs of nursing home care ($92 billion) and home health care ($32 billion).[1]

Those who provide this unpaid, loving assistance are generally referred to as *informal* caregivers, in contrast to paid agency or private caregivers, who are the *formal* caregivers. Most informal caregivers are women. The percentage of family or informal caregivers estimated to be women by the Family Caregiver Alliance (FCA), is 59–75%. The average caregiver, according to FCA, is 46, female, married, and working outside the home in addition to her unpaid caregiver job. At her paid job, she earns a paltry $35,000.[1]

More elders are alive today than at any other time in history, and the numbers, as everyone knows from baby-boomer media, are exploding. Advances in public health and the medical management of acute and chronic diseases have contributed to increased longevity and the graying of the population. The flip side of these medical advances is that they brought us a nation of elders with

chronic care needs that can last half a lifetime. With the fastest growing US population being those who are over 85 years old, this vulnerable group has greater needs for health care. The resulting building pressures on the acute and long-term care systems is escalating both logistically and fiscally, generating serious societal alarms. One major concern is the nature and scope of caregiving for elders has been ballooning. On average, chronically ill and disabled recipients need informal caregivers to the point where now one in four Americans is now an unpaid informal caregiver.

The development and expansion of the Medicare and Medicaid programs over the last 40 years have provided greater access to health care for the elderly. These entitlements, to a great extent, supported nursing homes and other long-term care services in their first two decades. However, over the last two decades, there has been a big shift from institutional care to more community-based and home health care. DRGs, or diagnosis-related groups, have been used to affect cost savings for Medicare and Medicaid. This has dramatically shortened hospital stays and thus shifted the responsibility and many of the costs for post-hospital management from paid hospital staff such as doctors and nurses to unpaid, largely untrained family members in the home. Gail Sheehy, in her new book on caregiving, suggests that DRGs and their sometimes abrupt and catastrophic effects on discharge should have the American public "following the money" and assessing how hospitals and the healthcare system benefit from DRGs and how care providers and patients suffer.[2] Even though at-home care is the preference of many seniors, there is little bolstering infrastructure to support older people who wish to remain at home. The result is most of older people's care is provided by largely unsupported, untrained, unprepared family members.

Given the dramatic increase in the numbers of frail elders, their increased need for care, and the budgetary constraints of public and private insurance programs and other funding sources, the role of the family in providing long-term care will inevitably continue its flood tide. With this swelling and overflow of care needs, informal family caregivers are seeking training, information, education, guidance, and emotional support and increased public and private providers to deliver these services. Geriatric care managers (GCMs) have an important role in building this desperately needed platform for drowning family caregivers.

Family structures today are more diverse than ever before; in addition to the traditional nuclear family, there are single-parent families, gay families, blended families, and grandparents raising grandchildren. Most women are in the workforce, seeking to financially support families and themselves. This is a sharp departure from the Depression era and the silent generations of women who stayed at home, available to provide child care and, when necessary, parent care. In the explosion of blended families, forged by remarriage after divorce or widowhood, there are often increased numbers of parents and grandparents who demand care.

Family caregiving is fraught with dilemmas. New roles and responsibilities are acquired, often unexpectedly, with no job descriptions, little preparation, and few, if any, role models. The caregiving duties are heaped on already full plates of work and family demands, piled on top of personal responsibilities and needs. For many individuals, caregiving is a long-term commitment, often lasting years—so long, in fact, that gerontologists speak of the caregiving career. The average woman today will spend more years providing parent care than she did child care.

This caregiving burden comes with substantial costs. There are adverse physical, emotional, and social effects.[3] In fact, research has revealed that caregivers experience excess morbidity and mortality. They develop stress-related illnesses and injuries. Depression is prevalent among them. They also suffer shrinking social networks. And there are consequences in the workplace—time lost, opportunities missed for advancement, and economic losses in terms of earnings, benefits, and pensions. These economic impacts will also have repercussions for the caregiver's own later years. Caregiving kin can face a mired swamp of legal problems through wills, trust, and inheritance issues involving the family members they care for. Caregivers can risk serious injury. The "sicker and quicker" DRG discharges in the American hospital system create a caregiving nightmare. Family caregivers then face older relatives discharged with pumps, IV lines, or wounds that require care needs that involve nursing skills. Most family caregivers are untrained and unprepared to render this level of medical care. They also risk personal injury through turning, lifting, and repositioning the client. Nancy Guberman, MSW, points out if family caregivers were paid and employed by a home health agency, they would be a worker's compensation nightmare.[3]

Untrained, undersupported, and emotionally stressed, family caregivers may, paradoxically, at times have a negative effect on their frail elder's well-being. Whether intentionally or inadvertently, the care they provide may be inadequate. Overburdened or burned out caregivers may become neglectful or even abusive to their care recipient. The strain of family caregivers can be overwhelming, a fact that the GCM needs to understand to deliver good care to our GCM client.

Other nations have seen this more clearly than the United States and we are, it seems, slow to learn this lesson. In 1995, the United Kingdom legislated the Recognition and Services Act, which afforded British caregivers a statutory right to ask for a caregiver assessment at the same time that a frail elder or adult with disability is assessed.[4]

■ WHO IS THE FAMILY CAREGIVER?

Generally, the family caregiver is a spouse, partner, child, or other relative who provides a range of assistance for an elderly or disabled person. They can be primary caregivers or secondary caregivers who give direct care or supervise the care given by someone else. Most are middle aged, and their ages range from 35–64 years old. Ethnicity varies but 21% are both white and African-American, 18% Asian, and 18% Hispanic.

One out of two caregivers are women.[5] Typically, the family caregiver is a daughter or daughter-in-law, but men are becoming increasingly involved. For some elders (about 20%), friends and neighbors fill this role. These informal caregivers may provide care in conjunction with others, paid or unpaid, and may live with or apart from the individual receiving care (i.e., the care recipient). The caregiver is often self-defined or identified by the care recipient, but even this is not so clear cut. Factors such as divorce, poorly blended family structures, estrangement, conflict, burnout, illness, disability, competition for being the favorite child, differing values, and unrealistic notions of the care recipient or caregiver are factors that may affect the actual care giving situation.

■ ASSESSING THE CAREGIVER

Although family and informal caregivers make up 78% of the long-term care system in the United States, geriatric care managers have not focused on the actual backbone that supports the care receiver, the GCM's aging client. Family caregivers' are overwhelmed by caregiver burnout, stress and overload. Geriatric care managers need to begin to see caregivers and care receivers as one organism. Caregivers are part of a homeostatic system including the care receiver and one cannot be separated from the other. If the caregiver's functional and psychosocial needs go unmet then the whole GCM care plan falls apart. So the GCM needs to take a whole-family approach and see that they have multiple clients, including the older person and the family caregivers.

Assessing the Family Caregiver

To meet the needs of the whole family, principally the care receiver and the caregivers, GCMs need to begin assessing the caregiver as well as the care receiver. A caregiver assessment is defined by the National Center on Caregiving at the Family Caregiver Alliance as a systematic process of gathering information that describes the caregiving situation and identifies particular problems, needs, resources, and strengths of a family caregiver. This new measure approaches issues from a caregiver's perspective and culture, focuses on what assistance the caregiver may need, examines outcomes the family member wants for support, and seeks to maintain the caregiver's own health and well-being.[6]

The National Center for Caregiving Alliance states that no one caregiver assessment tool fits all settings and situations. A suggested GCM caregiver assessment tool is offered in Exhibit 9–1. In general, a caregiving assessment tool should be tailored to the caregiving context, service setting, and program. The National Center for Caregiving at

Exhibit 9–1   Caregiver Assessment Tool for Care Manager

What triggered the caregiver assessment? _____

1. Basic caregiver information

    GCM assessors name _____   Date of interview _____

    In-person/phone/Skype/e-mail _____

    Caregiver's name _____   Care receiver's name _____

    Caregiver's telephone _____   Caregiver's sex   F   M

    Caregiver's address _____   Same as care receiver   N   Y

    Caregiver relationship to care receiver _____

2. Hours caregiver cares for care receiver

    All the time   N   Y

    Days (circle)   M   T   W   T   F   S   SU

    Hours per day   M _____, Tu _____, W _____, Th _____, F _____, Sa _____, Su _____

    How long has caregiver been caring for care receiver? _____ years   _____ months

3. Informal supports for caregiver (friends, neighbor family who help with ADLs IADLs)

    Help provided _____

    Name _____   Location _____

    Phone _____

    Relationship to care receiver _____

    Help provided _____

    Name _____   Location _____

    Phone _____

    Relationship to care receiver _____

    (Use back of page for more listings.)

    Is there anyone else that might help you with care receiver?

    _____

4. Formal supports (homecare agencies, adult day care, senior transportation, elder-law attorney)

    Present formal supports to help caregivers:

    Name _____

    Help provided _____

    Name _____

    Help provided _____

    Name _____

    Help provided _____

    Name _____

    Help provided _____

    (Use back of page for more listings.)

Exhibit 9–1   **Caregiver Assessment Tool for Care Manager** (continued)

5. Cultural needs

Language spoken by caregiver _____

Language spoken by care receiver _____

Informal or formal supports needed by caregiver if languages are different   N   Y

Describe: _____

Translator needed if caregiver does not speak care manager's language   N   Y

Name: _____

6. Limitations of care giver

Poor health   N   Y

Diagnosis: _____

Disabled   N   Y

Disability: _____

Doing tasks that are repulsive   N   Y

Describe: _____

Frail   N   Y

Describe: _____

Employed elsewhere   N   Y   _____ days   _____ hours

Providing care to others   N   Y   To whom? _____

Hours _____

Lack knowledge/skills   N   Y

Describe: _____

Poor relationship with care receiver   N   Y

Describe: _____

Long-distance care provider   N   Y

Lives where? _____

Alcohol, drug abuse   N   Y

Describe: _____

Unable to do ADLs   N   Y

Describe: _____

Unable to do IADLs   N   Y

Describe: _____

Financial strain   N   Y

Describe: _____

Dependent on care receiver for housing   N   Y

Describe: _____

7. Additional assessments for caregiver

Score on Zarit Burden _____

Score on GDS given to caregiver _____

continues

Exhibit 9–1   Caregiver Assessment Tool for Care Manager (continued)

8. Interventions needed for caregiver

   Formal supports needed by caregiver   N   Y
   Describe: _____
   Training needed by caregiver   N   Y
   Describe: _____
   Education resources needed for caregiver   N   Y
   Describe: _____
   Technology needed   N   Y
   Describe: _____
   Organizing tools needed for caregiver (e.g., calendar) _____
   Referral to physician needed for caregiver   N   Y
   Describe: _____
   Stress relief needed for caregiver   N   Y
   Describe: _____
   Respite needed for caregiver   N   Y
   Describe: _____
   Advocacy needed for caregiver   N   Y
   Describe: _____
   Family dysfunction impairing care   N   Y
   Describe: _____
   Emotional or mental health resources   N   Y
   Describe: _____
   Support group needed   N   Y
   Describe: _____

9. Caregiver care plan
   Problems = list
   Fill in what is needed if Y circled in section 8
   Formal supports needed _____
   Respite _____
   Education _____
   Training needed _____
   Impaired health _____
   Hours need reducing _____
   Depression _____
   High stress level _____
   Lives long distance _____
   Alcohol, drug abuse _____
   Family dysfunction _____
   Other _____

Use problems checked off in problems list above to create care management care plan for caregiver:

Caregiver Care Plan
Problems   *Interventions*
_____
_____
_____
_____

the Family Caring Alliance has suggested that no one approach to a caregiver assessment tool fits all.[7] This caregiver assessment tool is a suggested template to fit your particular GCM setting and situation. Carmen and Barbara Morano also suggest the stress and appraisal coping framework, developed by Perlin, in their article on caregiver assessment in the *GCM Journal*.[8] You can also use Zarit's Caregiver Burden in Exhibit 7 in Chapter 20 although it should be used along with a caregiver assessment tool.

The National Center for Caregiving states that seven domains should be measured in a caregiver assessment. These domains are:

1. The context of the caregiving rendered by the caregiver
2. The caregiver's perception of the health and functional status of the care recipient
3. The caregiver's values and preferences
4. The well-being of the caregiver
5. The consequences of caregiving
6. The skills, abilities, and knowledge needed to provide care
7. The potential resources the caregiver could choose to use[9]

What Triggers a Caregiver Assessment? When to Assess the Caregiver

One trigger for a GCM to do a caregiver assessment is at the initial GCM geriatric assessment and intake, when you start services with the client. However, generally, the caregiver should be assessed after the GCM has fully assessed the care receiver. All services should be in place for the care receiver initially because the caregiver will usually be totally focused on the care receiver and unwilling to be distracted to concentrate on their own problems. In a second visit the GCM can then assess the caregiver.

There can be many exceptions to this rule. If the family is so overwhelmed by the care that they are considering placement, this

threat should trigger the GCM to do a caregiver assessment immediately. If the GCM is called to relocate an older person and the underlying cause seems to be caregiver burnout, this can be another trigger for a caregiver assessment. If caregiver abuse is suspected, a caregiver assessment is a critical immediate tool. This is a situation where the GCM must contact Adult Protective Services, following their own state's laws. Elder abuse can be triggered by caregiver stress in some situations. Depression that reaches a clinical level in a caregiver can be predictive of elder abuse.[10] Hospitalization of an elderly client can prompt a GCM to do a caregiver assessment. If the medical condition that caused the hospitalization results in a decline in the older client's ADLs, the caregiver may have to have a higher skill level. As hospitalized patients are discharged sicker and quicker, caregivers may have to lift, give injections, change dressings, or complete care tasks they are unable and unskilled enough to do. This is especially true of elderly spouses, who can have back problems, vision loss, and be unable to care for an older husband or wife when the aging spouse is discharged.

The GCM should consider doing a caregiver assessment when he or she sees a change in level of care due to a hospitalization. This may prompt the GCM arranging training on the part of the hospital, increased community services to support care, or family intervention and support to identify another family caregiver or hiring paid caregivers.[11] A professional referral to a GCM can prompt a caregiver assessment. Any professional in the continuum of care may come in contact with your elderly client and their caregiver and discover problems with the ongoing care. This can range from Adult Protective Services to parish nurses to their care providers, neighbors, friends, or other homecare workers.

Caregiver assessment can be prompted by all these triggers. Caregiver assessment should also be built into the GCM's care monitoring on a regular basis. The caregiver assessment should be done periodically if the family or client agrees to this particular assessment. If the GCM is monitoring the client on a regular basis, the care manager can track changes in the caregiver's skill level, stressors, and physical health to see if there is a decline that warrants a change in a caregiver or support to keep that caregiver in place.

Where to Assess

Caregiver assessment is best done in the care receiver's home so you can actually observe the care. It is best completed out of earshot of the older person who is cared for so the caregiver can feel free to talk openly. As caregivers suffer high levels of stress, giving them a separate space to share their feelings is an important part of the caregiver assessment. However, the caregiver assessment should be done in a place that is convenient to the caregiver, which could be a donut shop, their home, or any comfortable venue. If the GCM must arrange respite, like bringing in another family member or paid caregiver to do the caregiver assessment, then that is another way to make this assessment go forward.

Connecting the Caregiver and Care Receiver Assessment

How are these two primary GCM assessments, a care receiver assessment and caregiver assessment, linked? Will there be duplication? The caregiver assessment is connected to the care receiver assessment through your care plan, which is the GCM's most potent tool. Your GCM care plan lays out the problems and solutions of the client. Many times the problem is the type of care the client is getting. So the care receiver's solution to a care problem can be suggesting a change in the way the care provider delivers that care or a change in the care personnel.

In our case study, caregiver Bertha has been caring for her partner Alfonso for about a year. She is burning out, and there is stress between his children from his former marriage and herself. The adult child Penelope has called you, GCM Ms. Goodhelp, to do a caregiver and client assessment. You use the caregiver assessment tool (see Exhibit 9–1) and find the following results.

Mr. Alfonso Paul

Problem

Mr. Paul's daughter, Penelope La Resto, agreed to work with the geriatric care manager because of her increasing concern about her father and his live-in companion Bertha. Penelope's aging father Alfonso is becoming increasingly dependent and caregiver Bertha is becoming overwhelmed by her caregiver role. The daughter is concerned that caring for Mr. Paul is too much responsibility for one person, and Bertha is becoming increasingly stressed and burnt out. The daughter who hired you to do the caregiver assessment walks a subtle line. She appreciates all that Bertha does for her father and doesn't want to put a hole in the tire. Caregiver and live-in companion Bertha, on the other hand, is sometimes suspicious of the adult children, who have no relationship to her, as Mr. Paul and Bertha are not married. Bertha feels that the adult children are judging her. Penelope would like someone objective, such as a GCM to come in and help prioritize her father's needs, get some additional help, and get confirmation that issues of concern are being addressed.

History

Mr. Paul was born September 22, 1924, in Atlantic City, New Jersey, but he has lived most of his life in Ventnor, New

Jersey, where he practiced law until he retired in 1986. He was widowed with four young children. He has lived in the same neighborhood for over 47 years, moving from his family home 14 years ago into a beautiful beach house that would accommodate aging in place with his best friend Susan. She was diagnosed with kidney failure and died soon after they both sold their homes and moved in together. Mr. Paul met Bertha Mully through the Internet. After a long-distance relationship of frequent visits, she relocated from a large city 1 hour away to share her life with him. They have not married, but live a married life. She almost left 2 years ago, but has stayed and has taken on increasingly greater caregiver tasks.

His children are spread throughout the country. Son Gino lives 1 hour away in the Franklin Lakes near where Bertha is from. Son Pete lives across the country in Arizona. Emily, the youngest adult child, lives in Great Neck, New York. Penelope is the adult child who lives locally, within a 10-minute drive from her home and workplace in Somers Point, New Jersey. None of the adult children have a warm relationship with Bertha and as result do not see their father very often.

Assessment of Client Mr. Paul

Mr. Paul suffers from short-term memory problems and poor hearing. He has increasingly limited vision. He has a deteriorating arthritic spine that now has him in a wheelchair. He has problems with IADLs, so he cannot write checks or pay his bills alone. The GCM performed a psychosocial assessment on February 7, 2010, using the following tools: a mini-mental state exam, a clock drawing test, the geriatric mood scale, a psychosocial assessment, a functional assessment, the geriatric depression scale, the Beck anxiety inventory, and a genogram.

Daughter Penelope has expressed fear about her father's failing memory. Penelope was concerned that her father may be depressed because of his increasing limitations and his social isolation. The geriatric depression scale did not indicate any evidence of depression. Mr. Paul expressed satisfaction with his life and expressed general cheerfulness, although Mr. Paul has said at times that feels he is a burden to care provider Bertha and wishes he saw more of his children.

Mr. Paul cannot complete most of his ADLs in a wheelchair and has a home-health aide to assist him with most activities of daily living. Bertha is his partner, caregiver, and the basis of his social network. Mr. Paul gets very anxious if Bertha leaves him with others. Bertha does all housekeeping, shopping, makes all appointments, administers medications, coordinates with a home care agency, which comes in to get him bathed and dressed. Bertha and Mr. Paul pay bills together. Bertha is his healthcare proxy. There is no durable power of attorney. At one point, the daughter Penelope had helped her father with his Excel spread sheets and QuickBooks when her father's vision started to fail. Bertha became suspicious when she discovered the daughter was intervening with Mr. Paul's finances. Some of the investments are controlled by son Pete. Finances have become a difficult issue. Mr. Paul is becoming less willing to expend cash, and Bertha is uncomfortable spending without his permission, even for increased services that would offer her respite and are covered by Medicare.

They no longer socialize with old friends and have become socially isolated. They no longer attend mass together, which they used to do every Sunday morning, followed by a coffee hour, which they really enjoyed. Bertha drives him where they need to go in his wheelchair van. The bathroom has been retrofitted with handrails, toilet adaptation, and shower seat that slides in and out of the tub area. However, he no longer has the strength to use the seat and is bathed standing up by the aide.

His poor hearing has increased his isolation, as he has a hard time hearing even when someone is sitting right next to him. He has stopped communicating to his out-of-town children on the telephone. Bertha also has an increasingly hard time talking with him and is frustrated by her need to frequently repeat what she has said. He sees the audiologist regularly. His audiologist has stated there could be improvements to his overall hearing with different adaptations, but Mr. Paul has refused to pay for these out of pocket as Medicare will not cover them.

Two years ago Bertha left Mr. Paul alone and came home to find there had been a break-in and the burglar had thrown Mr. Paul to the floor. Since then, Mr. Paul becomes very upset when she goes out, and she is too worried to leave him alone. He has refused to purchase a personal emergency system.

Caregiver Assessment

The GCM interviewed Bertha alone on February 8 to assess her caregiver strain and overload. Bertha appears to have a bad back, vision problems, and high blood pressure at 77 years old. She is overwhelmed, lonely, and without her old social supports. She needs help with his care, a support network, and a channel for her own interests. She has potentially serious health concerns that she has not dealt with. She needs to have an

MRI on her shoulder, which she has put off. She has noticed vision problems of her own and has had blurry vision and blood in her eye. She suspects macular degeneration but has avoided taking care of herself and going to the doctor. She has high blood pressure, which she takes medication for, but because she is stressed, it can rise. She also has family and property in Atco, New Jersey that she needs to take care of periodically. She takes Mr. Paul with her, but he gets very agitated when left with his son at a nearby motel in Cherry Hill.

There is a strained relationship between Penelope, the other children, and Bertha. There is financial suspicion on both sides. Bertha would like them to have a healthier connection. Penelope has had another stepmother and is deferential and thankful of what Bertha has done for her father. However, Penelope does not want to go as far as creating a loving relationship. Penelope's paying for the GCM caregiver assessment is a step she feels is offering support to Bertha. Penelope has offered to help in the areas that she can be most useful. She is a technical writer and writes yet unpublished romance novels on the side, so she has computer skills. She works full time and has three children of her own so cannot help with her father's personal care. She would like to take over her Dad's finances, as would her other three siblings. This is a conflict between the adult children and Bertha, the live-in girlfriend.

Care Plan

1. **Problem:** Mr. Paul has severe hearing loss and needs new hearing aids in both ears.

   Intervention: The GCM will follow up with the client regarding an appointment with audiologist. Then the GCM will follow up with getting new hearing aids.

2. **Problem:** Mr. Paul has impaired communications with all three of his children.

   Intervention: The GCM will set up a family meeting and facilitate between the three adult children and Bertha to discovers ways that Mr. Paul could communicate better with his children. The GCM will arrange visits of adult children to Mr. Paul on a monthly basis.

3. **Problem:** Bertha needs weekly respite from caring for Mr. Paul.

   Intervention: The GCM will arrange a trial day at the Frank Farley Adult Day Program. This solution would be for 2 days a week where they have bingo, a favorite of Mr. Paul.

4. **Problem:** Bertha has a bad left shoulder and should not be lifting.

   Interventions: The GCM will arrange weekly housecleaning by Merry Maids.

5. **Problem:** Bertha has been preparing all meals and assisting with some bathing and grooming. She has shown symptoms of caregiver overload.

   Intervention: The GCM will arrange for the private duty agency Livhome to provide aides 8 hours a day, 5 days a week, to offer respite to Bertha so she can attend to medical appointments and have time to herself. The GCM will coach Mr. Paul on the importance of care to lessen care provider burden on Bertha and risk that she would leave and increase care costs for him.

6. **Problem:** Bertha and the adult children have a remote, cold relationship and the adult children have not discussed this or their father's problems in depth with each other.

   Intervention: The GCM will arrange an initial family meeting with all the adult children via videoconference and facilitate the meeting to discuss working together as a team to help their dad. One goal of the team will be to develop a better, more trusting relationship with Bertha. The GCM will create the agenda for the family meeting, send it to all the children, record the family meeting, send minutes with agreements and goals to all the children, and have them sign off on the minutes. The GCM will coach Bertha to do a caregiving journal to track her feelings about caregiving, Mr. Paul, and her relationship with his children.

7. **Problem:** Mr. Paul misses attending religious services. He enjoys the mass and misses the sense of the Catholic community. There are also few opportunities for Penelope the daughter to spend time alone with her father.

   Interventions: Each Sunday, Penelope will come to their house and take her father to mass. If she is comfortable taking him out afterwards, they can go out for dessert to a handicap-accessible restaurant. Penelope will stay with her father until 1 pm.

8. **Problem:** Finances are becoming a constant worry for Mr. Paul and further stressing Bertha, making her feel uncomfortable spending money to make both of their lives more comfortable. Penelope has tried to address some of the financial issues but has been met with resistance.

Intervention: The GCM will arrange for a second family meeting via videoconference. Finances and who will handle them will be one topic on the agenda. Penelope will consult with Mr. Paul's elder-law attorney and accountant to find out what information the siblings can access. The GCM will facilitate the family meeting agenda, set rules, take minutes, and send the minutes to all adult children.

9. **Problem:** There is no long-range plan in place should something happen to Bertha.

   Intervention: The GCM will arrange a third family meeting via videoconference to create a future plan for what will happen if Bertha leaves Mr. Paul or is disabled. A plan will be discussed and made.

10. **Problem:** Bertha feels isolated from her own family and old friends, which have become a low priority.

    Intervention: Bertha will use her respite time on the weekends when the adult children visit to go and stay with her own family and friends in Atco.

11. **Problem:** Bertha needs respite.

    Intervention: The adult children of Mr. Paul who live on the East Coast will take a weekend each month giving Bertha respite to visit her own family in Atco. West Coast son Pete will visit every 3 months for 5 days and include a weekend in the visit. The GCM will set up a Google calendar to keep track of all visits of all the adult children, and all will share the calendar.

12. **Problem:** Bertha is in need of emotional support to bear the stresses of caregiving. She would benefit from a caregiver support group.

    Interventions: The GCM will refer Bertha to a caregiver support facilitator at Knucky Johnson Memorial Senior Center that meets weekly on Monday nights. A facilitator will make a home visit to introduce the group to Bertha.

13. **Problem:** Bertha may have serious shoulder problems.

    Intervention: New care providers from LivHome will do all Mr. Paul's transfers from out of the wheelchair and in and out of bed. Bertha will make an appointment with her doctor to have an MRI on her shoulder.

14. **Problem:** Bertha may have macular degeneration.

    Intervention: Bertha will make an appointment to have a full eye exam.

15. **Problem:** The relationship with adult children needs to be better developed and nurtured.

    Intervention: The GCM to set up a videoconference via Skype with each adult child except Penelope once a week. She will visit an hour before the first two sessions to coach Mr. Paul and Bertha how to better communicate their needs and experiences. The GCM will set up a Facebook site dedicated to Mr. Paul where all the adult children and Bertha can become friends.

■ BARRIERS TO CAREGIVER ASSESSMENT

The number one barrier to doing a caregiver assessment is whether the family will pay for this additional assessment process. In the initial intake process, the GCM agreed contractually to assess the older client. To take this extra step and assess the caregiver makes the process more nuanced and expensive. The caregiver may balk at both time and cost. One roadblock here is that many caregivers do not see themselves as caregivers but as family, so they may find the assessment confusing and unneeded. Often they do not see themselves as part of the client problem, but the major solution, so assessing themselves may be rejected. Caregivers also classically neglect themselves in favor of the care receiver and so may balk at spending extra money to repair their own safety net.

Selling the Caregiver Assessment to the Family

How does GCM sell this caregiver assessment to the family caregiver? The care manager will have to make the link between the needs and health of the caregiver and care receiver crystal clear. Underscoring that the caregiver cannot care for the client if they themselves are ill or unhealthy is often a good way to approach this. You can meet their resistance by emphasizing that this is all about making them strong enough to continue to render care. This means being convinced yourself as a GCM that the caregiver assessment is a needed product. You can't sell this to the caregiver or family unless you believe in it yourself. You have to understand that if your caregiver falls apart, your care plan also falls apart. Assessing the care provider means an intact care plan, no unnecessary placement, and less chance of hiring expensive private home care.

Integrating a Caregiver Assessment in a GCM Agency

A second major barrier to a caregiver assessment is making the paradigm shift with your GCM staff if you work in an agency. This transition in thinking needs to reach across all administrative lines from your mission statement down to the frontline geriatric care manager. Your organization must be in agreement that you not only assess the client but also the caregiver because only seeing the needs of both will create a care plan with true change. What does this take? It means meeting and reassessing your operations manual and deciding that this is an additional step you want to take in delivering client services.

If you can afford it, this may take revisiting your corporate vision. You may have to rewrite your business plan, your mission, and your operations manual to include this. Once you have agreed on the importance of caregiver assessments, it will mean having all your administrators, supervisors, and in-field care managers in full agreement that this is a shift you will make.

One major impact on a geriatric care management agency that a caregiver assessment can have is increased time spent by care managers, thus increased billing to the client. Another impact is that the organization itself will spend unreimbursed money to revise its entire operations. This will mean revising your operations to include caregiver assessments. This will trigger the creation of new policies and procedures to include a caregiver assessment, expanding client records to include the information from a caregiver assessment, and measuring the budgetary effects of making all these operational changes. You may also have to reassess case load size for an individual care manager as the GCM will have to spend more time with each individual client by doing a caregiver assessment.

The National Center for Caregiving at the Family Caregiving Alliance says that one of the biggest barriers for an organization adding a caregiver assessment is the length of the caregiver assessment tool. It behooves your GCM organization to add a brief but effective caregiver assessment tool so that it takes less time for the GCMs to do the assessment.

■ TRAINING THE GCM TO ASSESS THE CAREGIVER

If your organization decides to move forward and include caregiver assessment into its training curricula, you will have to educate your GCM staff to use this assessment tool. If you have a single private practice, you will have to educate yourself. One of the first steps you must take is to change the point of view of the GCM, whether it be yourself or an entire staff.

In the United Kingdom, where they have been doing caregiver assessment nationally since 1995, they advocate for the care manager to develop an entire new mindset. The English social service describes this new attitude as a "caregiver in partner approach."[12] In the United States, we have too long looked at family caregivers as secondary sources of problems or information when they are actually integral to our care plan. This new approach demands that we as GCMs look at the family caregiver as an equal partner in delivering the appropriate care for the client as described in the care plan. Training of the GCM must start with this shift in attitude.

After reframing the GCM attitude that caregivers are secondary in assessment, training for caregivers assessment must include specific training in the assessment tool your agency uses, caregiver skills, family and caregiving dynamics, and resources in your community to train and support caregivers.

■ THE GCM ASSESSMENT OF THE FAMILY TO HELP THE FAMILY CAREGIVER

The extended family of the care receiver should be assessed during the GCM's initial intake to find their strengths, weaknesses, and abilities to render caregiving services. Using a genogram suggested in Chapter 3 can be helpful in assessing the care receiver's family support network and each relative's relationship to the older client. The genogram, when paired with a psychosocial assessment, can help the GCM assess whether the older client is living with a helpful spouse or partner, living with a difficult spouse, has a relationship with an ex-spouse, has cooperative and supportive children or grandchildren, has fighting or alienated children or grandchildren, has fighting or alienated stepchildren or adopted children, or has several children but only one child who does all the caregiving The genogram also can help tell the GCM whether there are ex-spouses or partners who want to participate as caregivers and what their emotional relationship is to the care receiver.

An assessment through a genogram will help you assess whether any extended family and friends will make suitable and emotionally appropriate caregivers or not. For example, if a son has a historically strained relationship with his father, is he a good choice as a caregiver? The genogram will help to assess this old family tension and help the GCM make a decision with the family as to who can really be a good caregiver.

By doing a psychosocial assessment outlined in Chapter 3 the GCM can assess key abilities and availabilities for the extended network of family caregivers.. Your psychosocial assessment should tell you as a GCM the client's financial status, including income, assets, benefits currently being received, health and long-term care insurance coverage, and eligibility or potential eligibility for entitlement programs. This will help you assess whether outside paid care providers can be afforded if needed.

Your psychosocial assessment done at intake or updated as more care is needed should tell you about the family, formal and informal support network, present and potential caregivers, and cultural variables.

Family Meetings to Solve the Caregiver Issue

A family meeting is a gathering of the extended or immediate family to identify the older person's needs, create a plan to meet those needs, and implement that plan to increase the quality of life of the older person. The plan that comes out of the family meeting most often establishes a critical action list of steps to take for the immediate and long-term safety, health, and psychosocial well-being of the older adult.[13]

According to Dr. Rita Ghatak, in her chapter "Family Meetings and the Aging Family," there are many common reasons to hold a family meeting.[14] Ghatak states that a red flag that often generates a family meeting is caregiver stress and burden.[14] If caregiver stress is assessed at a very high level by the caregiver herself or the GCM, a family meeting can be called by the GCM to come up with a plan to deal with that caregiver stress. First, the caregiver assessment and care receiver assessments (both functional and psychosocial or more as needed), should be done by the GCM to assess caregiver stress levels and pinpoint what other formal support, such as adult day care, support groups and informal support can be used to support the caregiver and older client.

After those assessments, the family meeting can be convened by the GCM and the family to discuss whether the caregiver who is presently is charge of the care of the older person needs to be replaced, provided respite by

other family members, supplied paid caregivers to supplement the care he or she is giving, or supported in any way by the formal or informal continuum of care or the family itself. For example, a family meeting decision could be that a long-distance adult child will foot the bill to hire paid caregivers, giving respite to a caregiver sister. Caregiver stress and solutions can be a prime reason to have a family meeting.

The GCM can suggest the family meeting to the key members of the immediate and extended family, organize the meeting, create the agenda and distribute it, help set the meeting rules, and find a mediator if necessary. The GCM can also act as a facilitator but should not act as a mediator, unless she or he has that highly trained skill set.. See Chapter 22 on mediation to help make a good choice about whether you have the experience level and skill set to simply facilitate or can actually mediate a family meeting.

Gail Sheehy, in her book Passages in Caregiving, strongly suggests having a family meeting over caregiving issues and offers some guidelines for families seeking this tool.[15] Sheehy proposes not involving the care receiver at the first meeting. The first family meeting should be held to set your overall plan for caregiving and reduce immediate caregiver tension or family problems around caregiving. Jagged family issues such as sibling struggles and brothers' and sisters' lifelong battles need to be addressed at this point. If solutions like sibling forgiveness need to be settled before caregiving problems can be solved, the older client should not be present. Other strategies like a forgiveness system might be tapped into as a goal before caregiving could be shared by adult child siblings.[16]

The GCM should have a thorough background in midlife sibling issues before she or he tackles a family meeting. Sparks can fly because adult brothers and sisters are gathering as a team for the first time since childhood, at a family meeting, called to face a red hot aging parent problem. Organizing this first family caregiver and sibling team is a good reason to have a first family meeting. The GCM must know sibling dynamics, such as the parental caregiving patterns in midlife siblings, sibling aid and direct services, and sibling rivalry extended into midlife.[17]

The geriatric care manager should query all family members who will attend the family meeting ahead of time to talk about caregiving concerns and what they might be personally willing to do to solve these problems. The GCM should record all conversations in service notes, e-mails, and electronic records.

With this family member input on individual and group issues in caregiving, the GCM can then create an agenda for the family meeting, covering all the caregiver concerns and problems, from everyone's point of view. You as the GCM can facilitate the meeting. If you feel that the agenda with the family members requires a high level of negotiation (see Chapter 22), hiring a mediator should be strongly considered by the GCM as a suggestion to the family.

Rules need to be set for the family meeting and sent to all attendees ahead of time via e-mail or letter. These rules can include, as Sheehy suggests, letting everyone have a chance to speak, don't interrupt, stay in the present, don't go back to past events, and using "I messages."[18]

A sample agenda might include the following:

- Financial concerns in caregiving
- Caregiver burnout of the primary caregiver
- Adult child feelings about aging parental illness and caregiving
- Ways family members share the caregiving by being direct hands-on caregivers
- Family members providing respite to the main caregiver
- Financial ability to hire paid caregivers for respite of the main family caregiver

- Hiring paid caregivers due to the increase in level of care
- Moving the care receiver to a higher level of care because of caregiving issues
- What the caregiving trajectory or future time frame is
- What support does each member of the extending family want to play.

The agenda can be made up of any pressing issues at hand about family caregiving of an older family member. The agenda needs to reflect family problems in caregiving in real time, prioritized by the gravity of each problem.

The meeting should not be a one-time event, according to the Family Caregiving Alliance's guidelines for a family meeting.[19] The GCM will have many issues to cover to help the family solve, and they may not be covered in this first meeting. Scheduling a second meeting at the end of the first is an excellent idea.

The GCM should either record the family meeting minutes or tape it as a record of what every family member said. Julie Menack in her chapter "Working With the Long-Distance Family: Tools a Care Manager Can Use," covers family meetings and recording them with a digital voice recorder.[20] She then suggests saving them to e-mail and/or a CD and sending them to each family member as a record of what was said by each attendee and what each person agreed to do, plus group agreements.

Dividing Caregiving Tasks at a Family Meeting

The issue of how the family can fairly share the caregiving with the primary family caregiver may be a key issue that can be discussed as an agenda item. To offer the main caregiver respite, one family member could take the care receiver for a weekend periodically. Another may foot the bill for formal paid caregiving rather than do direct care; one may handle all bill paying, using an online bill-paying account and having the care receiver's mail forwarded to them. One family member could manage a social media group, like a Facebook site, or organize a chat room dedicated to the older adult where friends joining the site can be local and long-distance family members. One family member could set up a caregivers' sharing site like www.lotsahelping-hands.com. One may do a family newsletter summarizing the caregiving month. A family member or friend who is tech savvy, which could be a grandchild, could set up all caregiving websites, calendars and e-mails, and videoconferencing needed by the family. One family member could manage ongoing house repairs for the care receiver. The idea is to be creative, meet the care receiver's needs, yet divide tasks up so that long-distance and local family members can share the tasks according to their abilities, skills, time available, location, and preferences. This is called striking a balance in the family.

The End of the Family Meeting

At the end of the family meeting, the GCM should summarize the tasks that every family member has agreed to take on, dividing the caregiving more fairly. This should be the new family caregiving plan. The GCM should get everyone to agree to that plan. The GCM should use the recorded minutes of the family meeting to put together this written plan and send each family member the minutes and agreed-on planned tasks, then ask each attendee to sign off on that plan of action. This is the prime goal of the family meeting.

■ RESOURCES THE GCM CAN BRING TO THE FAMILY TO RELIEVE STRESS AND BURDEN FROM THE FAMILY CAREGIVER

The GCM role is to pinpoint the resources and part that family members can play in caregiving. Solving the care receiver's prob-lems is in many ways solving each caregiving family members' problems. If a long-distance daughter is guilty that she is not able to help her local caregiving sister, who does most of the care of their mother, the GCM could suggest that the long-distance daughter take on the role of managing all the finances and contracts. That assignment of a role may help to diminish her guilt. If you can pinpoint a way an adult son who does not want to do personal care of his mother can aid both his aging mother and sister, the main caregiver, such as by building a ramp and doing the grocery shopping, you are solving both the adult brother and sister's problems along with your client's.

Circle of Care

One resource that a GCM can bring to a caregiving family is what Gail Sheehy calls a circle of care. To create this supportive connection, the GCM needs to take her or his GCM coaching skills and put together a support system around the formerly isolated, solitary family caregiver. The GCM in this chapter's case study has begun that by reorganizing the family so adult siblings can share in the care of the older client. You, the GCM, are what Sheehy calls a compassionate coach who can help the beleaguered caregiver attract and assemble a platform to keep on giving the care she or he wants to give the aging person.[21]

Adding Adult Siblings to the Care Provider Circle of Care

A circle of care would include emotional resources for the direct family caregiver. These emotional resources could and should include adult siblings. Reconnecting midlife brothers and sisters, through the circle of care, is an important GCM task, as siblings are the longest and deepest relationship in any person's life. The GCM may have to depend on his or her clinical skills in helping siblings with forgiveness or reconnecting siblings who live long distances apart to add them to a circle of care. Midlife siblings have often spent the last 30 years tending to their own families, so the point of reconnection of midlife brothers and sisters often happens when they are in middle age in the midst of a crisis in parent care. This is where the GCM either needs to have clinical skills in midlife sibling work or find the resources for the family to help with this healing sibling reconnection.[22]

The GCM should use his or her coaching skills to help the main caregiver ask adult brothers and sisters for help. Often the communication between brothers and sisters involving parent care is very poor and weak. Sisters especially need help in asking assistance from brothers, and all need help in asking for assistance from estranged siblings. After the help is requested coaching siblings to say "Thank you, I love you" and then set up the new caregiving system, which is an expanded circle of care, is a primary GCM job.

Adding Caregiver Friends to the Circle of Care

Friends of the care provider need to be brought into the circle of care. The main caregiver often desperately needs respite from the unremitting stress of caregiving. Encouraging the caregiver to use their friendship network—to go out with friends to lunch and dinner, go to a movie, go away for a girls' weekend—may take the GCM arranging respite with either paid or family caregivers to tie this loop in the family caregiver's circle of care. Encouraging caregivers to use a social network like Facebook can help reconnect the caregiver with old friends and classmates, and have a way of feeling emotionally connected without leaving the care receiver can be a good GCM task. Encouraging the family caregiver to let friends know how to reach him or her and what his or her caregiving situation is presently can help the caregiver build a circle of support. As caregivers often do not reach out for support, this takes coaching by the GCM.

Adding Professionals to the Caregiving Circle

You, the GCM, are the primary professional in the caregiver circle for the main caregiver. But you can also include, if they are willing to participate, doctors, nurses, other social workers who are very involved in the care of the older person and willing to support the care provider. For example, if the older person is dying at home with hospice, the medical social worker, if she or he is willing, can be involved in the family caregiver's circle of care. A geriatrician, if they are willing, could join the circle of care.

Other Ways That a GCM Can Support a Primary Care Provider

The GCM can help a primary care provider by coaching them to take care of themselves. Care providers needs to replenish themselves and find ways they can be kind to themselves to relieve the stress of caregiving. Suggesting personal care such as having their nails done, going to a spa, getting a massage, or taking a yoga, exercise, or mindfulness class are just some of the ways that care providers can personally care for themselves.

Setting Up Communication Among the Circle of Care

Communications among the circle of care can be facilitated by the GCM using several methods. The GCM can set up teleconferences at an established time and provide attendees a number to call in. The GCM can establish a private e-mail group for the circle of care, a virtual care meeting place, a videoconference through Skype, and a virtual bulletin board where messages are posted and permanently saved for members of the circle of care. They can share information about the care with each other at any time day or night in any time zone. Several free Web pages are available that caregivers can use. There are also several free and many paid teleconferencing nks a GCM can use for family meetings.[23] Also refer to Chapter 11 and the section on videoconferencing.

Tools to Help a Family Divide up Caregiving Tasks

After the GCM has worked with the family to more equitably divide up caregiving tasks, the care manager can offer tools for the family to divide up the care more easily. There are a number of Internet-based tools available that the GCM can suggest. One is www.lotsahelp-inghands.com. The program gives extended family and friends who live both close and long distance a way to share the older clients status and give the family care providers a way to schedule taking on caregiving tasks from any location. For example an elder father needs to go the doctor every week. Family members nearby and even those who are visiting can go into the calendar, check to see what task needs to be done on those dates, and sign up. Everyone else in the family who signs on to the calendar can see that task is taken care of. According to Gail Sheehy, who recommends it in her book *Passages in Caregiving*, the main caregiver can set this up in 5 minutes.[24] This initial step can be guided by the GCM who can add themselves to the calendar.

The GCM can also suggest a Google calendar so that the family and friends can share caregiving tasks, helping long-distance and local caregivers to work together and share the older client's schedule. An online calendar system can also be used to remind older adults of an appointment or to take their medications. Tyze.com and Familylink.com are some examples of this technology. See Chapter 11 on technology for websites and more information.

Family Caregiver Alliance and Caregiver Advocacy Groups

Family Caregiver Alliance, a national center for caregiving, has a plethora of caregiving supports and tools. To help locate resources

for caregiving they have a technological tool called the Family Care Navigator, which is a site that allows the GCM to help the family caregiver find local resources. Especially in this era of budget cutting, the GCM can use this excellent resource to locate resources for the family caregiver in their geographic area and then add them to their continuum of care for other family caregivers.

Other caregiving advocacy resources nationally include AARP, HICAP, Caregiver Resource Centers, and the National Alliance for the Mentally Ill.

Other Technological Interventions to Help Caregivers

Other technological interventions can be added by the GCM to help the family caregiver. These technologies include communication devices like adaptive phones and cellular phones designed with older users in mind. This also includes telehealth technology, electronic personal and health records, residential monitoring systems, reminder systems, and medication dispensers. Please see Chapter 11 for details. As a GCM you can evaluate technology for the caregiver's use and decide which technology works best for each family caregiver. Also see Chapter 11 for an evaluation tool.

Real-Time Aides to Caregivers

There are many real-time tools that the GCM can bring in to help the caregiver. One is the simple old idea of the diary. The main caregiver can be coached to keep a caregiving journal as a form of self-care. All this takes is pen and paper, a typewriter, or a computer. The GCM can coach the main care provider to write down his or her thoughts, needs, and wishes on a regular basis and read it to themselves. This allows the caregiver to note patterns of need, such as more support, and patterns of wishes, such as more time to themselves. Over time, with the GCM's help, they can trace how interventions have changed their personal balance and caregiving life. They do not have to reveal this journal to anyone but use it as a way of charting their own caregiver stresses and relief through the GCM's efforts.

Support Groups

Another critical real-time tool for the GCM to use to relieve caregiver stress is support groups. For elder-specific resources, the GCM can contact the local Area Agency on Aging in the county where they work or the senior information and referral office and get a list of local support groups for the main caregiver. If you have a family caring network office near you, this group can help you as well.

These groups are often run by nonprofits such as the Alzheimer's Association and facilitated by private therapists or paid or volunteer staff. They can be paid for with private pay, be on a sliding scale, or free.[25] Caregiver support groups give a real-time, in-person circle of care for caregivers who are in a similar situation to share their thoughts, feelings, and many times their own creative solutions. Caregivers can ventilate in a safe space, share experiences in positive and negative caregiving, and get practical tips on how to manage their caregiving job. It is a regular place to gather with others who have a very similar experience. The groups are generally set up to help the normal adjustment to the caregiving situation. If there are complex underlying stressors, a psychotherapist leading the group or individual counseling should be considered by the GCM. Support groups can also be found online. The GCM can also suggest long-distance care providers join a support group where they live.

Counseling

Family caregivers can often be so frustrated and stressed that they can lose their temper. They can lose sight of the differences between being mad at the person they care for and the

older client's behavior. You, the GCM, are a resource to the caregiver to coach them to identify the difference. By having you as a resource they have taken the first step to changing their behavior. As a resource, you can direct them to many other sources in the continuum of care to deal with their inner anxiety, frustration, anger, and sometimes rage. The GCM can refer the caregiver to their own primary physician to discuss their level of stress. You can refer them to a support group or advocate for self-care resources. If the caregiver is losing their temper with the care recipient, has long standing parent–adult child issues, or show signs of depression that are accelerating and the GCM feels that a support group experience is not enough, then one-to-one counseling may be an answer. If the GCM, for example, used a stress test for care providers such as a Zarit Burden and the caregiver scored in the moderate to severe or severe burden range, one-to-one counseling would be an appropriate referral for the GCM. If the care provider hit, shoved, or threatened the older person after a stressful encounter, that would be another serious sign to get the care provider in one-to-one counseling. You may also have to consider adult protective services as a referral because you are a mandated reporter. Losing control and lashing out at the care receiver is a direct sign that the caregiver may need one-to-one counseling. If you see signs of mental illness of family members or if the family caregiver suffers from mental illness or psychiatric symptoms brought on or exacerbated by the caregiving role, then a psychiatrist or psychiatric intervention on a one-to-one basis should be facilitated by the GCM. As 71% of all family caregivers suffer from one symptom of clinical depression, one-to-one counseling is a needed choice.[26]

Counseling can be offered by a marriage and family therapist who specializes in aging issues, the clergy, a licensed clinical social worker (LCSW) who has a specialty in aging issues, a psychologist, or a psychotherapist with a background in aging.[27] You as the GCM need to help the caregiver assess whether they need counseling or at times if a psychiatric intervention is a better choice. You can sometimes arrange counseling under Medicare for caregivers over 65 through the Family Services Association in your community. If the individual counselor is able to take assignment from Medicare they can at times bill Medicare. This is something the GCM can check on with providers in their community. The GCM needs to use their continuum of care in their own community to develop a network of one-to-one counseling for stressed care providers who need this type of one-to-one support.

Educational Resources for Family Caregivers

Knowledge is power. Family caregivers need more of it since they are asked to do tasks without much or any training or education. They are often accidental caregivers. Healthcare literacy is the ability of the caregiver to acquire, process, and understand basic health information and use that data to make better healthcare decisions. Family caregivers who are not trained healthcare professionals do not know what questions to ask, let alone whom to ask. They are surrounded by a tangled web of nurses, social workers from many agencies, multiple doctors, prescriptions, and many illnesses suffered by their loved ones. Their questions are myriad, and who to ask is many times a mystery.

The GCM can be there to interpret health information and talk to healthcare providers to link them. But helping the family care provider educate themselves is also an appropriate GCM task.[28] The GCM can take the older client's diagnosis and go online or go to the local branch of the association that works with this type of patient. There are many national organizations plus local chapters, whose mission is to provide education and resources to local family caregivers. For exam-

ple, if the older client has congestive heart failure, the GCM can go to the local branch of the American Heart Association and pick up DVDs videos, brochures, and a list of websites to bring to the family caregiver. The GCM can also send the information to all family caregivers so they can go online from where they are and research the disease or visit the local branch office in their town.

The GCM can give the family caregiver a bibliography of books, periodicals, and websites that cover information about the client's diagnosis. The GCM can refer the family caregiver to local workshops and conferences about the older client's diagnosis and arrange respite to get there. Local libraries can be great resources too.

Making sure the educational information is in a language the family caregiver speaks and is on their reading level is important. The average adult in the United States reads at a seventh or eighth grade level, and it is estimated that the average adult over 65 has limited or marginal reading skills. Healthcare materials are mired in medical jargon that is barely understandable to the average reader. Make sure the information you bring to the care provider is health literate to the care provider. If not, the GCM can help them understand the material. Also give them user-friendly formats, which may not be printed material but be videos or DVDs.[29]

Legal and Financial Resources

The GCM should, through the psychosocial assessment, find out the formal support network of the older person and thus the family care provider. This includes elder law attorneys, accountants, financial planners, and conservators or guardians. If the family does not have these resources and needs one, the GCM's job is to suggest contacts out of their continuum of care. As noted, family caregivers deal with a hornet's nest of legal documents such as wills, powers of attorney, durable power of attorney for healthcare, power of attorney for finances, living wills, and having a "do not resuscitate" order. Whether all these documents are in place should be questions on your GCM psychosocial assessment, see Chapter 3. Your job as a GCM is to help the family care providers make sure the documents are in place, that they understand them, and have the appropriate legal or financial professional who can assist them as well.

The GCM can bring many other resources to bear to reduce the stress on family caregivers. They can use spiritual resources (see Chapter 8). They can bring respite resources, care provider advocacy resources, or public benefits resources like Medicare, Medicaid, the Family and Medical Leave Act, Social Security, or the VA.[30] All these resources and how to navigate through them should be in your GCM toolbox for the family caregiver. Whether they are eligible for these benefits should be tracked in your psychosocial assessments. How to help the family caregiver navigate through the maze of programs and resources is the key to being a great geriatric care manager. Your client is only as strong as your family care providers. It does take a village, and you, the GCM, need to nurture the village and both the caregivers and your clients who live in it.

■ REFERENCES

1. Arno PS, Levine C, Memmott, MM. The economic value of informal caregiving. *Health Affairs*. February 2002;18:2:182–188.
2. Sheehy G. *Passages in caregiving, turning chaos into confidence.* New York, NY: HarperCollins Publishers; 2010:282.
3. Cress CJ. Assessing the caregiver. In: Cress C, ed. *Care managers: working with the aging family.* Sudbury, MA: Jones and Bartlett Publishers; 2008:91.
4. Cress CJ. Assessing the caregiver. In: Cress C, ed. *Care managers: working with the aging family.* Sudbury, MA: Jones and Bartlett Publishers; 2008:92.
5. Cress CJ. Assessing the caregiver. In: Cress C, ed. *Care managers: working with the aging family.* Sudbury, MA: Jones and Bartlett Publishers; 2008:93.
6. Cress CJ. Assessing the caregiver. In: Cress C, ed. *Care managers: working with the aging family.* Sudbury, MA: Jones and Bartlett Publishers; 2008:94.
7. Family Caregiver Alliance. *Caregiver assessment: principles, guidelines and strategies for change. report from a national consensus development conference.* San Francisco, CA: Family Caregiver Alliance. 2006;1:13.
8. Morano CL, Morano B. Applying stress and appraisal and coping framework to geriatric care management, *Geriatr Care Manage J.* 2006;17(10):3.
9. Family Caregiver Alliance. *Caregiver assessment: principals, guidelines and strategies for change. report from a national consensus development conference.* San Francisco, CA: Family Caregiver Alliance. 2006;1:16.
10. Cress CJ. Assessing the caregiver. In: Cress C, ed. *Care managers: working with the aging family.* Sudbury, MA: Jones and Bartlett Publishers; 2008:102.
11. Cress CJ. Assessing the caregiver. In: Cress C, ed. *Care managers: working with the aging family.* Sudbury, MA: Jones and Bartlett Publishers; 2008:115.
12. Cress CJ. Assessing the caregiver. In: Cress C, ed. *Care managers: working with the aging family.* Sudbury, MA: Jones and Bartlett Publishers; 2008:115.
13. Ghatak R. Family meetings and the aging family. In: Cress C, ed. *Care managers: working with the aging family.* Sudbury, MA: Jones and Bartlett Publishers; 2008:157.
14. Ghatak R. Family meetings and the aging family. In: Cress C, ed. *Care managers: working with the aging family.* Sudbury, MA: Jones and Bartlett Publishers; 2008:167.
15. Sheehy G. *Passages in caregiving, turning chaos into confidence.* HarperCollins Publishers; 2010:152.
16. Cress C, Peterson KC. *Mom loved you best, forgiving and forging sibling relationships.* New Horizon Press; 2010.

17. Cress C, Peterson KC. *Working with adult aging siblings*. In: Cress C, ed. Care managers: working with the aging family. Sudbury, MA: Jones and Bartlett Publishers; 2008:199.

18. Sheehy G. *Passages in caregiving, turning chaos into confidence*. HarperCollins Publishers; 2010:154.

19. Family Caregiver Alliance. Holding a family meeting. Available at: http://www.caregiver.org/caregiver/jsp/content_node.jsp?nodeid=475. Accessed December 6, 2010.

20. Menack J. Working with long-distance families: tools the care manager can use. In: Cress C, ed. *Care managers: working with the aging family*. Sudbury, MA: Jones and Bartlett Publishers; 2008:63.

21. Sheehy G. *Passages in caregiving, turning chaos into confidence*. HarperCollins Publishers; 2010;50.

22. Cress C, Peterson KC. Working with adult aging siblings. In: Cress C, ed. *Care managers: working with the aging family*. Sudbury, MA: Jones and Bartlett Publishers; 2008:221.

23. Dybnis B, Barlam S. Tools to support family caregivers. In: Cress C, ed. *Care managers: working with the aging family*. Sudbury, MA: Jones and Bartlett Publishers; 2008:141.

24. Sheehy G. *Passages in caregiving, turning chaos into confidence*. HarperCollins Publishers; 2010:155.

25. Dybnis B, Barlam S. Tools to support family caregivers. In: Cress C, ed. *Care managers: working with the aging family*. Sudbury, MA: Jones and Bartlett Publishers; 2008:137.

26. Dybnis B, Barlam S. Tools to support family caregivers. In: Cress C, ed. *Care managers: working with the aging family*. Sudbury, MA: Jones and Bartlett Publishers; 2008:138.

27. Dybnis B, Barlam S. Tools to support family caregivers. In: Cress C, ed. *Care managers: working with the aging family*. Sudbury, MA: Jones and Bartlett Publishers; 2008:136.

28. Cress C. The care manager's role during the hospital stay. In: Cress C, ed. *Care managers: working with the aging family*. Sudbury, MA: Jones and Bartlett; 2008:15.

29. Cress C. The care manager's role during the hospital stay. In: Cress C, ed. *Care managers: working with the aging family*. Sudbury, MA: Jones and Bartlett Publishers; 2008:15.

30. Dybnis B, Barlam S. Tools to support family caregivers. In: Cress C, ed. *Care managers: working with the aging family*. Sudbury, MA: Jones and Bartlett Publishers; 2008:141.

Chapter 10

Supporting Clients' Quality of Life: Drawing on Community, Informal Networks, and Care Manager Creativity

Nina Pflumm Herndon and Victoria Thorpe

■ INTRODUCTION

This chapter provides concrete tools and examples to support geriatric care managers (GCMs) in focusing on developing and sustaining quality of life (QOL) for their clients that goes beyond physical comfort and includes emotional, physical, intellectual, and spiritual well-being.

■ WHAT IS "QUALITY OF LIFE?"

Providing clients with an exceptional QOL is an important goal for a GCM. Activities that encourage clients to foster their emotional, intellectual, physical, and/or spiritual QOL can help to address a client's physiological health. QOL comprises (1) social interactions and a general sense of connectedness (to other people, upcoming generations, affiliations with groups, pets, or whatever brings the person a sense of meaning); (2) engagement with activities that promote a sense of purpose and feelings of physical wellness; (3) stimulation of the mind in the form of learning, creativity, or idea exchange; and (4) a sense of spirituality. Most important, QOL is a deeply personal response to one's situation and circumstances based on what brings one purpose and meaning.

Addressing a broader scope of an older adult's QOL is an important goal for geriatric care. There is a tendency within the geriatric care community to focus efforts on improving a client's QOL as it specifically relates to quality of care, whether by providing support and comfort at the end of life, attending to healthcare needs, drawing on community resources, or simply ensuring that the client is treated with respect and consideration by care providers. As a result, care managers have traditionally been called on by families to help ensure their clients experience all-important "quality of care." However, recent experience in geriatric care, along with new research about the aging process, suggests there is a greater opportunity to affect an older adult's QOL by expanding the notion to include how older adults can stay fulfilled and engaged in their lives, despite cognitive or physical limitations.

Consider Abraham Maslow's hierarchy of needs: once the most fundamental physiological and safety needs are met, the next level of needs are for love and belonging, esteem (the desire to be accepted and valued by others), and ultimately self-actualization (the opportunity to reach one's full potential). A care manager's support of a client's improved QOL can thus be viewed as a fundamental component of the care manager's efforts to address a client's needs.[1]

Similar to the focus on holistic wellness among the general population, there is a growing understanding in the geriatric care community that it is imperative to incorporate a larger sense of "health" for older adults, and to consider more of the facets that contribute to their mental and physical well-being. Indeed, the World Health Organization has defined health as a "state of complete physical, intellectual, and social well-being and not merely the absence of disease or infirmity."[2]

Although the physical elements of QOL are of paramount importance, new evidence shows that holistic QOL, including emotional and spiritual health, can have as much, if not a greater, impact on an older adult's overall well-being. In reality, this is not an either/or choice because these more holistic aspects of a client's QOL are intertwined with his or her physical QOL. For example, if a client is disconnected from friends and family and lacking emotional QOL, this can lead to a sense of isolation, which can cause negative mental and physical effects. Similarly, if a client nurtures a strong spiritual foundation, whether through a religious institution or on a more individual level, this may result in positive physical manifestations, such as an increased desire to live and a stronger resiliency against depression.

Holistic QOL is defined as incorporating four distinct, yet interrelated areas: intellectual, emotional, spiritual, and physical. Intellectual QOL includes activities that engage clients mentally, including hobbies, learning, "brain aerobics," or any form of creativity. Emotional QOL includes structured social interactions or time with family, friends, and peers who have shared similar life experiences, or other emotional connections, such as with pets or grandchildren, or even a sense of being at peace with oneself. The physical aspects of QOL in this chapter focus on activities that help clients stay physically active, increase their sense of strength despite possible limitations, and provide a sense of fun. Finally, there is spiritual QOL, which delves into how clients can maintain or build spiritual connections, whether through a relationship with a church or temple or through other avenues, such as volunteering or spending time in nature.

As GCMs, we are in a constant struggle to minimize the factors that inhibit the client's quality of life and enhance access to that which brings each individual a sense of purpose and meaning. While the oft-relied upon resources of assisted living facilities, senior centers, and adult day programs have offerings that remarkably improve their participant's quality of life, there are those that do not address the individual interests of each client. It is not reasonable to assume that resources are readily available to implement such individualized activity plans in most settings.

Yet, regardless of the barriers and obstacles that we face, many innovative GCMs have the opportunity to implement just the right plan to succeed in providing a client with enhanced quality of life in a way that is uniquely suited to the individual client. To orchestrate a successful plan, it is critical that we recognize the *forces* that we are up against. In his landmark book, *What Are Old People For?* Bill Thomas, MD, identifies the three "plagues" of institutional elder care as:

- Loneliness
- Helplessness
- Boredom

Dr. Thomas then goes on to describe in excruciating detail a life, for many, that is devoid of:

- Companionship
- Intimacy
- Self-direction
- Meaningful activity

Although Dr. Thomas was referring to institutional elder care, in essence, what he has identified is the dearth of things that give many a sense of satisfaction with life. Conversely, when a person does have the benefit of companionship, intimacy, self-direction and meaningful activity, their experience is usually more positive—despite whatever functional limitations may be present. At the very core of our work, regardless of the setting, is a continual struggle to help clients avoid that which causes suffering such as that described above while fostering the elements that lead to fulfillment. Whatever the cause that exposes older adults to the three plagues, be it cultural barriers, sensory impairments, or dementia, the antidote is the same; engagement. We must reach even the most lost of our clients by finding that portal that leads to the source of their interest and enthusiasm for life.

WHY HOLISTIC QUALITY OF LIFE MATTERS FOR GERIATRIC CARE MANAGERS

Care managers who focus on improving holistic QOL for their clients can make a measurable, sustainable impact on overall health and well-being. Activities that encourage clients to foster their emotional, intellectual, physical, and/or spiritual QOL can help to address a client's physiological health concerns. For example, one GCM worked with a client who was depressed and withdrawn and had little interest in social activities or even visiting with family. The GCM decided to delve into the client's spiritual well-being and began talking to him about the things in his prior life that had brought him joy and meaning. When the GCM learned that nature was especially important for the client, she arranged for him to visit a local bird sanctuary with wheelchair access, where he could view birds through a specially designed set of binoculars. This experience gave the client new interest in life; his appetite subsequently improved, and he started asking to see friends and neighbors again.

GCMs are uniquely qualified to assess and address a client's needs in terms of holistic QOL. A GCM has a bird's-eye view of a client's needs without the obstacles (real or perceived)

that might cloud the perspective of an adult child or family member (e.g., "Dad never liked puzzles; don't bother even trying"). A GCM can also tap into community resources to address holistic QOL that a care provider may not be aware exists, such as finding an art class for elders at a local community college (e.g., "Mrs. K says she likes to paint, but I don't know how to do that"). And GCMs have a third, more practical reason to address their clients' holistic QOL—if their clients are more fulfilled and engaged, they will have better health and a more positive affect, which will result in positive feedback from all parties, more referrals, and a continued flow of new business. Plus, holistic QOL activities are an opportunity for GCMs to be creative and to bring a sense of playfulness to their client interactions.

Research Supports the Focus on Holistic QOL

Although there is a great deal of anecdotal evidence that holistic QOL, including emotional, intellectual, physical, and spiritual elements, has a strong effect on the functional QOL for older adults, these stories are also supported by a growing body of empirical, scientific research.

Benefits of Activities That Promote Emotional QOL

Much research supports the benefits of promoting emotional QOL for older adults, particularly in terms of social connections.

A study of 3112 elders in Missouri indicated that when older adults had visits with friends or relatives, had close friends for emotional support, or had the perception that help would be available if they became sick or disabled, they had better emotional health.[3] Because of these results, the Centers for Disease Control and Prevention (CDC) recommends implementing effective prevention programs for older adults to help improve emotional health among older adults who have little social support.[3] In particular, the CDC notes:

> Social support can promote health by providing persons with positive experiences, socially rewarding roles, or improved ability to cope with stressful events. Social support is critical for older adults who are at increased risk for disability associated with chronic disease or social isolation after the loss of a partner.[4]

Social support can come in the form of connections with other people—friends, family, peers, and so forth, but it can also come through relationships with animals, particularly with household pets. Studies have demonstrated that pet therapy can help to improve social interaction, psychosocial function, life satisfaction, social competence, and psychological well-being, while reducing depression in elder residents of care homes. It is also thought that interaction with these animals can help break the cycle of loneliness, hopelessness, and social withdrawal that is often seen in older adults.[5]

Another study that focuses on socialization and aging is the Seattle Longitudinal Study of Adult Intelligence. It has followed a target group of more than 5000 people since the program began in 1956. The participants in this landmark study were recruited from Columbia University, Johns Hopkins University, and Massachusetts General Hospital. Participants were tested at 7 year intervals for over four decades. The study has shown that a lack of social interaction accounts for 40% of age-related decline, and that a complex and intellectual stimulating environment, as well as a high intellect of a spouse, may reduce the risk of cognitive decline in old age.

Benefits of Activities That Promote Intellectual QOL

Although for many years scientists believed that the human brain inevitably deteriorates over time, there has been new research in recent years that refutes this assumption and shows that intellectual stimulation may help preserve key cognitive functionality for older adults.

In 2002, the *Journal of the American Medical Association* published a study by Rush Alzheimer's Disease Center and Rush-Presbyterian-St. Luke's Medical Center in Chicago, Illinois, which found a connection between frequent participation in cognitively stimulating activities and a reduced risk of Alzheimer's disease. The study, which followed more than 700 dementia-free participants age 65 years and older for an average of 4.5 years, measured participants' levels of cognitive activity and correlated these levels with the amount of time the participants spent on activities that stimulate the brain, such as reading the newspaper or books, or doing crossword puzzles and playing card games. The study found that although all of the participants experienced modest, age-related declines on memory and information processing tests, the rates of decline were lower for those who had engaged in more frequent activities that stimulated cognitive development.[6]

This research not only generated a lot of press, but it has also caused some people to confuse repetitive "brain activities" that are designed to help older adults preserve singular mental skills with activities that promote intellectual QOL. Activities that promote intellectual QOL involve more than just "training" clients to better remember a set of tasks; they encourage mental stimulation and deeper engagement, such as visits to museums, reading interesting books or articles, or learning new skills or knowledge. According to research psychologist Arthur Kramer of the University of Illinois, Urbana, "There is no doubt that older people can improve their performance on these tasks through training. What we don't know is whether this transfers to real-world skills and cognitive function."[7] The practical application of this information therefore relies in the specific relevance to each individual's quality of life. If one enjoys the challenge of "brain activities" and is compelled by the appealing notion of maintaining the brain, then activities such as crossword puzzles and brain training software from Posit Science and others are an appropriate part of a client's QOL plan.

Perhaps even more relevant to QOL than the findings outlined above is the research that indicates a discrepancy between the rate of decline in the degree of Alzheimer's disease neuropathology and the clinical manifestations of the disease among those who engage in cognitively stimulating activity. In fact, some patients whose brains had extensive Alzheimer's disease pathology clinically had little or no manifestations of the disease.

Specifically, Dr. Yaakov Stern, professor of clinical neuropsychology at Columbia University, is one of the leading proponents of the Cognitive Reserve Theory. The theory hypothesizes why some patients with full blown Alzheimer's disease are able to conduct normal lives right up to their death and others with the same Alzheimer's disease pathology display severe symptoms and are unable to care for themselves.

The term *cognitive reserve* has been defined as "the ability of an individual to tolerate progressive brain pathology without demonstrating clinical cognitive symptoms." Cognitive reserve is used to illustrate the mind's remarkable resilience and ability to perform in light of the brain's damage. In studies conducted in the late 1980s, it was suggested that some patients have a larger "reserve" of neurons and abilities that "enable them to offset the losses caused by Alzheimer's."

Dr. Stern offers *life experiences* as one justification for greater reserves of these neurons, particularly those experiences that engage the brain in fulfilling and meaningful ways like education, a rewarding career, or creative hobbies. He goes on to explain, "This is so because stimulating activities, ideally combining phys-ical exercise, learning, and social interaction, help us build a cognitive reserve to protect us."

Not all activities require strenuous physical activity; even moderately passive activity such as reading, watching a movie, and visiting friends were evaluated as having benefits towards building a reserve. One study indicated that for each additional activity the participant reduced their risk of developing Alzheimer's symptoms by 8%. Physical exercise alone has a very beneficial impact on cognition; research now indicates that physical activity promotes neurogenesis (the creation of new neurons) in the human brain.

Although Dr. Stern suggests that it is best to begin building our reserve earlier in life, he recognizes that it is never too late to begin and that the effects of greater activity are cumulative. Studies indicate that people who lead mentally stimulating lives may have between 35–40% less risk of ever manifesting Alzheimer's disease. In studies that focused on relatively healthy older adults and then conducted autopsies after their death, up to 20% of these elders had full blown Alzheimer's pathology in their brains without ever developing significant symptoms. In the years ahead, Dr. Stern is hoping to gain greater understanding on how older adults compensate for their brain's area of decline by exploring whether new areas of the brain become activated as others decline.

Benefits of Activities That Promote Physical QOL

It seems obvious to state that research shows the importance of regular physical activity in promoting holistic QOL. However, with clients who have moderate to severe physical limitations, GCMs may inadvertently overlook physical activities that go beyond goal-oriented physical therapy to support more overall functioning. Recent research about the effects of physical activity specifically focused on older adults gives compelling new reasons why this element of holistic QOL cannot be neglected in addressing an older adult's well-being, no matter what limitations may exist.

Researchers at the University of Illinois at Urbana-Champaign found that previously sedentary seniors who incorporated physical activity into their lifestyles not only improved physical function, but experienced psychological benefits as well. Kinesiology professor Dr. Edward McAuley, who led the study, notes, "The implications of our work are that not only will physical activity potentially add years to your life as we age, but the quality of those years is likely to be improved by regular physical activity."[8]

In addition to promoting psychological well-being and better health, physical activity also appears to help preserve brain functioning for older adults. According to the *Wall Street Journal,* interventions that indirectly target intellectual fitness through physical conditioning show promise for brain preservation. In a 2003 review of 18 studies, Professor Kramer and his colleagues of the University of Illinois, Urbana, found that strength training and aerobics keep high-level brain functions, such as planning, remembering, and multitasking, sharp. Professor Kramer notes:

> Cardiovascular fitness training improves cognitive function in the elderly in as little as 6 months. It increases the volume of gray matter [neurons] and white matter [which connects neurons] in regions that handle executive functions. It also improves the efficiency of networks that underlie some forms of memory and attention.[9]

Researchers are finding, however, that all physical activity is not the same; some types of activities have more benefits than others do. Although walking and other cardiovascular activities are wonderful for older adults, there is new information about the positive effects of strength training for this population. If the idea of an older adult lifting big barbells seems outlandish, consider the evidence about the benefits of strength training, no matter how low the weight or how adapted the activity is to accommodate physical limitations. Weight training not only helps prevent deterioration of the musculoskeletal system (something that aerobic exercise does not accomplish), but it has also been proved to help older adults build new muscle. Weight training has other positive physiological and psychological outcomes. A Harvard University study showed significant psychological improvements when older adults engaged in strength training programs. After 12 weeks of strength exercise, 14 of 16 previously depressed elders in the study no longer met the criteria for clinical depression.[10]

The wonderful part about focusing on physical QOL is that it can have a ripple effect on the other factors that affect a client's well-being. As documented earlier, physical conditioning can improve mental acumen and functioning. With improved mental and physical health, an older adult can also more fully participate in group activities (emotional QOL), continue learning (intellectual QOL), and pursue endeavors that give him or her meaning and purpose in life (spiritual QOL).

Benefits of Activities That Promote Spiritual QOL

Given the myriad ways that individuals may interpret the term *spiritual,* it is difficult to find empirical research that "proves" the importance of a focus on spirituality for older adults. Undaunted, researchers have been trying to tackle this dilemma to better support the case for spiritual practice in elder care.

Dr. Bill Thomas demonstrates an insightful division between the *doing* and *being* stages of life that provides a greater context for spiritual pursuits in later life. He describes the *doing* stage as coming during our adulthood where we are involved, and in some cases obsessed, with all that needs to be done in order to build one's life. From the moment we graduate from school, enter a career, get married, buy a home, and become parents, our lives are overflowing with a continual stream of activity. This stage of life is also highly favored by the social structure in which we live; people are rewarded by grades, degrees, positions, salaries, status, and recognition for the quantity and the quality of our doing.

Dr. Thomas refers to the *being* stage of life as coming in our elder years. It is here that the *doing* slows down considerably, and not always to our liking. Even the definition of the word *retirement* comes from the French word meaning *to withdraw from*; never suggesting, however, where we *withdraw to*. He suggests that this elder stage of life is often an unrealized opportunity for *being,* now that much of the *doing* has taken place; a time of inner exploration and self-realization; a time of spirituality and creativity.

Similar to the psychology of Eric Erikson, Dr. Thomas recognizes the need for elders to have as structured a life path as their younger counterparts, even though their focus may be significantly different than those who are in the midst of building their lives. Both Erikson and Thomas seem to agree that elders need to have an experience of fulfillment over a life well lived—a sense of satisfaction. It may require the assistance of a well-trained geriatric care manager to bring about the elements that provide the elder with just such an experience: the all important realization of a complete and successful life.

. However, this reflection and satisfaction is only a part of Dr. Thomas' *being* stage, it is not just about looking back; it also embraces looking forward but through a new lens.

There is much rich, ethnographic research about the ways that older adults respond to and appreciate connecting with a larger spiritual purpose, whether it is through a church or temple, volunteer work, or time with pets or nature. Nurturing spirituality may be as simple as encouraging gratitude and taking stock of life's blessings. According to Eugene Bianchi, who works with elder adults in Atlanta, Georgia:

A strong trait among creative elders is a spirit of gratitude toward life. They are able to receive the small and large gifts along the way as blessings that evoke thankfulness. . . . These elders do not deny the pain and hardship of negative events, but they seem to be able to learn from them or at least to accept them as they turn back toward life.[11]

In her groundbreaking book, *Co-Dependent No More,* author Melody Beattie says, "Gratitude unlocks the fullness of life. It turns what we have into enough, and more. It turns denial into acceptance, chaos into order, confusion to clarity. . . . Gratitude makes sense of our past, brings peace for today, and creates vision for tomorrow." Clearly positive attitude is one of the fundamental components of successful aging. It is not just a candy coating that one puts over the tribulations of life's pitfalls; it is an overall optimism that allows us to view the glass as being half full.

This attitude of gratitude and optimism goes beyond psychological benefits to improving one's overall health. Dr. Laura Kubzansky, professor of health and behavior at the Harvard School of Public Health, says, "Optimism—confidence and a positive outlook on personal experiences—may be as heart helpful as any drug or fat-free diet." It is important to distinguish between our knee-jerk reactions to daily upsets and the long-term effects of a negative outlook.

In small doses, negative emotion may actually benefit health when released in a productive manner, says Don Colbert, MD, board certified in family practice and anti-aging medicine. According to Dr. Colbert, when negative emotions such as fear, anxiety, and anger are prolonged, "These attitudes may cause this heightened state to lead to adrenal exhaustion, fatigue, anxiety and panic attacks, irritable bowel syndrome and tension headaches, a weakening of the immune system, and the final result can be severe illness." He goes on to say, "This emotional turmoil is the breeding ground for many physical diseases." This offers a compelling case for how a geriatric care manager's QOL recommendations can have clinical outcomes typically associated with quality of care.

HOW GCMs CAN IMPROVE HOLISTIC QUALITY OF LIFE

There are so many ways that GCMs can promote emotional, intellectual, physical, and spiritual QOL for their clients; the key is to find the unique formula that gives meaning for each client and to build a plan from there.

There are four steps to addressing a client's holistic QOL: (1) assessing his or her needs and interests, (2) prioritizing these needs, (3) developing and implementing an activity plan that will address these needs, and (4) evaluating success and refining the plan. Although this may seem complex and time consuming, in reality it is a fairly intuitive process.

For example, one GCM focused her holistic QOL efforts for one client on gardening:

> My client, Mrs. J, was an avid gardener until she had a massive stroke with frontal lobe damage. When Mrs. J became distressed that she could no longer tend to her garden, I worked with the family to put in raised beds with wide edges so she could still get her hands dirty and experience the beauty and wonder of growing flowers, despite her stroke. While Mrs. J may have planted some of her flowers upside down, her ability to still do the thing she loved—gardening—gave a tremendous boost to her quality of life
>
> —Michelle Boudinot,
> NorthBay Eldercare Solutions

ROADBLOCKS TO ADDRESSING HOLISTIC QUALITY OF LIFE

There are many real roadblocks that can prevent care managers from focusing on holistic elements of QOL. Care managers are often brought in when a client is experiencing more urgent health matters, such as compliance with prescriptions, recovery from surgery, or deteriorating physical and/or mental capacity, which need immediate attention and leave little room for any other kind of care in the short term. In addition, there are baseline physical and mental health issues, including depression, decreased physical or cognitive functioning, social isolation, and client apathy, which can cause care managers to inadvertently ignore the client's holistic QOL needs.

Also, the general public is largely unfamiliar with how an older adult's holistic QOL can improve physiological ailments. As a result, GCMs have had to educate family members and medical practitioners about the importance of QOL in overall care planning and about the value of spending care management dollars on QOL issues. Although these impediments are sometimes difficult, they are not insurmountable, and by using creativity and drawing on community resources, care managers can adapt activities and adjust expectations to facilitate emotional, intellectual, physical, and/or spiritual stimulation for almost any client. The best way to get started on creating a QOL plan is to figure out what will provide the client with an enhanced sense of purpose, meaning, or connectedness.

STEP 1: ASSESS THE CLIENT'S HOLISTIC QUALITY OF LIFE

Assessing a client's needs in terms of holistic QOL can be done either formally, informally, or through a combination of the two approaches.[12] Unlike other kinds of health assessments, understanding an individual client's "recipe" for enhancing holistic QOL is far from scientific. Although the GCM using an assessment tool is helpful, ultimately it is a nuanced, relationship-driven process that will enable the care manager to figure out what gives each client meaning and purpose. In this chapter, there are examples of both formal and informal assessments that can be used to identify both how well a client's holistic QOL needs are being met and which elements are still missing. However, each care manager will probably develop his or her own unique way of assessing this very personal, individual question for clients. Ultimately, it does not matter how GCMs explore the elements of emotional, intellectual, physical, and spiritual well-being with their clients; what matters is that they find a way that works for each person.

Formal Assessment of Holistic Quality of Life

Geriatric care advocates and researchers now propose that assessing QOL for older adults should include an evaluation of the older adult's mind, body, spirit, environment, and life experiences.[13] In terms of formal assessment, Rosalie Kane and her colleagues at the University of Minnesota have developed an assessment for QOL in nursing homes that focuses on 11 outcome domains that constitute "psychosocial" QOL, including individuality, enjoyment, meaningful activity, and spiritual well-being. For purposes of this focus on holistic QOL, this assessment has been adapted and shortened as Exhibit 10–1.

Some care management practices have their own ways to assess holistic QOL and may be able to provide care managers with useful tools for determining where to focus QOL activities. Sage Eldercare Solutions, based in San Francisco and San Mateo, California, has developed the assessment shown in Exhibit 10–2 to help GCMs better understand their clients' holistic QOL needs as part of a therapeutic activities program they offer to their clients.

Informal Assessment of Holistic Quality of Life

Conducting a formal assessment of a client's holistic QOL is helpful for establishing a baseline of the client's current situation and needs. This baseline will be useful when evaluating progress and refining the holistic QOL plan for the client. However, care managers also build rich relationships with their clients and assess their clients' needs through more informal observations and conversation. This type of informal assessment can yield excellent information from the client and the client's caregiver and/or family because the care manager can weave questions and inquiries into the conversation in a way that may be less threatening than a formal evaluation.

If the goal of a formal assessment is to determine the "when" and "how" in terms of integrating a focus on a client's QOL, then the informal assessment will help determine the "what"—which activities will resonate with the client and are most likely to bring him or her meaning and fulfillment. This "what" information will come into play during the next step, creating the plan for improving the client's holistic QOL. Exhibit 10–3 provides a framework for informal assessment of holistic QOL.

■ STEP 2: ANALYZE ASSESSMENT RESULTS AND PRIORITIZE CLIENT NEEDS

After the GCM conducts formal and/or informal assessments, the GCM will have gathered a great deal of information about the client's needs and interests in the areas of emotional, intellectual, physical, and spiritual QOL. In all likelihood, a few themes or key areas will emerge in looking through these data. Perhaps the GCM noticed many photos of pets and the client mentioned a love of animals during their conversations. Or maybe the client is completely sedentary, yet described in great detail the wonderful camping and hiking trips he took in his youth. Or maybe the care manager learned that the client was a teacher for many years and yearns to work with children again in some capacity. Or it could just be that the client is lonely and needs to see other people, including family and potential friends, more often.

Exhibit 10–1   Formal Assessment for Holistic Quality of Life

Holistic QOL Area	QOL Outcome	Outcome Indicators	How to Assess Client QOL in This Area
Emotional	Relationships	Clients engage in meaningful person-to-person interchange where the purpose is social.	• Ask client to list the people in his life that are important to him. • Check his schedule and/or ask him when he last saw any/all of these people. • Interview caregivers and family members to assess how often the client has social interactions.
Intellectual	Autonomy	Clients take initiative and make choices for their lives and care.	• Ask client to name one decision she has made in the last month. • Interview caregivers and family members to assess how much they engage client in decision making.
	Enjoyment	Clients express or exhibit pleasure and enjoyment, verbally and nonverbally. Conversely, they do not express or exhibit unhappiness, distress, or lack of enjoyment.	• Ask client what brings him enjoyment and to identify activities that have been enjoyable in the past month. • Interview caregivers and family members to find out what brings pleasure and enjoyment for client. • Determine how often the client gets to do the things he finds enjoyable.
	Meaningful activity	Clients engage in discretionary behavior, either active activity or passive observation, which they find interesting, stimulating, and/or worthwhile. Conversely, they tend not be bored with their lives.	• Ask client to name at least one thing she enjoyed doing in the past. • Ask client to name at least one thing she enjoys doing now. • Ask client to describe the last time she engaged in an activity related to her past or present interests. • Interview caregivers and family members about the client's interests and the types of activities she does that match her interests.
Spiritual	Spiritual well-being	Clients perceive that their needs and concerns for religion, prayer, meditation, moral values, and meaning in life are met.	• Ask client about his religious background and the level he is/was engaged in a religious community, for example, church, temple, mosque. • If he no longer attends any regular services in his religion, probe for the reason why, assessing whether it is a logistical issue or true choice. • If the client is not affiliated with any formal religion, ask what gives him meaning in his life. Is it time with friends/family? Nature? Volunteering? Pets/animals? • If client is religious, ask what aspects of the religion are most meaningful to him. • Interview caregivers and family to explore what may give the client deeper meaning in his life.

Source: Reproduced with permission from Oxford University Press.

Exhibit 10–2   Sage Awakenings Therapeutic Program Assessment

---

Personal Interest Inventory

Name: _____

Address: _____

Place of Birth & Past Residences: _____

Current Living Status: ❑ Single ❑ Married ❑ Separated ❑ Divorced ❑ Widowed

Titles Held: _____ Dates of Marriage/Divorce/Death: _____

Past Occupations: _____ Special Achievements: _____

Hobbies: _____ Interests: _____

Social Activities Enjoyed: _____

Sports Played/Forms of Exercise Enjoyed: _____

Veteran: ❑ Yes ❑ No   If so, dates served, posts and branch of military? _____

Dreams: _____

Work/Volunteer: _____ Pets (past and present): _____

Birth Family Structure: _____ Nuclear Family Structure: _____

Primary & Languages Spoken: _____ Education (highest grade level)
                                          & Field of Study: _____
                                          Religious Preference: _____

Culture / Ethnicity: _____ Literacy: ❑ Reads English ❑ Writes English
                                                       ❑ Reads / Writes in Spoken Language

Favorite Foods: _____

Family Traditions: _____

Daily Rituals: _____

Sensory Limits: _____

Functional Limits: _____

Most Memorable Experiences:

1. _____
2. _____

Three things I enjoy the most:

1. _____
2. _____
3. _____

Three Things You Should Know About Me (Values, Beliefs, Traditions, Achievements):

1. _____
2. _____
3. _____

continues

Exhibit 10–2   Sage Awakenings Therapeutic Program Assessment (continued)

ACTIVITIES CHECKLIST: (Care Manager to fill in based on information provided below; may also be helpful to read off several items to gauge client's interest level for each)

- Brain Aerobics
- Crosswords
- Memoir creation
- Quizzes
- Documentaries
- Scrapbook creation
- Memory exercises
- Life review
- Reminiscence
- Creative writing
- Exercise
- Yoga
- Tai chi
- Historical review
- Painting, drawing
- Flower arranging
- Dancing
- Singing
- Playing instruments
- Sculpting

- Collage
- Gardening
- Poetry
- Cooking
- Shopping
- Sending and receiving mail
- Computer research
- Listening to music; types of music

    _____
- Social engagements:

    _____
- Philosophical inquiry
- Animals, pets; specify area of interest:

    _____
- Performances; mediums of interest:

    _____
- Arts and lectures; topics of interest:

    _____
- Lifelong learning; topics of interest:

    _____
- Nature walks and hikes

Source: Sage Awakenings Therapeutic Services, Sage Eldercare Solutions. www.sageeldercare.com.

The point is for the care manager to prioritize the client's needs based on the information gathered and to create a holistic QOL plan based on these priorities. Given limited time and resources, this prioritization process should help the care manager rank the various areas of holistic QOL in order of importance for the client and give a clear understanding of which should be addressed first, second, and so forth.

Exhibit 10–3   Questions to Use for Informal Assessment

Emotional

- How satisfied are you with the frequency of social interactions (with friends, family, neighbors) in your life?

- How do you feel when you are getting ready to see family members? How do you feel afterward?

- Is loneliness an important problem in your life?

- Do you cultivate friendships as one remedy for loneliness?

- Are friends more or less meaningful in your life than immediate family members are?

- If you have friends of long standing, to what do you attribute the success of these relationships?

- Do you seek out groups or organizations where you might meet new friends?

- How do you feel when you are getting ready to see friends? How do you feel afterward?

Intellectual

- What was your career when you were working? Are you involved in this profession in any way now? Would you like to be?

- How important was work to you? Was it more important than other, nonwork activities or relationships?

- Please describe some of your greatest achievements.

- What kinds of activities do you or did you engage in to use your mind and intellect? Reading? Crossword or other word puzzles? Political discussions?

- When was the last time you learned something new (new game, new kind of information, new way to do something)? How did this feel?

- What are some interests that you haven't yet had the opportunity to pursue?

Physical

- Looking back on your life, what were the things you did to foster your physical health? How can you retrieve and adapt these activities for the sake of your health today?

- If you were physically active in earlier stages of your life, what did you enjoy most about it?

- Do you have any fears or stereotypes that are holding you back from engaging in physical activity?

Spiritual

- Do you consider yourself a spiritual person? If so, what were the most influential factors (persons, teachings, institutions, events) in shaping this spirituality?

- If the words *spiritual* or *religious* have no meaning or have negative connotations for you, how do you express your deepest philosophy of life? What are its principles, its virtues, its goals, and its actions?

- What are you grateful for? Can you make a brief list of the things for which you are most thankful—either small happenings (for example, the warm sun through the window) or major items (for example, a loving family).

- How important is being in nature to you? What places, elements, or environments (beach, mountains, parks, or birds) bring you the most enjoyment?

Source: Crossroad Publishing Company (1994). Bianchi, Eugene. pp. 199–222. Used with permission.

■ STEP 3: CREATE A PLAN FOR ADDRESSING THE CLIENT'S HOLISTIC QUALITY OF LIFE

Now that the care manager has a concrete understanding of what brings the client joy or sparks interest or boosts his or her energy and which areas are most likely to bring the client fulfillment and improved well-being, the question is how to get there. This next section includes examples of activities and programs designed to engage older adults in the areas of emotional, intellectual, physical, and spiritual well-being, along with stories of how GCMs have successfully affected their clients' lives in these areas.

A. Explore Ideas and Resources Related to Each Element of Holistic QOL

The list that follows is just the beginning of learning how to address holistic QOL. GCMs can gather other ideas by talking with colleagues, visiting local community or senior centers, or using the Internet. Ultimately, each care manager will use his or her own creativity, along with all the resources and ideas he or she has gathered (including input from other professionals—art therapists, recreational therapists, care providers—and community opportunities) to tailor a plan that meets his or her clients' needs.

Emotional Quality of Life

When care managers work to address a client's emotional QOL, they tend to focus on social interactions. One important source of interactions with others comes from members of the care team and especially from the care providers who provide hands-on care. Geriatric care managers are in a unique position to positively influence the quality of communication between the care provider and client, whether it's because the care providers are employed by the care manager or simply because the care manager has ample opportunity to model effective and compassionate communication with clients.

Communications that enhance QOL can come in the form of very short practical exchanges and the quality of communications has specific nuances in relation to clients with cognitive impairment. According to studies funded by the Alzheimer's Association and the National Institute on Aging, we will experience a rise in the rate of Alzheimer's of nearly 30% in the first two decades of the new millennium; 70% in the first three decades; and a full 300% in the first half of the 21st century.[14]

It is safe to say that we are facing a constant and increasing demand for care providers who understand that the quality of their daily exchanges with their clients is a critical ingredient in their clients' overall quality of life experience. Furthermore, it is important to recognize that by extension, care providers' satisfaction from the work experience also benefits when the interactions are positive and grounded in a real understanding of appropriate communication techniques for clients with dementia.

Teepa Snow, a dementia care and training specialist who began dealing with dementias at the age of 7 when she cared for her ailing grandfather, works to bring other healthcare professionals up to speed about dementia care and how to both emotionally and physically interact with patients.

Snow not only brings with her a plethora of practical experience, she also has a great understanding of the organic changes that occur in the brain with dementia. First, she explains that it is important for caregivers and care managers to understand that the afflicted brain is permanently damaged and cannot be fixed. A patient who does not call her own daughter by the correct name, says Snow, "Is not holding out; this is brain failure."

Snow goes on to advise her training participants not to pressure patients into getting their information correct, but rather to continue with their client's reality, whatever that may be. Rather than providing a truth-based experience for the client with dementia, Snow suggests it is better for the patient to feel connected to another person. If a client asks if you have seen her grandmother, Snow recommends drawing on the knowledge about her to diffuse anxiety and build a connection such as "Do you mean your grandmother who took you fishing in the creek and taught you to bake bread when you were little?" rather than saying "No, I haven't seen your grandmother," or "Your grandmother is in heaven. Don't try to correct," says Snow, "go with the flow. Being right isn't necessarily helpful. Empathy is more important than trying to impose a reality that is long gone."

Just as important as how we engage clients with dementia, it is also important how we physically approach them. Snow teaches that the golden rule is to "Greet before we treat." Respect their physical space, and be sensitive to how easily they may become startled or frightened when approached. She suggests a fresh new greeting at the beginning of each encounter.

In contrast, in Reality Orientation, the patient is continually reminded of current information with every interaction. The patient is always reminded of the correct time, place, and person with whom they are interacting. Reality Orientation is often used by care providers who have not been trained in an alternative approach, such as Naomi Feil's Validation Therapy.

Validation Therapy focuses on the emotional and psychological consequences of short-term memory loss. Feil grew up in a residential facility for the elderly in Ohio where her father was the administrator and her mother was the social worker. From her early experiences she became aware of the negative effects that reality orientation had on those with dementia. She later wrote, "I found that not only was awareness of reality intolerable for this group of aged whose reality held steady deterioration in functioning, loss of affectional ties, and whose future held death, but sudden insight into reality brought about pain, withdrawal and increased dependency."[15]

Disheartened by what she had witnessed, Feil developed her alternative approach, which did not emphasize the need for a grasp on reality but rather set as its goal the communication with those suffering from dementia in whatever reality they happened to be; the objective being the relief of the sufferer's distress and the restoration of their self-esteem. In her own words, "Validation means accepting the disorientated old-old adults who live in the past. The Validation worker helps them sum up their lifetime. The Validation worker helps by listening with empathy . . . Accept people where they are. The disoriented old-old finally struggle to resolve past conflicts. Their goals differ from the goals of their middle-age caretakers. Validation helps them reach their goal in this last stage of life."[16]

Another approach to dementia and Alzheimer's care was developed in the 1990s by Virginia Bell, MSW, and David Troxel, MPH, while working at the University of Kentucky Alzheimer's Disease Research Center. Bell and Troxel suggest that a person suffering from dementia will benefit greatly by having a "best friend." This person, whether it is a caregiver, loved one, staff member, or friend, takes on the role of a close companion who provides the much needed empathy and concern for the client. The Best Friend's approach incorporates robust knowledge of the elder's past to help people feel seen and understood. It is through this relationship that the elder is able to feel their own security and value. One important ingredient for this "best friend" is something that they call the caregiving "knack"; defined as "the art of doing difficult things with ease, clever tricks, and strategies." The Best Friends model has been adopted by many dementia care programs throughout the world.

It is important for care managers to establish an approach that best suits their client and enlist other members of the care team to deliver their services accordingly. Having the ability to relate to and communicate effectively with those who provide an elder's care is fundamental in providing a quality of life that helps a person navigate through this tumultuous life stage.

Social interactions with family and friends are of key importance in addressing a client's emotional QOL. Opportunities for participation in programs that forge intergenerational relationships or provide structured social opportunities with other elders are also valuable resources available in many communities.

If the client's family is nearby, it could be as simple as working to arrange a regular schedule for visits and marking the visits on the calendar or having visitors sign a guestbook when they arrive so the client knows when to expect company. This allows the client to look forward to these interactions instead of not knowing when or if someone is going to arrive.

If family is far away or unavailable for other reasons, the focus may turn to friendships, helping the client nurture or rekindle relationships by arranging the transportation or other logistics necessary for the client to see his or her friends on a regular basis. Since it is common that friends move away to be near their families or go to a care community, it can be helpful to establish a regular "telephone date" to help support continued connections even at a distance. It can be helpful for the care manager to work with the care providers to take responsibility for keeping these dates by initiating the calls at the designated time. Further, new technology such as Skype, a software application that makes videoconferencing easy and accessible on most personal computers, has potential for tremendous application in keeping clients connected. Indeed, the author's 5-month-old and 3-year-old children regularly "visit" their 100-year-old great grandmother who lives across the country. These virtual visits bring the conversations alive in a way that is more interactive and more personal than typically is the case across a telephone connection.

Senior centers, which provide drop-in opportunities and structured events, can provide other occasions for older adults to have social interactions that may lead to friendships. Many schools and day care centers also have intergenerational programs, where older adults can spend time with children, each enjoying the special gifts the other brings to the exchange.

One care manager put together an extraordinary event for the clients in her care, which honored their wisdom and beauty and provided a big boost to the emotional quality of their lives:

> As a Mother's Day event and gift, I planned a ladies tea and called it "Les Grandes Dames Tea." The party (complete with formal invitations) was held at one of the nicest senior communities in the area, where we arranged for wait staff to serve petits fours and fancy cookies and pour coffee and tea from silver tea services. The care managers and our "ladies" all dressed up in all manner of finery, including big picture hats, treasured wraps, and lace gloves. Each Grande Dame even received a wrist corsage and even a glass of champagne. We also enlisted the services of a tuxedo-clad handsome young man who played the piano and sang oldies to each and every lady. A film crew and photographer caught all of this on tape and each lady had a personal filmed interview session. It was the best of care management—a celebration for those Grande Dames whose lives are no longer filled with very many high spots.
>
> —Marsha R. Foley, RN, MBA,
> ElderCare Options, Ltd.

Another care manager organized a social occasion in her client's assisted living facility, which evoked the client's past history as a very social person in her community:

> When Mrs. R, a former garden club lady, was moved into an apartment in an

upscale assisted living facility, I decided to help her host a Christmas tea to meet her new neighbors. I arranged for some furniture from her old house to be delivered, sent out invitations to all of the residents, and took her shopping to buy a nice outfit for the occasion. Mrs. R. was thrilled to play hostess again and it really helped her feel comfortable in her new living situation.

—Sally Gold, MSW,
Geriatric Resource Services

Sometimes the relationship between the care manager and the client itself can produce measurable improvements in the client's emotional QOL (and, as in the following anecdote, for the care manager, too):

When I first started working with Mrs. D, she had advanced dementia, was striking her care providers and refused to take her medications. To assist her, I decided to accompany her on outings around the city—something I love to do. We began walking around her lively San Francisco neighborhood, talking with interesting people we met, and pausing to entertain onlookers. These experiences provided socialization outside of her residential facility and enriched her daily life. During my time with her, Mrs. D has transformed from threatening other residents in her facility to creating collages in expressive arts groups with a smile on her face. Her anti-anxiety medications have also been reduced to their lowest level in years. Our relationship has helped Mrs. D re-ignite with her inner spark, and has allowed me to do the same.

—Tara Bradley, MA, MFTI,
Sage Eldercare Solutions

Perhaps one of the most innovative examples of connecting elders is the Senior Center Without Walls founded by director Terry Englehart in the San Francisco Bay Area. Using the University Without Walls as her model, Englehart developed her program to bring informational sessions, entertainment, and a support network to those seniors who are not able to leave their homes. Through her teleconferencing programs the center's members are able to participate in an ever-growing network of Bay Area seniors. Recently, Englehart has introduced a phone-based game of Boggle that she modified and personally facilitates. Throughout the duration of the word game seniors can be heard to express their joy and laughter.

Besides the critical cognitive exercise in generating words, the "Bogglers" are gaining the benefits of socializing and interacting with others who are also homebound. Nannetta Washington, a member of the center's teleconferencing program, says, "It made me realize there's a lot to do in the world even though I'm confined to my home." At 83 years old, Washington is determined to keep busy despite the disability that prevents her from leaving her home. Besides Boggle, she has enrolled in several other programs including a spiritual group, Bible class, bingo, creative writing, and play reading.

"We've all become comrades in arms," says Washington. "We all have illnesses or suffer from different things, but we are connected because we're all in the same situation. You form a sort of kinship." Her sentiment is echoed by 80-year-old Frances Denny, one of the original members who says, "The program has given me a sense of not being totally isolated from other human beings." Englehart launched her program with just six seniors, and within the first 30 months it grew to over 100 members. "We want to be able to help them," says Englehart, "because we might be their lifeline and sometimes their only thing they're connected to."

These are wonderful examples of social interactions for clients, but there are other ways to positively affect a client's emotional QOL, such as through pet or massage therapies. One care manager had tremendous success in helping address her client's loneliness through the adoption of a pet cat:

> We had one client, Mrs. N, who was 90 and had been widowed for over 25 years. Since the passing of her husband, Mrs. N had few constants in her life; family was far away and many of her friends were gone too. She loved to feed the squirrels and birds in front of her house, and spoke fondly of her neighbor's cat. After discussing the idea with her, we brought Mrs. N to the SPCA on her birthday, where a volunteer spent several hours helping her select an older cat that had been waiting for the right owner. The new pet was named "Penny," and she became Mrs. N's closest relationship, a loving lap cat who could sit for hours on her owner's knees. Penny gave Mrs. N a sense of responsibility for another creature and helped motivate her to keep living. Her connection to Penny also mitigated the loss of control Mrs. N experienced as her body changed over time.
>
> —Nina Pflumm Herndon, MA, CMC,
> Sage Eldercare Solutions

Touch therapy or massage is another innovative way to help clients feel emotionally connected and improve their physical well-being. According to national statistics, about one-third of massage patients are adults age 55 and older, and this growing popularity is helping to dispel some of the negative misconceptions about massage among seniors. Elmer "Lee" Manning, an 81-year-old man who has been getting regular massages for 2 years, has become a convert to the healing benefits of the practice. "It sure helps me sleep. It helps me move," he said. "It helps about everything." Massage and other forms of touch therapy can also provide clients with tangible emotional well-being. Anita Booth, a massage therapist who works with many older adults, sees the impact of touch for her senior clients. "The elderly don't get loving touch. They might get medical attention, but they don't get loving

touch," she says. "Massage therapy is very special. It's a much more sustained and loving connection between human beings."[17]

Intellectual Quality of Life

The informal assessment data gathered in Step 1 are essential in helping the GCM figure out how to foster intellectual QOL for a client. Some clients, who were very attached to their careers, will resonate most closely with activities and events that provide an opportunity to use their professional skills, such as talking with a former colleague or reading (or being read to/from) books or articles related to their professions.

For example, one care manager tried countless strategies to mitigate her client's sometimes disruptive behavior until she tapped into his background as an architect:

> One client was a man with Alzheimer's who had major agitation but was also wheelchair-bound. He was in a facility and was always pulling things apart and driving the staff crazy. We tried several interventions—nothing worked. Then we recalled that he used to be a draftsman and bought him an Etch-a-Sketch. The device reminded him of his former career and he was so content playing with all those lines!
>
> —Michelle Boudinot, MA,
> NorthBay Eldercare

The role of creativity is also very important for intellectual QOL. This category is not limited to traditional art activities; anything that inspires an older adult to engage with mind and spirit and to enthusiastically participate can be seen as "creative." Creative activities include cooking, hobbies, interesting conversation, or even community work. Creative activities not only help bolster the intellectual QOL for clients, but they may also improve their physiological health. According to researchers, "Experimental studies indicate that creative activities and their consequent positive effect on mood and morale can lead to an increased production of protective immune cells."[18] Many senior centers and community colleges offer low-cost cooking, art, or writing classes for older adults, where they can pursue their creativity in a supportive, low-risk setting.

One care manager tapped into her client's creativity to stimulate her intellectual QOL through the photographs the client had taken throughout her life:

> One client had been an accomplished photographer who took many pictures, but none were in photo albums. I arranged for a high school student to get credit in her class for community service by working with this client. The student visited twice weekly to talk about the photos and put them in albums where she could show the client the pictures. Some days, the client couldn't tell anything about a picture, but she always recognized the image and loved seeing the photo again. This activity also connected back to the client's career as a teacher and her love of working with students.
>
> —Martha J. Brown, MSW, LISW, RG, Geriatric Care Management, LLC

Here is another remarkable example of what can be accomplished when a care manager is able to combine the needs and creative talents of the client:

> One of our first clients was a 55-year-old single woman with a history of chronic mental illness dating to her early 20s. She had graduated from college, but soon after, spent much of her life in and out of mental hospitals. By the time we met her, she was determined to live independently in a condo her trust had purchased for her. Money was no issue—the family trust could pay for her needs and for our care management. However, she was "institutionalized"—not really having any experience with "normal" social interaction. Her care manager discovered that she

loved poetry and introduced her to a poet who had specialized training in using poetry as a therapeutic medium.

> They met weekly or bi-weekly over a number of years to talk about poetry and write poems. The care manager arranged to self-publish two books of poetry that the client wrote and send copies to her extended family. This gave her family a new understanding of the client that went beyond her label as someone who was mentally ill. In addition, with this and other interventions (including going to a nursing home once a month and playing the piano and making dolls for Children's Hospital), this client had only one hospitalization in the 10 years we worked with her, until her death at 65 of cancer.
>
> —Phyllis Mensh Brostoff, CISW, CMC, Stowell Associates SelectStaff, Inc.

Travel to new or familiar places is another way for clients to stimulate past interests and improve their intellectual QOL.

> I had a client who was devastated when his wife died of Alzheimer's. He didn't want to leave the nursing home where the two of them had lived, and became completely passive, refusing to even get dressed without assistance. As he grew increasingly complacent at the nursing home and depression loomed, we suggested that maybe it would be fun for him to take a trip, as he had once been an avid traveler. He researched his options and chose New York City so he could take in a Broadway show and go to some great restaurants. Not long after, he decided to go to Las Vegas, where he saw "girlie shows" and Cirque du Soleil, stayed at the Bellagio, and ate wonderfully. These trips recharged his interest in life and he now uses a laptop computer, talks on his cell phone and reads voraciously, despite his low vision. He's very frail and uses a walker, but he's planning his next trip to Paris and taking French lessons to get ready. Despite his age and the loss of his dear companion, this

client is reinventing his life and in the process is stimulating his intellectual, emotional and spiritual quality of life.

—Sally Gold, MSW,
Geriatric Resource Services

Reminiscence and Storytelling

As Erik Ericson discussed in his Theory of Psychological Development, the eighth and final stage of development is one of intense reflection and evaluation. Older adults, when confronted with the prospect of their own mortality, become somewhat consumed with the need to determine if their life has been one well spent and that they have achieved their goals and objectives. If this self-evaluation reveals a positive picture of a life well lived then this eighth stage of development can be experienced with satisfaction and integrity. If, however, the picture is not one of positive results, it is not uncommon for the elder to experience a deep despair.

Dr. Robert Butler, physician and first director of the National Institute on Aging, echoes these theories in his work on *life review* where he suggests that all people nearing the end of their lives undergo a psychological process whereby they evaluate and attempt to resolve their past as a preparation for death. Dr. Butler further proposes that this process becomes particularly complicated for those with memory impairment. In these cases the process cannot be completed "unless a means is found for both generating the *forgotten material* and for providing a sense of self-identity"[19]

Based on these insights, it is no wonder that the role of storytelling and reminiscence is very important for older adults, especially for clients that are beginning to experience memory loss and dementia. There has been much documented success with writing programs for Alzheimer's patients, where the participants come together regularly to write down and share their life stories with one another. Alan Dienstag, who documented the group's work, notes, "The writing group gave

memory back to its members. They transformed in the experience of writing from people who forget to people who remember."[20] Although the members of the group struggled to continue to write and read their stories as time progressed and their illnesses worsened, they still found dignity and solidarity in the process of sharing their lives with each other.

A similar program for more independent older adults, the Illuminated Life workshop, is a comprehensive, structured life review program designed to help improve participants' psychological functioning.[21] Through the workshop, participants look retrospectively at their lives to consider creative postretirement roles and integrate the learning they have gathered throughout their lives. Created in 1987 by Dr. Abe Arkoff, the workshop has been presented at its home base, the University of Hawaii's Osher Lifelong Learning Institute, and in other venues, including retirement residences, senior centers, churches, Elderhostel, and several mainland sites. At each weekly session, the participants discuss a predetermined life question and work in small groups to share their answers. Research with older women completing the workshop in 2000 showed significant gain on a measure of psychological well-being in contrast to a control group that showed no change.[22]

Similarly, the Autobiographical Studies Program, at the University of California, Los Angeles, helps participants become aware of the lives they have lived and more confident and optimistic about facing the future.[23] Using five different courses, including Guided Autobiography and Family History, the program equips participants to use the gift of long life in productive ways. According to the program's research, participants report feeling empowered in their self-knowledge and use their newly honed empathetic skills to forge new friendships and pursue new interests.[24]

Time Slips is a program being replicated around the country that encourages older adults with dementia to tap into creativity and share their stories.[25] Using hour-long, group storytelling sessions with up to a dozen people in the middle stages of dementia, care manager facilitators encourage creative responses that downplay the importance of memory. Using an image to prompt responses, a facilitator asks open-ended questions and weaves together all the answers, from the poetic to the nonsensical, into a story. The participants are encouraged to laugh, sing, and move as they tell their stories, which are often difficult to capture in words.

Even if a formal group is not available nearby, care managers can foster the act of reminiscences through writing prompts that begin with phrases such as, "I remember . . . ," "The house where I grew up . . . ," or "The last time I saw . . ." If the client is unable to write, the care manager can record his or her words in a special journal and can read these words back to the client periodically as a way of preserving these memories for him or her and honoring the life that the person has lived.[26]

One care manager used poetry to help her client connect with past memories:

> One client had been an English and biology high school teacher, who wrote many poems. We copied them and put them in page protectors and in a three-ring notebook so visitors and staff at the care home could look at and read her the poems and on good days (she also has dementia), she can read the poems herself. She also illustrated them. Having someone read them and refer to them honors and validates this client, and gives her extra attention.
>
> —Martha J. Brown, MSW, LISW, RG, Geriatric Care Management, LLC

Another care manager worked with an art therapist and the client's caregivers to help the client develop a scrapbook of family memories:

> For one client, who had a moderate degree of dementia, I worked with both an art therapist and the client's caregivers to create a family history scrapbook. The art therapist, who started the scrapbook project and met with the client once a week, also trained the caregivers so they could continue the process between visits. The client's aides were able to facilitate reminiscences while they worked with her on the scrapbook by learning about her family members and reading letters from different periods of her life. These activities had a calming effect for the client, and helped her connect to her family's rich history. Within six weeks after working on the scrapbook, the client had improved remarkably. She had amazing eye contact and had totally changed from agitated mumbling to having lucid moments with greater clarity of speech. She was also more connected to her past interests, more calm and could relate better to her care providers.
>
> —Leonie Nowitz, MSW, BCD, Center for Lifelong Growth

The scrapbook activity, where the caregivers pick some of the client's favorite photos and letters, is an excellent way to begin building an individualized therapeutic activity kit or "toolbox" to improve intellectual QOL for clients with dementia. This type of box (or basket, bin, etc.) contains activities that can be implemented by the GCM, caregivers, or family members to stimulate mental processing and ease the side effects of dementia for the client. Examples of items that might go in a therapeutic activity kit include letters in plastic coverings that can be read and reread regularly, music CDs, art supplies, postcards from places where the client has traveled, playing cards, balls or fabrics with different textures to help stimulate touch, and photos or other items that trigger pleasant memories and cognitive response.[27]

Of course, some clients may not resonate with or have the capacity to engage in activities related to past careers, reminiscences, or creativity. For these clients, who need some form of intellectual QOL activity, traditional "mind exercises," such as jigsaw, crossword or word puzzles or other activities may work best. There may even be a level of comfort for clients in the repetition of mind activities and in working to meet new challenges in the exercises as they become familiar with the process.

Physical Quality of Life

As described earlier, there is a great deal of new research about the benefits of physical exercise for older adults and about the different kinds of exercise that this age group can continue to practice. Common forms of exercise for older adults include walking, yoga, tai chi, gardening, and specially designed exercise classes that focus on cardiovascular, stretching, and/or weight training. Senior day care and senior centers are wonderful resources for exercise classes and activities for elders, as are local recreation centers, YMCAs, and community colleges.

Interestingly, recent advances in gaming technology have created a new outlet for older adults to benefit from such vigorous activities as bowling, boxing, and batting—all from their living rooms. Specifically, Wii, released by Nintendo, is a new home video gaming console that focuses on player interaction. The distinguishing feature of this console is that it employs a wireless controller that can be used as a handheld pointer that detects movement allowing the player to become an active character in the game.

Rather than sitting stationary and manipulating buttons and levers, players now move their own body to engage the game's animation. In this way, seniors, and those who typically cannot endure very strenuous activity can engage themselves in just the right movements to gain healthful benefits without the worry of exhausting themselves. According to Dr. Ben Hertz, a director at the Medical College of Georgia, "Wii allows patients to work in a virtual environment that's safe, fun, and motivational." He goes on to explain that "the games require visual perception, eye-hand coordination, figure-ground relationships, and sequenced movement, so it's a huge treatment tool." Yet even more impressive than the physical benefits gained by the 20 Parkinson's patients who participated in Dr. Hertz's 8-week study was the dramatic reduction in their level of depression; the majority of the group experienced depression levels decreasing to zero.

Van Wert Manor, a nursing facility that has provided long- and short-term care in Ohio for over 35 years, has been raving about their results in using Wii-fit games, cleverly dubbed "Wii-hab." Administrator Jacque Welch has found benefits beyond the physical through the use of the Wii system as patients' social interaction have also improved. People are not only playing games that they otherwise would not be able to, they are competing and conversing about their related experiences, including those from their younger days. Studies continue to be done on the impact of Wii-hab on those managing Parkinson's Disease, arthritis, and even Alzheimer's.

On Lok Lifeways, which began as one of the nation's first senior day health centers and now has 10 centers throughout the San Francisco Bay area, introduced Wii as part of their innovative physical therapy program in 2009. The initial responses to the program from their physical therapists have indicated significant improvements in participant's posture, endurance, strength, movement, and balance, as well as enhanced hand-eye coordination, motor skills, concentration, and mental acuity.

One 75-year-old participant at Lifeway's Rose Center for the past 12 years says, "The Wii helps me to exercise, moving my arms and fingers. I sometimes feel numb in my fingers and I feel the Wii helps to prevent it." An 81-year-old participant has stated that "Before I couldn't use my left arm so much, but now I can use it better. I think the Wii really helped me." The positive physical outcomes were certainly predictable, but what came as a surprise to Lifeway's recreation therapy department was the considerable improvement in participant's self-esteem and sociability. The games that Wii has brought into these elder's lives has brought with them a rare commodity for those who require constant care; excitement, participation, and the sense of accomplishment. Even among those who choose not to participate but engage in the supportive role of cheering on the players report a marked elevation of their mood, even having an impact on those suffering from depression.

One last important outcome of this innovative system of elder engagement is that it often triggers a new strand of intergenerational connectivity between grandparent and grandchild. It seems that game technology has bridged the oldest and younger generations. Now that children, teenagers, and elders share a common bond for the fun and camaraderie of gaming, a new link of communication has emerged. One of the most critical social relationships in the family dynamic, the grandparent and grandchild, has found new opportunities to connect; this alone is like a dream come true for many families, particularly the isolated elders.

Physical engagement is an area where care managers often encounter resistance from some clients. After all, by age 75, about one in three men and one in two women do not engage in any physical activity,[28] so encouraging older adults to be physically active may require creativity and persistence from care managers and other care team members. One approach is to focus on a particular activity and how fun or interesting it may be rather than on the health or physical benefits of it. For example, if a client mentions that she used to love to dance with her husband, the care manager can probe about what kind of music they enjoyed while dancing. Then, on the next visit, the GCM can bring some samples of that music and encourage the client to get up and dance along. Once the client has connected back to her love of dancing with her husband, the care manager can then explore senior dance programs (e.g., at a local community center), where the client can get physical exercise while she has fun.

One care manager worked with a client's caregivers to use music and dance to encourage the client to walk to the bathroom, which she had been refusing to do:

> Since the client was a world traveler, we tried out a range of music. The aides started using jazz music to motivate her to get up and "dance" to the bathroom, which helped the client overcome her refusal to use the facilities.
>
> —Leonie Nowitz, MSW, BCD,
> Center for Lifelong Growth

Spiritual Quality of Life

When a care manager focuses on a client's spiritual QOL, he or she has an opportunity to explore what gives the client deeper meaning and purpose. For some people, spirituality may mean traditional religion, and, for these clients, care managers can help encourage contemplation about the role of religion and about the client's interest in rekindling or renewing an interest in religious faith. The care manager can also help tackle the logistics (e.g., transportation, wheelchair access), which may be preventing the client from participating in regular services, whether they are at a church, temple, mosque, or other house of worship.

For homebound clients, traveling to a religious service may seem overwhelming, but for those who still wish to connect with a larger spiritual community, the care manager may be able to connect to alternative ideas. Perhaps a minister or chaplain could visit the client in his or her home or care facility, or maybe there is a small chapel or scaled-down service available through a local assisted care facility designed for people of the same faith, such as a Jewish community center. Religious services that are broadcast via television or radio can also provide a way for clients with limited mobility to bond with rituals and prayers that carry significance and meaning.

One care manager worked for over a year to help her client reconnect with her faith community because, despite her advancing dementia, the manager knew how important this community was to her:

> One client was very involved in her church and had been part of a Sunday school group for more than 25 years. For a while, the Sunday school group used to visit her, but once her dementia progressed, the visits stopped. Knowing how important this connection was for my client, I provided information to the church about her dementia. Eventually, the group finally started visiting the client again, coming back for her birthday party. The client really responded and rose to the occasion. The visitors from the church enjoyed it too and saw that the residential care home was a welcoming place with really caring staff. Now, individual members of this group visit her regularly.
>
> —Martha J. Brown, MSW, LISW, RG, Geriatric Care Management, LLC

For some clients, the topic of faith may provoke some fear, especially for older adults who are unresolved about their feelings or memories of organized religion, and may be afraid of facing the end of life without clear beliefs about what will happen after death. If care managers encounter fear when discussing faith or spirituality with a client, it is important to not back away, but to let the client discuss and work through whatever feelings arise.

With other clients, for whom traditional religion does not have a lot of meaning, the care manager may need to use conversation and reminiscences to discover what activities, places, or people may provide each individual with a sense of deeper purpose.

One care manager in New Mexico found a way for one client to connect with the mountains, which had been a source of inspiration during his younger years:

> In our practice, we try to focus on what matters or mattered a lot in a person's life—especially for those clients with dementia. For example, we had a client who used to live in Alaska; he was a bush pilot and he loved the mountains. We arranged for a companion service with a wheelchair van to take him on drives twice a week where he could see the sky and the mountains. His dementia was advanced to the stage where he couldn't talk, but the staff said that after the drives, he was calm and content, and whenever the driver arrived, he would break out in a huge smile. By bringing this client close to the mountains, the sky, and to nature, we honored the elements that gave him meaning and improved his spiritual quality of life. While the landscape may not have been as dramatic as Alaska, it offered a hint of what this man knew and loved and lived all those years.
>
> —Martha J. Brown, MSW, LISW, RG, Geriatric Care Management, LLC

Another care manager used a "soft" approach to help a client reignite an interest in his religion and participate in meaningful rituals:

> I heard that my client had once been an Orthodox Jew, but was no longer practicing his religion. When I went to visit him during Hanukah, the caregivers had put up Christmas decorations all around the living space, but I did notice a Menorah tucked away on a shelf. I visited him at the time of day when a candle is normally lit, brought down the Menorah, and offered to read the accompanying prayer. He said, "You know I am agnostic." When I was quiet in response, he continued, "I was an orthodox Jew at one time." After a brief conversation, he asked me to proceed with reading the prayer, and I could tell that he was definitely tuned in.

At the Passover holiday, he insisted that the care providers light the Menorah each evening for eight nights. While this is not a traditional way of celebrating Passover, it was his way of acknowledging the passing of time and reaching out for a ritual that had previously been a source of meaning for him.

—Leonie Nowitz, MSW, BCD,
Center for Lifelong Growth

Rituals, Traditions, and Music

The previous example illustrates the importance of ritual and traditions, which can promote spiritual QOL, either as part of or outside of religious practices. For the preceding client, just lighting the candles was enough to evoke a sense of calm and well-being, even though this ritual was not officially designated by the religious holiday he was recognizing. Similarly, setting the table a certain way, eating or preparing certain foods, or singing songs can help older adults to connect with rhythms and routines from their past lives that bring comfort and meaning. Sometimes a client will be able to request these kinds of rituals when asked, but other times the care manager and/or care providers will need to make suggestions or even initiate these rituals (for example, beginning to sing a Christmas carol or Hanukah song) before the client will be able or willing to participate.

For example, one care manager tenaciously advocated on behalf of her client, an elderly Japanese woman, to be able to enact an important ritual by brewing green tea in her room each afternoon:

My client was yearning to brew and serve tea, which was important for her culture and also for her health. However, her assisted care facility told her she could not have a hotplate in her room for safety reasons. I negotiated with the care facility managers for months until they allowed her to have an electric teapot with a safety mechanism. My client was thrilled to once again participate in a daily ritual that had deep significance for her.

—Sally Gold, MSW,
Geriatric Resource Services

Other care managers have had great success with using food as a ritual that can be curative and restoring for clients by bringing pleasure and cultural connections:

We had a French client with whom we celebrated Bastille Day by making crepes and also arranged for the care provider to bring her to local French restaurants. Despite having lived in the U.S. for more than 50 years, she had a close connection to her native France. She often talked of moving home to France, so we facilitated her making a visit. A few months after returning home, she decided to move back to France, where she could share an assisted living apartment with a cousin. Similarly, we had a client who was born in Italy, but who had stopped going to the local park for bocce ball matches when he could no longer drive. We worked with the family to hire a care provider who could bring him back to the park, accompany him on long-forgotten Wednesday lunches at the Italian American club, and take him out for a cappuccino in the afternoons. These simple rituals seemed to mean the world to him, and resulted in marked improvement in his demeanor and helped mitigate the behavioral problems we were brought in to help address.

—Nina Pflumm Herndon, MA, CMC,
Sage Eldercare Solutions

Another example of how one care manager was able to help re-create a feeling of belonging to a community for her client:

Maria was a charming, exuberant, and colorful Cuban woman in her 90s. She lived in a town with a large Cuban population, and many friends visited her daily on the street near her row house. When she came outside there were always people on her block shouting to her across the street, "Hola, Maria! How are you? Maria had reverted to using only Spanish for communication, although she was able to comprehend English very well.

Due to her dementia it was determined that the best placement for Maria was in an assisted living specializing in working with clients having memory impairment. As there were no assisted living residences nearby that had a Latino population, Maria had a difficult period of adjustment.

With the consent of her guardian we hired Spanish-speaking aides to spend time with her during the day. We arranged to have the home health aides pick up Latin food a couple of nights per week to give her "a little taste of home." In addition, I took her out to a nearby Cuban restaurant. The restaurant was a beautiful reflection of Havana, called Cuban Pete's. The waiters loved to have Maria come for lunch, and they would dance salsa and merengue in the aisles with her after she finished her meal. She would not allow anyone at the table to send any food back to the kitchen uneaten, and was quite insistent that it be packed for her to take home.

After initially being hesitant to leave the confines of the assisted living facility, Maria came to relish her trips to Cuban Pete's. She was given an opportunity to enjoy some of the things she loved, and to dance her beloved merengue and salsa while reminiscing of her early life under the palms at the restaurant.

—Lisa Monday, MSW, LCSW, CMC,
Services and Resources for Seniors, Inc.,
Morristown, New Jersey

Another care manager found that music, particularly war songs, were helpful to her client in reducing the effects of his advancing dementia:

When I began music therapy sessions with Mr. Y at the local Veteran's Hospital, I was told that he could not communicate verbally and that he had a history of striking care providers. I quickly found that Mr. Y was able to sing old war songs clearly and that his agitation seemed to be immediately eradicated through the use of music and sound. I experimented with practicing scales, movement exercises, energy work, and acupressure, and engaging him in music therapy techniques. These approaches reduced his body twitches and improved his clarity of speech. The music also seemed to evoke something deeper in Mr. Y, as he would often close his eyes and cry when we would terminate a session. I trained his care providers in these techniques and they reported the same positive results.

—Tara Bradley, MA, MFTI,
Sage Eldercare Solutions

Countless studies have publicized the dramatic benefits of volunteering through the process of giving back to the community. It may seem counterintuitive to think of people who are loosing control over so much of their lives and their bodies to have the motivation and capability to do volunteer work; however for some, it may just work wonders. According to an article published in the *Journal of Health Psychology* entitled "Volunteerism and Mortality among the Community-dwelling Elderly," older adults who volunteer more than 4 hours per week are 44% less likely to die during their volunteerism.

This notion is echoed in a similar article, "Life Meaning: An Important Correlate of Health in the Hungarian Population," published in the *International Journal of Behavioral Medicine*, which states that older adults who feel their lives are meaningful have significantly lower rates of cancer and heart disease.

Researcher and New York Times best seller, Dan Buettner, has conducted extensive studies into the communities with the highest longevity; asking those important questions to determine what factors account for strength, energy, and vitality of those living well into their ninth and tenth decades. Why are some people able to avoid the typical pitfalls of aging and remain happy and fulfilled through their extraordinary life span? He calls these communities where people are living longer "Blue Zones" and within these communities are elders who continuously outlive people who live in other communities. One cause that continues to ring true with most all long-lived elders is a "strong sense of purpose—a reason to get out of bed in the morning" says Buettner. He further states that this is "a common trait in many older adults who live to be 100 years old."

Volunteerism embodies the fundamentals necessary for developing that strong sense of purpose that Buettner has identified as critical towards extended longevity. "Volunteer work improves the well being of individual volunteers because it enhances social support networks. People with strong social support networks have lower premature death rates, less heart disease, and fewer health risk factors," claims the Public Health Agency of Canada in an article entitled "Volunteering as a Vehicle for Social Support and Life Satisfaction."[29] According to Allan Luks and Peggy Payne, authors of *The Healing Power of Doing Good,* "Medical and scientific documentation supports that volunteering results in a heightened sense of well-being, improves insomnia, strengthens the immune system, and hastens surgery recovery time."[30]

Along with volunteerism is another interesting common thread among the long-lived elders: regular attendance in religious services. According to Dr. Daniel Hall, a surgeon at University of Pittsburgh Medical Center, "Weekly attendance at religious services accounts for an additional 2 to 3 life-years compared to 3 to 5 life-years for physical exercise." Clearly, for those frail elders who could not imagine participating in an exercise program, attending services might be a possible alternative.

Improving a client's spiritual QOL takes creativity and perseverance, but doing so can have tremendous impact on his or her physical and psychological well-being. To address spiritual QOL, the care manager must be open to helping the client explore whatever gives him or her meaning and must not be afraid to delve into the feelings that may arise from this exploration, both joyous and troubling. It is a highly individual, unique process, and one that has almost infinite permutations. As Victor Frankl wrote in his unforgettable book about surviving the concentration camps in Nazi Germany, "What matters, therefore, is not the meaning of life in general, but rather the specific meaning of a person's life at a given moment."[31]

B. Tap into Informal Networks: Caregivers' and Family Members' Information, Talent, and Willingness to Help

A client's caregiver (either at home or in a facility), neighbors, friends, volunteers, assisted living community staff, adult children, and grandchildren are all excellent resources for both understanding what the client needs in terms of holistic QOL as well as for implementation of ideas for addressing these needs.

Before beginning the process of assessing the client's holistic QOL, the care manager should meet with the caregiver(s) and family members to explain the assessment process and to clarify the goals of the process. The GCM can explain how the caregivers and family members will be part of the assessment, and how important their ideas will be when creating the plan for addressing the clients' needs and, later, implementing them. As mentioned earlier, both parties may have some conscious or unconscious preconceived ideas about what the client needs, wants, and is interested in, which may or may not be accurate, so it will be important to also use an assessment process to really get to know what makes the client "tick," beyond what others say or believe about him or her.

Once the assessment process is complete, the care manager can go over the results with caregivers and family members and start to gather their ideas about how to address some of the areas that the client needs the most, whether it is emotional, physical, or another aspect. Family members may have great ideas about activities that may evoke pastimes the client used to enjoy in his or her younger years, and caregivers will have experience about what kinds of activities tend to engage the client. It is paramount to engage the client's larger network (family, friends, neighbors) and care providers in implementing a holistic QOL plan because of budget limitations (it is not cost-effective to have the care manager carry out many of the interventions) and to ensure that the care providers are engaged in making a difference during all the hours that the client's specialists are not there.

One care manager, whose client had advanced dementia and was experiencing a great deal of agitation, worked closely with the client's aides to create activities that would improve her emotional, intellectual, and physical QOL:

> Through these conversations, the aides became incredibly interested in the client; they understood that they had an opportunity to develop their own special interactions and generated a range of ideas about things to do with her. One aide counted blackberries with her and they were able to reach number six (a big milestone). Because the client was once a school teacher, the aides also decided to take her to nearby parks, where she could watch the children play. By collaborating with the caregivers, I was able to help them learn how to use the client's environment as a tool for stimulation, and to develop ideas for outings and stimulating activities that meshed with her interests and past history.
>
> —Leonie Nowitz, MSW, BCD,
> Center for Lifelong Growth

For another client, her schedule included regular outings, visits from a dance and music therapist, as well as pastoral visits from members of the clergy. The next "frontier" was to explore how to make "down time" at home with her care providers more engaging. A customized therapeutic activity kit was created and the care providers trained on how to use it:

> Our 95-year-old client spoke six languages, demonstrated tremendous fondness for people, traveled extensively, and stayed updated on current affairs. She exuded warmth and an aura of loving kindness. She had regular visits from friends and extended family and it was evident that connections with others were very meaningful to her.
>
> Our client had significant cognitive impairment, particularly affecting her memory and judgment; she had been conserved due to extravagant gifting in a way that was deleterious to her. Her fine social skills remained intact and helped her connect with those around her yet she was frustrated that she now had restraints on her giving.
>
> The therapeutic activity kit we created was designed with her love of giving to others in mind. It honored the impulse to give to others but was based on her making simple yet sophisticated gifts. The therapeutic activity kit included fine paper with intricate rubber stamps to make note cards. By simply stamping the paper with the rubber stamps, she created lovely images of which she was proud. She also made pretty beaded necklaces. She enjoyed doing the activities and then had the opportunity to share her creations with others as she chose. The recipients of these handmade gifts were generally delighted at the love and thoughtfulness that went into making them. An excerpt of the training guide we used to familiarize the care providers with the therapeutic activity kit follows [see Table 10–1].
>
> —Nina Pflumm Herndon, MA, CMC,
> Sage Eldercare Solutions

| Table 10–1 | Therapeutic Activity Kit Components for Mrs. X | |

Activity	Purpose	Instruction
Creating greeting cards Kit components: • 1 box of 100 prefolded cards on fine Italian paper • 1 box of 100 matching envelopes made of fine Italian paper • 4 rubber stamps and 3 ink pads • Decorative stickers and ribbon	The purpose is to work on creating greeting cards that she can mail to people who are on her mind and/or those who stop by her home. By giving/mailing these cards, she may also receive increased contact from her friends.	• Have Mrs. X take the front of a folded blank card and decorate it with a rubber stamp or sticker to create a nice card. • Put cards in groups of 5 and wrap with decorative ribbon. These handmade note cards could be given to friends, relatives or others who visit as her way of saying "thank you." • You can also use the mailing list from Mrs. X's birthday party and send individual cards to friends. Name one of the people on the list and ask her to share a hello, a memory of that person or a word she would use to describe that person. Then, you can write a message saying: ▪ Simply "Hello," "Greetings," or "Love from Mrs. X" and have her sign it ▪ "Just thinking about the time we _____" [fill in the memory] ▪ "Mrs. X wanted you to know that she appreciates _____" [fill in the description] about you • Please address the cards and mail them.
Create beautiful necklaces Kit components: • Beading kits	The purpose of beading is to use Mrs. X's sense of beauty to create art that she is proud of.	• Take the beads out of the box and ask Mrs. X to sort them. Then, she can plan a design on the bead board and string the beads into necklaces.

C. Develop an Action Plan for Addressing Holistic Quality of Life

When putting together the actual plan for how to improve a client's holistic QOL, it can be helpful for care managers to keep in mind the 3 *Rs*:

- *Respectful:* It is essential to respect the client's comfort level with any given activity and to honor his or her desire to do it

or not. It may take many attempts before a client will be willing to try something that he or she perceives as "risky" and it is only through gentle, respectful communication that the care manager will be successful in overcoming these feelings.

- *Realistic:* The domains of holistic QOL—emotional, intellectual, physical, spiritual—may touch on some very charged and difficult issues for clients. As a result, care managers can expect a fair amount of resistance when introducing activities related to QOL and may need to take baby steps to help clients get past their negative feelings in some of these areas.

- *Responsive:* Although care managers need to keep an eye on their goals in terms of holistic QOL, it's also important to be responsive to the client, and follow his or her lead when planning activities. It is an interactive process, and the care manager will have a better chance of success if she keeps an open mind, adjusting plans and ideas in tune with the client's needs and desires.

There is no one right way to create a good QOL plan, and each care manager may develop an approach that works best for her. However, there are a few elements that should be included in any QOL plan, including the following:

- Specific QOL area focus
- Evidence from the assessment that supports the need to address this area
- Feedback from family and caregivers about the client's needs and interests
- Activities to try, with a range from introductory to more advanced, along with space to record client response and potential next steps

Exhibit 10-4 provides a sample plan for addressing intellectual QOL.

Exhibit 10-4   A Sample Action Plan for Addressing Intellectual Quality of Life

Client Name: Mr. G

QOL Area to be Addressed: Intellectual

Evidence from Assessment:
- Family members said he used to paint when younger
- Paintings he did are around the apartment
- Caregiver said she suggested painting, but Mr. G said his hands shake too much
- Mr. G listed art and museums as two of his favorite things

Activities to Try	Response	Next Step
1. Bring in some "coffee table" art books for Mr. G to look at, note level of interest and which types of art seem to engage him		
2. Plan outing to art museum—choose type depending on response to different art books		
3. Bring materials for painting at home with GCM and caregiver		
4. Enroll client in senior art class at local recreation center		

■ STEP 4: EVALUATE AND REASSESS

Implementing a plan for improving a client's holistic QOL is an iterative process—the care manager will try an activity, gauge its success, try something else, and keep going until he or she sees positive change for the client. The goal is to be respectful, realistic, and responsive throughout the process and to continually adapt to the client's needs, reactions, and physical and cognitive condition.

After a care manager has been implementing the holistic QOL plan with a client for a reasonable amount of time—6 weeks or so—it is time to reassess the plan and revise it depending on the outcomes through a care monitoring visit. Reassessing the plan involves talking with caregivers and family members to see what kinds of changes they have noticed and conducting an informal assessment with the client, which includes conversation and observation. During this process, the care manager is looking for signs that the client's QOL has improved in any or all of the areas targeted in the original plan, and if not, to rethink the activities and approach that has been used.

It's important to reconsider not only the "what" of the plan (i.e., which specific activities), but also the "how" (Who has been working with the client on these activities? Where?). Perhaps the reason a particular activity has not succeeded or the client experienced a negative reaction was because of how the activity was delivered. For example, if the client didn't want to work with the care manager on a reminiscence project, the care manager doesn't need to rule out this type of activity, but instead might see if it can be done with a caregiver who might have a closer relationship with the client, or with an art therapist who specializes in this type of work. Similarly, a client might resist going for a walk or engaging in other physical activity with his caregivers, but might be open to an outing with other older adults that is planned by a local senior center.

■ CONCLUSION

Addressing a client's holistic QOL is a process that does not have a specific end goal. There are almost endless ways that care managers can improve a client's emotional, intellectual, physical, and spiritual QOL and almost endless ways that clients may respond to these activities. For the care manager, the caregivers, and the client's family members, the process of considering these elements may itself provoke new understanding of the client and new respect for his or her unique and special gifts. As demonstrated in the examples throughout this chapter, holistic QOL activities can also be fun and can add a dimension of playfulness and joy to the work of geriatric care for all parties involved.

Most GCMs already have the skills they need to be successful in this area; it just takes willingness and a conviction to prioritize holistic quality of care concerns at the same level with more traditional care management objectives. Although it may require a shift in thinking for the care manager, family, and client to focus on holistic care, the benefits for clients are potentially enormous. Improving emotional, intellectual, physical, and spiritual QOL has been shown not only to improve a client's affect and attitude toward life, but also to literally improve physical health. To be successful in addressing holistic QOL, care managers need only draw on the attributes that probably brought them to the field of geriatric care in the first place: creativity, resourcefulness, and respect for the humanity of older adults.

Indeed, a focus on QOL can be a win for all parties involved: improved well-being for the older adult, measurable and positive impact from the care manager, and relief and support from the older adult's family members and caregivers. This focus is also life affirming for clients, who still yearn to connect with their whole selves. As one 90-year-old woman said, "The invisible part of me is not old. In aging we gain as well as lose—our spiritual forces expand. A life of the heart and mind takes over as our physical force ebbs away."[32]

■ REFERENCES

1. Maslow A. A theory of human motivation. *Psychol Rev.* 1943;50(4):370–396.

2. World Health Organization. *Preamble to the Constitution of the World Health Organization as adopted by the International Health Conference.* No. 2, p. 100. New York, NY: 1946.

3. Centers for Disease Control and Prevention. Social support and health-related quality of life among older adults—Missouri, 2000. *Morb Mortal Wkly Rep.* May 6, 2005. Available at: http://www.cdc.gov/mmwr/preview/mmwrhtml/mm5417a4.htm. Accessed June 5, 2006.

4. *Ibid.*

5. *Ibid.*

6. National Institutes of Health. Use it or lose it? *Senior Net.* [Press release]. Available at: http://www.seniornet.org/php/default.php?PageID=6796. Published February 12, 2002. Accessed June 7, 2006.

7. Begley S. Dementia studies confuse causes with effects. *Wall Street Journal.* April 28, 2006.

8. News Bureau, University of Illinois, Urbana. Exercise adds years to life and improves quality, researchers say. Available at: http://www.news.uiuc.edu/NEWS/05/1110exercise.html. Published November 19, 2005. Accessed June 1, 2006.

9. Begley S. Dementia studies confuse causes with effects. *Wall Street Journal.* April 28, 2006.

10. Westcott WL. Strength training for older adults. *Healthy Net.* Available at: http://www.healthy.net/scr/Column.asp?id=228. Published 1998. Accessed June 13, 2006.

11. Bianchi EG. Elder Wisdom: Crafting your own elderhood. New York, NY: *Crossroad;* 1994.

12. Frytak J. Assessment of quality of life in older adults. In: Kane R, Kane R, eds. *Assessing older persons.* New York, NY: Oxford University Press; 2000:200–237.

13. *Ibid.,* 214.

14. Malaz B, Reed P, Sloane PD, et al. The Public Health Impact of Alzheimer's Diease, 2000–2050: Potential Implication of Treatment Advances. *Annu Rev Public Health.* 2002; 23:213–231.

15. Feil N. *Summary of 1972 Research Data.* San Juan, Puerto Rico, 1972. Available at: http://www.vfvalidation.org/validation/FeilNaomi_GerontologicalSoc1972PuertoRico.pdf. Accessed August 13, 2010.

16. Morton I, Bleathman C. The effectiveness of validation therapy in dementia—a pilot study. *Int J Geriatr Psychiatry.* 1991;6(5):327–330.

17. Baker S. Massage therapy for seniors provides a "loving touch." *Copley News Service. Jewish News Bulletin of Northern California.* Available at: http://www.jewishsf.com/content/2-0/module/displaystory/story_id/17615/edition_id/349/format/html/displaystory.html. Published January 25, 2002. Accessed June 29, 2006.

18. Cohen GD. *The creative age: awakening human potential in the second half of life.* New York, NY: HarperCollins Publishers; 2001:61.

19. Morton I, Bleathman C. The effectiveness of validation therapy in dementia—a pilot study. *International Journal of Geriatric Psychiatry,* 1991;6(5):327–330.

20. Dienstag A. Lessons from the lifelines writing group for people in the early stages of Alzheimer's disease: forgetting that we don't remember. In: Ronch J, Goldfied J, eds. *Mental wellness in aging.* Towson, MD: Health Professions Press; 2003:350.

21. MetLife Foundation. MindAlert Awards 2004. Available at: http://www.asaging.org/awards/mindalert.cfmm. Accessed June 29, 2006.

22. *Ibid.*

23. *Ibid.*

24. *Ibid.*

25. *Ibid.*

26. Dienstag A. Lessons from the lifelines writing group for people in the early stages of Alzheimer's disease: forgetting that we don't remember. In: Ronch J, Goldfied J, eds. *Mental wellness in aging.* Towson, MD: Health Professions Press; 2003:350.

27. Conedera F, Mitchell L. Therapeutic activity kits. *Try This.* 2004;1(4). Available at: http://www.hartfordign.org/publications/trythis/theraAct.pdf. Accessed October 3, 2006.

28. Department of Health and Human Services. *Physical activity and health: a report of the surgeon general.* Centers for Disease Control and Prevention. http://www.cdc.gov/aging/info.htm. Published 1996. Accessed June 15, 2006.

29. Northbridge Hospital Medical Center. *Nine Steps to Better Health.* Available at: http://www.northridgehospital.org/Who_We_Are/Better_Health/185972. Accessed August 13, 2010.

30. Lukes A, Payne P. *The Healing Power of Doing Good.* Lincoln, NE: iUniverse, Inc.; 1991.

31. Frankl VE. *Man's search for meaning.* New York, NY: Washington Square Press, Simon and Schuster; 1963:171.

32. University of Kentucky Cooperative Extension Service. *Aging gracefully: quotes for aging wisely.* Available at: http://www.ca.uky.edu/fcs/aging/pdf/Quotes_for_Aging_Wisely.pdf. Accessed October 3, 2006.

Chapter 11

Technologies That Support Aging in Place

Julie Menack

Technology can be used to help the care manager's clients to age safely in their home and also to ease some of the challenges of caregiving. It has the potential to help older adults maximize their independence, support professional and family caregivers' needs, improve the quality of care and quality of life, reduce and limit the cost of health care, and increase efficiency of care. The care manager who is willing to try new innovations is in a position to recommend affordable technologies that will enable the client to live in the least restrictive environment for as long as possible. The market for technology in care management is driven by the combination of an aging population with longer life expectancy, a shortage of physicians and nurses, a mobile population in which families are no longer living in close proximity to one another, and the technological improvements that have occurred in recent years.

"Gerontechnology" is a term that was coined to describe the field that encompasses the design of technology and environment for independent living and social participation of older persons in good health, comfort and safety. This includes innovative technology that serves an enabling role for aging people by:[1]

- Maintaining their independence and equality including considerations of residence, mobility, safety, security, communication, activities, and quality of life;
- Supporting their well-being and health;

- Realizing their individual and collective/social ambitions and needs;
- Keeping them embedded in their changing socio-cultural environment;
- Enhancing their dignity; and
- Supporting their caregivers.

Technology can benefit all those involved in a client's care, including the client, the care provider, and the person or organization that pays for the care. The benefit to the client is prolonged independence created by a greater sense of security, improved health and quality of life, and opportunity for social interaction. The benefit to the care provider is greater peace of mind due to increased safety, more contact due to increased communication, and the opportunity for intervention before a crisis occurs. It is presumed that the benefit to the payer, whether it is the insurance company, family, or private fiduciary, is that overall cost of care is reduced.[2]

Recent studies indicate that most older adults are aware of commonly available technologies such as Personal Emergency Response System (PERS) buttons and alarms on doors and windows but are not aware of new and emerging technologies, many of which are described in this chapter.[3] The greatest obstacles to implementation, which are older adults' lack of awareness and usability challenges, will be less of a concern in the future as the baby boomers get older because the baby boom generation is typically more familiar with technology.[4] Increasing proof that there is value in technology to support aging in place will help to erode the other obstacles, such as the question of whether the technology will be covered by medical insurance or be paid for out of pocket, licensing issues across state lines, and the need to develop consistent standards across technology platforms.

The care manager is uniquely qualified to identify, recommend, implement and prioritize strategies including technology-based solutions that will support a client's unmet needs. This is because during the assessment, the care manager has identified deficits in the client's care and is expected to know about available products and services. As with all care management recommendations, no one solution fits all—there are many creative ways to meet a client's needs. The technologies that can support the care of aging individuals can be divided into the following categories, which is how technologies are subdivided in this chapter:[5]

- Health and wellness
- Safety and security
- Communication and engagement
- Learning and contribution

Figure 11-1 illustrates that these technology categories closely correspond with

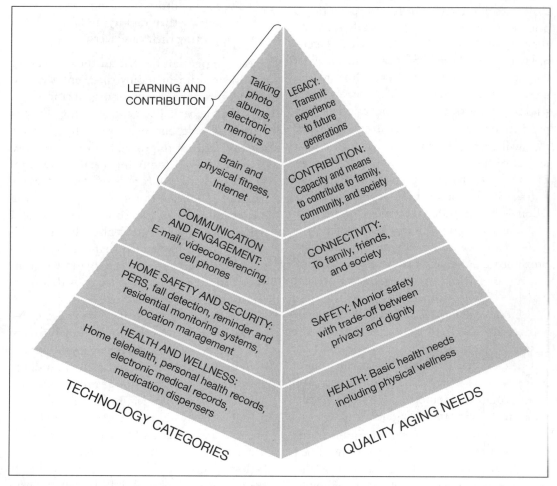

Figure 11–1   An Integrated Approach Toward Technology and Quality Aging

Source: Courtesy of Joseph Coughin, MIT AgeLab, 2006.

Maslow's hierarchy of quality aging needs of health, safety, connectivity, contribution, and legacy.[6]

■ STEPS TO SUPPORT A TECHNOLOGY SOLUTION

The care manager's job is to help the family come up with a solution that both supports the caregiver and empowers the care recipient. This should be done without losing "the human touch," as our clients need to feel connected, alive, and integrated so that technology is used to assist, and not replace human care. Steps that can be taken to support a technology solution include:[7]

- **Assessment:** Define the concern, including the physical, mental, and emotional issues that could be improved or stabilized using both functional and psychosocial assessment tools.
- **Investigation:** Research and identify technologies that fit the client's budget, lifestyle, cognitive abilities, and physical strength, while allowing the client to remain as independent as possible, making sure that the technology is HIPAA compliant.
- **Implementation:** Work with the care team to identify risks and concerns and determine how technology can be integrated into the client's home. Make sure that the home has the appropriate infrastructure (e.g., wiring, electrical systems, and Internet connectivity, as needed) and that any needed changes are made. Provide clear instructions and support for whoever is going to operate the technology to ensure a positive experience.
- **Follow-up problem solving:** Schedule follow-up visits at regular intervals to determine if the technology is being used appropriately.
- **Evaluation:** Determine whether the initial goal has been met, and if not, evaluate whether additional training is required or if the technology should be removed.

Potential impediments to technology implementation should be kept in mind during this process. The care manager should expect that many clients did not grow up with technology and may not be comfortable with it, may deny the need for care, or may resent the loss of independence that the technology signifies and try to sabotage or avoid using it. A client's limitations, such as physical impairment (e.g., vision, hearing loss), technical difficulty, and impaired cognitive ability may limit the use of some technologies, but support from a care provider can easily help overcome some of these limitations. Consideration should also be given to balancing a client's need for privacy, autonomy, and dignity with the usefulness of certain aging in place technologies.

An example of one day in the life of a client using technologies that are currently available, many of which are described in this chapter, is provided in Figure 11–2. This figure shows that many relationships can be enhanced by technology, including those of a client living at home with long-distance family, local family and care providers, and healthcare providers. The remainder of this chapter outlines the different categories of technologies and provides resources for the care manager, including a partial list of technologies that are available at the present time. This list may rapidly become obsolete, so it is hoped that the concepts also presented here will support future care managers to identify and consider technology options. (Table 11–1).

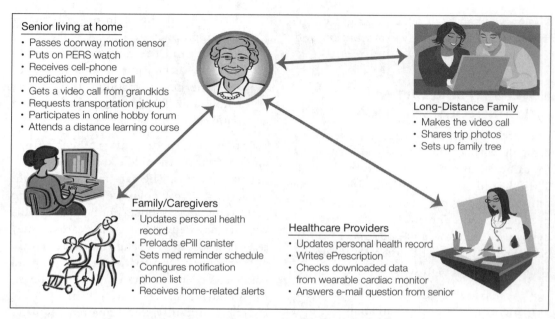

Senior living at home
- Passes doorway motion sensor
- Puts on PERS watch
- Receives cell-phone
  medication reminder call
- Gets a video call from grandkids
- Requests transportation pickup
- Participates in online hobby forum
- Attends a distance learning course

Long-Distance Family
- Makes the video call
- Shares trip photos
- Sets up family tree

Family/Caregivers
- Updates personal health
  record
- Preloads ePill canister
- Sets med reminder schedule
- Configures notification
  phone list
- Receives home-related alerts

Healthcare Providers
- Updates personal health record
- Writes ePrescription
- Checks downloaded data
  from wearable cardiac monitor
- Answers e-mail question from senior

Figure 11–2   A Day in the Life of a Client Utilizing Technology

Table 11–1 Monitoring Recommendations Based on Care Management Assessment	
Type of Monitor	**What the Monitor Detects**
Motion sensor	Detects activity patterns that can be evaluated to determine changes
Water monitor	Detects leaks or overflowing water conditions
Chair sensor	Monitors length of time in chair and detects fall out of chair or wheelchair
Toilet monitor	Detects altered urinary/bowel elimination pattern
Smoke detector	Detects cooking accidents, smoking in bed, gas leak
Heat sensor	Detects whether the stove has been left on for a potentially inappropriate amount of time
Door/window sensor	Sends alert if door or window opened at inappropriate time, or not opened at all. Also can detect when cabinets are opened.
Refrigerator and cabinet door monitors	Can identify dysfunctional eating patterns
Bed sensor	Detects sleep disturbance
Impact sensor	Detects falls
Temperature monitor	Measures room temperature and sends alert if out of range

■ HEALTH AND WELLNESS TECHNOLOGIES

Health and wellness technologies include systems that are embedded in the home to monitor and respond to the care recipient's ability to carry out activities of daily living and also make the collection of important health information possible. This enables the client to participate in maintaining their own health, provides an objective assessment of the client's ability to live independently, allows healthcare providers to identify the early onset of disease, and helps care managers to coordinate needed care and services.[2] These technologies include telehealth technology, electronic personal and health records, residential monitoring systems, reminder systems, and medication management systems.

Telehealth

Telehealth is defined as a service that allows the clinician the ability to remotely monitor and measure physiologic health data and information. Chronically ill care management clients are ideal for telehealth monitoring as telehealth can allow individuals to maintain independence and keep as healthy as possible through prevention, early detection, and self-management. Recent studies have documented that telehealth results in a significant reduction in unplanned hospitalizations and emergency room visits and can also reduce the need for intensive home health care and placement in skilled nursing facilities.[8,9] Telehealth also results in improved self-care because as patients get to know their own symptoms better, they become expert in managing their own condition. The care manager can be involved with setting up the parameters for each client's specific condition and can be alerted along with other members of the care team if the data collected deviates from the programmed parameters. The care manager can recommend either a product that offers a clinical call center service or one that provides alerts to just the care team.

Telehealth devices typically consist of a hub device that contains communication capabilities as well as wireless peripherals that collect physiologic data. These tools enable patient data to be transmitted to and from the home. A broad range of chronic conditions including asthma, diabetes, chronic heart failure, chronic obstructive pulmonary disease (COPD), hypertension, wound care, and mental health (i.e., anxiety and depression) can be monitored remotely in this way. Peripherals include weight scales, blood pressure cuffs, glucose meters, pulse oximeters, and peak flow meters. Some base stations allow patients to manually enter measurements and may also include a text screen that asks a series of multiple-choice questions about health status and behaviors. The monitoring and reporting can be done either by the client, if capable, or by a home care worker, depending on the level of care and supervision required.

In this way, the client's chronic medical condition can be monitored in real time by the family, the care manager, or the clinician so that any telltale changes in health can be addressed and responded to immediately. Patients and families like home telehealth as it provides a sense of security by consistently updating the client's health status and is an easy way to keep track of specific health data to prevent emergencies.[10] Telehealth devices are starting to be provided by medical providers such as hospitals to help monitor a patient during the vulnerable period after discharge. They are also becoming available as an option from some health plans, doctor's offices, home health and home care agencies, as well as care management organizations. Some products will also be available directly to the consumer market. Established telehealth device manufacturers include Bosch (Health Buddy), Intel (Health Guide), Philips (TeleStation), CardioCom

(Commander), Honeywell (HomMed Sentry), and Ideal Life (Pod).

Electronic Personal and Health Records

Resources are becoming available for the care manager and care team to share personal, financial, and medical information about the care recipient securely on the Internet. This can be particularly helpful when there is an emergency situation, as immediate access can be granted to others, such as a doctor in an emergency room. Two such services, Life Ledger and RemCare, are marketed to care managers on a subscription basis and can streamline even a small care management practice. Both provide an online secure location where important documents can be uploaded, lists of medications and dosages can be maintained, and progress notes and other information can be shared with the family and other professionals. Other free online tools that include a calendar, diary, and a place to store legal documents (e.g., Careminds and CareDiary) and applications ("apps") for the iPhone are available to track personal medical information (e.g., CareConnector and Polka, which also provides an Emergency Card application). Some of these systems can be linked to electronic health records, as described below.

The consumer marketplace has made electronic health records (EHRs) available. An EHR is a repository of information about a client's care, collected both by telehealth devices and by traditional visits with healthcare professionals. The care manager can make sure that the EHR contains accurate and up-to-date information about a client's medical history and current health status. Organizations offering EHRs range from employers, insurers and healthcare providers, as well as commercial enterprises. There are currently two types of EHR. Stand-alone EHRs act as sophisticated medical record databases where the data must be entered manually. Connected EHRs are Web-based databases and are able to receive data from many sources in electronic format including pharmacies, physicians, insurers, and home health monitoring devices (e.g., Google Health, Microsoft Health Vault). In addition, The U.S. economic stimulus law of 2009 put forth a goal of universal adoption of EHRs by 2014 with penalties for healthcare providers who do not establish "meaningful use" of EHRs. A simplified user guide to creating an account in currently available EHRs can be found in Peterka.[11]

Secure online portals, offered by many healthcare providers, can help the care manager to streamline their day-to-day practice. These portals allow the care manager to schedule medical appointments, e-mail securely with a client's medical provider, and view the results of laboratory tests and other medical records. Permission from the client or their healthcare proxy will be necessary in order to gain access to these portals, which are secure. Use of online portals can be an efficient way for the care manager to contact medical providers and reduces the time needed to make medical appointments. One of the most sophisticated online portals is the Kaiser Permanente HMO's Health Connect at Home portal.

Residential Monitoring

The smart home is defined as "a residence wired with technology features that monitor the well-being and activities of their residents to improve overall quality of life, increase independence and prevent emergencies."[12] Monitoring systems that track an elder's movement within the home or retirement community are becoming more widely available and are often labeled telecare systems. Telecare has been defined as "the continuous, automatic and remote monitoring of real-time emergencies and lifestyle changes over time in order to manage the risks associated with independent living."[13] Telecare systems are embedded in the home to monitor and respond to the care recipient and their home environment, and differ from telehealth (as described above), which is the remote exchange of physiological data between a patient and medical staff to assist in diagnosis and monitoring.

Telecare systems include a broad range of minimally intrusive sensor-based technologies that continuously, automatically, passively, and remotely monitor real-time emergencies, patterns of behavior, and environmental conditions. They can be strategically placed throughout the residence and can utilize a combination of sensor cameras and recording devices. They are often wireless and easily installed. In addition, they are often unobtrusive and inconspicuous due to their small size. The benefits of telecare systems are that they provide insights into the client's needs, enabling more person-centered care, and that they allow the care team to be proactive, noticing changes in the client's condition at an early stage, before there is a crisis.

Sensor systems can monitor when the older person's pattern differs from the routine, and send an alarm to a central monitoring location if movement patterns differ from a previously observed or programmed norm. Sensors can be placed at strategic locations throughout the home to record a person's activities of daily living. This includes, for example, whether a person opened the door of a cabinet to take their medicine, how often the refrigerator door is opened to monitor nutrition, how long or how frequently the person is in the bathroom, whether the bathtub is overflowing, the temperature of the home, when the care recipient is in and out of bed to monitor a possible sleep disturbance, whether they have fallen out of their wheelchair, or how long they are sitting in their favorite chair.

Alerts of patterns that differ from the routine are sent by phone call, e-mail, text message, or personalized Web page. Depending upon the system, these messages can be sent directly to the family member or care manager, or in some cases, alerts are first screened by a corporate call center. Some skilled nursing facilities and retirement communities are using this type of monitoring and provide access to information such as the location of the resident, the number of assistance calls placed to staff and staff response, the level of movement, restlessness, sleep habits, weight, participation in social activity, and percentage of time spent with others or alone.[14] Some currently available motion sensor systems that care managers might encounter include GE Quiet Care, Grand Care, Healthsense ENeighbor, WellAware, AFrameDigital, CloseBy and BeClose. A few of these are only available in retirement communities.

Another way to determine the care recipient's safety is with a camera-based system, which can provide direct visual confirmation of the client's status. Unfortunately, unless monitored constantly, having a camera does not guarantee that whoever is monitoring will see something going wrong as it happens. Video can be useful to determine for example, if a person is taking their medications or whether they have eaten. The spectrum of available camera systems ranges from the use of a teleconferencing system (as described in the section of this chapter on Communication) to wireless webcams, to coordinated systems such as Rest Assured, a telecare service that provides video monitoring and a remote care provider who can interact with the client via microphone. This allows a care manager to check in with clients who are situated in remote locations.

The care manager should supervise telecare system design, installation, and monitoring. As illustrated by Table 11–2, the care manager's functional assessment can be easily tailored to identify the type and location of sensors and video monitors, based on specific care recipient deficits. In this way, each system can be tailored to the particular need and want of the end users, the caregiver and the care recipient. There is a role here for a new

Table 11-2   List of Technologies and Product Categories That Can Be Used to Support Care Management Clients

Category	Product	Website
Health and Wellness Technologies		
Telehealth	Bosch Health Buddy	www.healthbuddy.com
	Cardiocom Commander	www.cardiocom.com/commander.html
	Honeywell HomMed Sentry	www.hommed.com/Products/Sentry_Telehealth_Monitor-Total-Solution.asp
	Ideal Life Pod	www.ideallifeonline.com/products
	Intel Health Guide	www.intel.com/healthcare/ps/healthguide/index.htm
	Philips TeleStation	www.healthcare.philips.com
Electronic Personal and Health Records		
Electronic Health Record	Google Health	www.google.com/health
	Health Vault	www.healthvault.com
Electronic Personal Records	CareConnector	www.strengthforcaring.com/careconnector/index.html
	Care Minds	www.careminds.com
	LifeLedger	agingwisely.lifeledger.com
	Polka Health iPhone App	itunes.apple.com/us/app/polka-health/id300156700?mt=8
	RemCare	www.myremcare.com
Health Portal	Kaiser Permanente HealthConnect at Home Portal	www.kaiserpermanente.org
Residential Monitoring	AFrameDigital	www.aframedigital.com
	BeClose	www.beclose.com
	CloseBy	www.closebynetwork.com
	GE Quiet Care	www.GEhealthcare.com/AgingInPlace
	Grand Care	www.grandcare.com
	Healthsense E Neighbor	www.healthsense.com
	Rest Assured	www.restassuredsystem.com
	WellAware	www.wellawaresystems.com
Reminder System	Cadex Watch	www.cadexwatch.com
	Care Call Reassurance	www.call-reassurance.com
	Dosecast	www.dosecast.com
	FineThanx	www.finethanx.com
	iPills App	www.iliumsoft.com/site/iphone/products_ipills.php
	Lifetime Talking Calendar	Various websites (search)
	Medicine Cabinet App	itunes.apple.com/us/app/medicine-cabinet-ipad-edition/id363479668?mt=8
	OnTimeRx	www.ontimerx.com
	Personal Caregiver App	www.personalcaregiver.com

Table 11–2	List of Technologies and Product Categories That Can Be Used to Support Care Management Clients (continued)

Category	Product	Website
Reminder System (cont.)	Remind Me App	www.smudgeapps.com/Products/RemindMe.html
	Timex Messenger Watch and Datalink Watch	www.timex.com
	Wellness Wizard	www.safetyandwellness.com
Medication Dispenser	Beep-n-Tell	www.epill.com/beeptell.html
	EMMA Remote Dosage Management	www.inrangesystems.com
	GlowCaps	www.vitality.net/glowcaps.html
	Maya from MedMInder	www.medminder.com
	MedReady	www.medreadyinc.com
	Philips Medication Dispensing Service	www.lifelinesys.com/content/medication-dispensing/service
	SentiCare Pill Dispenser	www.senticare.com
	TabSafe Pill Dispenser	www.tabsafe.com/Medication-Management-System.aspx
	Talking Rx Pill Bottle	www.epill.com/talkrx.html
	The Alzheimer's Store	www.alzstore.com
Home Safety and Security		
Fall Detection	My Halo	www.halomonitoring.com
	Philips Lifeline with Auto Alert	www.lifelinesys.com/content/lifeline-products/auto-alert
	Wellcore	www.wellcore.com/
Location Management	Aetrex Ambulator GPS Shoe	www.foot.com
	AlzGuard	www.alzguard.com
	Comfort Zone (Alzheimer's Association)	www.alz.org/comfortzone
	Emfinders EmseeQ	www.emfinders.com
	LoJack Safety Net	www.lojack.com/safetynet
	Medic Alert Safe Return	www.medicalalert.org/safereturn
	People Track USA MobileHelp	www.peopletrackusa.com/mobilehelp
	Pocketfinder	www.pocketfinder.com
	SentryGPSid	www.sentrygpsid.com
	Zoomback	www.zoombak.com
Stove Use Detector	CookStop	www.cookstop.com
	HomeSenser	www.homesensers.com
	Safe-T Element	www.pioneeringtech.com/safe-t-element.html
	Safe-T Sensor	www.pioneeringtech.com/safe-t-sensor.html
	StoveGuard	www.stoveguard.ca

continues

Table 11–2   List of Technologies and Product Categories That Can Be Used to Support Care Management Clients (continued)

Category	Product	Website
Programmable Thermostat	BayWeb Thermostat	www.bayweb.com
	Kelvin Voice Activated Talking Programmable Thermostat	www.accendaproducts.com
	Temperature Guard	www.temperatureguard.com
	Trane Remote Energy Management Thermostat	www.trane.com/residential/products/thermostats
Communication and Social Engagement		
Computers for Social Networking		
Shared Calendar	Google Calendar	calendar.google.com
Computer for Seniors	GO Computer	www.thegocomputer.com
Computer Peripheral	Big Key Keyboard	www.bigkeys.com
Social Networking	Care Diary	www.ecarediary.com
	Facebook	www.facebook.com
	Famililink Photo Sharing	www.famililink.com
	PatientsLikeMe	www.patientslikeme.com
	Tyze	www.tyze.com
Software for Seniors	Big Screen Live	www.bigscreenlive.com
	Connected Living	www.mywayvillage.com
	It's Never Too Late	www.IN2L.com
Software for Seniors; VIdeoconferencing	Pointerware	www.pointerware.com
Computer Training	Computer School for Seniors	www.cs4seniors.com
	Senior Net	www.seniornet.com
Social Networking Without a Computer		
Computerless E-mail	My Celery	www.myCelery.com
	Presto Printing Mail Box	www.presto.com
Computerless Printing	Hewlett Packard ePrint Center	www.hp.com/enterprise/us/en/ipg/HPeprint-solution.html
Internet Viewer	Chumby	www.chumby.com
	Sony Dash	www.sonystyle.com/dash
Internet Photo Frame	CEIVA Digital Photo Frame	www.ceiva.com
	EStarling	www.estarling.com
	Kodak Pulse Wifi digital frame with dedicated e-mail	www.kodak.com
Internet Films	Netflix	www.netflix.com
Internet Radio	Pandora Radio	www.pandora.com
Internet Video	YouTube	www.youtube.com
Cell Phone	ClarityLife C900	www.clarityproducts.com
	Consumer Cellular	www.consumercellular.com/aarp
	Doro PhoneEasy	www.consumercellular.com/doro
	Jitterbug Cell Phone	www.jitterbug.com

Table 11–2	List of Technologies and Product Categories That Can Be Used to Support Care Management Clients (continued)

Category	Product	Website
Videoconferencing	ASUS AiGuru SkypePhone	www.amazon.com
	AttentiveCare	www.caregivertech.com
	Family Virtual Visits	www.familyvirtualvisits.com
	Google Video Chat	www.google.com/chat/video
	iChat	www.apple.com/macosx/what-is-macosx/ichat.html
	Skype	www.skype.com
	Virtual Interactive Families and Friends	www.togetherwhileapart.com/
Learning and Contribution		
Cognitive Fitness	CogniFit	www.cognifit.com
	Dakim BrainFitness Program for Seniors	www.dakim.com
	Posit Science	www.positscience.com
	Brain Age for Nintendo DSI	www.brainage.com
Physical Fitness	Kinect for Xbox 360	www.xbox.com/en-US/kinect
	Wii Fit and Sports Pack	www.nintendo.com/wii
Digital Music Player	iPod Shuffle	www.apple.com/ipodshuffle
	Also see Internet Viewers above	
Electronic Book Reader	Amazon Kindle Wireless Reading Device	www.amazon.com/kindle
	Nook eReader	www.barnesandnoble.com/nook
	Sony Reader Digital Book	www.sony.com/reader
	iPad	www.apple.com/ipad
Television Viewing	Slicker Clicker TV Remote	www.kiscompany.com
	TV Ears	www.tvears.com
Legacy Building	Ancestry.com	www.ancestry.com
	Life Bio	www.lifebio.com
	PhotoNote	www.bananasdesign.com/photonote
	QuickVoice Recorder	www.quick-voice.com
	Talking Photo Album	www.toy4education.com, www.amazon.com
Resources for Recommending Technology		
Industry Group	AgeTek Alliance	www.agetek.org
	American Telehealth Association (ATA)	www.atmeda.org
	Center for Aging Services Technologies (CAST)	www.aahsa.org/cast.aspx
	Center for Technology and Aging	www.techandaging.org

continues

Table 11–2	List of Technologies and Product Categories That Can Be Used to Support Care Management Clients (continued)	

Category	Product	Website
Industry Group (cont.)	Center for Telehealth and E-Health Law	www.telehealthlawcenter.org
	Home Care Technology Association of America (HCTAA)	www.hctaa.org
	Smart Silvers Alliance	www.smartsilvers.com
	Technology Centre for Independent Living	www.trilcentre.org
	Telecare Aware	www.telecareaware.com
Market Research	Aging in Place Technology Watch	www.ageinplacetech.com
Product Catalog	Able Data	www.abledata.com
	Alzheimer's Store	www.alzstore.com
	AssistiveTech	www.assistivetech.net
	Epill	www.epill.com
	FirstStreet	www.firststreetonline.com

Note: This information is what was available as of August 2010 and serves as examples of the types of technologies and information that might be considered by a care manager. The future availability of any of these products and websites cannot be promised or predicted.

type of care manager who can oversee and notice particular patterns of alerts and worrisome changes and intervene before a crisis occurs.[15]

Concerns have been raised regarding how to protect privacy and autonomy when utilizing monitoring systems that gather information about an individual's daily life and health.[16,17] The care manager should determine whether the elder is willing to trade privacy for security and safety, including the ability to remain in their home. The following safeguards should be considered: (1) informed consent to the initiation of monitoring, (2) continuing consent to monitoring, (3) control over who has access to the monitoring data (including a privacy policy from the vendor), and (4) regular access to the monitoring data generated. Privacy can be assured through the use of login and password codes, encryption, and other security mechanisms designed to ensure that only authorized users access the system. Privacy is the reason that motion-sensor technology is more common than video surveillance.[18]

Reminder Systems

The care manager can suggest some simple reminder systems to prompt clients with custom messages appropriate to their schedule, such as medication reminders, doctor appointments, emergency contacts, and identification messages. Messages that will help to orient the client with regard to planned activities can help to reduce a person's anxiety and confusion and can provide the information needed to help them remain independent.[19] For example, a computer in the bedroom with a screen that states, "It is nighttime, stay in bed," along with a photo of a family member or caregiver might reduce the number of telephone calls in the middle of the night from someone with dementia. Various devices, including computers, telephones (both land lines and smart phones), and wristwatches, can be programmed to provide reminders. The care can determine whether the client is capable of operating the selected system and may need to post reminder signs to coach the client.

Reminder systems can send scheduled one-time or repeated automated voice or text/e-mail messages to a telephone for a fee. Examples of these systems are FineThanx, and CARE Call Reassurance, which can provide automated wellness calls, and OnTimeRx, a medication reminder system. Many cell phones can be programmed with reminder messages, including the My Calendar service offered with the Jitterbug cell phone. Multiple pill reminder applications have been developed for smart phones including Personal Caregiver, RxmindMe, iPills, Dosecast, and MedicineCabinet. Some watches, such as the Cadex digital watch and the Timex Messenger and Datalink watches, can also be programmed with text and/or bell alerts. One reminder system, the Wellness Wizard, is a device that is referred to by the manufacturer as an electronic caregiver assistant; it plays a prerecorded reminder message at a specific time and if the message is not acknowledged, the device automatically calls a remote care provider. A simple reminder system, such as the Lifetime Talking Calendar, provides a verbal reminder of that day's schedule. All of the computerless e-mail devices described in the computer section of this chapter, can also be used to automatically send reminders.

Medication Dispensers

Medication compliance is a major concern and is an area where a significant amount of reminder support is needed to prevent clients from missing or skipping doses, failing to complete regimens, and other noncompliant behavior. Recent studies have estimated that $290 billion of annual healthcare expenditures would be avoided if medication adherence were improved, particularly among patients with chronic conditions.[20] For an individual living alone, remembering to take medication at the right time and in the right order can make it possible to remain independent.[21] Taking medications on time can result in reduced levels of confusion and fall risk, and having a reminder also lowers the stress of having to remember to take the medication.

The care manager can help to identify the appropriate electronic medication dispenser for each individual client ranging from simple to complex. Simple technologies include a talking pill bottle (i.e., Talking Rx), which states the name of the medication, who it is for, and other information recorded by the pharmacist, a beeping pill bottle that sounds an alert when the medication should be taken (i.e., Beep-n-Tell), and an electronic cap that beeps and sends a phone alert when medications should be taken or reordered (i.e., Glow-Caps). High-tech pillboxes and medication management systems organize the pills into compartments, allow the proper dose to be dispensed, and have an alert when it's time to take medication (e.g., those sold by epill.com and alzstore.com). Some systems monitor when the pill container is opened or removed, and send telephone and/or e-mail alerts to the client and care providers when it is not (e.g., SentiCare, TabSafe, Maya from MedMinder, the Philips Medication Dispensing Service, MedSignals, and MedReady). A few have the ability to also connect to a personal health record so that information about compliance can be shared with health professionals. The EMMA can do all of this and additionally allows the care team to change the dosage remotely. Some home care and home health organizations as well as companies that offer PERS systems market electronic medication reminders as part of a medication management service.

Considerations for selecting an electronic medication dispenser includes: (1) the number of doses per day; (2) the number of pills each compartment can hold; (3) the frequency the pillbox needs to be filled; (4) whether the device is or needs to be tamper-proof; (5) whether a monitoring service is available and if notifications are made via phone or e-mail, (6) the initial and ongoing cost, and (7) whether a free trial is offered. A medication dispenser that is connected to a professional monitoring system can demonstrate whether the appropriate amount of caregiving support is being provided and is also a way to double check on the client repeatedly during the day. If the client is using the device with no alerts, the care manager can infer that medication compliance is occurring. The data can also be useful to support a recommendation for increased care to a client or family who denies medication noncompliance.

One great benefit of having a monitoring system is that this becomes a way to check on the person repeatedly during the day—missing a dose may indicate that a person is unable to reach the pillbox and may require immediate assistance. The care manager should be aware that it is difficult to confirm that a person has actually swallowed a pill even when it has been removed from a dispenser, so these devices are best used with a motivated client who may simply need a reminder to adhere to a complex medication regimen and not with clients with dementia. In the future, it may be possible to track whether medications are taken, as pills are being tested that contain tiny sensor chips that can provide an alert when the pill has dissolved.

■ HOME SAFETY AND SECURITY

Fall detection systems, wander management systems, stove use detectors, and programmable thermostats can all be recommended to increase safety for the client who is at risk of institutionalization due to deficiencies in ADLs and IADLs.

Fall Detection

Research indicates that 13 million, or over one in three people over the age of 65 fall each year. Nearly half of those are recurrent falls, with fall-related injuries accounting for up to 6% of all medical expenditures in the United States. Of these, nearly 10% result in serious injuries or death from hip fractures and head traumas.[22] While fall prevention is the ultimate goal, currently available technologies can only be used for fall detection. Research is currently being done on systems of the future to identify activity patterns that provide early warning of changing levels of exercise and balance. This will enable the care team, including medical providers, to help diagnose and/or differentiate movement disorders or other conditions that might require early medical intervention to reduce the risk of future falls.[23]

Traditional fall detection devices are personal emergency response systems (PERS), which rely on the wearer's ability and willingness to push the button. These lightweight, waterproof devices send a signal via the home telephone line to a response center. The response center staff maintains contact with the wearer and can call rescue personnel in the event of an emergency. Care managers are already aware that these systems are rendered ineffective when the client is not able (due to loss of consciousness), forgets (due to cognitive impairment), or is too embarrassed (to show their vulnerability) to activate the system during an emergency. This has been confirmed by a study of falls among elderly where a medical alarm was installed and in use, in which 80% of the seniors did not activate the alarm during the fall. Various reasons were cited for not activating the alarm, including difficulty activating it, not wearing it, or wearing and choosing not to use it mostly because of a fear of hospitalization or to avoid embarrassment.[24]

Recent advances in technology have resulted in enhancements to PERS detection systems. Some systems are GPS or radio frequency based so they can be operated outside the home and can locate the wearer (e.g., People Track USA's MobileHelp). An exciting advancement in fall detection is passive products that monitor and report when a fall has occurred, thus eliminating the need for the wearer to provide the alert by pushing a button. The technology behind these devices include accelerometers and tilt sensors which detect the difference between normal movement, such as when a person goes from sitting to standing, and potentially dangerous falls. Some simply report falls (e.g., Philips Lifeline with Auto Alert), and others (e.g., MyHalo, Wellcore, and AFrame Digital) can track user compliance and notify care providers via text message or e-mail. Features to examine include the following: the client's comfort with the device's style (e.g., wristwatch, pendant, belt clip, torso band, etc.) as this will influence compliance, and whether or not the device can provide scheduled recorded reminders, works outside the home, can record the wearer's vital signs directly, or has Bluetooth interface to compatible medical monitoring devices such as the ones described in the Telehealth section of this chapter. One important factor is that in order to be effective, fall detection systems must be worn at all times including in the shower and at night.

Location Management

Wandering is a prevalent and dangerous problem for persons with certain types of dementia, can occur at any time, and is difficult to predict. It can occur for a variety of reasons, including a response to pain, anxiety, the need for exercise, or a mistaken need to attend to a task from the past. Typically, a person with Alzheimer's will not request help and many will not respond to calls. Products are available for the home that will help to keep the person with dementia safe. The lowest tech systems include jewelry identification programs (i.e., Medic Alert Safe Return), which works well only if a person can get close enough to see the bracelet. Watch-like devices with radio frequency technology allow the person to be located (e.g., LoJack Safety Net, Emfinders EmseeQ). Global positioning systems (GPS) such as the Alzheimer's Association's Comfort Zone, the Pocketfinder, Zoomback, SentryGPSid, and AlzGuard all use online location mapping and are available 24 hours per day to identify the person's location. The selection of monitoring technology (GPS, radio frequency or cell-based) will depend upon the reliability of the service available in the area.

The care manager may consider recommending a system that has a monitoring center that will provide an alert to a telephone or the Internet when the person leaves an established safety zone, also known as a geo-fence, where multiple care providers can view the location of the person on a secure website and also stores medical and emergency information.[25] To avoid the problem of removal of a device such as a bracelet, watch, or item stored in a pocket or purse by the person with Alzheimer's, GPS shoes have recently become available. These shoes contain a tiny embedded tracking device that will work anywhere there is cell coverage (e.g., the Aetrex Ambulator GPS shoe). Whenever the wearer wanders off more than a preset distance, the caregiver will receive an alert by telephone and computer from a monitoring system that can pinpoint their location.

Stove Use Detectors

The kitchen has the potential to be one of the most dangerous locations in the home as cooking left unattended is the source of a large number of fires. A care management home safety assessment will typically identify the need for smoke and carbon monoxide detectors as well as fire extinguishers. When there is a care provider in the home, the care manager can recommend that the appliance be unplugged, knobs removed, or a circuit breaker or gas-shut-off valve installed, or in the case of newer appliances, utilize the existing "lock-out" feature. Electric cooking appliance shut-off technologies that do not require the ongoing presence of a care provider can be recommended for the more independent client who may forget occasionally that they have something cooking yet could use the stove independently with an automatic stove use detector.

Features of these devices include a timer, a motion sensor, and an automatic-shut off. Considerations for selection of a specific product include the following: (1) a timer that is either preset or can be set for how long the food can be left cooking unattended; (2) when the stove has been turned off, some units turn the stove back on when the person returns to the kitchen and others must be manually turned back on; (3) the placement of the sensor differs for each unit, either to the side or above the stove, with an unobstructed view of the user; and (4) some products may result in the person with dementia becoming further confused, requiring reminder signs instructing the person what to do. Available products include the Cook-Stop, the Stove Guard, HomeSenser, and the Safe-T element Cooking System. The Safe-T sensor is a similar product for microwaves that senses smoke from foods in the very early stages of combustion and shuts the microwave off.

Programmable Thermostats

Clients who are visually impaired or disabled may have difficulty adjusting a thermostat, or the air conditioner or furnace may break down and a client may not notice or may not be able to communicate the need for help.

The Kelvin Voice Activated Talking Programmable Thermostat will tell the temperature when asked, and can be programmed using talking buttons. Products are also available that allow remote care providers to operate a thermostat from a computer or web-enabled cell phone (e.g., the BAYweb Thermostat, the Trane Remote Energy Management Thermostat, and the Temperature Guard). Features of these devices can include: (1) temperature and power monitoring; (2) the ability to program both low and high temperature thresholds; and (3) the ability to provide notification by telephone or Internet. Some home monitoring systems described in this chapter, also include remote monitoring of ambient temperature.

■ COMMUNICATION AND SOCIAL ENGAGEMENT

Recent studies have shown that remaining socially and intellectually engaged significantly reduces the risk of age-related disability and cognitive decline, and can also extend life.[26] It has been shown that the use of technology improves older adults' quality of life by reducing boredom and loneliness and helping them feel more connected to those outside their homes. Technology can enhance social interaction, provide an opportunity for lifelong learning and personal engagement, support emotional and spiritual well-being, and create leisure activities.[27]

One important care management task is to encourage ongoing communication between the client and the care team to help reduce the feeling of isolation and also to monitor well-being. Increased communication can also promote independence and help keep a frail elder out of an institution.[28] Computer- and noncomputer-based communication devices, cell phones, and teleconferencing (i.e., virtual visitation) devices all provide technological support in this area.

Computers and the Internet

Computer usage provides a greater ability to connect to people, places, and ideas. This can be in the form of e-mail, chat rooms, health information gathering, news, and games, as well as a network of supportive relationships through online interaction. According to the Pew Internet and American Life Project, the largest percentage increase in Internet use since 2005 has been in the 70-to-75 age group.[29] Although only 7% of those 65 and older use social networks, Facebook's own research indicates that in 2007, in the United States, there was a massive, 1230% spike in usage amongst those over 64.[30,31] According to a recent study, after 3 months of using a simplified computer, older adults had significantly greater energy levels, participated more in social engagement activities, were less depressed, demonstrated great self-efficacy, and experienced a greater quality of life.[32] Social engagement can be enhanced both by the client directly using a computer and also from devices that can receive e-mails and other internet files that would interest the client. Both types of social engagement are described below.

Computers for Social Networking

A companion can be hired who can set the client up with appropriate Internet service and then engage the client to use the system. The Internet can be used to stimulate conversation about a topic of interest, and the pictures and sound provided by a website can stimulate conversation, as new information is being shared by the client and care provider.[33] Social networking technologies focus on building communities that help older adults communicate, organize, and share with others.[34] A Facebook site dedicated to the older adult can enable that person to connect with friends and younger family members, or a Google Calendar can be used to help coordinate the elder's schedule. Another form of social networking exists where members share treatment and symptom information on chronic diseases (e.g., PatientsLikeMe.com). Some platforms have been developed that provide scheduling, task planning, messaging, and storytelling around an older adult or person with disabilities where the care team can communicate and also program reminders and calendar items or send messages and photos to the client. Examples of these systems include Tyze, Famililink, and Care Diary.

The care manager can suggest local vendors who can set up a computer system and resources to train the older adult how to use the computer. Many local senior centers offer computer classes tailored to a senior's skill level and learning pace. Computer training programs available nationwide include SeniorNet.com, a nonprofit that provides computer training both online and at over 200 volunteer-staffed learning centers across the country. Another resource is Computer School for Seniors, a virtual campus offering online computer and Internet classes.

Because conventional computer technology can be a challenge for many, simplified interfaces geared toward this market include features such as touch-screen technology, large buttons, and scalable text. Standard computers can be set up so that the size of the font, icons, and mouse pointer are enlarged, and alternative input devices such as a keyboard can be provided with larger keys and marking to support those with more limited dexterity and vision can be provided (e.g., Big Key Keyboard). Communication tools including webcams and audio e-mail, simplified Web browsing and e-mail, games, and a place to store and upload photographs or create a memoir are typical options.

Products include both computers designed for seniors as well as software products that can be used with existing computers. The GO Computer is a stand-alone computer developed for seniors that has all of these features and provides technical support for an additional monthly fee. Some software products that can be used on standard computers (preferably with a touch screen), including IN2L.com (It's Never too Late), PointerWare.com, Connected Living, and BigScreenLive.com, are available either at senior living communities or for in-home use. Newer technologies in the future will increasingly aim to wrap social networking, emotional connectedness, reminders, and telehealth support into one package to support isolated elders.

Social Networking Without a Computer

Several products support communication via the Internet without a computer. Most require subscriptions and are connected to but do not generally interfere with regular phone service. Only designated individuals identified by the appointed "system manager" (i.e., someone on the care team who takes this responsibility) can participate, preventing the client from receiving unwanted spam. These systems allow people who are often left out of the online communication "loop" to be included and to receive messages and photos as well as reminders and documents in a non-intrusive way. Another benefit is that the client can receive something up to date and tangible that can be easily shared with others. Some currently available products need only to be connected to a regular telephone line, and others require Internet access.

Several services specifically designed for the senior market allow the client's home to receive e-mail printouts, including both text and pictures. MyCelery is a two-way service that utilizes a standard fax machine. This service would be useful for clients who either already own a fax machine or who wish to send outgoing handwritten messages to any of the designated individuals as a PDF file. Care managers might find this product useful for receiving documents in electronic format that are sent from the client's home (e.g., daily care provider notes or potentially important mail). The Presto Printing Mailbox, when combined with the Presto Service, is another e-mail printer that has pre-set special formats available so that documents arrive looking very professional. Presto also allows photos to be automatically delivered from a Facebook account, offers a selection of its own content such as daily puzzles and articles on selected topics including travel and news, and has a well-organized command center where reminders and to-do lists can be programmed to be sent to the client or care provider. Web-aware printers (e.g., Hewlett-Packard) have recently become available that will print from any remote e-mail device. Although not designed specifically for the senior market, these printers, which require Internet access to the home to be able to receive the files to be printed, will provide similar capability to the MyCelery and Presto services. These new printers allow members of the care team to send e-mails, calendars, articles, pictures, or content from an "ePrint Center" to the printer's unique e-mail address to be automatically delivered at scheduled times to the printer in the client's home.

Devices including Internet photo frames and personal Internet viewers that receive internet-based information in a digital format are also available. Internet photo frames can receive digital photos uploaded by family and friends from anywhere in the world. These include the CEIVA Digital Photo Frame, EStarling, and Kodak Pulse Wifi Frame, which all connect to the home's phone line and can receive new photos every night. Internet viewers such as the Chumby and the Sony Dash are designed to sit on a table and can be programmed remotely with all kinds of information that might interest a client such as their schedule (e.g., Google Calendar), the weather, Twitter feeds of local news, and a personalized Pandora radio station. These devices can also support Netflix and YouTube video, can receive e-mail, and include applications for many different types of activities and entertainment.

Cell Phones

A cell phone can be used to improve communication since it becomes easier for others to reach the client. It gives the client more freedom to go out because they are not sitting by the land-based phone waiting for a call. Cell phones that care managers recommend should be easy to use with a large and easy to read display, big buttons, simple navigation, and clear sound or hearing aid compatible. Several phones that meet these criteria include the Jitterbug, the Doro PhoneEasy, and the ClarityLife C900. Of these, the Jitterbug is a phone that comes bundled with services that are tailored specifically to seniors, including a unique personalized operator assistance feature, and as mentioned in the section on reminder technologies, medication reminder capability. Other phones come equipped with GPS tracking devices. Some of the major carriers offer cell phone service plans geared towards seniors and Consumer Cellular offers a senior-friendly service promoted by AARP. A clamp-on cell phone holder is one supporting device by Ableware that provides a convenient place to store cell phones on wheelchairs, walkers, bed rails, and other 1-inch diameter tubing.

Videoconferencing

Videoconferencing allows all those involved to both see and hear each other in the way that comes most naturally to everyone—traditional face-to-face communication.[35] Recent studies have shown that the frail elderly population is capable of participating in videoconferencing, including those residing in nursing homes.[36,12] It is a way to share favorite people (e.g., a new baby, the care recipient's favorite nurse's aide), places (e.g., photos or a video of a vacation), and things (e.g., a new home or animal). Videoconferencing has been shown to reduce the feeling of isolation and loneliness of the older adult.[12] Additionally, videoconferencing is also a way

for a distant care provider located anywhere in the world that broadband is available to monitor well-being and quality of care—grooming habits can be observed, as can the elder's ability to perform simple tasks such as sitting and standing.

Care managers can use videoconferencing to enhance their practice. Systems set up in the client's home can be used to enhance family relationships, by medical practitioners to connect with clients who are too frail to travel to appointments, and by the care manager to interact with the client remotely in-between home visits. A laptop or tablet PC with videoconferencing capability can also be used by a care manager during home visits to connect a client with other members of the care team.

Computer-based videoconferencing requires a personal computer, webcam, microphone, and speakers (typically included in new computer systems), high-speed Internet (cable or DSL); and a security solution like a DSL or cable router and firewall software. Free software such as Skype, Google Video Chat for PCs and Apple computers, or iChat for users of Apple computers are available. Users just need to create an account, log in, and download the software. For clients who do not wish to use a computer, a dedicated stand-alone video telephone (e.g., the Asus brand AiGuru Skype phone) device can take the place of a centrally located telephone.

In addition to using Skype directly, some clients may find it easier to utilize videoconferencing systems which have been designed as products specifically for the senior market. These include Virtual Interactive Families and Friends, AttentiveCare, or Family Virtual Visits in addition to systems such as Pointerware that have other capabilities as were described in the Computer section of this chapter. Each of these systems offers different features (e.g., controls being only at the caregiver's end, multiple simultaneous connections, multimedia support including voice and text reminders, slide show capability). The care manager can help the client and their family to select the most appropriate system.

■ LEARNING AND CONTRIBUTION

Making sure that our clients remain both mentally and physically engaged is an important care management task essential to our clients' quality of life. Brain fitness programs are a popular way to continue to develop cognitive skills and music is known to stimulate the brain. Fitness games enable the older adult to improve their fitness by playing their favorite games. Technology can help a client with limitations watch his or her favorite television shows as well. Care managers can support legacy building as well with technology-based tools.

Cognitive Fitness

There is currently an emerging cognitive fitness movement and debate regarding whether the new computer technologies can actually improve memory and delay the onset of dementia. According to experts in the field, brain fitness is the brain's ability to strengthen connections between neurons and to promote the growth of new neurons in certain parts of the brain to maintain important brain functions.[37] The more successful technologies are typically fun to use and have age-appropriate content. Games focus on long-term and short-term memory, language, executive functioning, computation, visuospatial orientation, and critical thinking. Useful questions to ask about a brain fitness product include: (1) is the product based upon scientifically-proven research and supported by other professionals in the field?; (2) have benefits been shown to be generalized beyond the directly trained skills?; (3) what specific benefits have published studies shown?; and (4) is the product fun to use and of interest to the client?

Brain fitness products are typically available as software packages for use on a computer with or without a touch screen. One such product, the Dakim BrainFitness Program for Seniors, uses content that the older adult is familiar with, adjusts as the elder plays, with new games downloaded automatically on a daily basis. Programs from CogniFit and Posit Science claim to be scientifically proven and validated. These products create systematic personalized training programs that improve verbal memory, visual memory, or skills. According to PositScience, their Brain Fitness Program increases auditory processing speed by 131% and memory by the equivalent of 10 years, and their InSight program improves visual working memory by 10% or the equivalent of almost 50 years, reduces medical expenses, prevents a decline in health-related quality of life and the onset of depressive symptoms. In addition, the Posit Science DriveSharp program has been scientifically proven in a study founded by the National Institutes of Health to reduce the risk of a car crash by 50%, increase the useful field of view by up to 200%, and significantly reduce the distance required to stop.

Physical Fitness

Participants at innovative adult day health programs, rehabilitation programs, and residential facilities as well as those still in their homes are enjoying what has been termed *Wii-hab,* or the use of the Nintendo Wii program for therapeutic exercise and rehabilitation.[38] Wii is a simulation gaming device utilizing natural movements that can be played on a television, and in larger facilities, is projected onto a screen. Wii Fit is a game that incorporates yoga, strength training, balance and aerobics and Wii Sports is a game that offers golf, tennis, bowling, boxing, and baseball. Other available games include those that simulate skiing, dancing, cooking, and playing instruments as well as those that provide cognitive stimulation such as "Jeopardy" and

Wheel of Fortune." The Wii My Fitness Coach can chart a client's progress over time.

All of the Wii games are interactive and most require the player to physically move. Some Wii games can even be played from a seated position. It can be used for group activities including competitive sports. Many of these games are reported to improve general fitness as well as strengthening the arms and legs, and promote dexterity, balance, reaction speed, memory, and coordination, while being fun and motivational to those who may have previously been reluctant to move. Since Wii is enjoyed by all ages, it is a wonderful intergenerational activity. Before recommending Wii, it is advisable to get approval of a medical professional such as a doctor or physical therapist. Additionally, to avoid injury when playing, the client should be properly supervised. A newer generation gaming system that is controller-free and is expected to compete with the Wii, will be available as of the date of publication of this book (e.g., the Kinect for Xbox 360).

Digital Music Players

Although a client may not remember the name of a song or why they know it, those with memory impairment remain very responsive and obtain great pleasure from music from their past.[39] By reconnecting with favorite music, the result is often increased attention, improved cooperation and mood, and reduced depression, agitation, and anxiety.[40] Anecdotal evidence that indicates increased cognitive function after music therapy has recently been confirmed by functional MRI studies where it has been shown that the area of the brain that associates music and memories is one of the last parts of the brain to atrophy with Alzheimer's.[41]

Simple digital music players loaded with customized playlists can be used as a form of music therapy. The care manager can support family members and care providers to identify a client's favorite music or preselected music lists from various decades. The iPod Shuffle has been used successfully because of its simplicity of use.[42,39] Alternatively, if a computer or an Internet-ready device such as a smart phone or TV with BluRay player is available, a Pandora Radio station can be created that is similar to a selected piece of music, artist, or composer. The following guidelines can be kept in mind when selecting music for a client:

1. Music from a person's teenage years through their early 20s is often a good selection, as is music that a person loved throughout their lives such as opera, classical, religious, or jazz.
2. Make the music available only as long as the person is interested.
3. Share the music if possible, as the music can be a starting point for engagement and communication—listeners can reminisce together about what the music reminds them of or just hold hands to be more connected.
4. Use the music to enhance intergenerational interaction, as young family members can drum along.
5. Be prepared that music can evoke a multitude of emotions and memories both happy and sad.

Electronic Book Readers

Electronic book (e-book) readers are compact portable reading devices that wirelessly download books, magazines, newspapers, and blogs, with subscriptions to magazines and newspapers automatically received. Since older readers are typically big consumers of the written word, e-book readers may have a great appeal to care management clients. E-book readers are relatively ergonomic (for example, the Kindle is 10.2 ounces and 1/3 inch thick), can typically store over 1000 books, have built-in dictionaries, and allow on-screen bookmarks and annotation. Books can be automatically downloaded from any-where in the world if an account has been established and books already in the public domain are free. Features to consider when recommending an e-book reader to a client include size of screen, ability to magnify font, type of multilevel gray scale display, which affects contrast and glare, backlighting, ease of navigation, ease of downloading (e.g., wire-less, wifi, or computer connection with decreasing preference), and battery life. E-book readers are now available from Ama-zon (the Kindle), Sony (Sony Reader Digital Book), Barnes and Noble (the Nook) and Apple (iPad). Each reader has different fea-tures, for example, the Nook allows the owner to share books with others, and the Kindle can download books wirelessly. Many of these devices are becoming more and more book-like and some even allow the reader to flip pages by swiping the page, as would be done with a regular book.

Television Viewing

The care manager can recommend various products designed to support clients with cognitive or physical disabilities to continue to enjoy television (TV). A TV remote designed for a person with memory loss called the Slicker Clicker has three simple buttons and can be set to turn to only those channels that the person watches regularly. TV Ears is a wireless headset designed for those with mild to moderate hearing loss and makes it easier even for those with hearing aids to hear the television. A high-definition TV advertised as "senior-friendly" is now available with a built-in transmitter for TV Ears, a simplified remote control, automatic sleep timer, and "white glove" delivery and set up.

Legacy Building

As described in Chapter 10 on quality of life, the role of storytelling and reminiscence is very important for many older adults, espe-cially for clients who are beginning to experi-ence memory loss and dementia. Many of the following technology-based resources and ideas can be supported by family members of different ages as well as care providers:

- Life Bio offers an ongoing digital scrap-booking service that includes over 250 thought-provoking questions. A PDF version of the scrapbook can be printed or ordered as a hardcover book.
- Family tree programs are available as software or online, such as Ancestry.com.
- Talking photo albums or photo juke-boxes allow the older adult to record a brief personal description of a photo, drawing, newspaper clipping, or text. The purpose might be to record autobio-graphical information, to facilitate daily conversation, to help order in restau-rants, and to facilitate memory, among other things.
- Creating a digital video of the older per-son's life that includes activities and peo-ple that they enjoy can be valuable; show it to them and send it to distant family members.
- Digital photo albums, blogging, and memoir-building tools may be incorpo-rated into previously described, com-puter-based communication tools.
- Applications are available for the iPhone, iTouch or iPad that allow members of the care team to record stories and remi-niscence of loved ones in their own voices (for example, QuickVoice Recorder), or to create notes that can be attached to photos (for example PhotoNote) that can then be e-mailed.

■ THE CARE MANAGER'S ROLE IN RECOMMENDING TECHNOLOGY

Care managers can challenge themselves to think about a new paradigm of caregiving for elders that includes technology-based tools. It s easy to see the benefits of the use of technology to support our clients to both enhance and stretch available resources. One advantage of technology is that those with chronic illness who need long-term attention but not necessarily continuous treatment, can be monitored and supported in their homes for a variety of conditions. Second, in emergency situations such as when a fall has occurred, monitoring will expedite support. Third, technology may be able to provide different types of social interaction and support.

To be able to recommend products for a client, the care manager should be aware of and be willing to experiment with available products or have a reliable resource who can make and support technology recommendations. It is also important for the care manager to have a process based on specific criteria to evaluate technology in a way that facilitates implementation in the caregiving routine or workflow. The following criteria can be considered:

- **Efficacy:** Does the technology perform according to expectations?
- Return on investment and cost effectiveness: Does the end result justify the means (for example, will it keep the person independent at home)?
- **Ease of use:** Do the care providers, family members, or elders using the technology day to day find it intuitive and user-friendly?
- **Low maintenance:** Does the solution require significant time and resources to maintain, or is there someone locally who can provide a service/maintenance plan?
- **Improved accountability:** Does the solution help the care provider to improve accountability and quality of care?
- **Connection, Contribution, or Legacy:** Does the technology support the client's feeling of contribution and connection to their family, community, or society? Does the technology allow the client to transmit their experiences to future generations?
- **Ethical Considerations:** Does the usefulness of the recommended technology adequately balance these factors of privacy, autonomy, and dignity?

The care manager can keep abreast of the latest consumer and healthcare technologies as they become more available and affordable to the general public by belonging to the Internet community of professionals in the field. Several websites, including those for the Center for Aging Services Technologies (CAST), a division of AAHSA, the Home Care Technology Association of America (HCTAA), the Smart Silvers Alliance, the American Telehealth Association (ATA), the Center for Technology and Aging, Center for Telehealth and E-Health Law, Aging In Place Technology Watch, TelecareAware, the Technology Centre for Independent Living, and the AgeTek Alliance follow available home-based technology and some send out regular e-newsletters or blog postings. An Internet search of "aging in place technology" will result in the identification of links to the latest products and articles on this topic. Product catalogs and websites such as First-Street, the Alzheimer's Store, Epill.com, Abledata.com, Assistivetech.net and others also provide products to consider. There is one book available, called *The Senior Sleuth's Guide to Technology* for Seniors that the care manager might find useful in their own practice or to recommend to clients[10] (although as with much technology information published in book form, much of it will not be current). The CAST Clearinghouse lists commercial products as well as pilot projects and projects under research and development. Websites of corporations and universities that do research on technology and aging also provide a wealth of information.

■ REFERENCES

1. International Society for Gerontechnology. http://www.gerontechnology.info. Accessed August 7, 2010.

2. Alwan M, Nobel N. State of technology in aging services: summary. http://www.agingtech.org/documents/bscf_state_technology_summary.pdf. Published 2007. Accessed July 24, 2010.

3. Barrett L. Healthy @ Home. AARP. http://assets.aarp.org/rgcenter/il/healthy_home.pdf. Published 2008. Accessed July 24, 2010.

4. Wang H. Digital home health—a primer. http://www.parksassociates.com/free_data/downloads/parks-Digital-Home-Health.pdf. Published 2006. Accessed July 24, 2010.

5. Orlov L. Technology for aging in place: a 2010 market overview. http://www.ageinplacetech.com. Accessed July 24, 2010.

6. Coughlin JJ, Lau J. Cathedral builders wanted: constructing a new vision of technology for old age. *Public Policy Aging Report.* 2006; 16(1):4–8.

7. Smith D. How to utilize technology with care management clients. *J Geriatric Care Manag.* 2010;Spring:22–24.

8. Veterans Health Administration receives grant to extend use of Bosch Healthcare's Health Buddy Telehealth System. http://www.healthbuddy.com/content/language1/html/6386_ENU_XHTML.aspx. Accessed July 24, 2010.

9. Philips announces release of National Study on home healthcare technology and telehealth. http://www.healthcare.philips.com/Resources/News.wpd&id=1736&c=global. Accessed July 24, 2010.

10. HealthTechWire (2007, October 8). Philips announces results of national study on the future of home healthcare technology. http://www.healthcare.philips.com/wpd.aspx?p=/Resources/News.wpd&id=1619&c=main. Accessed August 10, 2010.

11. Peterka D. The senior sleuth's guide to technology for seniors. Morrison, CO: Conifer Books; 2009.

12. Demiris G, Hensel BK. Technologies for an aging society: a systematic review of "smart home" applications. *IMIA Yearbook Med Inform.* 2008;33–40.

13. Hards S. What is telecare? http://www.telecareaware.com/index.php/what-is-telecare.html. Accessed April 23, 2010.

14. EliteCare. Elite care home technology. *New York Times.* July 1, 2007. http://www.nytimes.com/2007/02/04/business/yourmoney/04elder.html?ex=1328245200&e=ec63007ce80dfadc&ei=5088&partner=rssnyt&emc=rss.

15. Mahoney DF. The future of technology in mental health nursing—a nurse geropsychtechnologist? In: Melillo KD, Houde SC, eds. *Geropsychiatric and mental health nursing.* Sudbury, MA: Jones and Bartlett; 2007:392.

16. Cantor MD. No information about me without me: technology, privacy, and home monitoring. *Generations.* 2006;30(2):49–53.

17. Stevenson K. Elder Web: to watch or not to watch? Cameras, ethical considerations, sensors, systems in operation, what about the targets? http://www.elderweb.com/node/3001. Accessed August 10, 2010.

18. Mahoney DF. Linking home care and the workplace through innovative wireless technology: The Worker Interactive Networking (WIN) Project. *Home Health Care Manag Pract.* 2004;16(5):417–428.

19. Baruch J, Downs M, Baldwin C, Bruce E. A case study in the use of technology to reassure and support a person with dementia. *Dementia.* 2004;3(3):372–377.

20. New England Healthcare Institute. Thinking outside the pillbox: a system-wide approach to improving patient medication adherence for chronic disease. http://www.nehi.net/publications/44/thinking_outside_the_pillbox_a_systemwide_approach_to_improving_patient_medication_adherence_for_chronic_disease. Accessed July 23, 2010.

21. Horgas A, Abowd G. The impact of technology on living environments for older adults. In: Pew RW, Van Hemel SB, eds. *Technology for adaptive aging.* Washington, DC: The National Academies Press; 2004:230–252.

22. Rajendran P, Corcoran A, Kinosian B, Alwan M. Falls, Fall Prevention, and Fall Detection Technologies. In: Alwan M, Felder R, eds. *Aging medicine, eldercare technology for clinical practitioners.* Totowa, NJ: Humana Press; 2008.

23. Lohr S. Watch the walk and prevent a fall. *New York Times.* November 8, 2009, p. 4.

24. Fleming J, Brayne C. Inability to get up after falling, subsequent time on floor, and summoning help: prospective cohort study in people over 90. *BMJ.* 2008;337:a2227.

25. Kallmyer B, Cullen N. Aging safely at home: the use of technology to address location management and wandering for persons with Alzheimer's disease. *J Geriatric Care Manag.* 2010; Spring:14–17.

26. Rush University. Less frequent social activity linked to more rapid loss of motor function in older adults. http://www.rush.edu/webapps/MEDREL/servlet/NewsRelease?id=1237. Accessed July 24, 2010.

27. American Society on Aging. Existing and emerging technologies within the long-term care spectrum. Live web seminar presented by the Network on Environments, Services, and technologies for Maximizing Independence (NEST). June 11, 2009.

28. Span P. Old age, new gizmos. *New York Times.* January 6, 2010.

29. Fox S. Four in ten seniors go online. Pew Internet & American Life Project. http://www.authoring.pewinternet.org/Commentary/2010/January/38-of-adults-age-65-go-online.aspx. Accessed January 13, 2010.

30. Lenhart A. Adults and social network websites. Pew Internet & American Life Project. http://www.pewinternet.org/Reports/2009/Adults-and-Social-Network-Websites.aspx. Accessed July 24, 2010.

31. Roberts S. The fictions, facts and future of older people and technology. Intel Corporation. http://www.ilcuk.org.uk/files/pdf_pdf_112.pdf. Published December 2009. Accessed July 24, 2010.

32. Green House Project Partners. "It's Never 2 Late" and Mather LifeWays Institute on Aging in Pilot Study of Quality of Life in Green House Homes. http://www.in2l.com/index.cfm. Accessed January 30, 2010.

33. Lewis, B. (2009). Personal Communication on October 2009, Ben Lewis of www.engageasyouage.com.

34. Lindeman D, Steinmetz V, Ratan S, Redington L. Technologies for home and community-based services: considering the options. Paper presented at American Society on Aging, West Coast Conference on Aging, September 11, 2009.

35. Gough M, Rosenfeld J. Video conferencing over IP: configure, secure, and troubleshoot. Rockland, MA: Syngress Publishing; 2006.

36. White C, Rondeau S. Virtual visiting pilot program final report. Western District (Australia) Health Service. http://www.wdhs.net/agedcare/virtualvisiting/virtual%20visiting%20Pilot%20Program%20Final%20Report.pdf. Published 2007. Accessed July 23, 2010.

37. Van Pelt J. Brain fitness games: the real deal? *Aging well.* 2010;Winter:22–25.

38. Sager N. On-Lok Lifeways gets into "Wii-hab." *Aging Today.* 2009;November–December:6.

39. Beck M. A key for unlocking memories: music therapy opens a path for Alzheimer's patients; creating a personal playlist. *Wall Street Journal.* November 16, 2009.

40. Suggested top 10's for loved ones with memory impairments. http://www.bethabe.org/Top_10s_for_Memory327.html. Accessed July 23, 2010.

41. Janata Lab. Music, memories, and emotions. http://atonal.ucdavis.edu/projects/memory_emotion/index.shtml. Accessed April 18, 2010.

42. Well-Tuned. Music players for health program. http://www.bethabe.org/Aging_in_Place_Music289.html. Accessed July 23, 2010.

PART 3

The Business of Geriatric Care Management: Beginning, Expanding or Adding, and Managing a Geriatric Care Management Business

Chapter 12

How to Start or Add a Geriatric Care Management Business

Cathy Jo Cress and Jack Herndon

A new geriatric care management business must spring from the intersection of three streams: your passion, your competence, and market opportunity. To start a geriatric care management business, the adage to know thyself becomes critical. Are you passionate about geriatric care management? You will need passion to sustain you when the situation gets tough—which it does in the beginning of all businesses. You must have the core competence both to be a geriatric care manager (GCM) and to run a business. Good GCMs with no business acumen, which is often the case, frequently fail in business. You must also have the market opportunity. If no older people live in your community, you may not be in the right place to start a geriatric care management business. If 10 other GCMs are practicing in your town, that may limit your own market opportunity. Finally, you need to assess why you want to start this type of business in the first place. Are you motivated by the financial gains? By community recognition? By a need to make a difference? Use Exhibit 12–1 to assess your motivations, abilities, and personality to help you decide whether starting a geriatric care management business is a wise choice for you.

■ ENTREPRENEURIAL RISKS

There are several types of geriatric care management businesses. In 1999, the most common type was the owner-run business. However, new models have appeared, such as the corporate models of Senior Bridge, LivHOME, and ResCare, that integrate home care and geriatric care management practices. There are also GCM models pairing GCMs in business with physicians, attorneys, and accountants, as well as GCMs who specialize in such areas as relocation of older adults or death and dying.

This chapter focuses on starting a geriatric care management business and also discusses how to add a geriatric care management practice onto an existing business or not-for-profit agency.

■ STARTING A BUSINESS IN GERIATRIC CARE MANAGEMENT

According to a survey done by the National Association of Professional Geriatric Care Managers in 1997, 80% of all geriatric care management businesses were owner run, and 20% were run by nonowners.[1] Entrepreneurial people who do not mind some risk usually start owner-run businesses. Starting a geriatric

Exhibit 12–1   Know Thyself

Going into business for yourself requires certain personal characteristics. Not everyone is suited to be a business owner. Take some time to think about your motivations, personality, and abilities.

As a first step, ask yourself why you want to own your own business.

1. Freedom from the 9–5 work routine?
2. Being your own boss?
3. Do what you want when you want to do it?
4. Improve your standard of living?
5. Boredom with your present job?
6. Having a product or service for which you feel there is a demand?

Although no answer is wrong, some are better than others. Be aware, however, there are tradeoffs. For example, as a business owner, you can escape the daily 9–5 routine, but you may replace it with a 6 am–10 pm routine.

Do you have the personal characteristics typical to an entrepreneur? Try to be objective in the following self-analysis. Remember, it's your future that is at stake!

1. Are you a leader?
2. Do you like to make your own decisions?
3. Do others turn to you for help in making decisions?
4. Do you enjoy competition?
5. Do you have will power and self discipline?
6. Do you plan ahead?
7. Do you like people?
8. Do you get along well with others?

Think about the physical, emotional, and financial strains you will encounter when you start your new business.

1. Are you aware that running your own business may require working 12–16 hours a day, six days a week, and maybe even Sundays and holidays?
2. Do you have the physical stamina to handle the workload and schedule?
3. Do you have the emotional strength to withstand the strain?
4. Are you prepared, if needed, to temporarily lower your standard of living until your business is firmly established?
5. Is your family prepared to go along with the strains they, too, must bear?
6. Are you prepared to lose your savings?

Certain skills and experience are critical to the success of a small business. Since it is unlikely that you possess all the skills and experience needed, you will need to hire personnel or contract for services to supply those you lack. There are some basic and special skills you will need for your particular business. Identify your strengths and weaknesses with the following questions.

1. Do you know what basic skills you will need to have a successful business?
2. Do you possess those skills?
3. When hiring personnel, will you be able to determine if the applicants' skills meet the requirements for the positions you are filling?
4. Have you ever worked in a managerial or supervisory capacity?
5. Have you ever worked in a business similar to the one you want to start?
6. Have you had any business training?
7. If you discover you don't have the basic skills needed for your business, will you be willing to delay your plans until you've acquired the necessary skills?

care management business is not for the faint of heart. Many new businesses are started every day, only to be boarded shut within a few years.

People considering beginning a geriatric care management business should first find out whether they are comfortable with the level of risk inherent in starting a new business by honestly answering the questions in the self-assessment (Exhibit 12–2). Entrepreneurs share many personality traits, including high energy, aggressiveness, a love of ambiguity, a zest for problem solving, and monumental self-discipline.

After completing the general self-assessment, you should consider whether you are suited to own a business, even if you are an experienced and skilled GCM. In a presentation to the 1998 National GCM Conference in Chicago, Elizabeth Bodie Gross and Linda Fordini Johnson outlined the skills and personality traits GCMs should have as follows:[2]

- Has he or she worked as care manager? Has he or she worked with older adults or had education or training in geriatrics or gerontology? These experiences help prospective GCMs know what to expect and whether they like the work.
- Does he or she have a business background? Does he or she know accounting, has he or she ever had to meet a payroll, and can he or she tolerate not being paid the first few years? Can he or she do another job while also being a GCM? Many budding GCMs hold other jobs for years until their geriatric care management practice can make enough money to support them.
- Does he or she have the energy to run a 24-hour-a-day, 7-day-a-week business? Can his or her family tolerate calls night and day? Can his or her family accept this invasion of privacy and family life? Will his or her children suffer from receiving less attention?

In the beginning, running a geriatric care management business can be lonely. Often, the entrepreneur is the entire business, doing all the jobs, including billing, seeing clients, marketing, being on call 24 hours a day, and perhaps even running to the bank to borrow more money to cover operating expenses. Often, the entrepreneur sees much less of his or her family because the GCM is consumed by running the fledgling operation. Often, GCMs face initial criticism or rejection of their services if they do not have already established sources of client referrals. (Chapter 16 discusses marketing in more detail.) Finally, to be successful, the entrepreneur

Exhibit 12–2   Are You Entrepreneur Material?

- Are you a leader?
- Are you a self-starter?
- Do you make decisions easily?
- Do you like competition?
- Do you get along well with different types of people?
- Are you good at planning and organizing?
- Do you have the physical and emotional strength to run a business?
- Do you have the drive to maintain your motivation in times of trouble and slowdowns?
- Can your family survive on a more limited income the first few years of your business?
- Do you have self-discipline?

needs to seek out the advice of experienced professionals, listen to it, and be willing to adapt and change as needed.

So, what are the rewards of running a geriatric care management business? According to Kraus, the dividends for many GCM entrepreneurs are as follows:[3]

- Finding an outlet for their creativity
- Working on a flexible schedule
- Earning the respect of their community by offering a service that gives great support to older people and their families
- Doing a variety of tasks every day
- Interacting with many other professionals in a variety of disciplines, through assessment, marketing, and interacting with clients
- Meeting other like-minded people through joining the National Association of Professional Geriatric Care Managers and the Case Management Society of America (CMSA) and by exchanging new and creative ideas about geriatric care management and running a geriatric care management business
- Working in an up-and-coming discipline

Another way for people to find out whether they really want to start a geriatric care management business is to talk to working GCMs. Prospective GCMs can try one or more of the following options to learn from the experience of working GCMs:

- Attend a GCM or CMSA national, state, or regional conference to meet GCMs and talk with them about their practice.
- Go to the GCM or CMSA website to find names of nearby GCMs, and then make an appointment to meet with a GCM in person to discuss his or her business experience.
- Buy compact disks (CDs) and manuals that discuss starting a geriatric care management business.
- Buy products that help you start a professional geriatric care management

business such as the GCM Toolbox, offered through GCM Products on the website http://www.caremanagers.org. You don't have to reinvent the wheel, but instead use materials that have already been tested in the field and found to be useful.

- Hire a GCM consultant who can help measure your market opportunity and do a business plan to set up your GCM business.

Prospective GCMs can and should try to learn from the experiences of others who have been down the path before.

■ TYPES OF GERIATRIC CARE MANAGEMENT BUSINESSES

This section discusses three different ways to organize a geriatric care management business: solo practices, partnerships, and corporations. For more information, refer to the workbook *The Business of Becoming a Professional Geriatric Care Manager* offered in the GCM Toolbox on the website listed above.

Solo Practices

Most GCMs begin their business as a solo practice. They choose a legal entity known as a sole proprietorship, which means that the business is owned and controlled by a single party. In a sole proprietorship, the proprietor is always responsible for any legal or financial liabilities that occur during the course of business. In a 1997 survey of GCMs, Knutson and Langer found that 45% of all GCMs were organized as sole proprietorships.[1]

A sole proprietorship is probably the easiest and most common type of business to start. It is appropriate for an individual or one person. There are few legal restrictions (compared with those that come with partnerships and corporations) and few legal papers to complete, with the exception of a business license or a fictitious business license in some states.

Any profit is taxed at the individual's personal tax rate. There are no separate income tax forms to complete; the individual can put the business revenues and losses on Schedule C of his or her personal IRS Form 1040. Sole proprietors have relative freedom from government taxes and regulations.

There are many other advantages to starting a geriatric care management business as a solo practitioner. It is easier to maintain control and be flexible because the GCM makes all the decisions and is able to respond quickly to client requests and business needs. Another advantage is financial, in that 100% of the profits go to the owner rather than profits being split between multiple owners. In addition, solo practitioners can dissolve the business more easily if they decide being a GCM is not for them, which might be a distinct advantage if the owner decides to close the business.

There are also many disadvantages to being a solo practitioner. Multiple tasks are involved in running a geriatric care management business, including marketing, bookkeeping, managing human resources, counseling, and being on call. A sole proprietor must either do all of these jobs or outsource some of them, which can be expensive. Many times, sole proprietorship leaves a GCM exhausted.

Another negative aspect is that sole proprietors have to be on call 24 hours a day, 7 days a week because this is the nature of being a GCM; the only alternative is to outsource some time to an employee or another GCM. If the GCM becomes ill or cannot practice for any reason, there is no one else to bear the burden of the cases or to run the business. Having an agreement with another GCM who you can rely on is a possibility, but client service will be less consistent.

Sole proprietorship can also pose tough financial issues. In this business form, the owner has unlimited or 100% liability, so creditors can come after the owner's personal assets. The owner has 100% of the risk, so his or her personal assets are at risk. It is much more difficult to borrow money for this type of ownership, and few lenders are willing to make ongoing business loans to a sole proprietorship. Sole proprietors may have a hard time getting long-term financial capital, which can affect their ability to grow. However, because a sole proprietor is also the only one making the decision to spend money, it may be less necessary to seek loans or credit.

Finally, sole proprietors have no one to lean on in times of crisis. Having a colleague to bear the burden of care and decision making means that a GCM gets feedback, support, and respite from the pressure that is an inevitable part of being a GCM and being a business owner.[4] Future GCMs should consult with an attorney and an accountant before deciding whether to choose this form of business organization. An attorney can help with many issues, including a right of survivorship agency agreement in case of the GCM's death or disability. An accountant can explain tax requirements for recording business expenses and profits, Social Security, and employee wage withholdings.[5]

Partnerships

Some GCMs prefer to have a partner. There are two legal types of partnerships. First, there are general partnerships, where the business has two or more owners. All individuals are liable if the business defaults, no matter what percentage of the business each individual owns. Each partner must report income or loss in the business on their individual tax returns. Second, there are limited partnerships, where one partner simply invests in the business but does not make business decisions. In this case, the investing partner is liable for only the amount of the investment. Before deciding on setting up a partnership, you should see an attorney and an accountant to decide whether a partnership is the best option and which type of partnership to choose.

Partnerships have their advantages. Partners share financial, administrative, on-call, and emotional burdens. If you have to take time off, you should be able to rely on your partner to cover your cases and respond to new referrals. Compared with corporations, partnerships are relatively easy to set up and are flexible in that a limited number of people make decisions. Lending sources tend to prefer partnerships to sole proprietorships, although partnerships are still less appealing to lenders than corporations.

There are also disadvantages. Unlike corporation owners, partners have unlimited liability. Like sole proprietors, partners may still have an unstable business life, with fluctuating incomes and exhausting schedules. If something happens to one partner, the partnership may be dissolved. If a partner decides to leave, it may be hard on the other partner because buying out a partner can be legally and financially difficult.

Wendy Marks and Carol Westheimer gave a workshop at the 1995 GCM conference entitled "Partnerships: The Good, the Bad, and the Ugly. Why Do They Succeed or Fail? Or Everything You Wanted to Know About Marriage Without Sex But Were Afraid to Ask." According to Marks and Westheimer, partnerships are as delicate as marriage, and people need to think carefully before becoming partners. As Marks points out in her 1996 article about partnerships in the *GCM Journal,* people should first assess whether they are suited to be in a partnership.[6] Some individuals, according to Marks, have problems sharing tasks with other people, whether they are equals, subordinates, or superiors. People with this domineering personality type are probably not suited for partnerships. Partners are meant to bear a mutual burden and make mutual decisions. Some people have a hard time sharing leadership duties and think of

everything in terms of mine or yours, which can cause the same types of problems in a business partnership as in a marriage.

Marks also suggests understanding the relevant skills of both people considering a partnership. This list may include bookkeeping, care management, geriatric assessment, marketing, payroll, hardware and software support, administration, and human resources management. A skill map can identify which partner has which skills. Marks points out that areas that are not covered by either partner as well as areas that are covered by both partners are of concern in establishing a partnership.

Another step is to assess how long of a commitment each partner can make to the fledgling enterprise. If one partner plans to retire in 5 years and wants to stay in the partnership only for that long, and the other wants to make a 20-year commitment, the mutual venture may need to be reassessed. Does one partner want to have another child in a few years? Does one partner expect to relocate anytime soon? People should assess the present commitment to the partnership, and then anticipate what the partnership will look like 2, 5, and 10 years down the line. There may be a period where one partner would be running the business alone, and this may not seem agreeable to the other partner.

Next, the partners should list the tasks that their business will require to make it operate well. These tasks can include marketing, being on call on a 24-hour basis, paying bills, doing accounts receivable and accounts payable, and handling human resources. Both partners should decide what level of commitment they have to each task. One partner will have to do each task, or the partners will have to outsource the task. For example, if neither partner understands bookkeeping, the partners will have to hire a bookkeeper. If you are considering a partnership—or are already involved in a partnership—we suggest you refer to *The Partnership Charter* by David Gage (Basic Books, 2004), an excellent resource that includes a number of templates to help prospective partners identify compatibility in responsibilities, goals, and expectations.

According to Marks, the ideal partnership has two people who are equally committed. If there are differing levels of commitment, then partners may want to explore splitting the profits accordingly (i.e., a person who does 40% of the work gets 40% of the profits). This needs to be thought out and explored with an attorney.

What all this leads to is the importance of exploring whether the potential partners have a similar vision for the future of the business. In addition to writing a business plan, the partners each may also want to write down a 5- or 10-year plan for his or her involvement in the business, and then compare their visions. If the forecasts are similar, great. If they are different, the partners can negotiate and try to agree. Are both partners willing to share the evening and weekend responsibilities in this around-the-clock business? Resentment can build if someone is unfairly shouldering more of the burden.

The best GCM partners make decisions objectively and are comfortable with change. They learn from their mistakes and are not afraid to fail. If one partner cannot stomach failure, that person may blame the other partner, rather than see the errors as a way to learn what does and does not work in the business. Together, good GCM partners are prepared for and able to survive a crisis because crises are inevitable parts of new (and ongoing) businesses. An adjunct to this is the worst nightmare scenario; partners should consider what they would do if the business failed, because, realistically, this is not an unlikely occurrence. What contingency plans might be set up? Would the partners survive without blaming each other?

Being partners in a business also means spending many hours together working very hard. People considering a partnership need to make sure that they can comfortably spend that much time with another person. Many partners have tested the waters by going off and spending time with each other (e.g., taking a trip together). This helps them gauge their compatibility. Partners should also make sure they have compatible values, according to Marks.[6] If one partner believes that earning a profit is immoral and the other partner embraces capitalism, there will be problems. If one partner believes in spending all available funds and the other is fiscally conservative, there will be problems. Partners may complete some kind of values assessment and compare the results. Potential partners may also, as Marks suggests, interview friends, family members, and colleagues to see how their potential partner's values mesh with their own. An accountant can help partners assess their beliefs about finances (e.g., should you have credit cards, what the limits should be, what constitutes abuse of those cards), and then compare the responses for compatibility. If the responses are not compatible, the partners may try to negotiate, may rethink the partnership, or may decide not to proceed with the partnership.

As Marks points out, partners should also discuss their commitments to their families, because geriatric care management is such a time-intensive business. Are the family members on both sides willing to accept the partners' absences? This needs to be assessed before the partnership begins. Can each partner devote the same amount of time to the business? If not, should one partner get more money? If the imbalance cannot be resolved, the partnership should be reconsidered. Exhibit 12-3 contains a quiz that sums up many of the points discussed here. Potential partners should take the quiz before formalizing the partnership.

Exhibit 12–3
Partnership Quiz

- ❑ Do you both have the entrepreneurial qualities to survive the first 5 years of a business?
- ❑ Is either one of you unable to share tasks with anyone else?
- ❑ Can you both commit to this company for the next 7 years?
- ❑ Do you both have all of the following traits?
  - ❑ Honesty
  - ❑ Risk-taking ability
  - ❑ Ability to withstand failure
  - ❑ Ability to withstand rejection
  - ❑ Capacity to share
  - ❑ Ability to argue strongly and courteously lose
  - ❑ Ability to forgive
  - ❑ Ability to survive a crisis
- ❑ Do you both look at each other as someone with whom you could spend long periods of time?
- ❑ Can you both say "no" to a plan but "yes" to a person?
- ❑ Do you both have a similar vision of the future?
- ❑ Do you both have the finances to cover expenses until you turn a profit?
- ❑ Can you both survive failure?

Corporations

The third and most complex form of business organization is the corporation. If you decide to form a corporation, you need to hire an attorney or use third-party service, such as LegalZoom.

Setting up a corporation offers several advantages. Corporations are considered legal entities that exist apart from the shareholders. If a founder or stockholder dies, it does not affect the business's legal status. Liability is limited to the assets of the corporation; therefore, the personal assets of the share-holders are not affected if the corporation becomes insolvent. This is the advantage of establishing a corporation when starting a business. Ownership is easily transferred, so if the founder wants to relocate or retire, he or she simply has to sell his or her stock in the company.

Another advantage is that banks and lenders are more open to lending to a corporation that has a good track record or a new corporation that has sufficient equity and promise. However, as a precaution lenders will still most likely ask for collateral and possibly personal signatures from the stockholders. The corporate form of ownership can also offer certain advantages with regard to fringe benefits such as health insurance, stock plans, or pensions.

Choosing the corporation business form also has its drawbacks. First, it is more expensive to start a corporation than it is to start a sole proprietorship or a partnership because of the legal costs. And, unlike sole proprietorships and partnerships, corporations may be exposed to regulation by state, local, and federal governments and require more assistance from attorneys and accountants.

In a C corporation, another limitation is double taxation. Profits from a C corporation are taxed once to the corporation and again as income when the profits are distributed to the stockholders. The stockholder pays taxes on his or her salary and any share he or she might have of the distributed profits. Corporations are also required to have bylaws, may be required to hold stockholder meetings, and must keep records.

Another form of corporation is an S corporation. In an S corporation, both income and losses are passed directly to the individual shareholders, rather than the corporation; therefore, they are taxed at only the shareholder's rate. Because new businesses generally lose money in the first year, this can be a distinct advantage to the shareholder. Any loss can be applied against any other personal income, thus reducing the amount of income tax levied. However, it is necessary to consult an attorney to find out whether you can qualify for an S corporation status.[7]

Attorneys help with many essential corporate functions, including the following:

- Filing articles of incorporation in the state where the business is located
- Issuing stock
- Organizing the election of directors and officers as required under the laws of the state
- Drawing up bylaws
- Helping devise procedures for conducting stockholder meetings, keeping records of these meetings, and creating stock and buy–sell agreements

It is also essential to have an accountant to set up the corporation's books, ensure that all taxes are paid fully and on time, and provide other advice on the proper keeping of the corporation's books.

■ CREATING A BUSINESS PLAN

After choosing which form a business will take (sole proprietorship, partnership, or corporation), future GCM business owners need to write a business plan (see Exhibit 12–4). Writing a business plan clearly organizes all of the ideas about the GCM business in a focused description of the products the geriatric care management business will sell, who will buy these products, who the competition is expected to be, and how your products are similar to and different from that of the competition.

Why do this? First, a business plan makes ideas concrete and ordered, turning subjective dreams into objective goals. It also lists the obstacles that a business might face. It explains, step by step, how a person's entrepreneurial dream will become a reality.

In addition, a written business plan is required if you need to borrow money to start the business. Bank loan officers and other funding sources expect to see a fully developed, written business plan. Merrily Orsini, in her workshop titled "Doing Good Makes Cents: Advanced Business Practices," presented at the 10th annual national GCM conference in 1994, emphasizes the importance of having a business plan at every stage of a geriatric care management business, but particularly in the beginning.[8] A business plan makes you think through the whole business you envision, not just individual parts. It helps you evaluate whether you should be in business. It gives you a way to evaluate your daily business operations. And, finally, it gives you a tool you must have if you expect to find investors or seek a loan or line of credit with a bank.

Why Plan?

The future comes no matter what. Planning helps you to anticipate the future and make well-informed decisions. Planning is the first step in business management. Without it you may have no business. You should write this plan yourself if you expect to be successful in owning your own geriatric care management business based on your ideas and efforts. Of course, you may want to have someone else review your business plan, but the bottom line is that businesses that do not have a

Exhibit 12–4
Outline of a Business Plan

I.	Business
II.	Products and Services
III.	Industry
IV.	Location
V.	Market
VI.	Competition
VII.	Marketing
VIII.	Operations
IX.	Personnel
X.	Finances

written business plan have a much higher failure rate than businesses that have a written plan. Increase your chance of success in your geriatric care management business—write a business plan.

Prior to developing a business plan, you need to consider many personal abilities and skill sets. You should consider referring to the workbook *The Business of Becoming a Professional Geriatric Care Manager,* available in the GCM Toolbox on the GCM website, and answering the questions in the section titled "Prior to Developing Your Business Plan."

Courses on How to Start a GCM Business

Many universities and colleges now have classes, degrees and certificates in geriatric care management that teach how to start a GCM business. Some programs offer online classes. Contact these academic programs to see which one has a class in how to start a GCM business and is either near you or online. You can also take a small business class through a local college.

Your GCM Business Plan

When developing a business plan, several sections are key to making your plan successful. The first key section is value proposition.

Value Proposition

The first section of a geriatric care management business plan should state your value proposition. It begins by describing the business in general terms. Include a description of the background of the principals. Résumés of the principals can be included as an attachment to the plan. This section also explains how you plan to use your business plan and why the plan is being written (e.g., to attract investors, to show how the operation will work, to show that the business is financially feasible, to clarify your business operation, to create a guide for managing your business).

Start with your mission statement, which should state the core of your business in a few sentences. The mission statement should reflect the goals and values of your organization. It should be short, focused, perhaps only 20 words, written in the present tense, in positive terms and without qualifiers.

Industry

Next, describe the geriatric care management industry. It is a relatively new industry that must be described to bankers and other investors who may not be aware of it or the niche market it fills. Helpful information to describe the geriatric care management industry is available on the website www.care-manager.org, including what a GCM is, how many GCMs are in the country, how long the profession has been around, the financial performance of the industry, the role of government regulation, and so forth. You might add a history of the geriatric care management industry (see Chapter 1, "Overview and History of Geriatric Care Management") and describe the growth patterns of the GCM industry and of the GCM organization.

Current Situation Analysis

If you are already operating an existing and related business, for example, a home care company, you should describe that business, including key indicators such as revenue, profitability, number of customers, and so forth. Include a brief history of the existing business, why it has been successful, key points of the business's growth, profitability patterns, and how the existing business has changed over time. You should also explain how the addition of a geriatric care component will enhance or fit in with your existing business operations.

Market Assessment

Next describe the customers you intend to serve. Start with a definition of your ideal client. An example would be "Woman, 85 years old with chronic care needs who has an income or liquid assets of $500,000 or more." Again, you want to list the customers who will reward you the most financially. Please see Chapter 17 "Private Revenue Sources for the Fee-Based Care Manager: Need vs. Demand in the Private Eldercare Market."

How many of these ideal clients are in the area you wish to serve? You need do an analysis of the age and income levels. Generally, geriatric care management customers are over age 85 or are disabled younger people with incomes in the top 10% in your community. Your customers are also the local overstressed adult children of clients, long-distance caregivers with family members who need help and live in your community, and third parties who may hire you as a GCM, such as trust officers, attorneys, conservators, or guardians.

You need to do market research to define the size of the market in the area where your business will be located (e.g., how many people over age 85 live in San Luis Obispo, California, how many third-party target markets such as trust departments are in the town). This type of demographic information may be available from US Census Bureau reports, local Area Agencies on Aging, local chambers of commerce, local hospitals, and even members of the local media who have done their own surveys. You can use the Internet to retrieve US Census data in your area, and in addition you can search online for the state department of aging, find your local department of aging, and then find all senior services that may have data on older people in your area.

The market assessment section also contains all your target markets besides older people and their families. These would be defined as client representative or third parties. They include targets who you expect to refer older people and their families to you, including physicians, elder-law attorneys, trust officers, senior services information and referral agencies, hospital-based care man-

agers, and so forth. You can use the Internet or the yellow pages to track the number of third parties. For example, if you want to know the number of elder-law attorneys in your community, go online and search for *National Academy of Elder Law Attorneys* and enter the zip code of the location and border areas where you intend to start your business, and you will find a list of elder-law attorneys.

The market assessment section should also include your own research into the needs of the area. Who else is providing similar or related services in your target market? Why do you think the local target market needs this business? Will older people in the area be able to afford your services?

Finally, calculate the total market opportunity in your geographic area in terms of the expected total market and how much you believe your business can earn from that total possible market.

Problems Faced by Your Target Market

GCMs are problem solvers. What problems do you intend to solve in your market area? You need to describe the specific problems you are expecting to solve. For example, a problem you may expect to be a major focus of your care management practice is the needs of long-distance caregivers who live in your geographic area, but whose elderly family members live elsewhere. These long-distance caregivers may require help in managing their own burnout and finding resources where their elderly family members live. Another example could be the needs of chronically ill adults over age 85 who need supportive services arranged for them, and then monitoring of these referrals to ensure the best continuum of care. A third possibility is meeting the needs of trust officers who do not want to be available 24/7 and who want to contract with a trained care manager to visit their customers on a regular basis to monitor customer needs and report back to the trust officer. A final example would be the needs of elder-law attorneys who need a thorough geriatric assessment to present to court in conservatorship or guardianship cases.

Your Unique Solution to These Problems

This section of your business plan describes in more detail the geriatric care management products or services you expect to provide. Why should people buy these services from you? What makes your business unique and special? How do you intend to charge for your services? What do you expect your fees to be and how will they be organized; for example, will you charge by the hour or by the product? Even though the geriatric care management business sells services, you can think of services as products; for instance, geriatric assessment might be one product, and placement assistance another product.

Here is a real-life example of a geriatric care management product and how you would describe it in this section of your business plan:

> Care Management Plus is a weekly monitoring service for chronically ill elders. It includes a monitoring visit to the older person, a monthly report, phone support as needed by the family or client representative, and e-mail communication with family members, third parties, and client representatives (attorney, trust officer, conservator, etc.). Additional visits to solve a crisis or as requested by the family or family representative are also included in this package.
>
> Why should people buy it? Client representatives should buy this product to assure themselves, the courts, or other third parties or family members that all the older client's needs are met, any crisis is resolved, and all interested parties are communicated with daily, weekly, and monthly.
>
> What makes this product unique and special? Families in our town have no other services similar to Care Management Plus. Conservators, elder-law attor-

neys, third parties, and families have no other means to monitor ongoing care or the client's current status, or to solve emergencies as they arise.

> How much does it cost to provide Care Management Plus? We pay a GCM $25.00 an hour to cover a caseload of between 5 and 10 clients who each require on average 4 hours a week of the care manager's time.
>
> What does Care Management Plus cost for the customer? We expect to sell the care manager's time for $125.00 per hour, which covers payment of all required taxes, training and supervision, charting, and so forth.

The value proposition itself is arguably the most important statement you make about your services. The statement communicates to prospective clients and referral sources how you add value and answers the question, "Why should I pay for your services?" Few clients understand care management services, so a concise and informative value proposition is critical. Do your services save time? Do they save money? Will they enable quality of care that the older adults would not have otherwise? Remember, you're asking a family to pay $100 or more per hour out of their pockets, so they need to understand clearly what you will do for them and how these actions will help them.

You may want to use the following exercise to build your value proposition. Complete the following sentence: We provide *X* services that provide *Y* benefits. For instance, we provide community referrals that save you time and ensure high-quality providers for your family. Or, we facilitate all aspects of a hospital discharge coming back home to ensure your parents receive the care they need.

Competition

When describing your market and the total market opportunity in the area, you need to estimate the money you expect your business to earn. Next, you need to describe what share of that expected opportunity you believe your business can expect to attract. To do this you need to assess your competition.

Are there other geriatric care management businesses in the area? Do home health agencies in the area offer care or case management? Are there physician practices offering geriatric care management? You can do research into these issues in a variety of ways, including using the local phone book or the websites of CMSA or the National Association of Professional Geriatric Care Managers. Also, make sure to identify any providers who offer services to older adults, even if they don't appear to be direct competitors. For instance, non-profit organizations often offer information and referral programs; if older adults and their families are looking to these services for similar benefits to those that you offer, then you need to consider them as competitors.

You might consider doing a competition survey. This is a survey of other GCM businesses in your area. It is a process called mystery shopping. (See Chapter 16, pages 363–365.) This should give you an idea of what your competition is in your area, their services and products, and what clients and customers pay for each service or product. This will help you gauge whether the market can bear your new GCM business and if so, what your fees and services should look like, measured against the competition.

Setting Yourself Apart from Competition

Once you have identified the competition, you need to describe any traits you believe your new business shares with the current competition. What differentiates your new business from the competition? Do you expect the new business to woo customers or referral sources away from the competition? Do you expect to offer lower prices or better and different services? A competition survey is used to find out what your competitors are doing that is different, better or worse, and then use that information to your benefit.

To compare your geriatric care management business to others in your area and to describe your competition you can also make a comparison chart ranking your new business against the competition. You can do a competitive analysis with the help of any of the small business development centers throughout the country. When updating your business plan, you may also redo this competition survey yearly.

Sales Plan

GCMs rarely see themselves as salespersons. However, this is a fatal error. You may have a product, but to make money from that product, you have to sell it. In the beginning, you yourself may have to sell your geriatric care management product. To begin to put together a sales plan you need to identify who makes the decision to buy your geriatric care management products. With older adults over age 85, the buying decision is generally made by the adult children or the third party (trust officer, etc.). Many times young older adults (65–85 years of age) make their own buying decisions.

You then need to identify what criteria the person making the buying decision uses to evaluate your geriatric care management product. For example, you have to figure out whether the decision to purchase your Care Management Plus product is made by the adult child based on price, features, or availability. How will you give your customer, the adult child, enough information to say yes? Does this buying decision require personal contact in intake, GCM intake, a Care Management Plus sell sheet you dropped off at the parent's physician's office, word of mouth, paid advertising, or public relations such as a story about your services submitted and published by the local paper? Describe your sales plan.

Operations

Where will your business be located? This section of the plan discusses the place where the company will do business. Some beginning geriatric care management businesses start in the GCM's home office. Some GCMs prefer to rent an outside space. You need to make that decision. If finances are a critical factor, you might choose a home office. You have to consider whether location is a factor in getting customers. If you are going to have a business address, is the office going to be in a certain part of town because that is where the customers are? Perhaps the business will be near a hospital or a large assisted living facility that offers services for older people. Geriatric care management businesses are not like clothing stores or other merchandise-based businesses, which need to be located in areas with considerable foot traffic (e.g., malls, busy streets). Locating next to a long-term care discharge unit might increase business.

Describe where you will be located and what the square footage will be. Include blueprints that show accurate diagrams of the floor plan, including where staff, furniture, and customer access are located. Add photos of the location. Then describe the occupancy cost of the location by month and by year, listing rent, property tax, maintenance and repairs, insurance, utilities, telephone service, and other expenses that may apply to your location.

Next, describe how your geriatric care management product is created and delivered. Your product is created by your expertise as a GCM. Refer to your résumé or those of your GCM staff included in the value proposition for information on expertise and experience. Refer to your sell sheets, presentation folders, brochures, intake folders, case files, and all hard-copy descriptions of your products to describe how these products will be delivered. Describe which staff member will take these marketing tools out to your target market representatives (physicians, elder-law attorneys, discharge planners, etc.).

Who actually delivers your geriatric care management services? Your staff of GCMs or perhaps just yourself in the beginning? Create a flowchart that shows all steps of delivery from the time a customer calls to inquire about your geriatric care management products and services, through intake, and onto delivery of your products and services (e.g., employee Miss Help monitors 85-year-old Mr. Bottomly weekly as part of the Care Management Plus product package).

You might refer to quality control of your product—do you have customer satisfaction letters or surveys that are sent out on a regular basis or after a customer closes the case? If not, develop one.

Describe when the office will be open and when GCMs will be on call. Describe a typical day in your GCM office. Include a blueprint for the upcoming days, weeks, and months of geriatric care management operations, defining how and when the entrepreneurs will carry out the tasks necessary to run the business and serve the clients. Give a clear picture of how many people are needed to run the business. The section should also describe the following:

- All equipment and supplies to be used in running the business (e.g., software, hardware, a printer, a telephone, a pager, a cell phone, a BlackBerry device, PDA)
- The business's recordkeeping system and how much it will cost to operate (i.e., how client information will be tracked and whether it will be stored in case files, computerized records, on the Web or in another storage system)
- The business's accounting and billing system (is it manual? computerized? outsourced?), and how much it will cost to operate
- How stock is divided in the business agreements and the business succession in case of the loss of key personnel
- Which professionals the business will need to use (e.g., an attorney, an accountant, a cleaning person)

The Management Team

In this section, describe who the key players are in your geriatric care management business, both existing and new. The professional experience of the owner and key employees must be described. Each person's daily role in the business is explained. The business's organizational structure (i.e., sole proprietorship, partnership, or corporation) is also noted.

The next step is to describe the key players in your business. Is it just you or you and a business partner? Describe who is on this team and how they are uniquely qualified to make this business happen. Include a résumé of all people on the management team that shows the background that makes them qualified to run this business. For example, you may have 15 years of experience working with seniors and your partner is a certified public accountant with 15 years of small business experience.

Building a Financial Model

In building a financial model, start with the first year and project out 2 to 5 years. Estimate your annual revenue, and then calculate your gross margin potential (i.e., the selling price of your geriatric care management products. For example, Care Management Plus will be sold to the customer for $100 an hour, and cost of goods sold will be $25.00 an hour to staff plus employment taxes plus overhead expenses). Calculate your margin. You must make a profit and sometimes that means raising fees. Include how much money is needed to fund the venture and a history of the owner's finances. Also, mention people who will offer audits of the business's success or failure, such as an accountant. The financial planning template (Exhibit 12–5) provides a good place to start the planning process.

Sometimes it is helpful to get expert advice on these financial matters. The SBA has small business development centers all over the United States to help small businesses get started. Local chambers of commerce can provide information about where local small business development centers are located. The Service Corps of Retired Executives (SCORE) can also provide assistance. There are also consultants who specialize in helping geriatric care management businesses get started. The GCM and CMSA websites may be able to direct you to these consultants.

Funding Requirements

What cash will be available to launch the business? Does that include your own money? How much will be needed over the next 18 months? Are there already identified sources of funding? These are the first questions a lender will ask. If you are looking for investors, how much of the company are you willing to sell and at what price? Again, consult your local SBA center or SCORE counselors for help in this area. Don't begin your business without this critical financial advice.

■ FINANCING A GERIATRIC CARE MANAGEMENT BUSINESS

According to the SBA, 80% of new entrepreneurs start their businesses without any commercial loan or debt financing.[9] Banks are usually hesitant to make loans under $50,000 because the loan is not cost-effective for the bank.

Because small businesses often need less than $50,000 and frequently have difficulty finding banks to lend them money, they look for other financing. Serious lenders and investors want to finance new businesses with a track record and an excellent business plan. New business owners with some background in geriatric care management, social work, or nursing will probably have an easier time satisfying lenders and investors.

The SBA lists the following sources of financing that new care management practices often use:

Exhibit 12–5
Financial Planning Template

Revenue

	Jan	Feb	Mar	Apr	May	Jun	Jul	Aug	Sep	Oct	Nov	Dec	Annual Total
Number Clients Beginning of Month													
Clients Gained This Month													
Clients Discontinuing Services This Month													
Number Clients End of Month													
Average Revenue per Client per Month													
Reimbursable Client Purchase													

Expenses

	Jan	Feb	Mar	Apr	May	Jun	Jul	Aug	Sep	Oct	Nov	Dec	Annual Total
Salaries													
Advertising													
Office Supplies													
Computer Equipment													
Rent													
Utilities													
Purchases Made for Clients (reimbursable)													
Employee Expenses (mileage, etc.)													
Other:													
Other:													
Total Expenses													
Income													

This template is also available in Excel spreadsheet format on the catalog page for this book: http://www.jblearning.com/catalog/9780763790264.

- Personal savings
- Personal credit (including credit cards and personal lines of credit)
- Loans from friends and family members
- Loans from informal investors
- Home equity loans (especially in areas where home values have risen considerably)
- Financing from credit unions (which tend to be more open to lending to alternative or new borrowers)
- Financing through city and county economic or community development programs
- Bank loans or lines of credit
- Angel investors or venture capital
- Donors, such as nonprofit organizations

The SBA itself is another source to consider. It has loan programs of its own and lists of local economic development offices that may have loan programs for start-ups that respond to local economic development needs. Some of these programs offer loans and provide information and technical assistance for starting a business.[8]

Getting Funded

Now that you have written your business plan, you need to use it to get funded. Before you submit it to any bank, angel, or informal investor, you need to take several more steps. Prepare all the marketing material for your business opportunity. Write a letter of introduction, write an executive summary (limited to two pages in length), and create a presentation about your geriatric care management business opportunity (use Microsoft Office PowerPoint or another electronic slideshow application).

Then, identify prospective funders, make initial contact through personal referral if possible, and make an initial deal presentation using your business plan and all your marketing materials. If the investor is interested, secure a term sheet or loan agreement, which will form the initial framework for the transaction, and is usually prepared by the legal team. This document includes purchasing terms if agreed on and outlines how many shares you are selling and at what price, if this is your plan. You will then go through the long and sometimes painful process of due diligence and negotiate a final agreement. The last step is when you accept the check to begin your geriatric care management business. Do not go through these last steps without an attorney and accountant on board and make certain to use the help of your local SBA, SCORE, or other advisory source.

It's important that you understand the criteria that investors use to evaluate a prospective investment, as few GCM businesses meet these criteria. Investors typically look for rapid growth opportunities as well as leverage where revenue can grow without a significant increase in staff. For instance, a software technology company can (at least theoretically) increase sales of software without significantly increasing costs. A GCM firm, on the other hand, relies entirely on employees and owners to generate revenue. An additional hour of services requires paying an additional payroll hour. In all likelihood, you will be working on financing via personally secured loans as described above. The good news is that many GCMs have taken this route successfully.

■ PROFESSIONAL CONSULTANTS

Professional consultants are an important asset in setting up a geriatric care management business. Consultants help businesses grow revenue, avoid costly mistakes, and make better choices. Just as an attorney can help a new business avoid lawsuits and an accountant can help the business owner develop figures to help get funding from the bank, a geriatric care management business consultant can help a business owner come up with excellent geriatric care management services and products to make the business really grow. Similarly an IT consultant can guide you through technology choices to avoid purchasing the wrong expensive software and hardware. This section discusses the role of different professional consultants in helping establish a new geriatric care management business.

Attorneys

A new geriatric care management business needs an attorney, and not just any attorney. The attorney should have considerable experience in working with small businesses. The attorney can help set up the legal business entity, help the business decide how to register or get licensed, help the business meet Internal Revenue Service (IRS) requirements (e.g., whether the business needs an employer identification number), offer advice on whether the business should employ staff or independent contractors, and help the business obtain a fictitious business name. Attorneys can help you along the way to getting funded by making sure your business opportunity meets all legal requirements and reviewing any deal you are offered. An attorney is essential to managing and reviewing legal problems that may come up and monitoring the growth of your company.

Accountants

The business needs an accountant, possibly one that is a CPA. The accountant helps with setting up the business plan by assisting with the financial arrangements. Owners need help determining the funding requirements of the new business, including how much cash is needed to open the business, the terms under which the business will obtain the money, and the type of money desired (loans, personal savings, etc.). Business owners also need to decide with accountants what type of accounting system to use.[9] An accountant can also offer advice on what types of business records to keep, including a cash receipts journal, a cash disbursement journal, a sales journal, a purchase journal, a payroll journal, and a general ledger.

GCM business owners often find that accounting and handling money is not their skill set. There are many accounting software packages out there that can help you. Choosing the right accounting software should be something that your accountant can help you with. According to Lisa Moody, a care management software developer, the accounting software used by most business is QuickBooks Pro, which will track all billing payments, expenses payment to vendors. It also has a payroll module and can do a profit-and-loss statement. Unless the geriatric care management business owner is an accountant, has a degree in business, or has owned businesses before, getting help from a professional accountant is important. The purchase of accounting software is also critical to running a GCM business profitably.[14]

Consultants in the Geriatric Care Management Field

Most new geriatric care management businesses can benefit from assistance from a specialist in the industry. A professional consultant can help a business owner gain a thorough understanding of geriatric care management, which can help the business owner develop services or products to sell to future clients. The consultant can help with the business plan and be on call in case a crisis occurs. An operations manual, training manual, opening timeline, and feasibility study to find out if you should open a GCM business in your area can all be done by a GCM business consultant. Contact the National Association of Professional Geriatric Care Managers or CMSA for referrals to these consultants.

IT (Information Technologies) Consultant

Along with an attorney, accountant, banker and GCM business consultant, you will need an IT consultant. The framework of your GCM business is not only your skill as a GCM but the flow of information about geriatric care management, information about services, your clients, and random information in general. All this information must flow through hardware, software, and phones, including all the applications on them and be networked in a way that your GCM employees can use that information to help your clients. You may be a GCM expert but unless you are a technology expert, you need an IT or information technology consultant.

The IT consultant will advise you on the most efficient way to use the current technology and help you or your GCM business consultant create a plan for growth in your GCM company.[14] The IT consultant can also help you choose the correct type of computer for you and your staff (such as a Mac or PC) the right type of hardware (laptop or desktop), the right networking tools, and the best software to use in your business. It is also critical that your IT consultant help you integrate all your technology so that your GCMs can easily use them and can capture time and billing in the most effective and user-friendly way. You want the interface, from time capture to invoicing, to be easy and seamless so you can financially support your GCM business and yourself. Other hardware choices such as scanner setups, printers, answering machines, backup drives, and handheld computers can be selected with the help of an IT consultant.

Bankers

Bank representatives can help new geriatric care management businesses as well. Even though banks do not operate the way they used to, with one-on-one relationships between bank representatives and customers, some banks (especially small-town banks and credit unions) do have representatives that handle small business loans and can work with the business on an ongoing basis. Ted Turner, now famous for developing CNN, has many secrets to his success, including incredible energy, an ability to fail and pick himself

back up, and unbelievable vision. He also had an uncanny ability to work with bankers and borrow money. Owners who find a bank to loan them money should also try to develop a long-term relationship with a representative at that bank, for assistance with both future lines of credit and direct deposit for employees and payroll. Credit unions are sometimes a good choice and more open to a new industry such as geriatric care management. The financial meltdown of 2009 made bank loans difficult to negotiate. Checking with the SBA and SCORE or your local chamber of commerce on the present status of general funding availability in your community is a good idea.

Insurance Brokers

Insurance brokers also provide new geriatric care management businesses with an important service. See the section titled "Business Insurance" later in this chapter for more information on the contribution of these professionals.

Free Advice

Other sources of advice and assistance are free. One is the IRS. It offers new business owners many free materials and workshops, including information about record keeping, tax reporting, and hiring employees and independent contractors. (Business owners should, of course, also work with their attorneys and accountants in determining their tax reporting requirements.)

Another source is the local chamber of commerce, an excellent resource for information on what help is available to new businesses in a particular area. Chambers of commerce can point the way to local small business development centers. In addition to helping businesses get started, chambers of commerce can help businesses grow. Many case management services across the country, like other small businesses, have joined the chamber of commerce to develop relationships to further their business. Some chambers have newsletters that announce new businesses, and chambers usually have mixers where businesspeople can meet each other, talk, offer support to each other, and exchange business cards. Owners might ask local chambers if it would be possible to celebrate the opening of their businesses at one of these mixers.

■ PROFESSIONAL ASSOCIATIONS

Professional associations are another helpful resource. The National Association of Professional Geriatric Care Managers and CMSA, as stated previously, have a wealth of resources to help geriatric care management businesses get going. New business owners must seriously consider joining one or both industry-specific organizations and purchasing their start-up materials. These associations also put new business owners in contact with (1) more experienced professionals who can either act as mentors or simply offer advice about setting up a business and avoiding pitfalls, (2) other new business owners with whom you can form an informal support group, and (3) products to help you start and run your geriatric care management business.

These associations also have regional and local chapters that offer start-up information and information about ongoing areas of interest in the field (e.g., Alzheimer's). Owners should also consider attending the regional and national conferences of the National Association of Professional Geriatric Care Managers and CMSA. These events usually include pre-sessions that occur before a conference and are more intensive, covering issues that owners of fledgling geriatric care management businesses need to understand. CDs of presessions and regular sessions are also available, as are CDs that cover start-up business issues.

The National Association of Professional GCMs offers a Care Manager's Resource section on its website that can help you research other professional associations that might be

Exhibit 12–6 Professional Consultants and Groups to Help a Geriatric Care Management Business Get Started

- Individuals
- Accountants
- Attorneys
- Bankers
- Chambers of commerce
- Consultants specializing in geriatric care management
- Groups and agencies
- Insurance brokers
- IRS
- Professional associations
- SCORE

helpful to your practice. Exhibit 12–6 summarizes this section and lists the individuals as well as groups and agencies that can help a new geriatric care management business get off the ground.

■ DEVELOPING PROCEDURES AND FORMS

Any geriatric care management business needs procedures to run smoothly, efficiently, and legally. New business owners need to have many procedures in place, including how to do a geriatric assessment; how to open, manage, and close cases; how to store records; how to open and close the office; and how to set up and maintain a filing system. The business owner must write out how each procedure will be done. For instance, if the owner is unable to run the business for some time, someone else will need to take over, and unless procedures are written out, inconsistency and other trouble will result. (See Chapter 19 on preparing for emergencies.)

The National Association of Professional Geriatric Care Managers publishes procedure manuals (*GCM Policies and Procedures*) that can help new business owners get started. These general procedures need to be tailored to each business. A GCM business consultant can provide assistance to develop an operations manual, which is key to setting up a GCM business. This operations manual should contain an overview of each of your GCM services or products. It should describe how you operate your business; a case records section, which is how your office staff will open, maintain and close and store GCM cases; how you will manage miscellaneous records such as employment and training records; and how you will manage your office. It should also contain step-by-step descriptions of how your professional GCM staff will deliver direct GCM client activity (e.g., geriatric assessment, intake, care monitoring), how your GCM staff will take an inquiry, do an intake, set up, manage, and close a case using all the forms you have chosen. It should cover exactly how and who will be on call 24 hours a day using what kind of technology. It must cover how your professional and office staff interface to deliver your GCM products. The expense of using a consultant is worth it in the end because a successful business does not operate by trial and error but with a thoroughly considered, step-by-step operations plan.

A local chamber of commerce or GCM chapter can provide names of consultants who can help. A comprehensive GCM Forms Book and CD is available in the GCM store on the GCM website. You can take these forms and tailor them to your own agency and also adapt some forms suggested in this book for assessment tools. You can also take a course on starting a GCM business through the University of Florida Master's Program online.

■ BUSINESS INSURANCE

Business insurance is taken out to protect people from professional, business, and personal liabilities or risks created by a private practice. Both start-ups and mature geriatric care management practices need business insurance. It protects assets, prevents loss of income, covers expenses in case of illness, provides coverage for errors and omissions, and meets requirements for third-party reimbursement. As in legal and accounting matters, it is best to hire the services of an insurance broker to provide advice about what type of insurance coverage a business needs and to help the business with claims. Because geriatric care management is a new field, business owners should make sure to talk to an insurance broker who understands the needs of businesses in this field.

Beginning geriatric care management businesses need the following types of insurance:

- **Professional malpractice insurance:** This insurance protects a business and its employees for any (subject to the policy conditions) act, error, or omission that arises out of the performance of professional services to others. Policies may also be extended to cover independent contractors.

- **Business liability insurance:** This insurance covers bodily injury, property damage, product liability, and job completion in the general operation of a business. Personal endeavors are excluded. A business can also decide to insure the building in which it operates as well as improvements or personal property for either replacement value or actual cost. Other options include coverage for loss of business earnings, accounts receivable, and valuable papers and records.

- **Workers' compensation insurance:** This insurance offers disability coverage for work-related illness or disability for employees. All business employees must be covered under a workers' compensation policy.

- **Business overhead insurance:** This insurance, also known as disability insurance, is designed to cover loss of income caused by the disability of a principal in a business. It is based on the monthly expenses of the business, not its earnings.

- **Social Security Disability Insurance and other disability insurance:** Social Security Disability Insurance is paid through payroll taxes and provides a minimal income after a period of 6 months of disability if the disability is expected to last 1 year or more. In various states, short-term disability insurance is available. Long-term disability provides monthly benefits after the 26-week, short-term disability benefits are used up.[5]

◼ SETTING UP AN OFFICE

A geriatric care management business needs an office. Many GCMs start practicing out of their homes. In this era of telecommuting, running a home office may be even more attractive if space is available. Using a home office eliminates the expense of renting office space but may be too distracting. Crying babies, complaining children, and laundry that just has to be done can get in the way of running a GCM business out of your home.

Whatever the choice of office location, it is helpful to make a timeline listing all tasks that need to be completed before the business can open: renting office space or refurbishing a home office; buying office equipment; getting insurance; recruiting and hiring staff; ordering a system to handle telephone calls, voicemail, e-mails, texts, and paging; arranging for a security system and cleaning people; arranging for an answering service or setting up an on-call system; buying office equipment; making arrangements with suppliers of items such as office supplies; arranging for credit cards; ordering brochures; and so forth. The new business owner should estimate how long each task will take, put each task on a timeline, and give him- or herself a deadline of opening day. Exhibit 12–7 shows a sample timeline.

If there is no space for a home office or working at home seems too distracting, entrepreneurs need to contact a realtor and look for a small space to rent. They might want to consider renting 400 to 600 square feet with a small reception area, so clients are not walking

Exhibit 12–7   Sample Timeline of Startup Tasks

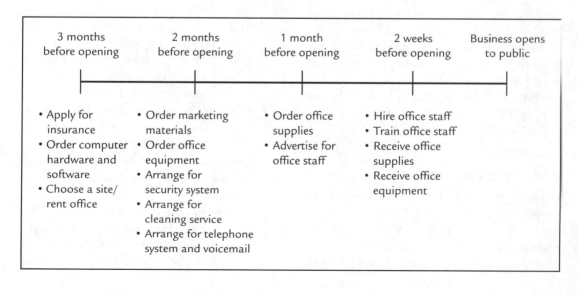

3 months before opening	2 months before opening	1 month before opening	2 weeks before opening	Business opens to public
• Apply for insurance • Order computer hardware and software • Choose a site/ rent office	• Order marketing materials • Order office equipment • Arrange for security system • Arrange for cleaning service • Arrange for telephone system and voicemail	• Order office supplies • Advertise for office staff	• Hire office staff • Train office staff • Receive office supplies • Receive office equipment	

right in on conversations with other clients. The realtor and an attorney can offer advice about how long of a lease to take and what terms the lease should have.

Offices should be as professional as possible. Having administrative assistants and other staff members helps. An administrative assistant answering the phone is much more professional than using an answering machine. An administrative assistant can also help process paperwork in a professional and timely manner. Good staff can actually help a business make more money. When an owner does everything alone (e.g., answering the phone, e-mailing, seeing clients, doing the billing, bookkeeping, responding to emergencies), a business may not make as much money as it would if some tasks were handled by others. The business makes money off billed GCM time, and if a GCM spends a lot of time away from clients, less time is being billed.

Also, doing everything alone can send a GCM into a cycle in which too many care managers find themselves—people with human services backgrounds are so accustomed to emergencies that they become "adrenaline junkies." However, when a business involves dealing with clients' emergencies, the business itself should not have daily emergencies of its own. An owner who does everything alone may eventually find him- or herself in this cycle.

Setting Up Technology for Your GCM Office

Your GCM Website

Your GCM website is among your best form of advertising. To set up and maintain a website, you will have to purchase a domain name. This is a web address for the website you or your IT person will create. An example of a domain name is the NAPGCM website of www.caremanager.org. You can acquire a domain name through a domain registrar. Examples are www.godaddy.com, www.netsol.com, and www.registar.com. Once you obtain your domain name, it will be your business property as long as you pay the annual renewal fee. The amount of money you pay for the domain name should be low in the beginning but increase over the years you own it. Coming up with a domain name that fits with the name of your GCM business takes creativity. Your domain name should be easy for your clients to remember. A website designer or IT consultant can help you here.[14]

Business Website and E-Mail

Once you have purchased your GCM domain name for your GCM business you need to arrange for a website hosting account and at least one e-mail account. Your domain registrar will also sell you website packages that include e-mail accounts. It is especially important that your GCM website's contact page have clear information on how to access your services. If older clients, aging families, third parties, or any new customer cannot easily access you through your website's contact page they will go to another GCM. You want your web designer to create a contact page that tells customers how to reach you easily.[14]

Business Equipment

Today, all GCM practices are technologically driven. Even if you chose not to use technology to its fullest, information will come at you in the form of e-mails, electronic medical records and text messages. When you set up your GCM office, you need to consider this information, how you will manage it, and how you will pass it on to others, such as clients, your staff, third parties, and client families. Setting up your GCM office means being smart about planning so that you save money over time. You are a start-up business, so being thrifty is important. You are a business person, so watching your bottom line is critical to your new business success. Your IT consultant can help you with highly effective yet money-saving hardware and software options. Your GCM business consultant can create an operational plan describing step by step how your office and professional staff will manage the care you are selling. They will assist you in making sure the technology you purchase, whether it be phones, computers or PDAs, is integrated so you and your GCM staff can work efficiently, easily, and effectively. This will allow you to give your paying clients the care you say you deliver as a geriatric care manager.

The GCM business you are creating makes money through billing customers. To generate bills and make money, you need to make sure the information flow from GCM home visits, phone calls, e-mails, and whatever you as a GCM bill for moves easily to billing. This allows you to invoice your customers quickly and accurately. This process needs to be fast and seamless so you can get paid and support yourself and your practice.

To set up a smart GCM office, you need to start by purchasing a good computer system and a backup system. This may include one computer or multiple computers. You may want to consider a laptop or a netbook for easier portability. In addition, you will need Internet access and most importantly, a reliable backup system for data storage. Your IT consultant can help you with these decisions. Other office equipment needs to be cost-effective too. You want to buy office tools that save you money and are HIPAA compliant. This may mean instead of a large copier, you would consider purchasing a small copier and a cost-effective multisheet scanner that will process photos and documents. Lisa Moody of Jewel Code suggests the Neat Scanner for the small GCM office and the Snap Scanner for the medium-sized office. For larger offices, GCM Heather Frenette of Arizona Care Management suggests a copier with a built-in scanner and electronic fax capability. Most of the large copier companies offer these systems. There are several options for receiving electronic faxes, so before investing in a fax machine, consult an IT professional.

You will also want a method for carrying your calendar and contacts with you. A PDA, iTouch, iPad, or other smartphone allows you to have an electronic calendar and contact book, access to the Internet, and the ability to receive e-mails. Most smart phones have a built-in camera as well. Your IT consultant or GCM business consultant can help you make informed choices about brands and the type and number of devices to purchase.

To set up a cost-effective, highly efficient office, GCM Heather Frenette, RN, MSN, CMC, suggested in her presentation, entitled "Technology and the (Almost) Paperless Office," that you create an office that is as paperless as possible. The advantages of creating a paperless office are many. By having less paper to store in your office filing system, you have more room and can actually rent less space. Having information accessible electronically allows you to access it from anywhere you have an Internet connection. This eliminates the need for paper forms with client information and protects you and your client from identity theft. Your IT consultant can help you secure your electronic data so it is protected from hackers while making it easily accessible for you and your staff. This not only reduces your chances of identity theft but also your chances of being sued. Storing your GCM information electronically also makes it accessible to multiple GCM staff both in the office and in the field. Another benefit is that you can quickly forward information, such as medical records, to family, other providers, or a facility via electronic fax or an e-mail. From a business point of view, the electronic office saves money because you have less cost in paper, postage, office supplies (e.g., file cabinets and file folders) and less rent for storage. Keep in mind, most of your records need to be saved for several years. These records can quickly add up to a large amount of space.

To create a paperless office, you need a good computer system with the ability to create a hierarchal electronic filing system with file folders, similar to the paper folders you may be currently using. To access the files remotely, you will need an Internet connection. Creating the paperless office will also require a scanner so you can turn your paper documents into electronic documents. Frenette suggests you start with one type of document, such as medical records, and work the bugs out of your system before starting with the next group. You will still need some file folders for original documents such as marriage certificates, birth and death certificates, VA paperwork, certified court orders, and original estate plan documents. This should be decided with your GCM consultant or your attorney and added to your operations manual. You can also set up levels of security for your staff so that people can only access files related to their job responsibility. Your IT consultant can help you do this. Finally, you need to decide what to do with documents after you scan them. This includes filing documents, shredding documents, or just throwing them away. Once you have devised a system for your office, it should be documented in your operations manual.

■ HIRING GOOD STAFF MEMBERS

Hiring staff members is an art. Well done, this art can help a business considerably. Poorly done, this art can lead to trouble, making the owner a care manager to staff as well as to clients.

Before advertising for employees, an owner should write job descriptions. A sample job description appears in Exhibit 12-8. The description should list the qualifications applicants should have and the responsibilities and tasks of the position. A human resources consultant can offer assistance in writing job descriptions. Sample GCM job descriptions are also available through the national association's website, in the GCM *Policies and Procedures Manual*.

Advertising for staff should occur at least 3 to 4 months before opening your office. You can use newspapers, but much advertising has moved to the Web and is more effective if placed there. If you do advertise in a local paper, an ad should run for at least a full week. It takes another week or two to interview staff. It then may take 2 weeks or a month until someone is on board as a new employee because he or she may have to give notice somewhere else. GCM staff can be advertised through Craig's List and Angie's List (see the list of websites at the end of the chapter). An ad can also be placed on an e-mail list that serves a professional association, such as CMSA or a gerontology or university e-mail list. For example, UC Berkeley's e-mail list advertises jobs, including GCM jobs in the entire state of California. Miseracordia University advertises GCM jobs because it has a GCM program. You then need to train your staff, which can take up to a month. Again, using the services of a human resources consultant can help you tailor your advertising timeline to your agency's needs. GCMs who belong to the National Association of Professional Geriatric Care Managers can now advertise for staff on some regional websites. There also may be gerontology or employment websites in your area on which you can advertise for staff.

A business owner might want to put together a professional policy manual, which includes policies and procedures regarding paydays, vacation, and time off as well as all policies required by the US Department of Labor (e.g., sexual harassment, nondiscrimination). Sample policy manuals are available in bookstores and through the SBA. Again, a GCM business consultant can help here or a business consultant that specializes in policy manuals.

Employers should take care that they are meeting the legal standards for employment. An attorney can help the owner draw up legal contracts to sign with employees. The employer–employee relationship should begin on solid ground, which means making everything clear in a contract.

Exhibit 12–8   Sample Job Description

ADMINISTRATIVE ASSISTANT

QUALIFICATIONS:

Minimum	**Desired**
Excellent Communication Skills	AA in business
Administrative Skills	Case management experience
Organizational Skills	Home health care experience
Typing/filing Skills	Desktop publishing skills
Computer experience/knowledge	
Dependable	
Self-starter	

SUMMARY STATEMENT:

The Administrative Assistant is responsible for general operations of office procedures:

Answers telephones

Opens mail

Prepares and distributes all monthly charting

Prepares and maintains client data books

Prepares and maintains all client charting books

Prepares and maintains all case site charting books

Prepares and maintains blank charting files

Prepares and maintains completed charting files

Opens and closes all new intake files

Opens and closes all CMP, PP, CA, and GA cases

Takes minutes at staff meetings

Inputs, copies, and mails all monthly reports

Retrieves messages from answering service twice daily

On-call every third weekend

Creates emergency list

Maintains filing system

Creates and edits Care Staff Newsletter and quarterly marketing Newsletter

■ FINANCIAL PLANNING, CASH FLOW ANALYSIS, AND BILLING

Financial Modeling

With your market and competitive analysis complete, you are now ready to start the financial planning process for your care management practice. The goal is to understand the following: (1) forecast profit or loss over the first 3 to 5 years; (2) plan for three scenarios (i.e., best case, average performance and worst case) to help you envision the different paths your expansion can take; and (3) manage your cash flow, which is distinct from your profit or loss. In fact, more companies fail due to cash flow constraints than from any other single factor. With this analysis complete, you'll understand the investment required to establish your business as well as the potential rewards and risks through the initial years of operation.

Financial Model

The financial plan will be your primary decision-making tool. This section will help you build a financial model to include revenue, expenses and cash flow management. Once completed, the model will show you the 3-year projected profit (or loss), the amount of investment required to get the business off the ground, and the cash flow produced (or consumed) by the company. The template in this section (see Exhibit 12–5) provides a simplified view of this financial model; the text will refer to this template for you to complete.

Revenue

Care management revenue will depend on a number of factors: (1) the number of new clients acquired; (2) retention of existing clients; (3) average fees per client; (4) hourly rates; and (5) whether you charge for travel or not. For simplicity's sake, the financial planning template (Exhibit 12–5) asks you to fill in the average fees per client per month. If your hourly fees are $100 per hour and the average client requires 7 hours of services per month, the average revenue per client would be $700 per month. For a more sophisticated financial model, you may want to consider three or more tiers of clients, the number of hours of service per month, and the acquisition rate per tier per month (i.e., the number of new clients for each tier per month). As discussed earlier, the rate you use may depend on your research of competitive rates in the market. Next, you will want to project the number of clients gained each month—the number of clients who have contractually engaged services that are starting in a given month. These are clients who are actively receiving services in a given month, not prospective new clients in the sales and marketing pipeline. Your new client acquisition rate will depend on a number of factors including your current contact database, relationships with key referral sources, marketing programs to inform and educate potential referral sources, and so on. You will also want to consider the number of clients discontinuing services. If you anticipate that the average client will require services from you for 9 months, the "Clients Discontinuing Services This Month" in September of year 1 would equal the number of new clients in January of year 1. This number is critical to your revenue planning, as you will need to acquire more new clients the shorter your average client retention.

Scenario Planning

We recommend you create three scenarios of your financial plan: best case, moderate case, and worst case. The assumptions you use may vary across each scenario; for example, for the worst case, you may want to use an hourly rate lower than the other two cases. This would address the situation where you adjust your hourly rate lower in response to market response. You may also want to use a number of clients gained this month for your worst case that is lower than best or moderate cases;

this could occur when your marketing and lead development take longer to yield new clients than you plan. Similarly, on the expenses side, you will want to adjust your expectations for the worst case scenario; perhaps marketing costs will be higher than anticipated, for example. Your goal is to create a worst case scenario that represents the most conservative outlook where you are confident the revenue and expenses could not be any less favorable. You'll use this scenario to ensure your financial viability in the event that the expansion doesn't materialize as you plan.

Expenses

Your goal is to capture the monthly expenses associated with your care management practice. You will need to determine the pay structure for the care manager and also consider whether the care manager is paid hourly or salaried. Generally, care managers are paid an hourly rate for time worked. Paying care managers on a salary can offer long term advantages to the organization and care manager and also requires a significantly higher initial cash investment and also stretches out the time to reach profitability. The care manager's hourly rate or salary will depend on your current hiring practices; if you need an indicator of salary ranges, you may want to check job postings in your market for similar roles in other organizations. We also suggest you consider two other roles in your organization: a sales and marketing function as well as an administrative assistant or office manager. You will want to estimate the number of hours required for each role on a monthly basis and then calculate the monthly expense for salaries in your financial model. If you offer benefits, you will also include these in your total salaries amount as well as your employer taxes on the salaries. Another critical consideration for your financial model will be the care manager use rate; this rate summarizes the amount of time paid to the care manager that is billable to a client. For

example, if a care manager is paid for 36 hours of work in a week of which 30 hours are billable to a client, the use rate would be 30 to 36, or 83%. The target use rate will depend on the administrative, marketing, and other requirements asked of the care manager that are nonbillable. Given that the care manager will likely have the highest hourly rate in the group, we strongly advocate that the administrative and marketing work be delegated to team members; this would allow you to establish a target use rate of 80–85%. We believe another significant expense worth including covers credit card processing fees, which will enable you to accept payment from clients via credit card. Banks and other merchant services (such as PayPal) will typically charge about 2.5% of the amount charged in processing fees. We believe these fees are merited, as you will be able to collect your fees paid via credit card on a predictable schedule and will minimize the risk of nonpayment. You will also want to consider expanding your workers compensation and liability coverage for the care manager(s) as well as the marketing expenses associated with printing materials, expanding your current website, and advertising (including purchase of search words on Google and other search engines).

Cash Flow

Cash flow refers to the timing of actual cash receipts and expenses. Cash flow does not always match your revenue from an accounting perspective, and the difference is critical to your business. For example, you may have delivered $2500 in services last month to a client who is under contract with you. You generate an invoice and record this as revenue. However, you have not yet been paid. If your payment arrives 45 days after mailing the invoice, you will already have paid your staff members for the time spent delivering those services. The biggest challenge companies face revolves around cash flow; you can't make payroll based on the unpaid invoices that you've sent to clients. The goal is to manage your cash flow as proactively as possible—to collect as quickly as possible on the revenue you've earned. To do this, you may want to consider the following:

1. Accept credit card payments (or even requiring clients pay by credit card, as some agencies do) to ensure you will be paid on time and in full each month.

2. Invoice twice monthly, and send invoices as close to the service date as possible. This typically means generating and sending invoices within 2–3 business days of the completion of service period. To do this, you will want to establish an effective means of capturing billable activities and then creating a rapid and accurate process for generating invoices.

3. Enforce the policy that you deliver services only after receiving a signed service agreement for care management services. Unlike home care, few people understand the role and services of care management, and many people believe these care management services are (or should be) free. As a result, the potential for confusion or refusal to pay is generally higher with care management than with home care.

4. Require a deposit or initial payment. Even a payment of $250 can help establish that these services are in fact paid and condition the client to the mindset that all care management activities will be billed.

Taken together, these best practices can help you ensure you optimize your cash flow management.

Billing

Billing customers is key to keeping a geriatric care management business afloat. A billing system needs to be set up and functioning well before a business opens. A good accountant can help a business set up portions of an appropriate billing system. Other pieces can be set up by your IT consultant. However, you will need to understand the overall process and flow of information. Unless you plan to remain an individual practitioner with few clients, we recommend designing a system that can grow as you expand your client base. If you do intend to limit your client base and remain a solo practitioner, an Excel spreadsheet tracking billable time may suffice. For the vast majority of care managers, however, a manual process relying on Excel will quickly become unmanageable.

Instead, we recommend you invest your time and financial resources in a system that can address the following: (1) capture of billable activities, (2) aggregation of billable information by client in an invoice format, (3) process for editing and finalizing invoices, and (4) account receivable management. Your objectives in the invoicing process are to include the appropriate amount of information (not more or not less), generate invoices quickly (within several days of service), and ensure accuracy (therefore minimal editing and rework).

Capturing Billable Activities

Financial success or failure of your care management practice will depend largely on your ability and commitment to capture all activities that are billable to a client. Whether you are attending a medical appointment with a client or answering a phone call from an older adult's family member late at night, you need to have a process for capturing both the amount of time spent as well as the actions completed. Because you will be capturing these billable activities in the field as well as in your home or office, you will need a system that can receive information via phone, PDA, e-mail, or as direct input. Three systems you may want to consider are Jewel Code, Care Manager Pro and TimeSlips. You may also want to consider a dictation service (e.g., CopyTalk) that will convert a voice message into an e-mail, which can then be copied and pasted into your billing software. Following these steps can significantly increase the capture of your billable time. If you work on billable activities 40 hours a week, you may only be able to capture 35 hours if using a manual tracking and billing process. Using the tools outlined above can help you capture all 40 hours. If you charge $100 per hour for your services, that equates to an incremental $500 in revenue a week, or more than $25,000 in incremental revenue per year.

Aggregation of Billable Activities by Client

You will also want a software solution that will aggregate all billable activities and expenses by client. Jewel Code, TimeSlips, and QuickBooks are three examples of solutions that provide this function. You will need to decide what information to provide on the invoices; some organizations provided detailed invoices that itemize each activity and associated cost (i.e., telephone call with Dr. Smith regarding medication changes; 10 minutes in length; $10.00) while other organizations simply list a single line item for all services and fees within a given month. If you choose the latter system, you will want to have the details available to provide the breakdown for clients, as you may eventually be asked to provide the makeup of a given invoice.

Successfully managing cash flow depends on the prompt distribution of invoices as close to the service date as possible. You may choose to invoice monthly or twice per month. If you invoice monthly, your goal might be to have all invoices sent to clients for prior month's services by the 15th of the following month.

Process for Editing and Finalizing Invoices

Your software system will generate an invoice for each client's billable activities and expenses (including purchases and mileage). You will need a process to review the invoices, provide edits, finalize the invoices, and distribute them to clients. Invoice review and editing can be an extremely lengthy process, particularly if you choose to issue detailed invoices. For instance, with 20 clients and an average invoice length of 3 pages, you would have 60 pages of invoices to edit. This editing time is unbillable, and easily falls to the bottom of the list of priorities. At the same time, prompt editing and distribution to clients determines your financial success and cash flow management. For this reason, we suggest you create a process that minimizes the need for editing and minimizes your time inputting the edits. By entering the information accurately at the point of origin, you'll greatly reduce the need for edits at time of invoicing. You may want to consider using sentence templates for activities where each entry follows the same structure (i.e., telephone call to inform daughter of doctor's recommendation). We suggest you find administrative support to generate drafts of the invoices, review them for accuracy, enter edits, and finalize what is sent to clients. This will help you ensure you follow a scheduled process each month. Finally, you may consider e-mailing invoices to your clients, which can help reduce paper as well as shorten the time before payment. JewelCode, TimeSlips, Care Manager Pro and QuickBooks all offer the ability to generate an invoice as a PDF, which can then be sent via e-mail.

Accounts Receivable Management

Finally, you will want a software solution for managing accounts receivable. Successful cash flow management also depends on the ease with which clients can make a payment. We suggest you encourage (if not require) clients to pay by credit card. Keeping a credit card account number on file, your clients agree to have you charge their card at a specified date for the previous month's services.

You will pay a credit card processing fee (usually 2–3% of revenue); this is money well spent and eliminates the risk of nonpayment and ensures that invoices are paid promptly.

Your software package will provide some important tools to manage your accounts receivable. The longer an invoice remains unpaid, the less likely you are to receive payment. You will therefore want to stay on top of the aging of your receivables. Your software will create a report for you showing you the amount and the age of the amount owed. We highly recommend contacting clients (or those responsible for making payment) for any invoices that have been unpaid for 30 days or more. You want to determine why the invoice hasn't been paid; in the worst case, the client is planning to discontinue services. In this case, you may decide to reduce or terminate services (while also addressing the client's well-being) so not to incur additional receivables that would likely go unpaid.

■ INTEGRATING A GERIATRIC CARE MANAGEMENT BUSINESS INTO ANOTHER PRACTICE, BUSINESS, OR AGENCY

Throughout the United States, geriatric care management practices are slowly merging with for-profit agencies and private practices, including law practices, trust departments, physician offices, accountant offices, and the practices of a myriad of other professionals who deal with the needs of older people. GCMs offer these practices one central and important skill: the ability to do geriatric assessment. GCMs assess the older client in his or her home and bring back to the trust officer, attorney, accountant, physician, or other professional helpful information about the client's health and psychosocial status as it is in the home setting. Other professionals may see the client in the home but do not assess the client's functioning based on the home environment.

Integrating with Physicians

Because older patients represent such a large segment of most physicians' practices, GCMs are naturally helpful to physicians. As the skills of the GCM are increasingly recognized as an important part of solving chronic health problems, physicians' practices may become more open to having GCMs on staff. In 1992, the John Hartford Foundation funded a 5-year initiative to come up with better approaches to caring for the frail elderly.[11] Part of the study looked at how case management became integrated into physicians' practices. In general, the study found that integrating a GCM into a physician's practice worked well. The GCM was able to work closely with the family and patients because the GCM had access to the patient that neither the staff members nor the physician had. The physician's busy office staff found it a relief to "hand off" the older patients when problems involved accessing the continuum of care in the community or dealing with complex family problems. Physicians in the study found the GCMs' home visits quite helpful; GCMs could alert the staff to potential patient problems early on, before they became a crisis, so physicians treated patients in half the time, an outcome that impressed the physicians.

The study found that integrating the GCMs into the physicians' practices initially required GCMs to overcome the resistance of the office staff by making a good first impression. Whether the physician accepted the case manager depended on the physician learning and appreciating the value of case management before the GCM was really integrated into the patient's care. GCMs had to build trusting relationships with both the office staff and the physicians before they were fully accepted into the practices.

Integrating with Attorneys

Attorneys have slowly begun to integrate GCMs into their practices. Elder-law attorneys in particular stand to benefit from involving a GCM in their practice. Both elder-law attorneys and GCMs serve aging clients, have long-term relationships with their clients, and address conservatorships, medical planning, elder abuse, powers of attorney, and geriatric planning. Attorneys understand law as it applies to older people, and GCMs understand psychosocial and health issues as they apply to aging, making these professionals a good match.

GCM time is not billed at as high a rate as attorney time. GCMs often see clients before attorneys do, reducing the amount of time that clients need to spend with high-cost attorneys. Few attorneys employ GCMs at this point, but many may look into employing GCMs because of the benefits of such an arrangement, including one-stop shopping for the client.

Benefits to the elder-law attorney are many. If the attorney handles conservatorships, the GCM can assess competency. This can be helpful when the attorney may suspect that a person petitioning for conservatorship has a questionable agenda for getting the older person conserved or whether the person should be conserved or make legal decisions. Financial abuse is often involved in these cases. GCMs also have valuable knowledge of the continuum of care in the community when cases need to be referred to psychiatrists or medical social workers. GCMs can not only assess the level of confusion but help create care plans to deal with the confusion (either the primary GCM or another GCM can then take on the older person's care).[12] GCMs employed by attorneys have also been helpful in making placement suggestions in cases where the attorney serves as guardian, attorney in fact, or healthcare agent.

Advance planning for times when the client is unable to make medical or personal care decisions is another area where having a GCM on staff in an attorney's firm can be helpful. GCMs can help clients formulate the ques-

tions to which they need answers. Older clients may be confused about the various options available to them. The GCM can have a discussion about the medical planning needs of the client before the client sees the attorney, thereby helping the older client be better prepared to work with the attorney. The specific needs of the client will determine how the GCM will be of assistance in this area. For example, if the client is fully capable of making decisions and is seeking assistance for the future, the discussion will be about hypothetical situations. If the client is already in poor medical health and needs assistance, the GCM can facilitate communication between the client (or family) and the attorney about these often difficult and private matters through precounseling. This reduces the time the attorney needs to spend with the client and raises the quality of medical planning. In a similar way, GCMs can help clients sort through personal feelings about will making and power-of-attorney appointment.

Caregiver education is another general area where the GCM can really benefit an elder-law practice. A GCM on staff can help to educate families, older people, and third parties about Medicare. Medicare benefits are little understood and, unfortunately, the majority of older people and their families still believe that Medicare will cover long-term care. Having a GCM educate clients about what Medicare will and will not cover is helpful to a law firm because the GCM's time, again, can be billed out less expensively. With a GCM, clients and their family members quickly come to understand Medicare's limitations and benefits and can do better long-term-care planning, saving themselves money and making smart choices. GCMs can also educate clients and their families about managed care. As more and more older people are going into managed care plans, this education can be helpful.

Some law firms have used GCMs as part of the general legal team helping an older client. GCMs can do telephone checks on older clients, make home visits, go with older clients to physician appointments, consult with physicians and other healthcare consultants about clients, consult with staff and caregivers in a client's facility, or serve as a liaison between the client and family and friends. All these standard geriatric care management tasks enhance the legal firm's services.

Integrating with Accountants

Accountants and GCMs have begun to work together in both formal and informal relationships. Accountants and GCMs both deal with older people, have clients who are in the upper income brackets, have long relationships with clients, have a strong ethical code, and can work with other professionals to meet their clients' goals. Unless accountants specialize in elder-care services, they do not always have extensive knowledge about entitlements such as Medicare and Social Security and can benefit from a GCM's understanding of these entitlements. Accountants understand taxes, long-range financial planning, and resolution of financial problems, while GCMs understand psychosocial issues and the continuum of care, especially in managed care systems. All in all, the professions are complementary.

Because long-term care is so costly and considerable financial planning must be done to make it affordable, accountants are a wonderful resource to older people facing long-term-care planning and decision making. Because long-term-care planning hinges on the client's ability to pay for his or her care or have it covered by insurance or third-party payment, accountants and GCMs can complement each other by helping the older client come up with options for long-term care based on the client's finances and the care options available in his or her community. This pairing will benefit the accounting firm and the accounting firm's clients, who will be able to do one-stop shopping.

The accountant and the GCM need to be able to work together, have open lines of communication, and have mutual trust and confidentiality, according to Rona Bartlestone and George Lewis, who have presented workshops on this type of collaboration.[13] The American Institute of Certified Public Accountants (AICPA) has encouraged accountants to move into the elder-care field. AICPA has established an ongoing task force to communicate with AICPA members about elder care. It offers five 8-hour courses on elder care (available in self-study or group-study formats) for accountants and is working on creating more. In addition, AICPA has published a guide called *Eldercare: A Practitioner's Resource Guide.* Another guide, *Guide to ElderCare Engagements,* is published by Practitioners Publishing Company. The AICPA also has an elder-care marketing kit for accountants. AICPA suggests that accountants create relationships with GCMs as well as other specialists such as elder-law attorneys. The accountants can then refer clients to the GCMs and the clients can hire the GCMs independently.

Like physicians and attorneys, few accountants have GCMs on staff. However, accountants are interested in expanding the relationship between the professions and have reached out to the National Association of Professional Geriatric Care Managers to speak at its conferences and begin collaborating.

GCMs and Trust Departments

Mellon, a well-respected financial services firm, discovered the advantages of having an expert on aging working with them and their clients. GCM Catherine C. Thompson worked in the Mellon Bank trust department for 21 years. Catherine served as the Social Service Consultant and Professional Geriatric Care Manager for Private Wealth Management of Mellon Financial Services. Ms. Thompson was responsible for each incapacitated person with a guardian account in conjunction with the trust officer for each account. She also worked with any trust clients referred by the trust officer. In addition, her expertise was solicited by the trust officers to handle unusual circumstances where the skills of a care manager are essential.

The use of a care manager by the bank is considered a good business decision. It embodies the bank's commitment to quality service to the community. It also saves time and money for the bank to have a person skilled and knowledgeable in the psychosocial area handle health- and care-related situations, leaving the trust officer to deal with the financial areas. Mellon found that caring for the personal needs of trust customers as well as financial needs is much appreciated by trust customers and their families. Providing that extra personal attention helps to keep the clients happy and increases business. The GCM is able to provide a care plan to the trust officer who is dealing with a client with incapacity or other issues. The care manager assists in providing an accurate diagnosis of a client's problems and recommends a course of care for the current and future needs of the client. Even experienced trust officers do not have the training and experience necessary to deal with the medical, psychological, and social issues when planning for the clients.

The costs of long-term care and the effect that longevity will have on clients have big impacts on clients' financial situations. Many people are now living into their 90s. The trust officer and the care manager together can consider the impact of the possibility of increased longevity on individual clients with particular types of healthcare issues and particular financial situations. The care manager can manage chronic illness and even save money for clients by protecting their health and well-being. Working within a trust department or as an outside consultant, the care manager and the financial officer can form an alliance that benefits the trust officer, the client, and the care manager.

GCMs and Corporate Models

In the past decade, two national corporate geriatric care management models, Senior Bridge LivHOME and ResCare, have emerged. These models have grown throughout the United States by acquiring smaller GCM businesses and integrating them into the larger corporate model. They are both geriatric care managed, home care models, employing care providers. The future may bring more corporate players into the geriatric care management industry.

GCMs Specializing in One Area

Geriatric care managers have also evolved into specialized geriatric care management practices in the past 5 years. GCM Peter Belson runs a nonprofit care management agency that provides care management to adult and adolescent (older than age 12) populations who have developmental, psychiatric, or traumatic brain injury-related disabilities (or combinations thereof). They offer geriatric care management for elders who have lifelong, severe, persistent mental illness, who have not been well served by other GCMs.

Many GCMs have begun primarily to serve dementia clients in their practice. Many GCMs focus their practice on elder move coordination (see Chapter 7). Some new GCM practices specialize in death and dying issues. This diversification of the geriatric care management field will probably continue in the next decade with even more specialties emerging.

■ CONCLUSION

Starting a geriatric care management business is no easy task. Many decisions must be made, many tasks must be completed, and many systems must be put in motion before the business's opening day. Once the business opens, the hard work continues.

In the future, many GCMs may find themselves no longer running their own businesses but integrated into the businesses of physicians, attorneys, accountants, managed care organizations, corporations, and other entities that can benefit from GCMs' great input.

REFERENCES

1. Knutson K, Langer S. Geriatric care managers: a survey in long-term/chronic care. *GCM J*. 1998;8:9.

2. Gross EB, Johnson LF. The development of a case management business: the changing paradigms. Presented at: The National Association of Professional Geriatric Care Managers Conference; October 22–24, 1998; Chicago, IL.

3. Kraus A. Before you leap: a start-up guide for the beginner. Part I: Do you have the soul of an entrepreneur? *GCM J*. 1993;3:2–10.

4. Brostoff P, Stewart H. Basic components of private geriatric care management, Part II. Presented at: The National Association of Professional Geriatric Care Managers; October 14–17, 1992; Tucson, AZ.

5. Dolen L, Rubin E, Charnow J, Cress M. The business of becoming a private geriatric care manager. Presented at: The National Association of Professional Geriatric Care Managers; October 17–19, 1992; Tucson, AZ.

6. Marks W. Partnerships: the good, the bad, and the ugly. Why do they succeed or fail? *GCM J*. 1996;6:6–9.

7. Burstiner I. *The small business handbook: A comprehensive guide to starting and running your own business*. New York: Prentice Hall; 1989.

8. Orsini M. Doing good makes cents: advanced business practices. Presented at: The National Association of Professional Geriatric Care Managers Conference; October 19–22, 1994; Paradise Island, Bahamas.

9. US Small Business Administration, San Francisco District. *Women's small business start-up information package*. Denver, CO: SBA Publications.

10. Thompson CC. Billing and invoicing options for geriatric care managers. *GCM J*. 1996;6:15–19.

11. Netting FE, Williams FG. Geriatric case managers: integration into physician practices. *Care Manag J*. 1999 Winter;1(1):3–9.

12. Miller AH, Karasov MA. Elder law and elder care. Presented at: The National Association of Professional Geriatric Care Managers Conference; October 21–24, 1999; San Diego, CA.

13. Bartlestone R, Lewis G. CPAs in partnership with care managers. Presented at: The National Association of Professional Geriatric Care Managers Conference; October 21–24, 1999; San Diego, CA.

14. Moody L. Managing your business with technology. *GCM J*. 2010;Spring:27, 28.

WEBSITES

- Alzheimers Association—www.alzheimers.org
- Angie's list—www.angieslist.com
- Care Manager Pro—www.healthhistory.com/cmpro
- CMSA—www.cmsa.org
- Craig's List—www.craigslist.com
- GCM store—www.caremanagers.org/storeindex. cfm
- LegalZoom—www.legalzoom.com
- LivHome—www.livhome.com
- NAPGCM—www.caremanager.org/storeindex. cfm
- Neat Company— www.neatco.com
- QuickBooks—www.quickbooks.com
- Res Care—www.rescare.org
- SBA Center—www.sba.gov/contactus/index
- Scan Snap—www.fujitsu.com/scanners.html
- SCORE—www.score.org
- SBA—www.sba.gov/aboutsba/sbaprograms/sbdc/index.html
- Senior Bridge—www.seniorbridge.com
- TimeSlips—www.timeslips.com
- University of California, Berkeley list serve—agingresources-request@lists.berkeley.edu
- University of Florida distance GCM program—http://gcm.dce.ufl.edu
- US Chamber of Commerce—www.uschamber.com/default

Chapter 13

After the Start-up: Issues for Mature Care Management Organizations

Phyllis Mensh Brostoff

■ INTRODUCTION

As Chapter 12, How to Start or Add a Geriatric Care Management Business, made clear, the new geriatric care management business has very particular concerns. It must define itself, decide who it serves, and establish its place in the community. After this flurry of start-up activities, methods of operation have been established and relationships have been initiated. Eventually, the business comes to a point at which initial premises are reexamined, systems are refined, and directions are reconsidered. If the owner decides to go beyond a one- or two-person business model, new organizational systems must be developed. If the owner decides to expand significantly, he or she begins a period of adding staff and working him- or herself out of jobs they previously had done. To decide how to proceed, the mature geriatric care management business begins a process of periodic reassessments and adjustments that should continue as long as the organization exists.

■ DEFINING A NICHE

The organization's niche is defined by the services it provides and the population it serves. When contemplating growth, the maturing geriatric care management organization may be ready to consider expanding or changing the population it serves and the services it offers. Just as a functional assessment of a new client guides a geriatric care manager (GCM) in planning initial services, and periodic reassessment keeps GCMs responsive to changing client needs. A reassessment of the type of clients served and the services provided can offer guidance in developing a plan for growth and development for the organization.

Organizations finding themselves at this crossroads will review the following data about the clients they have served and the services they have provided:

- The geographical location and pattern of the population being served (e.g., within a given city, which neighborhoods have the highest density of older people or older people in certain income brackets), by zip code if possible
- The average income of the clients served
- The living arrangements of the clients (e.g., primarily living at home alone, with spouses or family members, or in facilities)
- The level of functional dependence of the clients
- The focus of service: one-time consultations or long-term care management, or a mix, primarily aimed at arranging in-home care or finding appropriate alternative living arrangements in assisted living or skilled facilities

- The average length of service to clients
- Is the primary focus of service aimed at the elderly individual or at family members?
- Are services provided in assisted living or skilled nursing facilities?
- Are fiduciary services such as bill paying, guardianships, or conservatorships provided?
- What services has the organization actually provided to the clients it has served since it began?
- What services have proved to be economically viable and which ones are money losers?

Understanding the demographics of the clients and families served and the patterns of the services actually provided, the care management organization can assess the success of its service mix to its clients, and begin a process of deciding whether services should be added, dropped, or shared with other providers.

■ MODELS OF GERIATRIC CARE MANAGEMENT

Geriatric care management has evolved largely as a private professional practice shaped by the unique skills and orientation of the GCM conducting the practice and the identified needs of the clients served. The GCM practicing alone may continue indefinitely or as long as the individual's strength and health allow. Some GCMs practice with other professionals such as elder-law attorneys, certified public accountants, or physicians (as described in Chapter 12).

In the late 1970s, when geriatric care management was beginning to be recognized as a distinct practice specialization through the federally funded community option Medicare and Medicaid waiver programs, care management was defined as a broker model. The care manager employed by a gov-

ernmental unit or nonprofit organization was expected to assess the client, define the service mix the client needed, order those services for the client from vendors with whom the organization had contracts, and then monitor the quality of care provided by those vendors.

In the early 1980s, when private pay care management services began to develop as stand-alone businesses, it was the expectation of the entrepreneurs who opened up these private practices that they would be paid directly by their clients. In fact, when the National Association of Professional Geriatric Care Managers was founded in 1986, it was called the National Association of Private Geriatric Care Managers, reflecting the expectation that all of the members would be providing care management as a business, on a fee-for-service basis. The association's name was later changed to National Association of Professional Geriatric Care Managers when membership was opened up to care managers working in nonprofit organizations.

As this private care management model matured, a major service the private care manager found herself providing to clients was finding competent, reliable caregivers to work in the client's home. Care managers typically screened and recommended these caregivers, charging their regular hourly rates for this service. However, hiring private caregivers required families to pay the required taxes, obtain needed liability insurance, and other payroll-related expenses. Care managers found that it was sometimes difficult to supervise the caregiver she had screened and recommended to the family because she was not the employer and could not discipline or fire the caregiver. In addition, families and third parties (e.g., trust companies, attorneys) did not want to bother with the payroll-related tasks. Care managers began to hire their own caregivers, and the care-managed home care agency model was born. An example of a care-managed home care business is Stowell Associates SelectStaff Inc., which began in 1983 in Milwaukee, Wisconsin, and almost immediately added caregivers, at the request of clients (www.elderselectstaff.com). A multistate company that provides care-managed home care is LivHome (www.livhome.com), headquartered in Los Angeles, California.

Brokerage or Free-Standing Care Manager Model

In the brokerage or free-standing care manager model, the care manager service is the only service provided. All of the assistance needed by and arranged for clients, including caregivers, are provided by other businesses or organizations. The GCM assesses the client's level of functioning and living situation, explores options, develops a plan of care and recommendations. If the case goes beyond the assessment and recommendation phase to ongoing care management, the GCM arranges for whatever service the client needs, which might include caregivers, shopping, transportation, emergency response, and so forth. The GCM monitors and coordinates the care that is provided by all of these independent providers. The care manager's job is ongoing monitoring of the services clients are receiving, advocating for clients so that they obtain the best quality of care from the service, and revising the service package in response to the client's needs. An example of a stand-alone mature care management business is Proeger Associates, in Sarasota, Florida (www.proegerassociates.com).

Care managers who provide only care management services sometimes find that they specialize in short-term consultations. Other care management practices find that clients come to them to research and recommend alternative living arrangements when they no longer can remain in their own homes. Another specialization of a mature care management practice is working with the probate court, trust, and estate attorneys in disputed guardianship cases, where the expertise of a care manager can assist in untangling complex family disputes such as "dueling" powers of attorney. Finally, mature care management-only practices generally have long-term monitoring roles with clients whose care they may oversee for many years. A mature care management-only practice may also find that it is asked to do presentations to local civic organizations, or teach a class in gerontology or services to the aged at a local university. These opportunities may provide some additional income to the sole practitioner as well as provide an excellent means to market the care manager's expertise, even if there is little or no compensation for the work.

Service-Integrated Models

There are a number of integrated models of mature care management practices paired with one or more related services. The most common one is the care-managed home care practice, which employs caregivers directly, as described above. However, there are also mature care management practices that combine care management with selling insurance-related services, usually long-term care insurance. An example is the practice of Jerie Charnow in New York and Florida (www.ltcamerica.com). Another combination of services is care management and employee assistance or eldercare in the workplace programs, for example the practice of Mary Lynn Pannen in Tacoma, Washington (www.soundoptions.com). These services may be provided primarily via the telephone, or they may be combined with in-person assessments and family consultations, or "brown bag" programs in workplaces to provide education and support to employees. Combining care management and becoming a corporate guardian or conservator has also proved to be a successful model for the expansion of mature care management practices. These practices vary greatly across the country because guardianship and conservator systems are governed by each state or municipality, rather than with a uniform system throughout the country. A long-time provider of care management and guardianship is Gordan Wolfe's in Denver, Colorado (www.humannetworksystem.com). Some care managers provide emergency response services through one of the national systems, such as LifeLine or ResponseLink, or a combination of a number of these services such as SeniorBridge, headquartered in New York City (www.seniorbridge.com).

However, no matter what other service the care management practice also operates, the GCM still begins with a client assessment, identifying options, and developing a plan of care. All care managers who provide more than care management services need to be familiar with the NAPGCM *Standards of Practice* including Standard 13 (Disclosure of Business Relationships) and Standard 9 (Undertaking Fiduciary Responsibilities), to guide their practice in an ethically sound manner, adhering to the national standards of practice this organization has developed.

Choosing a Model

After a geriatric care management business is well established, the owner is often confronted with a dilemma—if she has been successful, she may find herself with more business than she can handle on her own. Or she may find clients asking her to provide one of the other services mentioned earlier. The business owner must then decide if she wants the business to grow, usually by hiring another professional GCM. This is a relatively easy decision to make because it does not require building an organization. However, even this decision requires the care management business owner to develop some additional business expertise, including developing a job description and often a contract for the care manager employee, setting expectations regarding productivity, agreeing

on reporting systems, providing equipment, and supervising the employee. For some care managers, this is clearly not what they want to do. One-person care management businesses can thrive without employees. These practitioners have found creative ways to allow themselves vacations and time off, usually by pairing with another sole practitioner with whom they have developed a collegial relationship.

However, for care managers who want to build an organization, any of the service combinations identified earlier can be chosen, based on the care manager's own interests, background, and expertise. Because the care-managed home care model is the most frequent model for growth chosen by GCMs, this model will be the one that is most extensively discussed in this chapter. However, no matter which model is chosen, much of the following information is relevant.

■ MAINTAINING A CONSISTENT ORGANIZATIONAL IMAGE

As an organization grows beyond a single person, maintaining a consistent philosophy and approach to service is essential. The chief executive officer (CEO) must convey to all new employees—whether they are caregivers, administrative and clerical staff, or professional GCMs—the guiding philosophy and values of the organization. Defining and maintaining the image of the organization is an ongoing task for the CEO of any growing organization.

The image of the organization is based on everything the public sees and hears about the organization, including the following:

1. The expectations for personal grooming of the people who work for the organization
2. The appearance and location of the offices occupied by the organization
3. The observable behaviors of all the employees of the organization
4. The reputation of the organization

5. The collateral material (e.g., logo, letterhead, brochure, print advertising) produced by the organization
6. The training and experience level of the staff

Reputation depends partly on the professional training and orientation of the organization's leading GCMs. GCMs may have been trained as social workers, nurses, gerontologists, psychologists, health administrators, or educators. Whatever their professional background, all GCMs should project their competence as seasoned professionals capable of conducting autonomous, independent practices in which the welfare of the client is the highest priority. This image can be projected by having well-organized protocols, an attitude of caring and helpfulness, and respect for the client's need for autonomy and self-determination.

However, every member of an organization contributes to the image of that organization, and it is the responsibility of each person to project an image congruent with the mission of the organization. Although appropriate professional behavior is the most important factor, it is also important for employees themselves, their cars, and the organization's offices to look clean and neat. The organization's reputation will be enhanced by all employees looking and behaving in a professional manner.

Credential and Skill Guidelines for Hiring Geriatric Care Managers

In mature geriatric care management organizations that employ several GCMs, it is a good idea to employ professionals with different backgrounds, skills, and strengths. This will allow the agency to assign cases to professionals who can serve a variety of clients. Most mature agencies will need a care manager with expertise in such specialty areas as chronic mental illness, medication management, chronic disease management, complex family

issues, and court-related expertise, to name some of the most frequent specialists needed. Of course, regular, consistent, supportive supervision is critical to ensure high-quality service, so the mature care management agency will need to develop the role of clinical manager or director. The clinical manager will have the responsibility to hire and supervise the care managers. At a minimum, GCMs should have the following credentials, skills, characteristics and attitudes:

- At least a bachelor's degree in social work, nursing, psychology, gerontology or another human service field such as speech, occupational or physical therapy
- Specialized training or experience in working with the elderly
- Be licensed and credentialed by a professional organization (such as the National Association of Social Workers [www.naswdc.org] or the American Nurses Association [www.nursingworld.org]) and the licensing and certification bureau of their state or have one of the certifications approved by the National Association of Professional Geriatric Care Managers (see www.caremanager.org and search for "certification")
- A presentation of self that is friendly, caring, and cooperative
- An approach to client needs and problems that is organized and thorough
- A flexible and creative approach to clients and care plan development
- The ability to assist clients and families in making decisions without imposing their own opinions or being judgmental
- An understanding of their value as professionals and feeling comfortable in charging fees for their time and expertise
- The ability to delegate tasks that are appropriate to paraprofessionals or non-professionals
- Demonstration of their ability to be an integral part of the community by participating in community organizations

- An understanding how to use regular, consistent, supportive supervision

Guidelines for Hiring Paraprofessionals

Hiring paraprofessionals, aides and caregivers needs to be done as carefully as hiring professional geriatric care managers. They need to have the same type of personal characteristics as a care manager—flexibility, ability to use supervision appropriately and a positive manner that inspires trust. In addition, when hiring paraprofessionals the agency should consider the following:

- Require at least a GED.
- Seek individuals already trained and certified as nurse aides.
- Check in the state registry of nurse aides for any violation (this can be done online).
- Check police and driving records both locally and nationally (most states have online record checking available for a fee, and there are national online services also).
- Check at least three work references

In care-managed home care agencies, the CEO needs to develop a variety of ways to assure that the paraprofessional caregivers appreciate that their work for the organization is crucial. They are the eyes and ears, heart and hands of the care management organization. As the mature geriatric care management organization grows, and, in care-managed home care businesses, the number of caregivers increases, regular and ongoing training must be planned. A thorough orientation to the agency's policies, procedures, protocols, safety precautions, and care guidelines should be required for all new employees. The care managers usually supervise the caregivers, so the role of care manager must also be thoroughly explained and understood. The management team of the organization needs to develop a variety of team-building methods that are used throughout the year, such as an agencywide newsletter, sending birthday cards, remembering hiring anniversaries, yearly performance reviews, and periodic agency parties or celebrations.

■ MARKETING

To thrive and grow, mature care management organizations must refine their marketing approach by examining their marketing philosophy periodically and updating their marketing plan. If the organization has an annual strategic planning meeting, marketing is an appropriate topic for discussion. If the organization is a smaller business, choosing a new marketing strategy may simply mean deciding to develop a new brochure and update marketing materials. In larger organizations, additional marketing materials may be needed, targeting specific segments of the community. Developing a good website is a must today, when more and more people use Internet searches to find needed services. There are many competent website developers and the growing care management business needs to invest in building and maintaining a good Web presence.

Marketing Philosophy

Three strategies can provide a good marketing program for geriatric care management agencies: providing educational programs, building goodwill in the general community, and developing positive relationships with other professionals. Developing and offering educational programs to older people, their families, and professionals who serve older people is an excellent marketing strategy because it is useful and appreciated. In the course of a program on, for example, Alzheimer's and other dementias, the care manager can explain the spectrum of services geriatric care management provides to ameliorate the challenges these dementias present to families. Building goodwill in the community through, for example, participating in organizations like

Rotary and serving on nonprofit boards, establishes the agency's reputation as a responsible community citizen, keenly interested in the welfare of others. Finally, building positive relationships with professionals throughout the area is vital to developing the trust that encourages these individuals to refer their clients, and their own families, to the care management organization. Prospective clients choose providers of elder care whom they trust, with whom they feel safe, and whom they view as competent professionals. It is through a relationship of trust that prospective clients become actual clients. These three approaches—education, building goodwill, and developing relationships—form the fabric of a positive and effective marketing program, based on the philosophical belief that good acts are the basis for a good organization.

Marketing Plan

The marketing plans for mature geriatric care management organizations build on their previous marketing plans, which must have been at least successful enough for the agency to grow. However, most start-up organizations lack the financial and human resources to invest in the development of a full-blown marketing plan. As the organization grows, new challenges and opportunities appear. Additional resources may become available. An annual review of the marketing plan and assessment of the organization's functional capacity are critical to an organization's success.

Here are seven elements in developing a marketing plan in a mature organization:

1. Definition of services and target profiles
2. Market research
3. Community development
4. Advertising
5. Public relations and developing an Internet presence
6. Inquiries and the intake process
7. Tracking and learning

Definition of Services and Target Profiles

A marketing plan for a mature geriatric care management organization begins with a review of its services and a profile of its target markets. The organization that clearly defines the features and scope of its services can differentiate itself from other providers in the community. The demographic information that is gathered in the course of providing services to clients can be used to build the marketing plan that targets clients directly. It is important to develop a clear explanation of the services the organization provides directly to clients and how they are different from other service providers in the community.

Since adult children or relatives of the older person are frequently the ones who initially request service, it is important to understand how to reach these families as part of the marketing program. Although geriatric care management as a professional service has been in the marketplace for more than 25 years, many families do not know it exists, until a crisis occurs that compels them to seek help. The care management organization needs to understand the demographics of this target audience including their level of education, income, age, family constellations, and if they live out of town or out of state.

A third target market is other professionals who serve older people and their families. These professionals are valuable potential referral sources and frequently participate as members of the support team for the older person. This group includes trust and estate and elder-law attorneys, financial planners, geriatric physicians, psychiatrists, trust officers, private fiduciaries, hospital discharge planners, members of the clergy, and other community organizations providing services for older people. The care management organization needs to understand the profile of these professionals in their community—a geriatric care management company serving an upper-class suburb will target a different kind of professional than a nonprofit agency providing care management services to low-income older people.

Market Research

The second step in updating a marketing plan is to develop a market research strategy to clearly define the needs of those residing in its market area. A sense of the character and lifestyle of the older people in the community will guide the practitioner so that services are tailored to appeal to the individual community's older residents and their families.

Demographic information can often be obtained from the Area Agency on Aging. Census data can be obtained on the Internet. The local chambers of commerce and other planning bodies may also have valuable information.

When looking at broader demographic data, geriatric care management organizations should ask a number of questions. How many older people reside in the organization's service area? In what zip codes are they concentrated? How many of them are between the ages of 70 and 85 years? How many are older than 85 years? How many live alone? How many need assistance with the activities of daily living? What is their income level? What is their level of education? In addition to research pertaining to older clients, the organization will also want to research area families and professionals, the other two target audiences. This demographic information can inform future marketing decisions such as where and how advertising dollars would be most effectively spent.

Developing Community Relationships

Developing and nurturing good relationships with referral sources is important in growing a care management business. The mature geriatric care management organization will have a group of referral sources. The key is developing an ongoing strategy to keep in touch with these referrers and others who the organization can add to its list. Some organizations employ marketing professionals to do relationship development, but experience indicates that GCMs employed by the mature organization play a key role in this effort.

It is important for each GCM working in the organization to understand their role in nurturing positive community relationships and marketing the organization. One technique is to provide GCMs with information packets and small gifts to take with them when they are likely to meet other professionals in the process of assisting their clients. For example, an information packet and small gift (such as a pen or pad of post-its) given to a hospital discharge planner as the GCM is taking a client home from the hospital can result in ongoing referrals. Staff training focusing on how to talk about the services provided by the organization and how to encourage referrals should be part of the organization's ongoing marketing strategy.

A GCM who accompanies a client to an appointment can educate the physician about geriatric care management in general and the organization's services specifically. The GCM can illustrate the services by talking about how the client's sundown symptoms have been tracked in a logbook that is kept in the client's home or how the GCM is training and supervising the caregiving staff to carry out the physician's instructions. If the GCM works with an attorney on behalf of a client to arrange estate planning, the GCM can again take the opportunity to inform the attorney about the full range of the organization's geriatric care management services. The attorney will encounter other older clients who need the services of a GCM and will refer them, provided he or she understands what geriatric care management is and what services it can involve.

Experience has shown that community relationships take time to evolve. Repeated encounters and firsthand experience with geriatric care management services are often required before other professionals understand the scope of service provided by a comprehensive geriatric care management organization. It takes time for the professional to trust the GCM. In short, relationships are rarely established in one visit. Social workers and many nurses are trained to start any relationship where the client is. When the desired relationship is with another professional, the principle remains the same. Professionals have a particular point of view; they are trying to accomplish some goal for their client. If geriatric care management organizations can focus on these professionals' goals and learn how to make their work easier for them, the relationships between the care management organization and other allied professionals will flourish.

Although community relationship building can happen in the course of geriatric care management activities, an approach that combines both organized, concerted efforts and spontaneous encounters will yield the best results. The marketing plan must articulate the targets for community relationship development, identify who is responsible for developing the relationships, and how these contacts will be tracked. Community relationship activities can be divided by profession (e.g., one GCM is responsible for developing relationships with all the elder-law attorneys in the community). GCMs then attend the association meetings and network within that one group of professionals. Alternatively, one community relationship development representative can be responsible for a particular neighborhood or geographic area. Within that area, the GCM networks, educates, and develops relationships with physicians, elder-law attorneys, trust officers, hospital discharge planners, assisted-living residence administrators, and so forth. How community relationship tasks are divided is not important. What is important is that they are divided in a manner that clearly defines who is responsible for fostering which relationships. For example, a GCM serving a suburban area encounters a supervising trust officer during a routine call to a trust department. The GCM follows up with a letter and an information packet. He or she alerts the person in charge of marketing, who then follows up with a call to the supervising trust officer in the regional office, thereby expanding the company's opportunity to broaden its influence throughout the trust departments in the region.

Advertising

A marketing plan for the mature geriatric care management company should address what advertising will be done. Depending on the local market, different advertising options may be appropriate to achieve the business's marketing objectives. Advertising options for the mature organization include but are not limited to print advertisements, broadcast (television or radio) advertisements, Internet sites and links, billboards, booths at senior health fairs, and sponsorship of community events. Common print advertising options appropriate for geriatric care management organizations include general-interest newspapers (many newspapers have a senior section), senior newspapers, local civic magazines, local business journals, community newsletters, Better Business Bureau consumer guides, elder-care directories, and local professional newsletters. A geriatric care management organization may want to be listed in several categories (i.e., home care, geriatric care management, elder care, senior services) in local directories. The mature organization should budget for some paid advertising, but advertising to the general public may not be a good use of the agency's money. Advertising that reaches the most people in the target market at the lowest cost is of course the best choice. Many cities have specialized directories of senior services and advertising in these assures reaching the target audience. Being an underwriter of the local public radio station (WUWM) has been a good marketing strategy for Stowell Associates SelectStaff because this station reaches the agency's target market of mature, educated, and more affluent people.

Public Relations

The mature geriatric care management organization looking to grow will want to focus on public relations. Major relevant public relations activities can include creating media kits, sending regular press releases, building relationships with media contacts, publishing newsletters, holding open houses, participating in speakers bureaus, attending health fairs, and giving seminars and presentations at conferences. These activities are part of educating the public about the organization's services and building goodwill toward the organization. (See Chapter 16 on marketing.)

The mature geriatric care management organization will want to continue to use media kits to keep the press aware of the organization's history and provide information that is in the public interest. Media kits are used to educate media representatives about the organization and to solicit media coverage of the organization's services, activities, and events. Media kits can include the following items:

- Company background and fact sheet
- Company brochure
- Appropriate press releases
- Biographies of the executive team, board of directors, advisory board, and GCMs
- Client testimonials
- Reprints of articles on or about the geriatric care management agency or about geriatric care management in general
- Literature on the National Association of Professional Geriatric Care Managers or Case Management Society of America (CMSA)
- Photos with captions
- A sheet of frequently asked questions and their answers
- A sheet with common questions and answers or explanations for these questions

- Newspaper articles about the mature GCM agency
- A narrative of one client's experience with the organization (with the client's name changed for confidentiality).

Press releases can be sent for a variety of reasons: to announce an upcoming event (for inclusion in a newspaper's listing of events), to launch a new service, to announce a new office location, to announce a new contract or affiliation, to announce awards and achievements (awarded to either the company or an employee), or to announce a client's achievements. One organization was able to place a story about a 100-year-old client who flew cross-country to visit her childhood summer home with her caregiver in a feature article in a metropolitan newspaper. (Of course, this type of story requires prior approval from the client.) Press releases should be sent to contacts such as local press, trade press, business and financial press, investors, and prospective investors. Press releases should be sent on a regular basis by the mature geriatric care management organization because they can build and maintain awareness of the organization. Many organizations providing home care are springing up; a good human interest story can highlight the important differences between professional geriatric care-managed home care and other approaches to home care.

Relationships with media contacts begin by sending or delivering the company's media kit. Relationships are fostered by sending regular press releases, monitoring editorial calendars for media opportunities, pursuing appropriate opportunities with the media representatives, inviting editors and advertising representatives to visit the company, and working with media representatives on feature articles and interviews. The more these relationships are nurtured, the more often the organization will be mentioned by the local media, or called when there is a breaking story and a comment from a professional is needed.

Company newsletters that educate people about geriatric care management can offer a valuable service to the professional community and serve significant public relations functions simultaneously. A well-written, regularly published newsletter, hard copy or e-mail, can establish professional credibility and community presence. See the news, articles, and books section of www.elderselect-staff.com for a series of e-blasts on topics of special interest. Holding open houses to celebrate a new office or a significant anniversary can also serve a public relations function if professional and media contacts are invited.

Every mature care management company needs to have a robust website that they review and update at least yearly. Looking at other care management company websites can provide useful ideas and perspectives on how to approach this type of marketing. It is worthwhile for a growing care management organization to use a professional to develop their website. There are many technical issues such as SEO (search engine optimization) and paying for Google ads that require obtaining professional advice. In addition, many care managers are now using social media outlets such as Twitter, LinkedIn, and Facebook to market and network. These outlets will continue to evolve and change and the mature organization will need to evolve their use of social media as well.

Inquiries and the Intake Process

Targeted advertising and public relations activities help geriatric care management companies make the public aware of their services. But after an organization does the expensive work of getting people to pay attention, then what? In a marketing (and clinical) model in which relationships are primary, the focus is on educating and creating lasting relationships, not creating instant impressions.

Inquiries are the information-seeking contacts made by family members, older people, or professionals about the organization's services. The intake process is developed to respond to these calls, from the initial greeting at the reception desk to the information exchange, to the point when the caller chooses to work with the organization (as a client, as a relative of a client, or as a source of referrals) or chooses another organization. A critical element of the mature geriatric care management organization's marketing plan is ongoing analysis and improvement of the inquiry and intake processes so that as many inquiries as possible lead to new clients. A monthly summary and analysis of intake calls received, the referral source, and the outcome of the call is a vital management tool. If the research, community relationship building, advertising, and public relations are working, a steady stream of prospective clients will be calling.

These prospects have varying degrees of information about the organization's services. One caller's friend may have heard an ad on the radio. That caller may know nothing about geriatric care management and not be certain that an older aunt wants or needs assistance. Another caller may have heard about the organization from three different respected sources, may have done extensive research on how best to provide care for his or her aging parents, and may be seeking information about some of the fine points of the services. How does the organization handle these various calls to maximize conversions from callers to clients?

The mature geriatric care management organization has already designed an inquiry and intake process; however, periodic review and analysis are vital to organizational growth. Several elements are involved in designing and refining the inquiry and intake process. These elements include making sure clear information is provided, making sure the information packet is sent on a timely basis, following up on the initial call, referring when appropriate, and refining the intake process itself. Are the first contacts primarily phone calls, e-mail inquiries, written inquiries, or walk-ins? Who fields the first contact? Is it the receptionist? Does he or she convey a good image for the organization? Is he or she warm, inviting, professional, and knowledgeable? This is one of the most important positions in the organization. Does he or she have a script of what to say? Is there an established protocol of how to field inquiries? If not, the organization needs to design a script that includes the initial greeting, the question, "How may we help you?" and the assurance that the intake GCM will respond within the hour if he or she is not immediately available. This initial response tells callers how important they are to the geriatric care management organization. The protocol should include recording of the caller's name and phone number because lost calls are costly.

■ INFORMATION PACKET

Geriatric care management organizations will need an information packet of materials describing their services. The materials should accurately convey the organization's identity and be of a high quality, to reflect the quality of the services themselves. Remember that relationships are primary and the focus is on educating prospective clients about the organization's services. The material can be as simple as a brochure or as sophisticated as a presentation folder containing multiple pieces (e.g., a brochure, a description of geriatric care management, a sheet of frequently asked questions, a sheet of common objections and answers or explanations for the objections, information about the National Association of Professional Geriatric Care Managers or CMSA, reprints of articles about the organization or about geriatric care management in general, newsletters, and a narrative of a client's experience with the organization). It should always include a written fee schedule.

■ INTAKE

The intake process itself is very important. This is where the greatest opportunity exists to educate prospective clients and referral sources about the organization's services. The caller is giving the care management organization his or her full attention. The potential to convert the relationship from caller to client is great. It is critical that the intake coordinator keep the caller's full attention. The best intake coordinators have both strong clinical skills and an understanding of and comfort with sales principles. The intake coordinator will want to use a consistent format to find out as much as possible about the caller's situation and needs. Questions to be asked include the following:

- Who is the client?
- What is the caller's relationship to the client?
- How did the caller hear about the organization?
- How is the client's overall health and well-being? Where and with whom does the client live? How independent is the client in caring for him- or herself?
- What was the precipitating event that resulted in the phone call?
- What services does the client want?
- What does the caller know about geriatric care management?
- Does the caller understand the geriatric care management model?

It takes time to educate the caller. While seeking answers to these questions, the intake coordinator must spend ample time listening. It is here, in this sharing of information, that the relationship between the caller and the organization is being formed. Some callers request services immediately, whereas others require a number of follow-up calls before becoming clients, and some are not appropriate for the organization's services at all.

There are many ways to handle these intake and inquiry calls. One person may be the desgnated intake coordinator, or each GCM working in the organization can be trained to handle intake and inquiry calls. If the organization chooses to use each of their GCMs to handle these calls, it is best to have them scheduled in the office on a regular basis to handle the calls because multiple GCMs with widely varying schedules cannot field incoming inquiries in a consistent manner. The organization that responds most promptly to the inquiry is the most likely to be the chosen service provider when the caller has been given the names of several organizations to call or is calling from a list. Whichever system is put into place, it is vitally important that the intake coordinator or designated GCM intake worker offer information and referrals to callers who are not appropriate for the organization to serve.

The intake worker must be familiar with community resources. Disseminating information and appropriate referrals is an important community service and good public relations. It provides valuable education and builds enormous goodwill in the community toward the organization. In addition, clients who are not a good fit for the organization are weeded out at intake, including individuals who do not want to pay for services.

Tracking and Learning

The follow-up process is almost as important as the intake process. Intake coordinators at mature geriatric care management organizations can use lulls in the incoming inquiries to follow up on previous calls. A tickler system can be set up to follow up on callers who indicate that they need to talk to others in the family or who are not immediately interested in initiating services. Numerous computer software programs are available to assist in following up on prospects. It is important to know that "no" is not always a final answer in this situation; in fact, marketing experts suggest that it usually means "maybe" or "not

just yet."[1] Remember, if people have contacted the organization, they are serious prospects. Organizations that choose to use the intake coordinator model are in a better position to pay special attention to nurturing these relationships because one person is in that position and following up on calls should be included in that person's job description.

The geriatric care management organization, desiring to build equity, must be a learning organization across the board. According to Peter Senge, who developed the concept of the learning organization, a learning organization is a new source of competitive advantage.[2] Nowhere is this learning organization approach more important than in marketing efforts. At a learning organization, people are constantly researching the existing business, tracking every dollar spent on marketing, tracking every response, measuring and analyzing the data, and making modifications to the marketing plan based on those data. Learning organizations continually measure, learn from what they measure, and make changes according to what they learn.

Computer software can help manage the tracking of key information such as the number of intake telephone calls and e-mail contacts received, how many inquiries became active clients, what referrals were made to callers, and perhaps most important the source of the referrals. This and other information will allow the organization to refine its advertising and public relations plans, community development efforts, and intake process. Careful tracking is part of the vital feedback loop guiding the marketing plan and the organization as a whole.

■ ORGANIZATIONAL DEVELOPMENT

The information in this section is derived from direct experience building a geriatric care management organization and many discussions with colleagues struggling with the same issues during the course of more than 25 years of providing geriatric care management services. You are encouraged to borrow whatever is useful but ultimately to do whatever works best in your organization. This discussion of organizational development addresses four areas:

1. Defining the organization's identity
2. Assessing and tending the organization's culture
3. Developing leaders and staff members
4. Developing systems

Defining the Organization's Identity

To thrive and grow, a mature organization must have a clearly articulated identity. Organizations can begin the process of defining themselves by focusing on four elements: mission, purpose, values, and culture. (These elements are discussed in the following sections.) Most geriatric care management organizations develop mission and purpose statements when they start. However, as organizations mature and expand, it is useful to revisit these statements, refining them with the participation of the newer members of the organizational team.

Mission

A mission statement tells the community what the organization strives to accomplish through its work. In 2000, the mission of Stowell Associates SelectStaff of Milwaukee, Wisconsin, was "to maintain the safety, security and independence of our elderly and disabled adult clients by providing the highest quality of professional care management and caregiving services." In 2008, the agency rethought its mission and defined it as "The mission of Stowell Associates SelectStaff is to improve the quality of the day-to-day lives of our clients and their families in ways both small and large."

Ideally employees from the various levels of the organization participate in crafting the mission statement. When employees participate in creating the statement, they understand it and are more committed to it than they would be if it were developed solely by management or the owner. Once the mission statement is written, it becomes a guide for decision making at all levels of the organization. Placement of this statement on business cards, brochures, and other informational materials serves to remind the staff of their mission and educate the community.

Purpose

Whereas the mission statement speaks to the organization's community, the purpose statement (sometimes referred to as a vision statement) is an internal statement the staff make to themselves about how and why they do their work. According to Collins and Porras, the "core purpose is the organization's reason for being. An effective purpose reflects people's idealistic motivations for doing the company's work. It doesn't just describe the organization's output or target customers; it captures the soul of the organization."[3(p68)] Purpose should not be confused with specific goals or business objectives. The purpose statement answers the question, "Why is what we do important to us?" The purpose statement of the beginning geriatric care management organization may be suitable for the mature geriatric care management organization, but a periodic review of the statement helps staff to maintain focus. As with the mission statement, staff will feel more committed to the purpose statement when they participate in creating it.

A complete purpose statement reminds staff members about how and why they do their work. It can also guide decisions that impact the culture and work environment. Management can ask, "Would implementing this new policy be in keeping with our purpose statement?"

The purpose statement can help management and staff assess how they are doing.

individuals can ask themselves, "Are my unique strengths and talents being nurtured?" and "Am I respecting and nurturing the strengths of my fellow workers?"

Stowell Associates created a much more succinct purpose (vision) statement in 2008: "Stowell Associates SelectStaff is the provider of choice for individuals, families, and professionals who seek superior care for disabled adults and elders."

Values

The third element for the organization to articulate in its process of self-definition is its values. Core values are the essential and enduring tenets of an organization. According to Collins and Porras, "A small set of timeless guiding principles, core values require no external justification; they have intrinsic value and importance to those inside the organization."[3(p66)] These core values are what the organization stands for. The core values of the geriatric care management organization may have been defined and articulated at the start and may have remained unchanged; however, the mature organization will do well to revisit these values as part of new-employee orientation and renew them periodically to remind and refocus all staff. The following questions can be posed to staff to help them define or review the core values of their organization:

- What core values do you personally bring to your work? (These should be so fundamental that you would hold them regardless of whether they were rewarded.)
- What would you tell your children (or grandchildren) are the core values that you hold at work and that you hope they will hold when they become working adults?
- If you awoke tomorrow morning with enough money to retire for the rest of your life, would you continue to live by those core values?

- Can you envision those core values being as valid for you 100 years from now as they are today?
- Would you want to continue holding those core values even if at some point one or more of them became a competitive disadvantage?
- If you were to start a new organization tomorrow in a different line of work, what core values would you build into the new organization regardless of its industry?[3(p68)]

For a geriatric care management organization, core values might include the centrality of relationships, the belief that clients are best nurtured by staff that are respected and supported, the acceptance of and respect for the uniqueness of every human being, and the acceptance of growth and change as a part of life and of death as its natural end. Defining values as an organization when it begins is important. To remain effective, the mature geriatric care management organization should revisit its statement of its core values periodically to include new staff in value development, ensure their commitment to these values, and revise its value statements as the organization evolves and changes.

Many successful organizations publicize their values. For example, three core values of the Nordstrom's retail stores are:

1. Service to the customer above all else
2. Hard work and individual productivity
3. Excellence in reputation

Stowell Associates SelectStaff's 2008 value statements are:

- **Respect:** We are respectful in our encounters with colleagues, clients, and families.
- **Integrity:** We follow rigorous national professional standards through our accreditation by the Council on Accreditation.

- **Trust:** Trust is at the core of the relationships we establish with our staff, our colleagues, our clients, and their family members.
- **Excellence:** We are committed to excellence in every aspect of client care and service.

Assessing and Tending the Organization's Culture

Work cultures are made up of a variety of elements. These elements, which range from encouraging innovation to maximizing client satisfaction and providing secure employment, can be prioritized so that organizations can begin to determine both their current and their ideal cultures. The new organization must assess and define its culture. The mature organization should redefine its culture periodically. The following questions can be helpful in the process:

- What is the overriding strategic intent of the organization? The strategic intent refers to how the organization does what it does. The strategic intent answers such questions as these:
  - What do customers want?
  - How does the organization deliver what the customers want?
  - How is the organization different from other organizations?
- How is the organization structured (e.g., hierarchical, flat)?
- How is work organized (i.e., teams versus individual contributors)?
- How do teams and individuals interact?
- How are decisions made?
- What behaviors are encouraged? What behaviors are discouraged or prohibited?
- What kind of people work for the organization?
- How do they think?
- How do they act (e.g., in a task-oriented way)?

- How much power do they have?
- How much risk are they allowed—and do they wish—to take?
- How are they selected and developed?
- How are they rewarded?
- How is pay viewed? Is it seen as an investment or merely a cost of doing business?

An organization that has clearly articulated its mission, purpose, and values and assessed its culture, can more effectively continue the dynamic process of improvement. If an honest review of the organization's current reality does not match the desired state, efforts to improve can be planned and implemented. Development is not a one-time event but a continuous process. A dynamic organization always believes that improvement is possible and acts on that belief. Attention must be paid to the organization's culture if the organization is going to remain robust and dynamic. Cultures differ from organization to organization. There is no one right answer. Whatever works is what is right for that organization.[4] However, the centrality of relationships appears to be one value that is essential to the culture of a healthy geriatric care management organization.

It is the quality of the relationship between the GCM and the client (and the family) that makes geriatric care management a unique service and is, perhaps, the key for its success. It is, in part, the absence of positive human relationships in bureaucracies, medical systems, and elsewhere that creates the need for geriatric care management.

If relationships are the lifeblood of the organization, what is the organization doing to foster them? This element of the culture must be focused on, nurtured, and developed for the organization to continue to mature. If management wants the GCM to develop mastery in his or her relationships with clients, managers must develop mastery in their relationships with the GCMs and other staff members. If the organization wants

GCMs to nurture their clients, the organization must nurture the GCMs. If the organization wants to support the autonomy and self-determination of older people, it must also support the autonomy and self-determination of its employees. Examples of organizational practices that foster staff autonomy and self-determination include participative management and self-managed teams.[5]

Developing Leaders and Staff Members

Geriatric care management organizations focused on growth must attend to leadership and staff development. Fostering professional development improves individual and team performance, strengthens an organization's effectiveness, creates a more cohesive culture, and encourages staff loyalty. An organization's plan for professional development should be based on an assessment of the organization's needs and the needs of the staff. Leadership and staff development based on an assessment can include training in building teams, conducting meetings, resolving conflicts, supervising, balancing work and life, managing time, making presentations, and handling the inevitable challenges the organization's staff experiences in working with each other, the clients, and their families. Table 13–1 lists different kinds of staff training and their impact on business, leadership, and clinical skills.

A key challenge to the leader of a mature geriatric care management organization is delegating tasks to others. Leaders who are accustomed to being solo practitioners may experience difficulty in delegating and supervising others. For an organization to grow, the leader is actually hiring staff to assume roles that she had done herself. A clear job description, well thought out in advance of adding a new position to the organization, helps the leader to clarify what is expected from this new employee. Delegation, to be successful, confers on the new worker the authority to carry out the assigned responsibility. This is a basic tenet, often overlooked as geriatric care management organizations grow. Regular supportive supervision (a set day and time each week) is a way to ensure that the new employee will have opportunities to ask questions and provide feedback. As the numbers of staff increase, it is vital to divide the work into professional or clinical functions and business or support functions, thereby always ensuring that every worker has a supervisor. Adequate delegation frees the organization's leader to have time to continue to provide leadership. Remember, it is not possible to play all the instruments at the same time one is conducting the orchestra. Also, delegated tasks create opportunities for staff growth and development.

Caregiver Training

In geriatric care-managed caregiving organizations (which is the model adopted by Stowell Associates SelectStaff), it is essential to develop orientation and training programs to educate the caregivers in the mission, purpose, and culture of the organization. This training should focus on how to work as a team to foster the client's well-being. It should address these issues and more:

- The caregiver's role and responsibilities
- The organization's guidelines
- Communication skills

Basic caregiving duties must be addressed (e.g., nutrition, hygiene, grooming, exercise, medications). Universal safety training is important to prevent caregiver or client injury. Safety training may include body mechanics (positioning, transfers, lifting), environmental safety (slips, trips, falls), disaster preparedness (earthquake, fire, utility outage), universal precautions (infection control), crime prevention (home security, weapons, theft, loss), and what to do in case of an injury to a client or caregiver. Training that addresses problems of caring for clients

Table 13–1   Impact of Staff Training on the Development of Business, Leadership, and Clinical Skills

Type of Training	Business Skills	Leadership Skills	Clinical Skills
Team Building	Teaches process skills that enable staff to work together to achieve business objectives.	Teaches leadership skills within the team context. Shared leadership is experienced.	Teaches people to work with family "teams" and caregiver teams.
Conduct of meetings	Teaches business leadership.	Teaches how to get results in teams.	Teaches people to handle family meetings and caregiver team meetings.
Conflict resolution and mediation		Teaches this core leadership competency.	Teaches how conflict resolution skills improve clinical effectiveness with clients, families, caregiving staff, and allied professionals.
Supervisory skills	Teaches communication and relationship skills. Teaches legal responsibility and laws affecting supervision.		
Annual company retreat		Encourages personal and professional renewal.	
Renewal	Anchors individuals in personal values and a sense of purpose. Results in increased motivation and professional commitment.	Encourages personal and professional renewal.	Results in work/life balance and an increased connection to one's sense of purpose.
Time management	Improves overall business effectiveness.	Increases the awareness of what is important.	Assists with prioritizing competing client demands. Assists with work/life balance.
Presentation skills	Improves business presentations and professional image and credibility.	Improves communication and leadership skills.	
Countertransference			Increases clinician's awareness of his or her own issues. Teaches strategies for skillful interventions.
Continuing education. Allows staff to customize learning according to personal goals.			

suffering from dementia, depression, diabetes, arthritis, Parkinson's, and other conditions gives caregivers the skills to provide excellent care.

Developing Systems and Adding Expertise

Procedures, policies, processes, and systems must be documented as organizations mature so that institutional wisdom is preserved and processes and procedures become reproducible and transferable. A number of care management-specific computer software programs with electronic client records are available for lease or purchase. There are several proprietary care management software programs that are widely used at this time and are available at Jewel Code (www.jewelcode.com), Life Ledger (www.elderissuespro.com) and Care Manager Pro (www.caremanager-pro.com). Any growing care management organization should be investigating and investing in computer software as a regular part of their budgeting process so that needed updates of both software and hardware will help maintain competitiveness in a marketplace that increasingly relies on technology to improve both efficiency and maintain effectiveness.

In addition to using care management software, the agency will need to develop documentation that includes personnel, policy and procedure manuals stating the organization's policies regarding holidays, vacations, sick leave, health insurance, job descriptions, etc. Growing organizations are not static; therefore, it is vitally important to periodically renew and update policies and procedures manuals. An annual review of the personnel policies should be a part of the human resources function. If there is a human resources manager, this should be part of his or her job description. If human resources is not a separate department, the review and update can be outsourced to a consulting firm. However updating is done, it is imperative that personnel policy manuals reflect current legal requirements. In the mature geriatric care management organization, timely revision of the procedures manual is generally the responsibility of each department head and the overall concern of whoever is in charge of operations.

A growing care management agency must also add depth to its organizational structure, including hiring a comptroller or financial officer, bookkeeper and accounting clerk. Developing and maintaining excellent financial records, sending bills out on time and with a high degree of accuracy, managing the payroll efficiently and effectively, and keeping a close eye on expenses and cash flow are all extremely important functions that require a well-trained specialist to oversee. Usually these are not the areas of expertise of the founder of a geriatric care management company. Part of the growth strategy is to make sure that the business office is well staffed, with individuals of absolute integrity, who are as devoted to the mission of the agency as the care managers themselves.

■ ESTABLISHING WORKING RELATIONSHIPS WITH KEY ORGANIZATIONS IN THE COMMUNITY

The care management organization's CEO serves an extremely important function by being known in many circles in the community and being perceived as a leader. In a larger mature geriatric care management organization with many employees, the CEO should make the development of these kinds of relationships a priority. No matter what size community the organization is in, the CEO should network through volunteering with community groups and joining civic organizations.

This type of networking helps to grow the organization's position in the community through demonstrating a willingness to be helpful and generous. Relationships, to repeat again, grow only with time and nurturing. Simple gestures such as sending thank-you notes for referrals and offering volunteer assistance will help maintain and nurture good relationships.

The CEO of the mature geriatric care management organization may want to consider the following avenues to expand the organization's presence in the community:

- Memberships in service clubs (e.g., Rotary, Kiwanis, Lions): The business-people in these groups may not know what care management is, but they often have aging parents. Membership gives the CEO an opportunity to educate key decision makers about geriatric care management. From these diverse contacts may come invitations to speak and other opportunities to share expertise. Referrals of clients often follow from nurturing these types of business relationships.
- A seat on the board of directors of advisory committees and community organizations (e.g., the Better Business Bureau, Community Chest or United Way, YMCA/YWCA). Participation by the CEO on community boards can widen the organization's involvement in the community and enhance the organization's image. Participating in advisory committees for the planning of neighborhood, city, or county services is also an excellent way to extend one's involvement and make a difference in the community.
- Active involvement in the religious community: Active involvement in the religious community can provide the CEO with opportunities to educate volunteers and clergy working with older people. Religious organizations in every community in the United States are grappling

with the problems of serving a rapidly aging population. Older people tend to look to their religious communities for support. By building a role in the ecumenical conference of churches, synagogues, and other places of worship, the CEO can often educate those who are attempting to guide the efforts of volunteers. By supporting or training volunteers who serve older people, the CEO can contribute to the well-being of many older people. Religious leaders can be a valuable source of referrals of clients who need more services than volunteers can provide.

CEOs may also want to take the following steps:

- Attend attorneys' community meetings. A significant group of professionals serving older people are attorneys specializing in wills and probate, estate planning, or other elder-law issues. Elder-law attorneys are becoming aware of the invaluable services GCMs can provide. Educating attorneys by attending their community meetings, providing information on health or psychosocial issues affecting older people, and making referrals to them when appropriate can foster relationships with this group of professionals who can become valuable referral sources for a growing care management organization.
- Call regularly on trust officers, trust departments, and accounting firms. These professionals are seeing the number of older people they are serving increase rapidly. Many of them become trusted counselors to their clients, but frequently there comes a time when the client's ability to make safe and sensible personal decisions diminishes or he or she becomes physically dependent and requires more personal care from others. These professionals are not trained in

assessment of need, provision, or supervision of home care. The mature care management organization's reputation for cooperation and service can be built by making personal calls, speaking at group meetings, and providing educational information regarding the role of geriatric care management.

- Call regularly on senior centers and when possible give presentations or host an event. In almost every community, senior centers provide education, recreation, and socialization programs vital to the well-being of active older people. The activity directors of these centers are often the first people to see signs of deterioration or disease. Adult day centers providing support and activities for special groups such as people with Alzheimer's or muscular dystrophy serve a very vulnerable group of older people who can often benefit from care management services. Ongoing contact, occasional talks to groups, and sponsorship of special events build awareness and trust of the geriatric care management organization.

- Maintain contacts with support organizations. In larger cities there are organizations providing counseling, specialized information, and referrals for older people and their families. These may be regional caregiver resource centers, Alzheimer's Association chapters, or associations organized for the education of people with other diseases and their families. The area agencies on aging provide information and referrals exclusively focused on the needs and issues of older people. Keeping these agencies regularly supplied with printed material describing the care management organization can be an important way to increase awareness of the care management organization expertise. Occasional talks at in-service training programs are

also helpful to keep new staff updated about the organization's services.

- Attend coordinating councils. In most areas, associations of professionals come together to share information, give mutual support, and network. These are often known as councils on aging or coalitions of elder services. Attendance and participation can foster good relationships with people in a wide circle of related service organizations.

In fact, there seems to be no limit to opportunities for networking with allied professionals. Tracking of referral sources will yield clues to which activities result in the best referrals. Measuring the goodwill engendered by the active participation suggested here is harder to measure. Building community awareness and good relationships is, for the mature care management organization, not only building the business but also building the perceived value of the organization in its community.

■ JOINING ORGANIZATIONS AND NETWORKING NATIONALLY

National organizations dealing with the concerns of aging have grown significantly since the mid-1980s. Many professionals who are still active in the field participated in the formation of these associations. Gerontology is a new field of study, less than 50 years old. The National Association of Professional Geriatric Care Managers celebrated its 25th birthday in 2010, but it is still unknown to many. Media coverage of aging issues in general and care management specifically has increased markedly in the past few years because of a growing awareness that the baby boomers are aging, which is creating new interest among business people, healthcare providers, and politicians.

Participation and networking in national organizations can inform the growing care management organization of legislative trends in health care, the results of scientific studies, and developments in clinical practices. As geriatric care management develops beyond a specialization within other professions such as nursing and social work into a profession of its own, new knowledge is developing and interaction with colleagues through these national organizations is enriching. Mutual support and open dialogue can be invaluable. The mature organization has the opportunity to present material to educate and mentor newer colleagues. Opportunities to participate in the development of professional organizations inform efforts to develop the individual geriatric care management organization. Here is a list of some of the leading national organizations of interest to the mature geriatric care management business:

- National Association of Professional Geriatric Care Managers (NAPGCM) and CMSA are both membership organizations for geriatric care managers that a mature organization's CEO should join (www.caremanager.org and www.cmsa. org). Consider getting involved in the organization's activities and perhaps run for office. This level of participation allows the leader to develop a broader understanding of national trends in aging policy, the policy development necessary to ensure supportive care for older people. It provides opportunities for the national organization and its members to strengthen and expand the services that will be needed.

- The National Council on Aging (NCOA) is one of the older associations addressing issues relating to aging. The National Council on Aging (www.ncoa. org) focuses on the issues and concerns of service providers, but its scope is much broader than that of organizations focused on provider issues. The needs and concerns of many different groups serving older people, such as

home care providers, senior centers, activity programs, or housing projects, to name a few, are addressed. This association also provides legislative advocacy.

- The American Association of Retired Persons (AARP) is the largest of all the geriatric associations (www.aarp.org). Its financial base is insurance and other business ventures. It exerts a strong legislative advocacy presence and ensures the participation of older people through volunteer groups at the local, state, and national levels. It publishes *Modern Maturity,* a magazine that addresses a wide range of geriatric issues and targets older readers.

- The Gerontological Society of America deals primarily with research and the interests of academia (www.geron.org). There are four primary sections: biological, psychological, behavioral, and policy. Emphasis at the annual meetings is on the presentation of research findings.

- The American Society on Aging puts emphasis on training at the undergraduate level and sharing information regarding advances in the field (www.asaging. org). The American Society on Aging has developed a strong program of seminars, often clustered around annual or regional meetings as preconference educational opportunities. The focus is on a wide array of services provided to older people, including care management.

- The National Association of Elder Law Attorneys is open for membership to attorneys only (www.naela.com). The National Association of Elder Law Attorneys and the National Association of Professional Geriatric Care Managers have held several joint conferences. Opportunities to participate on panels and to promote cooperation between the professions can work to the benefit of both organizations.

The mature geriatric care management organization can benefit from participation in the conferences and activities of numerous national organizations. Choices are clearly necessary. Membership in national organizations can be costly in terms of money, time, and energy. Establishing priorities for national participation and sampling conferences can help determine the extent to which the mature care management organization involves itself in networking at the national level.

ACCREDITATION

Obtaining accreditation from a national accrediting organization is another strategy that mature care management organizations may decide to pursue as part of their strategic planning. Accreditation demonstrates to clients that the organization has achieved a level of excellence based on national standards that can set the organization apart from its competition. Accreditation can also substitute for state licensing when a client has long-term care insurance—many of these contracts called for state-licensed care providers, but many states do not require any licensure for either care management or the caregiving services provided by many care management companies. The mature care management organization can explore the following organizations if it decides to seek national accreditation:

1. Council on Accreditation (COA)
   120 Wall Street, 11th Floor
   New York, New York 10005
   (212) 797-3000
   www.coanet.org

The COA was started in 1977 by the Child Welfare League of America and Family Service of America. It accredits 38 different services, including care management and home care. COA standards are based on a social service model, consistent with the point of view of care management. Stowell Associates Select-Staff has been accredited by COA since 2000.

2. The Joint Commission
   One Renaissance Blvd.
   Oakbrook Terrace, IL 60181
   (630) 792-5000
   www.jointcommission.org

The Joint Commission (formerly known as JCAHO) began to accredit healthcare organizations, primarily hospitals, in 1951. It has expanded its standards to include accreditation of medical equipment, hospices, home care, nursing homes, and other organizations. Joint Commission standards are based on a medical model, and most of the home care agencies it accredits are state-licensed organizations that provide Medicare and Medicaid services.

3. Accreditation Commission for Health
   Care, Inc. (ACHC)
   4700 Falls of Neuse Rd., Suite 280
   Raleigh, NC 27609
   (919) 785-1214
   www.achc.org

The ACHC began in 1985 in Raleigh, North Carolina, through the efforts of members of the state home care association, and it accredited its first organization in 1987. The company began offering services nationally in 1996. It accredits home care services, as well as other health-related services such as medical equipment and specialty pharmacies.

4. Community Health Accreditation Program
   (CHAP)
   1275 K Street, NW, Suite 800
   Washington, DC 20036
   (202) 862-3413
   www.chapinc.org

CHAP was established in 1965 as a joint venture between the American Public Health Association and the National League for Nursing. In 2001, it became an independent, nonprofit corporation. It accredits 10 services, including home health, private duty services, home care aide services, and supplemental staffing services.

5. Commission on Accreditation of
   Rehabilitation Facilities (CARF)
   4891 E. Grant Road
   Tucson, AZ 85712
   (520) 325-1044
   www.carf.org

CARF was founded in 1966. It is a private, not-for-profit organization that promotes quality rehabilitation services, aging services, child and family services, behavioral health, employment and community services, and medical rehabilitation. It also accredits continuing care communities under the Continuing Care Accreditation Commission.

■ CONCLUSION

As the geriatric care management organization matures, it will revisit many of the steps it undertook in its infancy and take new steps on new pathways. These steps begin with redefining the organization's niche, confirming or changing the model of practice, and strengthening or adjusting its image in the community. The mature organization will need to rethink its marketing program and its strategy for organizational development through ongoing strategic planning. In addition, the organization will need to solidify its working relationships with key organizations in the community and reassess its involvement with national professional organizations. Finally, the mature care management organization may decide to seek national accreditation as a way of distinguishing itself in the marketplace and ensuring it meets the highest quality of national standards.

■ REFERENCES

1. Taylor W. Permission marketing. *Fast Company*. April–May 1998;198–212.
2. Senge P. *The Fifth Discipline: The Art and Practice of the Learning Organization*. New York: Doubleday; 1990.
3. Collins J, Porras J. Building your company's vision. *Harvard Bus Rev*. 1996;74:65–77.
4. Wheatley M, Kellner-Rogers M. *A Simpler Way*. San Francisco, CA: Berrett-Koehler Publishers; 1996.
5. Anderson B. *Pathways to Partnership*. Whitehouse, OH: Soulworks; 1998.

Chapter 14

Fee-for-Service Care Management in Not-for-Profit Settings

Stephne Lencioni, Kathleen J. McConnell, and Cathy Jo Cress

■ INTRODUCTION

The growth rate of the world's older adult population represents the most dramatic demographic shift in history. Projections are that in 2030, more than 20% of Americans will be 65 years of age or older, with the fastest-growing segment being the oldest-old, those 85 years and older. Increased longevity can produce an array of specialized needs, ranging from services such as health care, housing, home care, and nursing facilities to opportunities for recreation, leisure time activities, and education. Older adults may face health, cognitive, financial, legal, and housing problems with little or no idea of where to get help. Family members who care for older relatives also struggle with these same issues. To address these unique needs, a senior services industry has developed that has become big business and has enormous potential for profit.

One of the important components of the aging business is care management. Many older adults and their families are willing—and able—to pay for assistance with care planning and service selection. The growth of for-profit care management business has demonstrated the fact that there are customers to purchase these services. Picking up on this trend, the presence of fee-for-service (FFS) care management in the not-for-profit (NFP) agency has been slowly but steadily growing.

Probable reasons for the slow growth lie in both philosophical and operational issues. As NFPs have considered adding FFS services, agency leaders have found themselves in debates about their organizations' missions. Some struggle with what they see as conflicting goals. Traditionally, NFPs focus on service and meeting community needs, whereas the for-profit culture often measures success in terms of profitability. Others resist the new emphasis on the market. However, many large NFPs have taken the position that if there is no profit margin, they cannot continue their primary mission of serving people in need. The debate is not a simple one nor has it been resolved.

Contrary to the past, today NFPs and government agencies are no longer the only trusted providers of services for older people. Quality services are now found in the for-profit sector as well. As funding sources shrink, NFPs are at risk of being left to serve only the poor and to operate at a deficit. Thus, to expand the client base and to offset the expenses of serving those who cannot pay, many NFPs are competing with private for-profit entities for clients who can afford to pay for service.

Initial interest in establishing FFS case management programs within NFP agencies was twofold: to develop the capacity to meet the needs of multiple income groups and to generate revenue. FFS case management evolved very slowly within NFP agencies during the mid- to late 1980s, and then picked up during the 1990s. Knutson and Langer, in a survey of geriatric care management practice, found that by 1997, NFPs made up 16% of the membership of the National Association of Professional Geriatric Care Managers, an organization formerly accepting only for-profit practices as members.[1]

This chapter explores the development of FFS case management programs in NFP settings. It draws on the experiences of three agencies that have successfully implemented such programs: the Council of Jewish Elderly (CJE) in Chicago, Illinois; Huntington Hospital Senior Care Network (SCN) in Pasadena, California; and Older Adults Care Management (OACM), a division of the Institute on Aging (IOA), in Palo Alto, California. The Council of Jewish Elderly, a large NFP agency, has always provided some form of case management services. Fee-for-service care management was started in 1995 to address the need for producing revenue from services to offset budget deficits. By the late 1990s, FFS care management was a part of CJE's continuum and a self-supporting service. Huntington Hospital Senior Care Network developed FFS case management in response to a clear need; namely, people with higher incomes had no access to case management services even though they experienced the same problems as people with lower incomes. Another objective was to generate revenue. The program grew from one to six care managers and incorporated a variety of care management services, including long-term care insurance underwriting and claims assessments, elder care services for employed caregivers, and other fee-based contract services. In contrast, OACM began as a for-profit agency in 1982 and only later became an NFP after being gifted to the nonprofit IOA in 1999. OACM was originally conceived as a case manage-

ment business but soon added a licensed home care component to meet the identified need for hands-on assistance to elderly clients. Its history as a for-profit agency along with the coexistence of care management and home care services created both opportunities and challenges for OACM.

■ TERMINOLOGY AND DEFINITION

Historically, social workers were caseworkers. The term *case management,* which implies that people are "cases" with their lives to be managed, has come to seem both negative and paternalistic. Despite numerous potential alternatives (e.g., care coordination, service management, service coordination), *case management* continues to be a commonly used term. However, *care management* is gradually becoming the preferred terminology, especially among FFS professionals. But, as pointed out by Bodie Gross and Holt, "From a consumer's perspective, there is no difference between a care and case manager. The sole standard of judgment is one of satisfaction with the services being delivered."[2(p23)]

For the purposes of this chapter, *care management* is most frequently used, especially when referring to fee-based services. However, *case management* may be used when referring to a particular program or where that is the common terminology.

Just as no one name or title is used for case management, there is no single agreed-on definition of *case management or scope of services.* However, there is consensus on the key tasks performed by the case manager: assessment, care planning, coordination, follow-up (including monitoring of client status and service delivery), reassessment, and termination or case closure. Although the focus here is on care management for older people and their families, it is important to note that care management is used in a wide range of settings for a variety of populations.[3]

■ BRIEF HISTORY OF CASE MANAGEMENT

It is difficult to trace the beginnings of case management definitively because many disciplines lay claim to inventing at least some element of it.[4] Its principles can be found in the early 1900s in the social work settlement movement, but public nursing, mental health, disability, and other fields can all point to historical beginnings of case management within their own discipline. Clearly, identifying and solving problems by assessing needs, linking people to needed resources, and coordinating the delivery of services are central themes of case management throughout the history of human services.

Geriatric case management grew popular as a means of reducing public costs of long-term care. Case management programs of the 1970s and early 1980s were largely funded with public dollars—specifically through the Medicaid program—and targeted the low-income, frail elderly population at risk of institutionalization. The goal of case management was to decrease the use and expense of nursing home care by keeping individuals at home with supportive services. Through these and other national demonstration projects, case management became an important part of long-term care programs.[5] Many of these projects were implemented in NFP agencies as part of a continuum of services provided for older people. They all used case management, which rapidly became a popular approach to linking clients with needed resources.

By the mid-1990s, some form of case management could be found in virtually every service setting: geriatric care management was delivered in public government agencies; in private not-for-profit settings that used a combination of public funds, fundraising, grants, and FFS dollars; and in FFS private practice. In fact, the private practice business was enjoying enough success that professionals and paraprofessionals from a wide range of educational and disciplinary backgrounds were opening FFS care management businesses catering to families of means. This trend continues and is expected to grow.

■ THE DEVELOPMENT OF FEE-FOR-SERVICE CARE MANAGEMENT

With the proliferation of publicly funded case management programs that focused on low-income populations, private FFS care management was a logical development. The need for help solving problems associated with aging is not linked to income. Families at all income levels share the same sense of helplessness when crises occur, and often lack knowledge of available resources. Parker delineates the reasons why families hire care managers:

- The need for a professional assessment
- The need for an objective opinion regarding service options
- Help with the feeling of being overwhelmed
- The inability to resolve family conflicts
- Help in transitioning a relative to a nursing home
- Long-distance caregiving issues
- The need for respite care
- Help with filling out forms[6(pp4-5)]

Higher-income families ineligible for income-based case management programs provided the ideal market for the for-profit care management business. These families had the means and the willingness to pay for services they wanted.

Doing Market Research to See Whether Your Nonprofit Area Can Support a GCM

Does a for-profit geriatric care management business fit into your nonprofit organization? To make this decision, it is best to do a market feasibility study before you decide to add a GCM to your present service mix. Have you weighed the chances of a for-profit succeeding in your present nonprofit culture? Have you studied the competition in your area? Have you evaluated the number of customers and potential demand for these care management services? All these steps should be taken in evaluating the opportunity to add a for-profit geriatric care management arm to your existing nonprofit agency. Hiring an outside consulting firm to do this market feasibility study is a good business move and may save your nonprofit many dollars and regretted decisions. (See the Chapter 12 section, "Professional Consultants.")

An informal survey done in 2010 of seven large nonprofits who added a GCM component found that only two had been profitable, and none of them had done a survey of the market opportunity before launching the care management practice. The mix included care management practices within an Area Agency on Aging, Visiting Nurse Association, Jewish Family Services, and two long-standing former Medicare waivers who had all added GCM services at some time in the last 30 years. Only two had achieved profitability after 25 years. They stated their success could have been increased by several good business decisions, which will be covered in this chapter. In retrospect, the nonprofits polled believe they could still have gone forward and would have been profitable sooner, if they designed and marketed their services differently including care manager roles, marketing, and infrastructure. A feasibility study can guide a nonprofit in evaluating the investment required, the critical success factors, and the growth objectives that create a roadmap for a successful implementation.

Defining Your Customer Base and Referral Sources

The first thing that a nonprofit would be wise to do is to define the customers they wish to serve with a new care management practice. These aging customers and their adult children will buy your product of geriatric care management services. You start by defining the ideal client who will pay for and can afford your GCM services. In essence this will take creating a new business plan for your GCM for-profit business, to complement the business plan for your existing nonprofit agency. The market analysis includes a definition of the target client's age, income, family structure, and level of chronic care needs. Income becomes an important criteria as care management services are almost entirely private pay, which is a significant difference for most nonprofit organizations. We can't overstate the importance of this shift, as your nonprofit would now be providing care management services to a clientele largely made up of households with income greater than $100,000, and your new GCM business would need to attract clients who have an average income level in the top 1%. (Refer to Chapter 12, How to Start or Add a Geriatric Care Management Business.)

Next you need to determine the geographic footprint of the market you wish your GCM for-profit arm to serve. You should look at your entire nonprofit services area. For example, if your nonprofit serves the whole state of Rhode Island, the entire city of San Diego, the zip code 33023 in Hollywood, these are the areas you would examine. You are searching for the section in your nonprofit service area most likely to yield older clients and their families who can afford GCM services.

If you cover all the counties in Rhode Island, select all those counties. Create a market survey of those counties to find out which counties have the highest number of seniors with the highest income described as your ideal client. You will be using the US census figures and other metrics. (See the section on targeting your audience in Chapter 16, Marketing Geriatric Care Management.)

Finding the Highest Number of Internal and External Referral Sources

Your care management practice will rely (and can thrive) on referrals both internally as well as from your existing partnerships and networks. You will be looking at all the areas your nonprofit serves for the one section that contains the highest number of third-party referral sources for your GCM add-on business. To do this you need to outline all the third-party GCM referral sources, like elder-law attorneys, physicians, and trust officers who will refer your GCM clients to your new GCM business. (See the "Targeting Audiences" section in Chapter 16, Marketing Geriatric Care Management.)

Following the survey, you should do a competition survey of all GCMs who serve the areas your nonprofit covers. You are surveying who your competition is and discovering if you can achieve market share in the area you choose to serve.[7] You want to create a survey that tracks the individual GCMs in your service area, and find out what their fees per hour are, do they now include home care, and what geriatric care management services does each competing GCM offer. For example do the local GCM businesses offer care monitoring, do they offer home care or any of the standard GCM services and products? Next you want to survey what geographic areas your potential GCM competitors serve. You can use this to set your home care agencies' hourly fees, choose competitive geriatric care management services and products, and make all your fees competitive in the area you finally choose to serve. It will also tell you if the local market is too saturated for your nonprofit to compete with the other care management agencies. This will also help you position yourself in your market and decide what new innovative GCM services you can offer that other geriatric care managers do not sell.

You should also identify and survey other direct GCM competitors like the area agency on aging, which may have a GCM arm or for-profits like accountants or elder-law attorneys who include geriatric care management in their service mix.

Identify substitute providers (i.e., agencies or private providers offering assessments, medical advocacy, and residential care guidance), and record their services offering and pricing structure. These can also be part of your competition to take market share.

All these competition surveys will recommend marketing and positioning alternatives in your competitive landscape.

Identifying Potential Referral Sources in Your External Market

You also should evaluate existing eldercare providers in the external marketplace to determine your potential GCM referral sources. You are again measuring the degree to which the market currently would support your private FFS GCM services. You would want to look, for example, at the number of Alzheimer's Association chapters and Older American Act programs in your market such as friendly visitors and senior transportation. You can also look at services like adult day care, home care agencies, and assisted living facilities if located in the service area county and may refer to your new geriatric care management arm.

You should also identify your targeted audiences. This is broadly older people who have an income over $100,000 and their adult children who buy GCM services for their loved one. It also includes third parties who refer to geriatric care managers. To establish who your target audience is for your new GCM agency, see Chapter 16 about marketing to targeted audiences.

Looking at Your Existing Nonprofit for Potential Internal GCM Customers

After you have completed these investigations, you want to look internally and survey your own nonprofit services for potential referral to your new geriatric care management business. If you have a home care agency, hospice, or a skilled nursing facility, they are an ideal source of referral to GCM services. You would begin by listing all of the services you offer, such as home care, independent living, hospice, information and referral, or counseling could generate and refer GCM clients who can pay for your new GCM service. You need to identify which of your existing services would produce clients and customers to your new for-profit geriatric care management business.

To begin this internal investigation, start with an introductory meeting with key internal groups or divisions to explain what geriatric care management is. Many human service professionals do not understand geriatric care management. That internal meeting should cover what geriatric care management is and why your staff should buy into adding this program to your mix, if it is feasible. Social workers and nurses many times see themselves as delivering care management services already and can be very threatened by adding GCM services to your nonprofit services. They may see you taking away what they give away for free because that is what clients deserve. They may also see their own jobs threatened by this new service. You need to demonstrate how the GCM program will benefit all clients in your nonprofit services such as home care, counseling, or skilled nursing. Then you need to demonstrate how each staff member will benefit by the addition of GCM services. This is critical so your nonprofit staff can see the advantage of incorporating GCM services into your program and will make referrals. You are in effect priming the well of internal referrals. After you do this, you could begin surveying your staff to measure whether you have potential GCM clients in your present services who would pay for geriatric care management services.

Following that internal needs assessment, you can design a survey of which internal clients in your nonprofit could use GCM services and have a meeting with the managers of each service to discuss how to do the survey. You want to tally the number of potential GCM customers in your existing nonprofit customer base. You would want to find out which service could refer GCM clients. As an alternative you could send out the survey to measure approximately how many clients each service feels they could refer to a for-profit GCM service. You will want to set up a means for tracking and rewarding internal referrals, and also for providing feedback to referral sources when prospective clients weren't a good fit (and for what reason). This closed-loop feedback of both the successful and unsuccessful referrals will help educate your internal partners and improve your lead-generating relationships.

■ FINANCIAL MODELING

With your market and competitive analysis complete, you are now ready to start the financial planning process for your care management practice. The goal is to complete the following:

1. Forecast profit or loss over the first 3 to 5 years
2. Plan for three scenarios (best case, average performance, and worst case) to help you envision the different paths your expansion can take
3. Manage your cash flow, which is distinct from your profit or loss

In fact, more companies fail due to cash flow constraints than from any other single factor. For a detailed financial modeling analysis, see Chapter 15, Combining a Home Care Agency and a GCM Practice.

■ PUBLIC NOT-FOR-PROFIT AND PRIVATE SETTINGS

Geriatric care management has similarities that are independent of the setting in which it is provided. The same tasks are performed with regard to assessment, care planning, referral, service coordination, and monitoring. Care managers must have the educational background, professional skills, and training to handle the challenges they will encounter when called into difficult and complicated situations. There must be some provision for after-hours emergencies. Caseload numbers are limited to enhance the quality of service delivery. Forms, procedures, and billing may be similar in both NFP and private agencies; however, the NFPs may have federal, state, or local regulations; external funding requirements; and internal policies and guidelines because of their nonprofit status that may affect their practice and procedures.

Overall, FFS practice has the major advantage of being free of constraints, thus enabling a customized, intensive, and personal relationship that is important to clients looking for a surrogate family member. This may be even more true for an FFS private practice as opposed to an FFS program within an NFP setting. Parker explains how FFS private practice is different from public and NFP geriatric care management:

- **Eligibility.** Whereas there are strict eligibility requirements to participate in a publicly funded program, the ability to pay a fee is usually the only criteria for becoming an FFS client.
- **Availability.** Private practitioners will typically be on call or actually available 24 hours a day and on weekends.
- **Staff turnover.** Unlike the public agency with higher caseloads and more frequent staff turnover, the private care manager is more likely to be able to offer a more stable, long-term relationship.
- **Conflicts.** There appear to be fewer conflicts about providing direct services in addition to care management, including home aides and companions.[6(pp4–5)]

■ FEE-FOR-SERVICE IN A NOT-FOR-PROFIT SETTING

The FFS geriatric care management program within an NFP agency offers different kinds of advantages. Many NFPs provide other services in addition to care management, giving clients served by the agency more choices and an opportunity for more closely coordinated services. NFPs often employ a multidisciplinary staff, enabling cross-training and collaboration that may result in a better-quality product for the client. A case in point is the OACM client who chooses to take advantage of both the case management and home care programs. The client will receive coordinated care by a team consisting of the care manager, a nurse, a home care coordinator and scheduler, and a home care aide. Additional services of the parent IOA NFP may also be considered and coordinated. A well-established NFP can also offer greater fiscal security to a fledgling FFS care management program. Unlike many of the smaller for-profit companies, a well-funded NFP is more financially secure and therefore able to support the care management program in times of slower business.

Another advantage of the NFP is its standing and perception in the community. Through its established community relationships and reputation, the NFP brings immediate credibility to the geriatric care management program and can help it grow. Many potential referral sources come from social service settings with cultures that are more comfortable with NFP programs than with private for-profits. Geriatric care managers have an entire agency behind them and great support in the beginning of the program when many crises are to be faced and much is still to be learned.

In addition to positives, Vocker discusses some negatives of integrating FFS geriatric care management into an NFP agency.[8] Many NFPs receive case management funding through the Older Americans Act (OAA) and are thereby subject to certain requirements and criteria. To be a recipient of OAA-funded case management services, a client must be at least 60 years old and live in the geographic area served by the agency. Through OAA funding, an agency is also required to be open 8 hours each weekday and never closed for 4 or more consecutive days. When the agency is closed, alternative assistance must be offered. This could include access to staff pager numbers or arrangements with police and fire departments. In addition, the agency must meet the needs of non-English-speaking and physically challenged clients. Other types of requirements cover case assignments, care plans, and supervision.

Geriatric care management is an around-the-clock business, and it can be hard to get staff to participate in after-hours service. Also, because of its time-intensive nature, FFS geriatric care management typically means smaller caseloads; thus, keeping track of client caseloads is especially important. In some NFP settings, FFS clients are not the only clients served by any one care manager in the agency, so it is important to monitor the GCM's ability to respond to the intensive expectations of FFS clients.

If the NFP offers both publicly funded and FFS case management programs with separate staffing, friction may arise between the different care managers. Because geriatric care management is so labor intensive, staff in the public program, invariably working with a low-income population with fewer available resources, may feel that they are in the trenches doing the hard work and may resent the disproportionate amount of time spent with the paying clients. It is critical that an NFP create an internal culture that is mutually respectful of both case management programs.

■ NOT-FOR-PROFIT FFS PROGRAM DEVELOPMENT CHALLENGES

In making the decision to implement FFS care management, NFP boards and staff address many questions. Will FFS alter our commitment to serve those most in need? Will revenue-seeking activities compromise other social service involvement? If building the business means selling services, how can client interests come first? Are we being driven by profit motives? Should services be different if people are paying? What would it mean to have a two-tiered system? How can we work with demanding customers when we went into this to help the needy and vulnerable? Will we be asked and have to do things that seem unprofessional yet are therapeutically appropriate and within the scope of case management such as escorting someone to the opera?

NFPs continue to struggle with these fundamental questions as they develop FFS programs and must consider and resolve them if programs are to succeed. Among the biggest hurdles is overcoming the reluctance to charge fees. Other major challenges include developing a customer orientation and marketing FFS care management services.

Overcoming the Reluctance to Charge Fees

Charging fees in exchange for services remains one of the most difficult challenges in developing FFS care management in an NFP setting. Generally, charging for services has been considered inappropriate for the NFP sector. The reluctance to charge for services most likely stems from traditional attitudes that the NFP sector's mission is to provide access to those who are unable to pay or to meet other criteria such as need, status, condition, location, race, ethnicity, or religion. In many cases, services are given to clients who are not eligible for public-sector case management or prefer not to use it. But decreasing opportunities to acquire public dollars and private donations for direct care have led more NFPs to generate revenues through fees.

Although there are clinical as well as fiscal and operational reasons to collect fees, there has been significant resistance within NFPs to implementing FFS programs. This resistance has come from all groups: staff, volunteers, administrators, and clients who have been receiving free services for many years.

Many human service professionals who have worked in publicly funded social services and the NFP sector appear to suffer from a type of fee phobia. For example, when SCN first developed its FFS program in 1985, it was difficult to find professionals who were comfortable with charging for care management. These professionals felt that social services should be free to clients and that clients would not pay or would refuse help if they were charged. The professionals were inexperienced in setting rates and did not feel confident about negotiating fees. Many of them objected to the idea of selling services, stating that they did not choose to become a social worker (or nurse or other human services professional) to work as a salesperson.

Charging a reasonable fee for GCM services is problematic for many people in the helping profession. Case managers often undervalue the expertise and commitment they bring to their profession. They set their hourly fee too low or are alarmed at the hourly fee established by the sponsoring agency.

This may occur because in previous positions, case managers have been paid a salary and are unaware of the many costs associated with running a business. The charge for hourly case management looks large when compared to the hourly rate received by the care manager, but it must be recognized that salary is only one portion of the cost of doing business.

A more perplexing aspect of this concern over fees is the guilt that people feel over charging specialist fees. GCMs act as if anyone could do what they do. This is simply not true. Case managers need to acknowledge their expertise in geriatrics, a process that has involved years of preparation. Their emotional resilience, even in the face of the most heartbreaking situations, a GCM persists and crafts a care plan for the best outcome possible.

A GCM exhibits good judgment, professional commitment, and an understanding of what is possible. These are attributes that are extremely valuable in providing care to the elderly. They are not available in the public at large.

GCMs need to focus on their unique skills and acknowledge that because of those abilities they should be compensated as a specialist in geriatric care. It is money well spent!

The Council of Jewish Elderly struggled with many of these same issues. This organization began its FFS private geriatric care management service with a few interested staff members who took on cases. The intake worker who responded to initial inquiries played a significant role in engaging callers to view the service as viable. An after-hours call system was developed, and only supervisory staff responded, to protect staff time. As the number of cases grew, the staff became excited, particularly by the positive feedback they received from clients. Staff members were soon sold on the idea and requested beepers so they could respond to their own after-hours calls. The few specialists' enthusiasm was infectious, and other staff members became interested in providing care management services.

Most practitioners who provide care management in NFPs have backgrounds in helping professions in which revenue is not discussed. Many of these practitioners believe that older adults have no disposable income and should be taken care of because they are needy and frail. It is difficult for these practitioners to 'see their services as products and think that older people should pay a fee for those services. The OACM experience was different in that they did not encounter fee resistance from the case management staff. The OACM model used clinical supervision from a licensed clinical social worker (LCSW) in private practice who was used to selling services. One of the case managers also had a background with a large assisted living chain and was quite comfortable with marketing activities. These two factors combined with the fact that OACM has been in the business of selling home care services for many years created a culture where fee-for-service was the norm.

Early in SCN's FFS program, staff noticed that clients also created barriers to selling care management as a service. Many clients said that they should not have to and could not afford to pay for this kind of service. Others thought that because they had already donated to the organization, they were entitled to get free services. Still others believed that if they did pay for both case management and a service provider, they would spend more money than necessary.

In his study of nontraditional in-home services, Hereford reports that older people did not see case management as a distinct product worthy of a fee.[9] Prior to implementing its FFS care management program, CJE conducted market research that reinforced this perspective. It was found by CJE that fees of $50 to $100 per hour were considered too high; a few older adults would pay $20 per hour, but most wanted to pay nothing. Family members, on the other hand, supported the concept of paying fees for this service.

Many of today's older adults still have what is known as Depression-era thinking—the desire to preserve every penny to save for a rainy day. Many services to seniors have been based on entitlement, and consequently, many seniors expect services to be provided for them. Older adults also find it distasteful to pay for something they could previously do for themselves. Others resist outside involvement by a professional because they fear a greater loss of control than they already experience as a result of aging. The OACM experience has found that it is easier to deliver quality service when the bill paying is done by someone other than the older adult (e.g., an adult relative, a bank, a trustee, a conservator).

A reorientation of practice philosophy is necessary to shift staff members' thinking about charging fees for these services. An NFP needs to help staff see the need for revenue to offset deficits and survive in a time of more limited resources. Full-paying clients are needed so the agency can continue to serve those who cannot afford to pay.

Sales training sessions, sessions to increase understanding of NFP funding mechanisms, and sessions teaching about marketing and appreciating the value of care management as a professional service were all held for FFS staff at SCN. Letting staff members articulate their objections and do role-playing helped them be comfortable with charging fees. Care management program managers at SCN focused on establishing a business mentality, paying attention to changing attitudes as well as language. Figure 14–1 shows an example of training materials used to help achieve this shift.

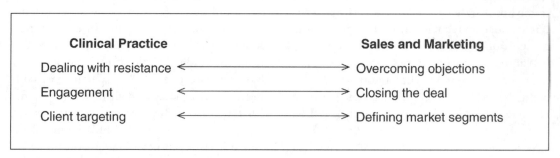

Clinical Practice		**Sales and Marketing**
Dealing with resistance	⟷	Overcoming objections
Engagement	⟶	Closing the deal
Client targeting	⟷	Defining market segments

Figure 14–1   Clinical Practice with Sales and Marketing

Source: Reprinted with permission by Lynn Hackstaff, LCSW, Downey Kaiser Permanente, Orchard MOB Family Medicine & Orchard Urgent Care HealthCenter (OUCH).

In response to similar issues, CJE spent considerable time defining care management so that staff could comfortably articulate the benefits of the service. Then staff could better help older adults and families understand the value and necessity of care management when it was indicated. Staff worked on increasing their comfort with fees through outlining and challenging staff biases and paternalistic views about what older people could understand and afford. Discussions were held with private practice GCMs about their views, which helped staff members realize the value of their services in the marketplace. Role-playing was used to increase everyone's comfort level. Once again, OACM's experience was different in that the hourly rate was set at $100, which included charging for visits, phone calls, and e-mails. The client was told of this up front, and a contract was signed. The main challenge that OACM faced was getting its care managers to keep careful track of billable time. A weekly time sheet was developed that motivated staff to keep better track of time spent. In addition, a monthly revenue report is done where the case managers can see how much they billed, both in regards to individual clients and also in relationship to their coworkers.

This type of a practitioner paradigm shift takes time. The reality is that some care managers have an easier time with charging fees than other care managers do. To integrate a private care management philosophy into NFP structures, an organization needs to allow for some anxiety and sadness about the change. It is important, wherever possible, to create mechanisms for staff input into the development of the service. One way to begin is to identify staff who are comfortable with fees and create specialist positions. They can then act as champions as the program develops. The organization's leaders should think about similar changes from the organization's past and what helped ensure staff commitment as those changes were taking place.

DEVELOPING A CUSTOMER ORIENTATION

Care management, for a fee, provides many of the case management services traditionally offered by senior and social services agencies at no cost to clients. When an NFP decides to develop an FFS care management model, it must also develop a customer orientation rather than the traditional client orientation. Customers expect to have choices and to be treated in a special way, with privacy, flexibility, control, quality, and a personal touch. This customer orientation begins with the first phone contact. In a customer-oriented approach, the phone call will be answered quickly, by a pleasant human being as opposed to a recording and menu, and the caller will be efficiently directed to an employee who can knowledgably discuss case management services. Whereas best practice dictates that the client should be involved in the decision-making process whenever it is feasible, there is usually an increased expectation on the part of the paying client that they will have ultimate say over their plan of care and what services they will use.

In traditional case management, the case manager identifies what he or she thinks the client needs, and then tries to ration services to meet those needs, when possible still relying on the support of family members, neighbors, and other people in the client's life. This is very different from the "surrogate child" or "substitute family member" model associated with private geriatric care management. Private GCMs are available weekends and evenings to provide the personalized touch that accommodates requests above and beyond just client need.

At CJE, every effort was made to develop an FFS geriatric care management business that reflected an integrated practice model. This model balances customer wishes with assessed needs and priorities to maximize independence, reduce risk, and strengthen family support. For both paying and nonpaying older people, the values and goals were similar.

A major goal at SCN was to develop a true care management continuum with a full range of opportunities for older people to receive services regardless of income or condition. Centered on a triage model with professional telephone screening, consultation, information, and referral, SCN established case management programs with several public and private funding sources. The addition of FFS care management made the service available to virtually anyone. It also created a customer service approach that eventually permeated the other programs. Although OACM provides strictly fee-for-service care management, its parent organization, IOA, provides services to those who cannot pay.

■ MARKETING

A critical factor in creating an FFS geriatric care management business in an NFP is the image of the organization. A marketing plan needs to be developed that communicates that the agency is broadening its program. To seek services from an organization viewed as serving lower-income clients, FFS customers must realize that FFS services are being offered and trust the organization to provide high-quality services. Conversely, residents of the community may well be drawn to the NFP's care management program because they view the NFP as having no profit motive. Outreach and marketing staff must be prepared to deal with both perspectives. In either case, the reputation and credibility of the NFP organization are the most important factors in the success of the new program.

Marketing of FFS care management is rarely focused directly on the person who will receive the service. Rather, it is aimed at adult children and other individuals (e.g., attorneys, physicians, financial planners) who help older people make decisions. Different marketing strategies are needed to reach these different audiences. An NFP can look to the for-profit business sector to learn about successful marketing and, at the same time, build on the NFP's history and tradition of service to set itself apart from the for-profit business sector.

Before developing FFS care management, an NFP's leaders must consider whether there are enough potential customers in the community. The leaders should also consider whether the community already has enough organizations providing these services. The OACM experience was able to capitalize on the strong reputation of the agency as a home care agency. This level of respect fostered respect for the case management program based on reputation.

The success of the services will depend on a network of trusted, caring service providers committed to quality and open to suggestions for improvement. A trusted provider network is an important part of what is being sold. The case manager continually needs to be marketing. Key referral sources need to be reminded frequently of the services. Marketing of case management services isn't a one-step process, but rather it needs to be ongoing and is a series of collaborative activities. Helping an assisted living facility with a talk or health fair is more effective than giving a fancy holiday gift. Marketing for case managers involves developing long-term relationships with referral sources and always delivering excellent services.

■ COSTS, RATES, AND BILLING

One of the first questions typically asked by potential clients is, "How much will it cost?" Setting rates takes a good understanding of direct and indirect agency expenses. Profits can be built in but must be reasonable, keeping prices competitive with those of similar service providers in the community. Many NFPs are able to keep their prices somewhat lower than those of for-profit businesses because of their size and funding from other programs. However, FFS care management fees are billed by the task or hour; thus, staff productivity becomes an important element in the program.

Productivity in an FFS program most commonly means the number of hours each care manager can bill. This is a strange concept to those unaccustomed to billing and requires training and experience to become second nature. As noted by Bellucci and her colleagues, productivity can be raised through methods such as objective feedback.[10] A study in an NFP's FFS case management program serving human immunodeficiency virus and acquired immune deficiency syndrome clients showed a 13.4% increase in billable hours after an expected number of billable hours and weekly reports were provided to each team of case managers. These findings show the importance of good supervision, target setting, and ongoing staff development.

■ SOFTWARE TOOLS

There are software programs available that are specifically designed for fee-for-service geriatric care management. Among other features, they can offer tools for assessment, a concise way to store client demographics, and other important client information and billing modules. They can also record client contacts and progress notes. Many care managers express that these software programs help capture billable time that can otherwise get lost in handwritten notes. Two specific software programs are JewelCode (www.jewelcode.com) and CareManager Pro (www.caremanagerpro.com).

■ CONCLUSION

Many decisions must be made prior to implementing an FFS care management program in an NFP setting. Choices must be made about the program's purpose, staffing, struc-

ture, rates, relationship to other programs, and marketing strategies. In the years to come, there will probably be more questions than answers as NFPs further develop for-profit enterprises. These debates will help ensure that the mission and values of NFPs can be maintained while paying customers are accommodated. Moving into the FFS world will enable NFPs to survive and to serve a broader range of people.

■ REFERENCES

1. Knutson K, Langer S. Geriatric care managers: a survey in long-term/chronic care. *GCM J.* 1998;8:9.

2. Bodie Gross E, Holt E. Care and case management summit—the white paper. *GCM J.* 1998;8:22–24.

3. White M. Case management. In: Maddox GL, ed. *The Encyclopedia of Aging.* 3rd ed. New York: Springer; in press.

4. White M, Gundrum G. Case management. In: Evashwick C, ed. *The Continuum of Long-Term Care: An Integrated Systems Approach.* 2nd ed. Albany, NY: Delmar Publishers; 2000.

5. Austin CD, McClelland RW, eds. *Perspectives on Case Management Practice.* Milwaukee, WI: Families International; 1996.

6. Parker M. Positioning care management for future health care trends. *GCM J.* 1998;8:4–8.

7. Cress C. *Handbook of geriatric care management.* Gaithersburg, MD: Aspen; 2001:103–105.

8. Vocker M. Care management from the perspective of a not-for-profit agency. *GCM J.* 1996;6:11–15.

9. Hereford RW. Private-pay case management: let the seller beware. *Caring.* 1990;9:8–12.

10. Bellucci M, Tonges MC, Kopelman R. Doing well by doing good: the case for objective feedback in case management. *J Case Manage.* 1998;7:161–166.

Chapter 15

Combining a Home Care Agency and a GCM Practice

Cathy Cress and Jack Herndon

■ WHY COMBINE GCM AND HOME CARE?

Why should you add a GCM component to your home care agency or nonprofit? First, a care management practice can be an important differentiator for agencies that offer home care. An assessment and care plan can be a valuable way for families to understand care needs and recommendations and to consider options for providing this care. This care planning process can be vital to families particularly in the early stages of caregiving, as most families do not understand the needs of the older adult, the options for meeting these needs, nor the costs associated with these options. Providing a care plan and opportunity for discussion and buy-in among family members can therefore be an important step in initiating, modifying, or continuing home care services.

Among the other reasons to add GCM to your home care mix are financial considerations. You may be able to capture billable hours in home care that were previously unbilled by your social worker and nursing staff who are doing many of the GCM tasks for free in your existing home care business. Having a geriatric care management component will help you better manage people with complex care needs, keep them at home and out of hospitals, and from cycling through the emergency room. A GCM component

offers support and education to your home care workers, giving them more skills, including professional one-on-one problem solving expertise, so that the paraprofessionals do not feel like they are alone and can better work as a supported team member.

■ FEASIBILITY AND PROFITABILITY OF ADDING A GCM

Is adding geriatric care management to home care a good business decision? Does a for-profit geriatric care management business fit into a home care agency? Or into a nonprofit? Have you weighed the chances of the cultures of home care and geriatric care management succeeding together? Have you studied the geriatric care management competition in your area? Have you done a market survey? To make this business decision, it is best to do a market feasibility study before you add a for-profit geriatric care management model to your home care service mix. Launching a feasibility study to measure whether a GCM would really be profitable in your geographical area is a critical move before you add a for-profit GCM. Whether you complete the analysis yourself or hire an outside consulting firm to do this market feasibility study, this evaluation is a good business move and may save your business many dollars and regretted decisions.

Defining Your Customer Base and Referral Sources

The first thing that a home care company should do when considering the addition of a GCM component is to define the customers you wish to serve. Similar to home care clients, geriatric care customers are aging consumers and their adult children in your area who need your geriatric care management services. You start by defining the ideal client who needs to purchase and who, most importantly, can afford your GCM services. In essence, this will take creating a new business plan for your new GCM for-profit business to complement the existing business plan for your present home care agency.

You will need to define your ideal client's age, income, family structure, and level of chronic care needs. Income is very important because by adding a for-profit GCM agency arm, you will need to make a profit. Given that care management is almost always paid privately (i.e., not reimbursed) you need to work with clients who have an average income level in the top 1%. (Refer to Chapter 12, How to Start or Add a Geriatric Care Management Business.) Next you need to explore the size of the market your GCM for-profit arm might serve. You should look at the entire geographic area your home care agency serves. For example, if your business serves the whole state of Maine, you are looking for which counties in Maine will yield you the most profitable geriatric care management clients.

If you serve all the counties in Maine currently, start with all the counties. Create a market survey of those counties to find out which counties have the highest number of seniors, with the highest income described as your ideal client. You will use the census, hospital admissions, and other data to quantify the size of the market. See the section on market assessment in Chapter 12 on how to do this. Your goal is to determine the total available market for care management services within your service area, considering the total number of older adults, the income of that population, and the number of hospital discharges of patients 65 and over (which indicates the number of medically complex cases potentially requiring care management).

Finding the Highest Number of Referral Sources

Next, you will also be looking at locations in your home care services area to select the locales to target for your GCM business addition. You want the geographical area that has the highest number of third party referral sources who would refer geriatric care management clients to you. To do this you need to outline all the prime GCM referral sources, such as elder-law attorneys, physicians, and trust officers who will refer your GCM clients to your business.

Next you should do a competitive survey of all GCMs who serve the target segment of your home care territory. It's critical to identify all individuals and agencies (for-profit and nonprofit) that offer services that are directly competitive or substitutes for care management. For instance, a hospital's information and referral service may be partially competitive to care management. You are identifying who is your competition and if you can achieve market share in the area you choose to serve.

You want to create a survey that tracks the individual GCMs in your services area and find out their fees per hour, if they now include home care, and what geriatric care management services each competing GCM offers. For example, do the local GCMs do geriatric assessment, offer care monitoring, offer home care themselves, or any of the standard GCM services and products? Next you want to find out what areas your competitors serve geographically. You can use this information to set your home care agencies' hourly fees for all geriatric care management services, making your fees competitive with the area you serve. The survey will also tell you if the local market is too saturated to compete with the other geriatric care management agencies or if combining home care and GCM services is actually a competitive edge in your service area. This will also help you position yourself in your market and decide what new innovative services you can offer that other geriatric care managers do not.

Competition

An important factor in your decision to add care management services will be the extent to which competition already exists in your market. In looking at possible competitors, you will want to understand their geographic coverage, background and training of care managers, and the fee structure of potential competitors. Very few markets in the United States are currently saturated with care managers, so the fact there is an existing practice in your market is not necessarily a reason to abandon your expansion plans. Even if there is a large number of care managers in your market, there are likely areas that are not served by existing providers. In addition, existing providers may not focus on medically complex cases, for example, if they do not have a nurse on staff; these may represent an opportunity for your practice. In fact, you may even consider a partnership or referral relationship with this group to refer you medically complex cases (assuming you include a nurse in your practice). Finally, pricing of existing care managers in your market can indicate the range of care management services for you to include when considering the financial attractiveness of your expansion.

Examining Existing Home Care Services for Potential Care Management Customers

Next you want to look internally and survey your own home care services for potential referrals to your new geriatric care management business. In doing this survey, you will

be introducing the geriatric care management concept to your professional and administrative staff. These professionals are often not experts in geriatric care management, as is the general public. This meeting gives you a chance to educate your staff and begin the important process of having your staff buy into the concept of adding GCM services to your home care agency.

Professional home care staff can often believe they already deliver geriatric care management to their clients. They can be territorial and then threatened by the new GCM program. Your professional staff has probably been giving GCM services away for free and may feel defensive, threatened, or frustrated that you will now bill for what they may believe should be given at no charge to the older client and their family.

At the meeting of your home care staff, introduce the concept of GCM services. Your staff needs to understand how GCM services work and feel that adding those new services to their plate is a win–win situation for them. If you expect the staff itself to assist you in doing the survey of how many potential GCM clients they may have in their home care caseloads, you must educate your staff on exactly what this new GCM service is and have them buy in. This education can come with handouts and power points, so the staff can see all the agency and personal benefits of adding GCM services to your home care mix. After you have the meeting or perhaps several meetings to introduce the GCM concept, if you feel your staff has bought in, distribute the survey to the managers of each service who could personally refer a client to a GCM service.

Your home care agency may have already done a survey of your home care clients. If so this survey should act as an easy resource. If not you can design a questionnaire to survey your home care clients, tapping into potential geriatric care management clients. One design may be drawn from Chapter 13 in the section about defining a niche. You are looking for home care clients in the service area you want to serve who have an average income of over $100,000, need long-term care, would benefit from coordinated care, have long distance family members, and have health and or psychosocial issues that would benefit from geriatric care management.

At the end of your market feasibility study, you want to choose the geographical area that serves those with the highest income, has the most consumers who can afford geriatric care management, the least GCM competition, plus the greatest number of referral sources. So say of all the counties in Rhode Island served by your home care agency, two counties have all these factors. This is where you would choose to launch your new GCM for-profit business.

■ FINANCIAL MODELING

With your market and competitive analysis complete, you are now ready to start the financial planning process for your care management practice. The goal is to complete the following:

- Forecast profit or loss over the first 3 to 5 years
- Plan for three scenarios (best case, average performance, and worst case) to help you envision the different paths your expansion can take
- Manage your cash flow, which is distinct from your profit or loss

In fact, more companies fail due to cash flow constraints than from any other single factor. With this analysis complete, you'll understand the investment required to establish your business as well as the potential rewards and risks through the initial years of operation.

Financial Model

The financial plan will be your primary decision-making tool. This section will help you build a financial model to include revenue, expenses, and cash flow management. Once completed, the model will show you the 3-year projected profit (or loss), the amount of investment required to get the business off the ground, and the cash flow produced (or consumed) by the company. The financial planning template shown in Chapter 12 (Figure 12-1) can help guide you through this process. (A full version of Figure 12-1 is available for download as an Excel spreadsheet online at http://www.jblearning.com/catalog/9780763790264.)

Revenue

Care management revenue will depend on a number of factors, including the number of new clients acquired, retention of existing clients, average fees per client, hourly rates, and whether or not you charge for travel. If your hourly fees are $100 per hour and the average client requires 7 hours of services per month, the average revenue per client would be $700 per month. For a more sophisticated financial model, you may want to consider three or more tiers of clients, the number of hours of service per month, and the acquisition rate per tier per month (i.e., the number of new clients for each tier per month). As discussed earlier, the rate you use may depend on your research of competitive rates in the market. Next, you will want to project the number of clients gained per month, meaning the number of clients who have contractually engaged services that are starting in a given month. These are clients who are actively receiving services in a given month, not prospective new clients in the sales and marketing pipeline. Your new client acquisition rate will depend on a number of factors including your current contact database, relationships with key referral sources, marketing programs to inform and educate potential referral sources, and so on. You will also want to consider the number of clients discontinuing services. If you anticipate that the average client will require services from you for 9 months, the number of clients discontinuing services per month in September of your first year would equal the number of new clients in January of your first year. This number is critical to your revenue planning, as you will need to acquire more new clients the shorter your average client retention.

Scenario Planning

We recommend you create three scenarios of your financial plan: a best case, a moderate case, and a worst case. The assumptions you use may vary across each scenario; for example, for the worst case, you may want to use an hourly rate lower than the other two cases. This would address the situation where you adjust your hourly rate lower in response to the market. You may also want to use a number of clients gained per month for your worst case that is lower than the best and moderate cases; this could occur when your marketing and lead development take longer to yield new clients than you plan. Similarly, on the expenses side, you will want to adjust your expectations for the worst-case scenario; perhaps marketing costs will be higher than anticipated, for example. Your goal is to create a worst-case scenario that represents the most conservative outlook—where you are confident the revenue and expenses could not be any less favorable. You'll use this scenario to ensure your financial viability in the event that the expansion doesn't materialize as you plan.

Expenses

Your goal is to capture the monthly expenses associated with your care management practice. You will need to determine the pay structure for the care manager and also consider whether the care manager is paid hourly or salaried. Generally, care managers are paid an hourly rate for time worked. Paying care managers on a salary can offer long-term advan-tages to the organization and care manager and also requires a significantly higher initial cash investment. It can also stretch out the time to reach profitability. The care manager's hourly rate or salary will depend on your current hiring practices; if you need an indicator of salary ranges, you may want to check job postings in your market for similar roles in other organizations. We also suggest you consider two other roles in your organization: a sales and marketing function as well as an administrative assistant or office manager. You will want to estimate the number of hours required for each role on a monthly basis and then calculate the monthly expense for salaries in your financial model. If you offer benefits, you will also include these in your total salaries amount as well as your employer taxes on the salaries. Another critical consideration for your financial model will be the care manager use rate; this rate summarizes the amount of time paid to the care manager that is billable to a client. For example, if a care manager is paid for 36 hours of work in a week, 30 hours of which are billable to a client, the use rate would be 30/36, or 83%. The target use rate will depend on the administrative, marketing, and other requirements asked of the care manager that are nonbillable. Given that the care manager will likely have the highest hourly rate in the group, we strongly advocate that the administrative and marketing work be delegated to team members; this would allow you to establish a target use rate of 80–85%. We believe another significant expense worth including covers credit card processing fees, which will enable you to accept payment from clients via credit card. Banks and other merchant services (such as PayPal) will typically charge about 2.5% of the amount charged in processing fees. We believe these fees are merited, as you will be able to collect your fees paid via credit card on a predictable schedule and will minimize the risk of nonpayment. You will also want to consider expanding your workers compensation and liability coverage for the care manager or managers, as well as the marketing expenses associated with printing materials, expanding your current website, and advertising (including purchase of search words on Google and other search engines).

Cash Flow

Cash flow refers to the timing of actual cash receipts and expenses. Cash flow does not always match your revenue from an accounting perspective, and the difference is critical to your business. For example, you may have delivered $2500 in services last month to a client who is under contract with you. You generate an invoice and record this as revenue. However, you have not yet been paid. If your payment arrives 45 days after mailing the invoice, you will already have paid your staff members for the time spent delivering those services. The biggest challenge companies face revolves around cash flow; you can't make payroll based on the unpaid invoices that you've sent to clients. The goal is to manage your cash flow as proactively as possible by collecting as quickly as possible on the revenue you've earned. To do this, you may want to consider the following:

- Accept credit card payments (or even requiring clients pay by credit card, as some agencies do) to ensure you will be paid on time and in full each month.
- Invoice twice monthly, and send invoices as close to the service date as possible. This typically means generating and sending invoices within 2–3 business days of the completion of service period. To do this, you will want to establish an effective means of capturing billable activities and then creating a rapid and accurate process for generating invoices.
- Enforce the policy that you deliver services only after receiving a signed service agreement for care management services. Unlike home care, few people understand the role and services of care management, and many people believe these care management services are (or should be free). As a result, the potential for confusion or refusal to pay is generally higher with care management than with home care.
- Require a deposit or initial payment. Even a payment of $250 can help establish that these services are in fact paid and condition the client to the mind-set that all care management activities will be billed. Taken together, these best practices can help you ensure you optimize your cash flow management.

If you now believe the market can sustain GCM services and financial opportunity looks attractive, then proceed with implementation.

■ IMPLEMENTATION

If you decided to proceed and add geriatric care management to your home care mix because you now believe that the financial opportunity looks attractive, then you are going to proceed with implementing your new program. You have chosen to create an integrated model of geriatric care management, which is to combine home care and GCM services (see Chapter 13 for information about integrated models).

Integrating the Two Models of Care

The next step you need to take is to integrate your home care agency model with your new geriatric care model. You must get on the same page philosophically and culturally and decide who leads what area of care and who follows. This means revisiting the present business plan for your home care agency. You need to take the time to do this at a retreat or contemplative day, talking and revising your model to include key staff and owners. It may be helpful to employ an outside consultant to help your staff do this business revision. You are moving to an incorporated model of care so you need to create a combined model by updating or changing your company's mission, purpose, and values. You are growing, so you need to articulate your new identity.

An organization's identity is defined by four elements: mission, purpose, values and cultures.

Revising Your Mission Statement

Your mission statement tells the community you serve what you want to accomplish in your work and thereby sell it to them. You now have to redefine what you want to achieve and what you want to sell. If your mission was to provide excellent professional home care services to your community in Santa Cruz, California, now that new mission is to additionally provide excellent care management services to your community. Care managed home care may now be your mission. You need to combine these in a new mission statement as your mission statement is key to your marketing effort. When Cresscare Care Management for Elders was a geriatric care management agency, the mission was to serve older people's needs. When Cresscare combined with home care, the mission was to meet the needs of care providers, older clients, home care staff, geriatric care management staff and customers.

Revising Your Purpose Statement

As you are adding care management to your mix you also have to redefine your organizational purpose. Your mission statement says what your organization does for your community. Your purpose statement says what your organization does for your staff. You will now have a home care staff and a geriatric care management staff. A good purpose statement tells your staff your company's idealistic motivation. The purpose statement describing your company's work may be to nurture your community's family caregivers and older people by helping them stay at home. It may

also be to nurture the staff that delivers that care. Your purpose statement should remind both your GCM staff and home care staff why they come to work each day (see Chapter 13, and the section on purpose).

Revising Your Values

The third part of an organization's philosophical identity is their values. You may have had one set of company values when you were just a home care company, but those values will change when you integrate your GCM component. Values are what your company stands for. A value for a home care company may be keeping older or disabled people at home for as long as possible. But a geriatric care management value may be to give service to a customer above all else. How do you combine these two values (see Chapter 13, values section)?

Hiring Geriatric Care Management Staff

The first thing you want to do is decide what the staffing will look like in your new GCM office. How many GCMs will you hire? Will you add a salesperson? Who will be your office staff and how will you recruit all these personnel?

Geriatric care managers are frequently human service professionals, nurses, and social workers who have never billed for anything in their professional career. If they come from a Medicare background they have never billed the private market. Choosing a GCM to add to your home care agency means adding someone to your culture that cannot be adverse to billing or who finds for-profit business toxic. Designing both a job description and recruitment ad to find a GCM will mean adding language that draws someone who has GCM skills, clinical skills, and an openness to billing hourly and charging for services. This is a difficult combination. It is as if the left brain was mixed in with the right brain. Few people have both strengths.

Next you need to create your job description to find a GCM. Do you want them to do sales presentations and public education seminars about your new services? If sales is added to the GCM's job description, you will most definitely want to seek a geriatric care manager with both a clinical and a sales or marketing background. This is a hard combination as most human service professionals have never been trained in sales and have no idea how to see the client as a geriatric care management customer nor their GCM services as products they sell and charge for. They do not understand closing a sale, a sales pipeline, or making a sales presentation. All this must be done to market your new GCM business to the external public and the internal staff, including your home care staff.

Social workers and nurses have traditionally been trained to give their services away or have not seen an hourly fee attached to them. Hospital and home health agencies bill for their hours, but the nurses and social workers never do and thus are not involved in any billing loop. Many human service professional are adverse to billing for services and have been educated and acculturated to give services away.

You also need to look for a geriatric care manager that has a master's degree in social work, nursing, physical therapy, or any one of the allied health fields. A master's in geriatric care management is preferred but hard to find (see Chapter 1, section on academic programs in geriatric care management). You want to hire someone who is left- and right-brain oriented, compassionate, and caring yet able to prioritize work and follow up on minute details. You need someone who can juggle multiple complex clients all at once, is willing to be on call, and is highly literate in software, hardware, social networking, and technology.

The geriatric care management position should be an hourly one directly based on hours billed. Compensation should be tied to performance. The salary should be based on the average hourly salary for a social worker or registered nurse in your area.

There is a potential roadblock in asking the GCM to do marketing. This can be avoided by hiring a part- or full-time salesperson who will do sales calls to all your GCM targets, such as doctors and elder-law attorneys (see Chapter 12, section on market assessment), and make presentations about your new GCM agency to community agencies and social services agencies who may refer you clients. This salesperson can make presentations internally to your home care staff, who are excellent sources of referral but who will have to be educated about GCM services and sold the advantages in referring GCM clients to the new GCM component. You may have someone already in your home care agency who does marketing and could take the extra hours to do this. This is critical because without a sales force you cannot sell GCM services, but without a clinically skilled GCM you cannot offer great GCM services or accrue the billable hours to make this GCM addition profitable. So you need to decide if you combine the GCM sales and GCM clinical job or break it out.

You should consider making the salesperson part-time to reduce start-up expenses. You should have created a sales plan in your business plan for your new GCM business and the hours, salary, and job description should be created according to your business plan (see Chapter 12, section on creating a business plan).

Setting Up the Business

Your geriatric care management agency needs its own office and own staff to make money and serve your home care agency. You need to rent or lease office space. A small space with 400–600 feet is necessary, as well as ordering office equipment, phones, and computers, including software, hardware, PDAs, laptops, smart phones, and bringing in case-related records. Insurance, including business insurance, needs to be purchased. See Chapter 12 for more information about setting up an office and insurance.

Geriatric care management forms need to be designed, including forms for intake, care monitoring, geriatric assessment, and for opening and closing cases.

Procedures and Operations Manual

It is a very good idea before your opening to write a geriatric care management operations manual including forms so there are procedures, forms, and steps for all GCM staff to follow. McDonald's famously refers to this as how to fry the hamburger. You are dealing with someone's mother not hamburgers. All the more reason to have a step-by-step manual before training staff and opening.

Outside consultants can be hired to design this to get your operations up to speed quickly (see Chapter 12 in the section about professional consultants). In some states, such as Florida, this is required. You can consult the National Association of Professional Care Managers GCM store for their forms, books and CD. You need to tailor the outside forms to your particular GCM and home care business and services. You need to create your own procedures, which will include designing all your GCM services. These services could be geriatric assessment, care monitoring for heavy 24-hour cases in your home care agency, geriatric care monitoring for light cases (5–7 hours a week), or a service of monitoring for long-distance care providers and adult children. Whatever you decide for your GCM services and products, you need to map out procedures for each one from setting up the case, intake, managing the case, and closing the case. This needs to be airtight because you are selling this product, and people will complain when it does not work. They will especially complain and may just not pay you because that product is for their mother. To

have each service work, it has to have written procedures or a manual, just like software or hardware. An operations manual with a companion form is key.

Training

You will need to design a training program to educate your new GCM, office, and sales staff. Training is key to your new geriatric care managers to educate them in your procedures and system to deliver geriatric care management. This includes GCM intakes, opening cases, closing cases, care monitoring, and delivering all services for each GCM service you plan to provide. You have to train them to write monthly reports, bill for their time, and capture their time to both get paid and make a profit for your business. You can't train them to be a geriatric care manager. So hiring someone with a GCM background or degree is key. You do, however, have to train them on your own individual GCM system. Designing a training manual with that training program in mind is a good idea, and again, looking into hiring outside consultants is a good idea. The GCM training program should be approximately 40–50 hours for your new GCM staff.

Organizations to Join

Your home care agency and GCM program should join professional associations locally, statewide, and nationally to help your business learn GCM services to help your community grow and prosper and to stay educated on geriatric care management issues (see Chapter 12, professional associations).

■ ADDING A HOME CARE AGENCY TO YOUR GCM AGENCY

Adding home care to your geriatric care management agency can significantly increase revenue, but it also involves a number of changes to your operations, marketing, hiring, and overall agency management. The process follows many of the steps outlined in the section on adding geriatric care management to home care. This section provides additional steps specific to adding the home care business. The addition of home care staff gives you ultimate control of the care management process because you have control across the entire relationship with the client, from geriatric care managers down to home care staff, if your client chooses home care. You do not have to depend on the integrity, safety, and reliability of outside care management agencies to deliver high-quality care to your customers. However, this means adding a large burden of creating that safe reliable home care staff yourself.

Rewriting Your Business Plan

Your present geriatric care management business plan must first be reviewed, and key staff and owners, whether in a partnership or corporation, should meet and appraise the plan together. Again, hiring an outside consultant is a good idea so you can make this business integration in a way that benefits your care management practice rather than hinders it. If you are a sole proprietorship, a business plan can be invaluable in setting the direction to follow. You will have to create a combined model including a new mission, purpose, and values to reflect both your old GCM model and the addition of a home care model.

Rewriting Your Mission

If your mission was to offer the best geriatric care management services in San Mateo County, California, your revised mission would be to provide those geriatric care management services plus a new product, home care. In fact, you will now be selling geriatric care-managed home care services. You need to define this new mission with a rewritten mis-

sion statement, which you will use for your new marketing campaign after the integration. This updated mission statement will also help to define exactly what you are providing to your community with your new GCM and home care agency.

Rewriting Your Purpose

In adding home care to your GCM practice, you want to rewrite your agency purpose. Your purpose communicates how your new agency benefits your staff. Your agency's purpose tells the people who work for you why they come to their job every day, week, and month. It may be that you offer excellent family and employee health benefits. It may be that you have technology systems that improve the quality of care-managed home care and also make it easy for staff to use. To help you articulate your new home care and GCM agency purpose see Chapter 12 in the organizational development and purpose sections. You will also need to revisit the statement of values for your practice to ensure compatibility with the addition of home care services.

Changes to Operations

Adding home care will require a number of additional processes and roles within your organization. You will need to augment your forms to include documents that track activities in the home, such as home care daily sheets or daily charting. Your intake process will also need to include an understanding of many factors such as scheduled days and hours, client dietary restrictions, quality of life, social interests, as well as individual preferences that could be important in determining which home care aide to staff and how to individually orient that staff to the particular case. You cannot legally discriminate according to race or creed, but a preference of a quiet home care provider can be accommodated.

Hiring A Home Care Personnel Coordinator

You will need to hire a personnel coordinator who handles recruiting, screening, orientation, placement and management of your home care staff. This person can also do staffing placement when you are a small agency, but as you grow you will need a staffing coordinator to handle cases. This will again mean designing a detailed job description and creating a large section of your operations manual. This person should have human resources and home health experience with highly competent computer skills and be highly organized.

Recruitment and Screening of Home Care Staff

Home care staff employees will be the face of your new combined organization, so you will want to ask detailed recruitment questions, involve multiple employees in the process, and complete a thorough background and reference check. You are only as strong as your weakest link, so you need to make your home care staff dependable, safe, and trained.

You will need to design and set up an entire recruiting and screening process in your operations manual to draft home care staff. This will include advertising for home care staff through the Web and devising a community resources database to recruit through employment sources in your community. You will need to create a screening process for home care staff that will include the application process, interviewing, checking references, and a background check including fingerprints if you choose or if the law in your state requires this. Home care staff safety is an important marketing tool for your agency. For background checks, we recommend using a reputable vendor such as Intelius or Kroll Background Screening, which provides an Internet interface to initiate screenings. In addition, you may choose to have all employees fingerprinted. You should consult your employment attorney for a recommendation about background checks and fingerprinting policies. Finally, you will need a complete employee handbook that includes materials relevant to caregivers (i.e., job responsibilities). Nolo Press publishes a valuable guide called *Create Your Own Employee Handbook: A Legal and Practical Guide.* You can also use your consultant to help you design this handbook.

Then you will need to input all home care staff into a scheduling database and set up physical or electronic home care staff files.

Scheduling of Home Care Staff

Next, you will need staff members and a clear process to handle the home care team scheduling. Several programs, such as Home Trak, are able to partially automate the process. At the same time, you or your staffing coordinator will need to identify the changing availability for each home care worker and then match demand against availability. You will also need to have additional home care workers available to cover shifts in the event of sickness or no-shows and a database to track all this.

Home Care Staff Supervision

Next, you will want to provide for caregiver supervision. You can have your personnel coordinator supervise the home care staff. You need to devise a plan in your operation manual for the personnel coordinator and your care management staff to use to guide their supervision. For example, if your GCM makes a home visit and the home care provider is not carrying out the care plan, what are the joint steps the GCM and personnel coordinator take to change the home care worker's actions? Often, agencies employ another medical professional in a supervisory role to handle medically complex cases. Also, you will likely need to add or expand the care coordinator role in your organization, as clients receiving home care may need a higher level of coordination such as grocery or medication delivery, home maintenance, or other tasks.

Designing an On-Call Process for Your Home Care Staff

You will need to greatly expand your on-call process that ensures immediate response 24 hours a day, 7 days a week. The process will ensure your home care clients, their families, and your staff are able to reach help when needed. You will also need to establish emergency procedures for your home care staff when they are unable to make a shift. The person on call will have to handle staffing and care management or have the ability to reach care management staff for emergency questions. You will have to include an augmented procedure for on-call situations in your operations manual that outlines step by step how your staffing coordinator, the on-call person, and care managers work together after hours. You will also need to prepare procedures for your on-call staff, including disaster preparedness for each client.

Orientation of Home Care Staff

Introducing geriatric care-managed home care will require tight integration between your care managers and home care staff. Clear distinction of roles and responsibilities will help ensure the highest possible quality of care and also ensure that you capture billable activities performed by your care managers. You will want to build agreement from care managers and home care staff that the assessment and resulting care plan will provide the guidance for what and how care is provided. Ensuring caregivers are able and willing to read and follow the care plan is essential. This will take developing a section of your care provider training program that is included in your operations manual, covering initial orientation to each care provider and group training of new care providers. This will include scheduling care provider training, conducting orientation for care providers, doing group training for new care providers, and doing individual orientation on specific cases for care providers. All this should be in your operations manual.

Making Your GCMs' Time Billable When Supervising Home Care Staff

Next, you want to ensure that your geriatric care managers' activities are spent on billable activities, and not handling transportation, scheduling, or coordination for caregivers. These tasks, which are essential to everyday operations, need to be addressed by care coordinators.

Changes to Sales and Marketing

You will need to update your marketing materials to reflect the addition of home care. You may decide that your practice will only provide home care to those clients who are care management clients (i.e., all home care clients must have some level of geriatric care management). If you choose to accept home care clients who aren't care management clients, we don't recommend planning that these clients will eventually become care management clients, as families who start with home care alone tend to stick only with home care. For marketing purposes, we suggest developing several case studies that show how care management can enhance the quality of home care; otherwise, families will often opt for the lower cost option of only home care—and assume you (as their agency) will provide care coordination and perhaps care management included in the home care fees. This will be an effective tool in competing against home care agencies who will likely position themselves against your practice as a low-cost option. You need to be able to show the incremental model that geriatric care-managed home care offers versus stand-alone home care.

Managing Home Care Staff

Employing home care staff means managing home care staff. This should be done by your personnel coordinator. This includes counseling and discipline, replacing care providers on cases, terminating or firing care providers for cause, contracting with care providers, filing incident reports if a patient is injured, and training. Your personnel coordinator needs a human resources background. You need to design forms and procedures in your operations manual for all of these steps for management of home care staff. You must also follow state and federal employment law to the letter. Consult with your attorney regarding all of these human resources procedures.

Risk Management

Adding home care to your care management practice will introduce several business risks that you will need to address. The first is employee status. Technically, caregivers can either be compensated as independent contractors or as employees. The advantage to an agency of paying caregivers as independent contractors is that the agency is not responsible for the employer taxes (i.e., contribution to Social Security, etc.) that can total 7.5% of gross wages or more. However, state laws have strict definitions that determine whether an individual can qualify as an independent contractor. If an audit is performed and the state determines the caregivers did not qualify as contractors, the employer becomes responsible for back taxes. The next caregiver issue relates to the number of hours worked. Employees are entitled to overtime pay after a certain number of hours. For live-in staff, a threshold also applies, above which caregivers are entitled to overtime pay. In California, this issue is addressed by Wage Order 15;[1]

unfortunately, the legal precedent regarding this issue has not been established. We strongly recommend you consult an attorney familiar with home care employment issues and follow your state and federal laws.

Insurance

Adding home care to your practice will also require you to expand your insurance coverage. You will need liability and workers compensation coverage; you may elect to have your employees bonded to cover against theft or other financial losses within a client's home. Given the nature of home care, which may require caregivers to transfer clients to and from their beds, toilets, chairs, and so on, you will want to adapt your training to minimize risk of injury to caregivers and risk of an insurance claim against you.

Home Care Organizations to Join

You may want to consider joining the following home care associations:

CAHSAH (California only):
www.cahsah.org
(See also other state home care associations)
American Association for Homecare:
www.aahomecare.org
National Association for Home Care and
Hospice: www.nahc.org
National Private Duty Association:
www.privatedutyhomecare.org

■ WEBSITES

- www.intelius.com
- www.krollbackgroundscreening.com

■ REFERENCE

1. California Department of Industrial Relations. Wage order 15: regulating wages, hours and working conditions for household occupations. Available at: http://www.dir.ca.gov/iwc/WageOrders2006/iwcarticle15.html

Chapter 16

Marketing Geriatric Care Management

Merrily Orsini

■ OVERVIEW: MARKETING TO THE GERIATRIC CARE POPULATION

Although the concept of marketing may initially seem complex for the average geriatric care manager (GCM), an understanding of integrated marketing communications is an important component of building a thriving practice. Taking the time and resources to understand basic marketing strategy and to develop and implement an integrated, strategic marketing plan helps the GCM to increase visibility, credibility, and knowledge of services.

Because geriatric care management is an as-needed service that consumers seek only when the need arises, it requires a specific approach to marketing. The key to marketing for a GCM is to first educate consumers about what a GCM is and does, and then to get the company and GCM name known so when a potential client has a need, he or she will inquire, and then a request for service will follow.

According to traditional definitions, a *marketing communications mix* is described as follows: "Marketing communications, sometimes referred to as 'promotions,' involve marketer-initiated techniques directed to target audiences in an attempt to influence attitudes and behaviors."[1(p375)] Together, advertising, public relations (PR), sales promotions, social media, social networking, personal selling, networking, and direct marketing communications constitute the marketing communications mix, often referred to as the promotional mix. The three major objectives of marketing communications are (1) to inform, (2) to persuade, and (3) to remind the marketer's audience.[1(p375)]

Understanding the mix of marketing communications can assist the GCM in deciding what to do when, how to budget for marketing, and how best to reach desired targets. Overall marketing strategy is necessary to understand how best to use which tactics and for the best usage of resources, time, and money. Marketing is the overall strategy used and is based on thoughtful understanding of the environment, competition, and services provided. Sales are activities that are used to actually get clients to sign up for services. Public relations strategy influences public perceptions, whether in face-to-face communications or through targeted media relations, whether in articles, radio and TV spots, or on the Internet. Advertisements are paid and placed in relevant media outlets. Social media and social networking fall somewhere in between marketing and public relations, and the interactive nature of these communications makes them especially helpful for the GCM.

Beginning GCMs might have less money to spend on marketing activities, yet marketing is essential to starting and growing a business. A seasoned GCM still needs to use marketing strategy to grow the business, but the tactics are different because the GCM has a client base and is better known in the community. Being a salesperson for oneself is not intuitive, and only practice and experience make sales a comfortable practice for the GCM.

Consumers have many choices to make when they already know about available products and when they use products on an ongoing basis. Consumers may not know about geriatric care management and the differences between providers. Because using a GCM is usually based on a specific triggered need or an event, education becomes an important part of marketing. Understanding the marketing mix and how to use education as a significant part in the sales, marketing, and PR efforts is not unique to care management, but it is incredibly important.

In regards to marketing and sales, note that most GCMs are uncomfortable with the idea that profitability is positive. The concept that a profitable business is a healthy business, and only a healthy business can survive and grow, is crucial for the GCM to comprehend and embrace. Understanding and getting better at sales and marketing are key ways to make a business healthy.

■ CREATING A MARKETING STRATEGY AS THE BASIS FOR SPENDING MARKETING DOLLARS (BEGINNING AND MATURE)

Before the business can start generating revenue, a marketing strategy and sales techniques must be in place. The message communicated to the public about the business is of primary importance. Geriatric care management sells solutions to aging and end-of-life issues, including assistance with decisions for housing and medical and personal care, and support that family members cannot provide, and on a level that a non-GCM cannot provide.

Geriatric care management is better known today than when the profession got its start in the mid-1980s. In some areas, there is even fierce competition between providers. Reaching the elderly themselves, their trusted advisors, and their families takes a combination of education, careful design of marketing materials, a targeted database of potential referral sources, consistent and pertinent communication over a variety of Internet-based communication channels, and lots of positive public relations. Inherent to business success is that the GCM is educated, experienced, and truly provides a value-added service to clients and their families and loved ones.

Potential clients must have the ability to pay for geriatric care management services, and thus are a very small segment of the general population. Furthermore, they must have a need that family, friends, physicians, and trusted advisors are not meeting.

For the seasoned GCM as well as the beginner, most new clients will come from referrals, both personal and professional. The marketing strategy must revolve around positioning the GCM for reaching potential referral sources and educating contacts about the benefits that a GCM brings to a complicated or underresourced situation. How the GCM presents services and how clients are managed and serviced are critical to the GCM's ongoing success.

When creating marketing strategy and material, the following messages resonate with clients and referral sources: security and comfort, peace of mind, solutions, appropriate care, choices in care providers, and access to resources. The other component of marketing strategy is the educational component that a GCM can bring to the table, related to aging and care needs. Educating the consumer as to when care at home is appropriate, what one can expect from certain diseases common to aging, and which resources are available along the spectrum of care also places a GCM in the consumer's mind when the need arises for services relating to aging or health issues. These issues are all perfectly suitable for inclusion on a website and for ongoing updates via social media outlets.

DEVELOPING A STRATEGIC MARKETING PLAN

When it comes to distinguishing a geriatric care management business, nothing compares to a solid and well-thought-out marketing plan. A strategic and successfully executed marketing plan has the power to shape a geriatric care management business and how it is to be perceived by current and potential customers. It forces the GCM to take the time to define the values and unique benefits they offer and to develop various, affordable (time and money) ways to communicate those things to a specifically defined target audience.

The long-term benefits of marketing are obvious. A GCM can have the best product or service imaginable, but if no one knows about it or buys it, no business is generated. It's wise to invest time and resources in creating and implementing a results-driven marketing plan.

The classic four *P*s of marketing (product, price, place, and promotion) have been updated for the 21st century to include the four *A*s:

- **Accountability:** Marketing must prove its contribution to the business and be accountable for measurable results; that is, new clients.
- **Analysis:** Marketing requires both art and science, and analysis must no longer be an afterthought. Instead, measurable results will drive strategy; that is, if it works, do more of it.
- **Accuracy:** Performance metrics must be consistently and accurately measured across all marketing initiatives; that is, tracking results.
- **Action:** Optimization is only successful when it's an ongoing process of leveraging your analysis to take decisive actions toward improving results; that is, change tactics to do more of what is working.[2]

Focusing primarily on opportunities that bring face-to-face interaction, whether one on one or in a group setting, is the best marketing strategy for the GCM, but also the most time consuming. Twitter, Facebook and LinkedIn, however, allow a close facsimile to one-on-one interaction, but reach a wider audience. Targeting the right audience is easier on the Internet as the audience is looking for the resource, making the educational component an even more important factor in the marketing effort.

A strategic marketing plan should include descriptions of the following:

- **Target audience:** Prioritize who is most receptive to your services and keep track of those who use your services. This measurement will enable you to refine your target audience as the business progresses.
- **Sales and marketing objectives:** How many clients can a geriatric care management practice handle, and how many new referral sources does it take to generate enough business? What gets measured gets managed, so setting objectives and measuring against them is one sure way to achieve success.
- **Product benefit overview:** What benefits do you and your geriatric care management practice bring to the clients and your target audience? This is the crux of why clients would want to use your services and what problem you are solving for them. Understanding this is crucial to selling services.
- **Positioning strategy:** How do your business model or service offerings differ from the competition's? Is your background or experience different from that of other GCMs'? Are you specific about that and why a client would choose you over someone else?

- **Lead sources:** Who do you know now? Where can you meet others that you need to know to get more business?
- **Selling and lead generation tactics:** What can *you* do that will start you on the road to (1) selling your services, and (2) making certain that you are always gaining more information on those to which you can present information to start the selling cycle?
- **Communication strategy:** How will you reach these leads? Phone calls, follow-up letters, visits, seminars, a website, social media?
- **Creative and promotion strategy:** What collateral materials are you using that work with your positioning strategy and that also speak to your target audience? Is your website designed with organic search terms throughout so your targets can find you?
- **Recommended activity:** This includes the one, two, or three activities that you do today, tomorrow, weekly, monthly, quarterly, and annually to achieve the business you want to achieve.

■ UNDERSTANDING BRANDING AND BRAND DEVELOPMENT

What is a brand? "A product is made in a factory; a brand is made in the mind," says branding expert Walter Landor, founder of Landor Associates. Taking the time to understand branding and how it is important to your success can mean big rewards for you and your geriatric care management business. Although often associated with just advertising, branding is essential to everything a company puts in front of current and potential clients including business cards, brochures, websites, trade show booths, letterhead, and so forth.

Branding is about managing people's image of a company and making sure that image is in line with your company values and the benefits your company provides. By taking the time to manage expectations and build positive gut feelings about your company, you establish yourself as a trusted leader in your market.[3]

Your brand identity is built on your key messages and position, the unique customer benefits that you provide, and the expectations you set for your target audience. By consistently delivering the same symbols, messages, and design, you are reinforcing those messages, creating a link to your brand, and building an identity for your business that people will remember. You want to create a consistent look and feel for everything related to you and your business.

Logo creation is the single most important part of the design branding process. The logo sets the stage for colors and for the overall look and feel of your specific identity and marketing collateral. When developing a logo, let your key messages guide the design. Develop a stand-out image that plays on the benefits and messages that you want to communicate to your potential clients. Keep in mind that a logo must be easy to see and interpret on the smallest intended usage, such as a giveaway pen, and on the largest, such as a business sign or trade show banner.

Through consistent use of the same logo, tagline, even company colors, you'll create a cohesive identity for your business and help drive home the messages that you want people to know about you and the business.

For example, if your tagline is "Understanding Care Needs; Delivering Options," then use it whenever you send anything to anyone. If it is "Resources for Aging," use that tagline on all materials. If you are specializing in some aspect of information, such as Alzheimer's disease, note that on all correspondence. Keep it simple and repeat it. You want people to remember the one thing you do best and for them to make a connection with it.

■ TARGETED AUDIENCES

The target audiences on which geriatric care management marketing should focus encompass personal, group, and networking contacts. The geriatric care management market is a very narrow market because only those who can afford to pay can access services, and the client must be at a point in life to need assistance with some aging- or disease-related issue, but might not necessarily be ill or injured. Some clients come out of rehabilitation facilities, hospitals, or nursing homes, but many simply have gotten to a point in their aging process where they really do not know where to go for assistance. They may need housekeeping, meal preparation, or assistance with walking and not falling. They may need 24-hour supervision, but not hands-on care. They may simply need someone to provide balanced meals, medication monitoring, and assistance with money management. Although the range of needs can be broad, the primary requirement is assistance with determining resource allocation for assistance to maintain the quality of life that they desire and can afford.

Thus, geriatric care management marketing targets those who may buy services for themselves or a loved one, as well as anyone along the spectrum of care services who works with seniors and could be a referral source, such as the following:

- Seniors themselves
- Adult children of aging, frail, or demented parents
- Trust officers
- Certified public accountants
- Elder-law attorneys
- Trust and estate attorneys
- Hospice nurses or volunteers
- Long-term care insurance agents
- Funeral home directors
- School social workers
- Human resources departments

- Home care and home healthcare agencies
- Retirement communities
- Assisted living facilities
- Hospitals
- Rehabilitation facilities

Additional referral sources and audiences to educate about geriatric care management services include Alzheimer's Association personnel and volunteers, clergy, and any community or disease groups and associations serving seniors. In short, the target market for geriatric care management services is anyone who has a need for care or anyone who knows or works with seniors and can provide referrals. The following section describes specific strategies for reaching these targets.

Reaching Desired Target Audiences

Because there usually isn't any specific way to identify the adult children of aging, frail or demented parents using traditional psychodemographic research, the Internet has allowed for them to find you. Using educational resources targeted to your audience and placed on a website will increase the likelihood that the adult children can find the resources when they need them. The website should be optimized for terms those targets search on, and incorporate the usage of Facebook and Twitter to send out helpful tips, as well as writing articles on a blog. Additionally, the placement of news articles in industry-specific as well as general publications, and media attention focused on aging and related issues are also good tactics and deserve additional time and resources. Some other suggestions are to find a spot on an early-morning or a noon talk show as an expert in elder care, and you can use senior centers as a place to give talks. You can also sponsor events (if finances allow), and generally get your name out as a resource and expert on aging or disability issues. It is this getting the word out that has to be done to effectively reach the masses. The use of the Internet, social media, and public relations are simply the best ways to reach the general consumer successfully. Media relations will also build third-party credibility for a geriatric care management business.

Trust officers can be targeted with direct mail. Updating your list of trust officers regularly and sending them information on geriatric care management issues can introduce the GCM name to banks. Asking to present to a bank to discuss using a GCM for planning of care for bank clients can also get the GCM name recognized. Establishing a relationship with a trust department can be the best referral source available to a GCM for long-term clients. Mining those relationships, keeping in constant contact, and keeping the GCM name in front of them in a variety of ways are the best marketing tactics for this group.

Reaching the certified public accountant (CPA) as a referral source may be more difficult because the target audience is wider. It might be helpful to see whether there is a division of the local association for CPAs that deals with elderly or aging persons or trusts and estates. Apply the same tactics for this select group as used for trust departments. Getting the GCM name in front of this group is the key. Education is one way to do this, in addition to direct mail. The CPA group is not known as a good source for referrals for GCMs because they are not trusted advisors, as attorneys are, to a family. This is due to the annual or quarterly nature of tax work, as opposed to regular, ongoing contact for legal issues. However, if a GCM does some good work in relationship building, CPAs can become referral sources in the GCM's informal network as well.

You can easily obtain a list of long-term care insurance (LTC) agents in an area by finding all local agents for all companies that provide LTC. These agents will need a referral source for their clients who have questions about which services they need for their long-term care needs. Also, insurance agents may have clients who do not qualify to buy LTC insurance, have an elimination period that excludes those who waited too late to try and purchase, or do not want to use their benefits unwisely. Find the local chapter of the National Association of Insurance and Financial Advisors (NAIFA) and ask to be a speaker. This group is usually very interested in continuing education, and most agents do not understand the differences in the care their policies cover. Giving a presentation is the most effective way to get in front of this audience.

The key to all referrals is to never take on a client unless you can provide assistance in solving that person's problem. Keep all of these referral source lists updated and communicate with contacts regularly. Let your contacts know when you are presenting somewhere so they can provide your name and engagement as a useful resource for their clients.

Educating the home care and home healthcare agencies about the value a GCM brings to elder care enables these agencies to work with you and establish an ongoing relationship. As the care manager, you can supervise a difficult case and alleviate time and cost that is not reimbursable for the agency. Plus, home health agencies can learn a lot from a GCM relating to elder care and aging issues. You can also offer to copresent with quality agencies for more public exposure.

Hospital discharge planners are a fluid group. Continually update this list of contacts so it is always current. One strategy to introduce yourself to a new set of clients is to provide community resource guides stamped with your logo and contact information to discharge planners to be disbursed to patients with geriatric care management needs when they are being discharged from the hospital. When a call to assist following patient discharge does come in, follow up with the social worker or nursing case manager. Try to take this contact to lunch; the time and expense is usually worth it. Offer to do in-service presentations on the spectrum of care, how a GCM's services fit into other services available, and when it is appropriate to make a referral to you. Educating the discharge team as to when GCM intervention is appropriate creates a trust level that turns into referrals. A website or blog with helpful resources and pertinent care and chronic disease questions answered is also a great way to get the discharge planners to send their patients to you. If you can provide resources that make their job of explaining care to a family better or easier, then you will provide an added value to the discharge team, and they will start to see you as a resource.

Estate and trust attorneys need to understand the services and advantages a GCM brings to their clients when care and resource needs become apparent. Clients of these attorneys are usually long term because a responsible family member may not be available to provide any care or ongoing support that frail, elderly persons so often need. Also, their clients usually are financially well-off and have the potential of becoming long-term clients. Many times, estate and trust attorneys remain as a point of contact in addition to the GCM when problems arise. Making an attorney's life easier on weekends and holidays is just one additional value a GCM brings to the situation. When a relationship is established with an attorney, try to do a joint seminar so both of you can promote your businesses and educate potential clients.

Many times, physicians truly do not understand appropriate resources and options for care. They are programmed to refer to Medicare skilled care and Medicaid. The best way to get the information about geriatric care management services to a physician is either to form a relationship with the doctor's nurse or to accompany a client to physician appointments and discuss with the doctor the geriatric care management services available and how the client benefits from them.

Always send an introductory letter to a client's physician introducing yourself as a part of a care team. Offer to educate physicians on geriatric care management services and the spectrum of care available to their patients. Physician relationships and referrals are worth their weight in gold. If the doctor orders it, then patients usually will comply.

The assisted living and retirement community population sometimes has clients with needs that cannot be met in these nonmedical, non-one-on-one living arrangements. Establishing rapport with the administrative staff can be accomplished by offering to hold special events or other kinds of activities with the facility personnel. Offering to educate on aging-related topics and activities can also provide an initial way into the facility. Consistent visits and participation in activities, such as health fairs, are essential.

Rehabilitation centers also discharge patients back to their homes, and sometimes the patient is not ready for 100% self-care. To get referrals, try to get to know the therapists, and keep them apprised of the geriatric care management business. Share with them how you can assist their patients at the time of discharge, or even while patients are in therapy and trying to make decisions about living arrangements when they are discharged.

A Medicare-certified agency may be willing to refer clients to you when a need arises, if they understand what a GCM does and how a GCM can assist their clients. The agency may want a referral agreement in place so all skilled care is referred to them; that is, when the client is hospitalized and then discharged with home health. As a part of the care team, it is possible for you to influence the selection of a Medicare-certified agency at the time of discharge.

Joining the Alzheimer's Association or other associations dealing with chronic diseases is one way to spread the word about your geriatric care management services. In addition to joining and working on committees, you can sponsor events, write for the newsletter, and present at educational conferences.

Dementia is one of the leading issues faced by the elderly population. Specializing in the best options in care for persons with dementia can position a GCM as a leader, and referrals will come. Consider providing training on how to work with dementia patients and giving assistance to the home care agencies to help them understand what staff characteristics are best, such as patience and kindness. A website is the perfect place to house resources that are helpful to one concerned with the dementia of a loved one.

Keeping the GCM name out in front of trusted advisors is one way to get referrals. Pastoral counselors oftentimes have access to families and need more in-depth resources when their congregation has needs. Also community groups serving seniors can be a source of referrals.

Using a Website for Marketing

You must have a website that is easily found, informative, and easy to use. When it comes to creating a website, design and easy navigation are top priority, followed closely by relevant content. Understand that the Internet is a fluid medium, interactive and fast. Users must be able to find what they want quickly, get the information they seek, be able to find the site again, and return to the site while involved in a search.

Start with a good site design that matches your other marketing material. Make it uncluttered and easily navigable, and use only relevant content. Be sure to include plenty of easy-to-use resources. Give the visitors to your site what they want:

- Information, including specifics
- Resources that are helpful
- How they can contact you

Website text should not be traditional marketing brochure content. The information must be concise and easily readable in a short time. All pages should have headers and bullets. The content should be conversational, current, and engage the user. Make certain to maintain and update regularly, adding any articles written and any information that is new and pertinent. Use established conventions for website design so there is nothing unusual or odd about your site.[3]

■ SALES AND MARKETING OBJECTIVES

Starting a geriatric care management business starts with one client. Sales and marketing objectives will vary depending on your location and the population density. The most crucial elements to growth are continuous learning, updating of resources and options, keeping clients happy, and serving them beyond their expectations.

Benchmarking business growth and tracking where business is coming from are essential for a start-up GCM as well as for seasoned professionals. Keeping monthly track of referrals, who made them, and what kinds of clients turn out to be longer term can enable a geriatric care management business to set realistic sales and marketing objectives.

Marketing tasks should be divided into passive tasks (advertising, direct mail, birthday cards) and active tasks (visits, presentations, posts on blogs, updates on Twitter and Facebook, and thank-you and follow-up notes). Objectives need to be set, based on a budget, as to how many tasks are done daily, weekly, and monthly.

Sales is the conversion of demand into orders.[4] The sales process is sometimes called a sales cycle. The following are the definite steps in this cycle:

- Prospecting (lead generation)
- Cold calling (by phone or face to face)
- Initial questioning (can be phone inquiry)
- Sales meetings (face to face)
- Rapport building (face to face or by phone)

- Needs analysis (strategic and tactical questioning, usually using an inquiry form)
- Solution presentation (positioning, what the GCM can do to solve the problem or meet the need)
- Closing (signing on a new client or referral source)

These steps are described in the following paragraphs.

Prospecting, or lead generation, is the act and process of actually collecting names and contact information of those people or businesses who would make a good target for services or for referring services. It is logical that, to make sales, you must know to whom you could possibly sell. The more names on this prospecting list, the better the chances of making a sale.

Cold calling is making a call, either on the phone or in person, to someone you do not know, but who is a good target person for using geriatric care management services or for making a referral for services. Sometimes a cold call can be made to someone you already know, but who is not aware of your business and what you could do for them.

Initial questioning of a potential target is not unlike performing a needs assessment on a client. You question the target to see what need the person has that you can fill. Because a GCM offers a wide range of services, different people will want to use different components of what you offer. For example, a physician may want assistance with resource listings and appropriate placements so her patients have to move only once when they leave their homes. A bank trust officer may want assistance with transportation to doctors' appointments for a frail client. Only by questioning potential clients or referral sources will you know which services you offer will fit their need.

A sales meeting is best if it is face to face so you can establish credibility and a relation-

ship. It is best not to call this encounter a sales meeting, and for the GCM who is "salesperson phobic," it is best to think of this as a relationship-building meeting. You are presenting yourself and your services to a potential customer or referral source. If you were selling widgets, you would have some various sizes of widgets to show. Because you are selling geriatric care management services provided by you, it is good to know what your audience is interested in (you have questioned your target already and know this information), so you can take this wonderful face-to-face opportunity to focus on the services this particular target wants to know more about or wants to purchase.

Building rapport is a natural outgrowth of the face-to-face sales meeting process, and it will continue by phone (as you follow up when a referral is received), e-mail, and additional face-to-face meetings.

The needs analysis is a more in-depth questioning about ways you can assist. It is an extension of the inquiry process and simply occurs during the natural evolution of a relationship as the client uses services and wants to learn more about other services you provide.

You can present the solutions you offer to meet the specific needs expressed by the target verbally and with collateral marketing materials. Usually, testimonials, case studies, and real-life examples are the best ways to present geriatric care management services to the public and to interested referral sources. For example, describe a real-life scenario similar to the target's situation in which you had a positive impact. Geriatric care management services are not understood by many, so presenting real-life examples is a wonderful way to explain what you bring to the situation and to present yourself as a useful component in the relationship.

Closing the sale is when you get the contract signed, accept the initial payment, and start to work. Simply presenting and talking with a potential client does not bring money in the door; you must close the sale with a specific plan of action in place. And, as Peter Drucker was fond of saying, there is no business until money changes hands.

GCMs traditionally might be shy about performing all the sales steps. However, understanding that a needs assessment and a phone inquiry are natural parts of the sales cycle and that the GCM brings genuine assistance to a family in need should help new GCMs get over any fears of the sales cycle.

One well-known theory of persuasion—the Elaboration Likelihood Model—can work for the GCM and should help in the sales process. "Specifically, when consumer motivation and ability are high, persuasive message arguments are more thoroughly processed, and the strength of the arguments influences persuasion in what is termed 'the central route' to persuasion."[1(p409)]

Because geriatric care management services are only sought after when a need arises, the likelihood of the client being receptive to your sales approach is greater if the person inquires about services. The National Association of Professional Geriatric Care Managers (NAPGCM) sells a forms book that contains several initial inquiry and assessment forms that make the inquiry process less painful as a sales technique.

When someone inquires about what you do as a GCM, the main point to remember is to ask the question, "What is it you are looking for?" Then, clarify what it is the person is looking for, and tailor your response to fit that person's specific need. As a GCM, you can either meet the need or make a referral to someone else. That way, you meet people's needs and also build referral relationships.[5]

■ PRODUCT BENEFIT OVERVIEW

Identifying key benefits of service helps shape communications. Generally, geriatric care management businesses benefit the client by assisting in choosing arrangements, including best living choices, in what can be thought of as "frailty to the grave" care.

The peace of mind that results from contracting for professional geriatric care management services benefits the older person's family and support system. Frailty is usually unplanned and often occurs when family members do not have the time to learn all they need to know about care and aging issues. It's important for an older person's support system to understand that there are options for care, that some are better than others, that each person has individual needs, and that there are resources available to meet those needs. The downside to geriatric care management services is that most options for care are private pay and cost the consumer. The benefits of care management must outweigh the costs, so GCMs must continue to show ongoing benefits to clients and referral sources.

■ POSITIONING STRATEGY

A positioning strategy is simply a statement of how the GCM should be viewed (e.g., caring, intelligent, hard working). The positioning strategy essentially defines the GCM's personality and how the clients, prospects, and referral sources perceive services offered. Usually, it is based on the personal nature of the relationship between the GCM and the client.

A positioning statement should be brief and emphasize one or two points. Your positioning statement will help guide the direction of your marketing material. For instance, this is a positioning statement: Specializing in Alzheimer's Care. This positioning informs the consumer that the GCM understands dementia and the demands made on the family and care staff of Alzheimer's patients, and also assures that care will be taken to match and train care personnel used or to assist with placement in a facility where dementia care is the specialization.

LEAD SOURCES

As identified earlier, geriatric care management marketing has three key target audiences: individual clients who need care, referral sources, and children of aging parents. The following are some key ideas for lead sources for individual prospects and referral sources. The source of existing customer leads will come directly from clients.

Use a contact management database. GoldMine, ACT!, and SalesForce are the best known, but a Microsoft Office Excel spreadsheet also works. Get as much contact information as possible to insert into the database. If you use Excel, make certain that you use separate columns for last name, first name, street address, city, state, zip code, phone number, fax number, e-mail address, type of business, source of inquiry or identification, notes, and dates for follow-up. Track all inquiries by getting at least the person's mailing address, e-mail address, and phone number. Note when a person calls and for what reason he or she is calling. Follow up on a regular basis with those who have not yet become clients.

Referral sources should also be tracked in a contact management database system. Additional items to add for referral sources are the numbers of calls received and the numbers of referrals actually received, plus the types.

SELLING AND LEAD GENERATION TACTICS

This section provides details on selling strategies and tactics for reaching client goals. Creating an actual written plan for sales and lead generation tactics can ensure success. Table 16–1 shows an example of a suggested format. Break down tasks into weekly, monthly, and quarterly activities.

Lead Generation

Lead generation is finding new targets for business. For example, you are at a luncheon for the Chamber of Commerce and meet an attorney who works with estate and trust clients. Get the person's business card, add the attorney to your database, and include the attorney in your regular communication. Or, while you are driving, you see that a physical therapist has set up a new office. Stop in, get the name of the manager, and make certain the staff know that you provide assistance to the frail elderly so when they see a client who is in for therapy, you can become a resource. Add the manager's name and information to your database, and keep in contact with the office through regular communication.

Tactics for lead generation include the following:

- Record all inquiries and calls for assistance coming into the office.
- Keep a contact management database of all inquiries, and follow up at set intervals.
- Respond immediately with information via a direct letter and other marketing information.
- Send a hand-written thank-you note to those with whom you have had meetings.
- Follow up monthly with articles of interest or news on the business.
- Optimize your website so it can easily be found by interested searchers.
- Submit aging-related articles to targeted print and online publications.
- Use all communications to drive traffic to your website.
- Do volunteer work with local senior, aging-related, or chronic illness organizations.
- Join local elder-law, guardianship, and trust department groups.
- Develop a seminar series that discusses choosing care options, caring for an aged parent, or the "sandwich" generation (those who are caring for children at home as well as for aging parents).
- Hold seminars at churches, hospitals, and community organizations, at various

Table 16–1	Quarterly Activity Tracker	
Objective	**Description**	**Getting It Done**
One seminar focused on dementia.	Create a 20-minute lecture focused on care needs for those with dementia. Offer this seminar to bank trust departments and senior centers. Goal: 15 attendees (keeping it small enough so individuals get attention but large enough so they don't feel singled out).	Use some outside assistance in planning and communication of the event.
One article written for the aging network newsletter.	Use a "case study" example to showcase how a GCM can assist a family in need. Write one 1500-word article to be submitted to appropriate publications.	Contact and send to all aging network newsletters in area, one at a time, and follow up with a call to ensure publication. First come, first published.
Send reprinted article to referral sources on contact management list.	Reprinted article to use as educational tool for referral sources and keep name in front of them on a regular basis.	Mail merge contact list with a cover letter stating this reprint can be used for educational purposes.
Referral source appreciation luncheon.	Have at least one referral source appreciation luncheon each quarter to serve as a cross-networking event for aging related referral sources.	Find an inexpensive but quiet place to offer a lunch and ask each referral source to describe his or her business to all in attendance.
Community involvement.	Promote or attend at least one aging or care continuum related community event.	GCM responsible for selecting and attending.

times of the day and evening, to capture all potential prospects.

- Create an e-mail newsletter to stay in front of those with whom you have had contact. Search for these contacts on Facebook and Twitter, and request to be added as friends, to allow for additional communication through social media tactics.

Consider Strategic Alliances

Strategic alliances are mutually beneficial alliances; for instance, consider aligning with Alzheimer's Association staff and volunteers.

Other ideas for strategic alliances include the following:

- **Form partnerships with other businesses related to yours.** Home care and home health agencies are a natural fit. Most need geriatric care management services and do not provide them. These agencies can be wonderful cross-referral sources because they also need clients. Durable medical equipment stores also have clients with geriatric care management needs and could use a referral source for assessments. Elder-law attorneys can find a GCM partner incredibly helpful when trying to determine next steps with frail clients.

- **Work with universities.** Use students from nursing or social work programs as interns.
- **Identify one or two Web presences.** Chronic disease associations all have websites, some with local chapters. Having your web link as a referral source and cross-linking from your website to theirs can bring you credibility and also serve as an educational resource for clients visiting your website. Home care companies with whom you have referral relationships can also serve as good reciprocal links.
- **Partner with school groups or community service groups.** This is a way to offer something to the community. Perhaps you can partner with a group to host a fundraiser that will benefit seniors in your community.
- **Retweet information from others, and become fans of others on Facebook.** This is a way to grow your base of followers, attract new friends and fans, and to reach more people who have an interest in your topic.

Don't Forget Your Current Customers

Frequent and useful communication with customers is essential to maintaining and growing your business. With the variety of communication vehicles available today, not only do clients (and prospects) expect immediate answers—they expect them to arrive in many different ways.

Use e-mail effectively for those who like to communicate this way. Possibly once a week or once every month, send clients brief communications with a link to an interesting article or with the status of their account.

Consider creating a monthly newsletter delivered via e-mail and regular mail that keeps clients up to date on what's happening with recent home care legislation and care options, provides answers to frequently asked questions, and gives information on other pertinent topics. This can also be used as an opt-in tactic to communicate with prospects on a regular basis. Plus, teasers to articles can be included in the newsletter with full text appearing on your website. This format also can easily be turned into a print newsletter for general prospecting for those who prefer to receive a hard copy.

Let your clients know that you are on Twitter and Facebook. Studies show an increasing number of seniors accessing the social media sites.[6] In fact, the third most popular online destination for people over 65 in November 2009 was Facebook. Overall, the number of unique visitors who are 65 or older on social networking and blog sites has increased 53% in the last 2 years alone. Of all visitors to social networking and blog sites, 8.2% are over 65, just one tenth of a percent less than the number of teenagers who frequent these sites. If you are giving out helpful information and sharing it, then your clients will appreciate it and be able to spread the word to their friends about the good work you do for them.

Don't underestimate the power of taking time to recognize holidays, birthdays, anniversaries, and so forth. This helps show your clients that they really are your priority.

■ COMMUNICATIONS STRATEGY

Your communications strategy provides a clear guide to be used when developing all communications. It lists key messages that need to be considered in all communications from collateral materials, to e-mail, to website copy.

A communications strategy can help you create consistency among your key messages. You can then create a connection with potential customers and referrals by reiterating those messages again and again to your target audiences.

■ CREATIVE AND PROMOTIONAL STRATEGY

To maintain a consistent look and image for a geriatric care management business, it is important to define and document creative guidelines, including graphic and copy standards. This helps keep anyone who works on your creative materials informed of the specifications to be used in creative development and keeps your business looking professional and consistent to the public.

Develop graphic standards for your business that require use of the same images, font colors, and typefaces for every communication. Standards provide clear directions on when and how to use your logo and messages for anyone who may be working to promote your business. Carefully consider which fonts, colors, and styles to use and how your look might be interpreted by the public. Fonts with seraphs (little feet on them) are more pleasing and easier for older people to read. Red text is easier for the older eye to read. Large print size, at least a 12-point font, is also easier to read.

In an industry such as the aging-needs industry with many messages competing for notice, the use of a consistent logo and tagline on all materials is a must. This helps drive home those messages you want to communicate, creates a personal connection, and helps set you apart from the competition. Contact information on *every* page of communication is a must. You are striving for recognition and development of subliminal relationships that show that you are in the business of providing information and resources to frail elderly persons, and you are the best available at providing these services. Consistent communications and design state this without many words.

■ MEET YOUR MARKETING GOALS: RECOMMENDED ACTIVITY

Marketing goals need to be specific and measurable. Include specific weekly, monthly, and quarterly activities that you will ultimately use to meet the goals set forth in your marketing plan. Constantly watch for client demand; then, talk about it with your core staff. Listen to what the client needs and meet that need. The marketing plan should prioritize lead generation tactics and face-to-face opportunities and include joining the best local and national organizations to increase business. The local Rotary Club is a great organization with which to be involved because the membership is older and because members are community leaders who have accumulated some wealth. Not only may your local Rotary Club use your geriatric care management service, but the members may recommend you to others.

When considering which media to use to reach potential targets and referral sources, use every method available and affordable: Internet, mail, phone greeting played when a client is on hold, e-mail tagline, social media, stationery, signage, and so forth.

Every contact needs to be a positive contact. If you have staff, consider using a mystery-shopper service to perform regular checks on your staff's customer service performance. (See additional information on mystery shopping under "Setting Yourself Apart From Competition" on next page.) Answering the phone is probably the most important sales tool because the call may be an initial inquiry from an interested party. Excellent customer service and engaging the inquirer with questions about his or her situation and needs can lead to a new client. Always ask if you can send the caller information. If yes, send it *that day*. Ask the caller if he or she would prefer mail or e-mail as the method to receive your information. As always, record the contact in the database. One caution is not to solve the problem in one phone call. Decide on a timeframe—15 minutes is suggested—for listening and responding to the caller. Also, explain that geriatric care management services are professional services for which there is a fee, just like for the services of an attorney or an accountant.

Measure referrals and client sources and assess monthly where business is being generated. Track referrals to identify those sources who refer repeatedly. Each caller should be asked, "How did you hear about us?" Send thank-you cards to every referral source, or at least make a phone call or send an e-mail to thank them. Ask previous clients if you can use them as references.

Make the most of current referral prospects. Use note cards and give out business cards. Send press clippings to interested people. Use a contact management tool such as SalesForce, GoldMine, Act!, Outlook, or Microsoft Access. An Excel spreadsheet of contacts can work in a pinch if the file is set up correctly to capture the necessary information.

When it comes to media interest, make sure that you respond immediately if you receive a call from a reporter. Be clear about the services you offer and use your key messages and positioning statements to guide how you describe your business. Add reporters to your contact management tool, and code them as media as the type of group.

A Yellow Pages listing is also a source for phone inquiries. List small ads under several sections rather than using one large ad. Sometimes there is not an established category for care management, so people will search for assistance under the categories of geriatric consulting, nursing, sitters, companions, home health, and senior services, to name a few. Also use YellowPages.com listings so families from afar can find your service.

Search for online directories that list care management or aging services, and make certain that you are in each and every directory listing possible.

■ SETTING YOURSELF APART FROM COMPETITION

With so many aging resources available, the key to success is to use a specific strategy to decide on which messages, targets, and specific goals will accomplish the business growth you desire. Setting your business apart from the competition occurs only after you have assessed the competition and implemented a strategic plan that includes providing an excellent service, good customer relations, good referral relations, and using contact management tools effectively.

Mystery shopping is a term used to describe the act of surveying the competition while acting as a consumer making an inquiry. Conducting this type of competition survey is one way to look at the competition and find out what they are doing that is different, better, or worse, and to use that information to your benefit.

Your first step toward completing a competition analysis for your business is to create a scenario for mystery shopping. For example, you pretend your aunt is going to need some help because she is confused. You do not know what to do for her at this point. You are checking available options and are responsible for reporting back to the other family members.

Make a list of the competitors who do business in your area and include their phone numbers and website information. Then, make the calls to the competition. Use your predetermined mystery shopping scenario, ask the following questions, and track the answers as you go. Make certain to ask that a brochure or any other marketing information be mailed to you. In this way, you can compare not only what services are provided and the prices, but also how your inquiry is handled and the time it takes the business to respond.

Finally, take all of the information you have compiled and summarize it, along with your comments regarding the information your competitors sent to you, as follows:

Name of Agency
Phone number:
Website:
Spoke with:

How long in business:
Services offered:
Cost:
Advance notice needed to begin service?
Can they send information?
How did the staff person handle the call?
(1 is excellent service, 5 is poor service)
How well did the staff person meet your
needs about the information you
requested?
Did the staff person present the company
appropriately?

Overall impression:
Date material received:
Comments on materials:

Secrets of Marketing Success

The number one secret for marketing success is being where the customer can find you when he or she has a need. A close second is listening to customers when they do find you and providing excellent service. Setting very high standards for responsiveness can also contribute to success.

Table 16–2   Start-up GCM PR/Marketing Checklist

Description	Services Needed to Complete
Brand Identity, including logo design and collateral material design	Research competition, develop key differentiating factor, develop "brand positioning" statement, develop business name, graphic design for logo, colors for business communication
Business Identity (i.e., coordinated business cards, letterhead, envelopes, note cards, and folders)	Graphic design, printing, and delivery
Product Sheets and/or Brochure	Copywriting, graphic design, printing, and delivery
Identified and Defined Prospects, including a prospect profile	Identify prospects, research, develop prospect profiles, mailing lists, key factors for specific communication messages per targeted group
Testimonials captured in usable format	Identify procedures for obtaining testimonials
Targeted Referral Sources	Plan, design, and develop a system; data maintenance and administration; fulfillment
Website	Obtain URL, establish hosting account; develop content; maintain updated site
Blog	Use Word Press or another blog software, and set up an account to start posting information
Desktop & Industry Reminders (promotional items sporting your logo, brand image, and contact information)	Brainstorm and select items to be used, decide how to "brand" item with product logo, when to distribute
E-Mail Newsletter	Design format, write content, publish on a regular basis; create system for obtaining e-mail addresses and updating data

Table 16–2   Start-up GCM PR/Marketing Checklist (continued)

Description	Services Needed to Complete
Regular Newsletter	Design format, write content, publish on a regular basis
Twitter, Facebook, and LinkedIn Accounts	Sign up and learn how to play in social media; use Twitter for snippets of information and to grow contacts; use Facebook to educate and spread the work on speaking and events; use LinkedIn as a professional referral source
Charitable and Volunteer Work	Research for a match with key marketing factors; use publicity
Seminars and/or Workshop Presentations	Create text and presentations and use publicity; create evaluation form; use system for retrieval of attendees for marketing purposes
Trade Show Participation	Selection of appropriate shows, coordination, design of booth, design of materials, selection of giveaways for targeted attendees, preshow and postshow communication
Marketing and Promotional Packets (containing a variety of materials depending on their use)	Printing, assembly, mailing
Follow-Up Marketing Campaigns	Implementation strategy and execution
New Product Advertisements (could be as simple as tear sheets and PDF files to download off of the website or include in marketing kits)	Design, developing content, printing
Methods of Feedback/Measurement	Interviews, surveys, research, development of measurement methods
Direct Mailer/Response Cards	Design, printing, mailing
Press Kit (including company and principal backgrounder, press releases, articles, FAQs)	Develop key messages, refine media targets, develop press kit, preparation and distribution
Ongoing Press Releases	Writing and distribution
Current/Former Referral Communications	Client communication, follow-up phone calls
Website Integration (all press releases, newsletters, and publicity posted on website)	Website content updates/maintenance

■ CONCLUSION

The most important thing to remember about marketing a geriatric care management business is that services of a geriatric care manager are as-needed, and consumers seek a GCM only when the need arises. Being where the client or referral source is looking when the need arises is the goal. Secondarily, the GCM must, in many cases, educate consumers about what a GCM is and does. Projecting a professional image and a well-designed and thoughtfully considered message that resonates with the consumer is necessary to deliver your message to consumers in need and turn them into clients.

■ REFERENCES

1. Bearden WO, Ingram TN, LaForge R. *Marketing Principles and Perspectives*. 4th ed. New York: McGraw-Hill/Irwin; 2003.

2. Orsini M. Marketing private-duty home care services. *Home Health Care Manage Prac.* February 2006;18(2):114–123.

3. Orsini M. Branded! Use branding to cement image, gain referrals. *Success in Home Care.* July/August 2005; 9(4).

4. Kotler P. *According to Kotler; the world's foremost authority on marketing answers to your questions.* New York, NY: AMACOM: 2005:90.

5. Orsini M. *Private duty business manual.* Marketing module. http://shop.markethomecare.com/products/private-duty-business-manual-with-forms. Accessed August 27, 2010.

6. Horrigan, John. *Home Broadband Adoption 2009.* June 19, 2009. http://www.pewinternet.org/Reports/2009/10-Home-Broadband-Adoption-2009.aspx?r=1. Accessed August 26, 2010.

Chapter 17

Private Revenue Sources for the Fee-Based Care Manager: Need versus Demand in the Private Elder Care Market

Robert E. O'Toole

The independent professional practice of geriatric care management has continued its steady growth for more than 20 years. Private care management, however, continues to serve a small niche market and has yet to achieve the growth potential that many have been predicting for the past 2 decades. The National Association of Professional Geriatric Care Managers (NAPGCM), which is the national membership organization for our profession, has grown from 200 members in 1990 to more than 2000 members in 2010. Given the often cited needs of a growing frail elderly population and the millions of family caregivers who can benefit from skilled professional support, membership in this specialized multidisciplinary elder-care profession should be growing at a much faster rate. Prior to taking the bold step of developing an entrepreneurial, fee-based alternative to the largely third-party financed, long-term care service delivery system, most geriatric care managers (GCMs) worked in non-fee-based settings, such as private hospitals or healthcare systems, nonprofit agencies funded by grants or the United Way, church-supported organizations, or tax-supported public or quasi-public agencies.

Regardless of the care setting, the money to pay for the services provided to frail elders usually does not come directly from the recipient of the service. Neither do family members of the care recipients make significant financial contributions in most cases. In hospitals, outpatient health clinics, certified home health agencies, or nursing homes, the primary source of funding is likely to be various forms of third-party insurance. This most likely is from a federal insurance program such as Medicare or the joint state and federal insurance program known as Medicaid, as well as some funding from the federal Administration on Aging (AOA) through its nationwide network of Area Agencies on Aging (AAA).

■ DECLINING PUBLIC FUNDING AVAILABLE TO PAY FOR ELDER CARE: A CRISIS OR ESTABLISHED PUBLIC POLICY?

Most of the first decade of the 21st century saw an unprecedented rise in the national debt:

> On Inauguration Day, 2009, the debt stood at $10.626 trillion. During the Clinton administration, it took over 2 years for the national debt to increase a trillion dollars. But by the time former president George W. Bush left office, he had run up the deficit by a record amount: $4.9 trillion over 8 years.[1]

The Congressional Budget Office (CBO) estimates that the federal budget deficit for 2010 will exceed $1.3 trillion.[2] Federal spending on wars in Iraq and Afghanistan, steep tax cuts, a costly Medicare prescription drug program,

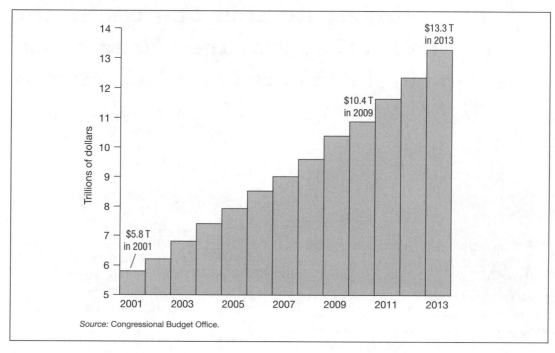

Figure 17–1 Building a Wall of Debt: Gross Federal Debt Soars

and finally, the near collapse of the country's largest banks and financial institutions in 2009 has largely depleted the pool of funds available to pay for services to frail elders.[3]

At a press conference in February 2008 on President Bush's FY 2009 budget, Senate Budget Committee Chairman Kent Conrad (D-ND) said:

> . . . I would suggest to you the debt is the threat. Why? Because . . . while the deficit goes up over $400 billion, the debt will go up over $700 billion in one year. The big difference, of course, is Social Security money that is being used to pay other bills. It doesn't get included in any deficit calculation, but every penny of it gets added to the debt.[4]

See Figure 17–1.

Further reductions in publicly funded services to frail elders will result from similar fiscal problems at the state level:

An already storm-tossed economy is about to receive a thorough drenching, as states across the nation face a collective budget shortfall of $140 billion this summer. The details, contained in a new report from the Center on Budget and Policy Priorities, are sobering, not the least for what they suggest about the fragility of the national recovery. Tax receipts—property, income, you name it— have dwindled and dwindled some more, the federal stimulus gas tank is near empty, and as many as 900,000 workers could lose their jobs as a result of state budget-cutting in the coming fiscal year. Nor is there much help on the way.[5]

These serious financial crises have occurred just when the first of two age waves is about to crest. The size and impact of our rapidly aging nation is like two tidal waves, one very close to shore, and the other visible, but far off in the distance.

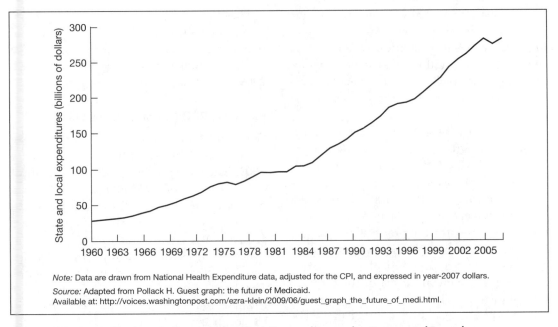

Figure 17–2 Inflation-Adjusted Medical Expenditures by State and Local Governments Between 1960 and 2007

The first tidal wave of frail elders needing care has now arrived with an unprecedented number of people living into their 80s and 90s. Currently, people age 85 years and older are almost six times more likely to need chronic, ongoing health and social services than those in their 60s.[6]

This first age wave is already taxing the available resources, which met the demand when the Administration on Aging and federal and state programs to provide long-term care to frail elders were initially developed.[5] Medicaid, the joint, federal- and state-funded health program for the poor, is now the largest and fastest-growing segment of most state budgets (Figure 17–2). The largest portion of Medicaid budgets pays for nursing home bills for both poor and middle-class persons who are ill prepared for the staggering costs of care.

The other major government healthcare program for those over age 65 is the Medicare program. The CBO has warned about the funding of Medicare:

> The Congressional Budget Office cast doubt . . . on claims that the healthcare bill currently before the United States Senate would help Medicare remain solvent. The nonpartisan agency, which is charged with determining the cost of proposals before Congress, said in a letter that proponents of the bill were in effect double-counting the impact of the savings the legislation would generate. The $246 billion the CBO estimated the legislation would save Medicare "can't both finance new programs and help pay future expenses for elderly covered under the federal program."[7]

Seventy-eight million baby boomers will start to turn 65 in 2011. They will continue reaching retirement age over the next 20 years, doubling the population covered by Medicare in the 1990s.

Moreover, these baby boomers will live longer than their predecessors. Almost as importantly, their generation is followed by the unusually small baby-bust generation, resulting in a smaller base of available workers for an even larger group of dependent retirees.[7]

The response by state and federal governments to this growing demand for long-term health care, so far, has been to tighten eligibility rules for the Medicaid program, reduce the amount of care available, and require elders and family caregivers to pay more out-of-pocket expenses for long-term illnesses. The Medicare program has been capping fees for a growing number of medical procedures, resulting in financial hardship for primary care physicians. The reimbursement rate for geriatric physicians is so low that many are refusing new patients. Because of this, a medical specialty that was expected to grow has instead declined with fewer geriatric physicians in 2009 than in 1990.[8]

The second age wave will make the first wave look like only a ripple by comparison. The large number of baby boomers, who will begin to reach age 65 in 2011, will swell the ranks of the elderly because life expectancy is expected to continue to increase in the 21st century. The baby boomers are likely to live longer than their parents did. Seventy-six million people were born during the postwar years of 1946–1964. Add the number of immigrants who have come to America since the end of World War II, and the result is that the population of those over 85 will grow by nearly 150% by the year 2030.[9]

In many ways, aging policy has become a major dilemma for our society. Benefits for the elderly command an increasingly large share of the budget, putting the squeeze on other programs. Yet many elderly suffer severe deprivation, and the social safety net fails to catch them; meanwhile long-term care costs have been growing faster than the rate of inflation.[10]

The cost of long-term care services not covered by publicly funded sources can easily run to more than $100,000 a year in some parts of the United States, according to the Genworth 2009 Cost of Care Survey.

Financial 2009 Cost of Care Survey

Genworth Financial commissioned the cost of care survey for the sixth consecutive year in 2009. The survey is believed to be the most comprehensive of its kind and includes data points from over 14,000 nursing homes, assisted living facilities, and home care providers across the country.

Following is a breakdown of the average costs of various services in the United States. These rates vary widely, with higher rates on the east and west coasts, and lower rates in the south and Midwest.

Home Health Aide Services
(Non-Medicare Certified)
(Also known as private-duty aides)
National median hourly rate: $18.50

Home Health Aide Services
(Medicare Certified)
National average median hourly rate: $46.22

Assisted Living Facility
(private one bedroom)
National average median monthly rate: $2825.25

Nursing Home (semiprivate room)
National average median daily rate: $183.25 or $5497 monthly[11]

Families that are faced with finding suitable care for an elderly family member are often surprised at the high cost of care or the fact that most of this care is not covered by public insurance programs. This sticker shock can make the decisions about care options all the more difficult.

Frequently, there is little understanding of how existing elder-care programs actually operate, what they cost, and who benefits. For this reason alone, the demand for the types of skilled elder-care services provided by geriatric care managers should be growing at a rapid rate as family caregivers struggle, trying to navigate their way through a maze of publicly funded services, health insurance programs, and an array of service options, as well as state and federal regulations that can seem impossible to fathom.

On February 8, 2006, President George W. Bush signed the Deficit Reduction Act of 2005 (DRA) into law. When the DRA was passed, the Congressional Budget Office predicted the new law would reduce federal Medicaid spending by $11.5 billion over a 5-year period and by $43.2 billion over the next 10 years.

For many families, the law suddenly changed the way that long-term care, especially nursing home care, is paid for by placing more monetary responsibility on those needing care. The National Academy of Elder Law Attorneys (NAELA) issued a statement saying that the DRA creates "a healthcare crisis of unprecedented magnitude for our most vulnerable citizens." Nearly 5 years after the DRA was signed, the impact on elders' eligibility for Medicaid and the savings produced by this law have yet to be determined.[11]

IS THE DEMAND FOR ELDER CARE LARGE ENOUGH TO SUPPORT FEE-BASED ELDER CARE PROFESSIONALS?

Today, after more than 20 years of specialized elder-care professionals providing skilled clinical services to frail and disabled individuals and their family caregivers, geriatric care management is still a cottage industry. Although a few corporate chains have been buying GCM practices that offer both care management and private-duty home care services under one roof, the vast majority of the profession's membership consists of either solo practices or very small business ventures with only a few owners and employees.

While growth in this profession has increased steadily, the growth of private, for-profit elder-care enterprises has been modest when compared with the growth of the aging population over the past 20 years.

Why is it then, that, in a nation that is aging rapidly, with unprecedented numbers of people living into their 80s and 90s, fee-based geriatric care management is still a cottage industry after becoming an established professional discipline more than 20 years ago?

Numerous for-profit enterprises, from small care management businesses to larger corporate enterprises offering an array of elder-care services targeted to a nationwide market, have failed after only a few years. It appears that many of these enterprises made a faulty assumption when developing their business plans. When they looked at the large volume of research and demographic data published in dozens of studies funded by groups such as the American Association of Retired Persons (AARP), the MetLife Mature Market Institute, and the Brookings Institute, among others, they saw a well-documented need for the services provided by private care managers.

Looking at this large and growing need for services, they confused "need" with "demand." The fact is that the services of private fee-based geriatric care managers, private duty homemaker agencies, and most assisted living facilities are only affordable to a very small percentage of the population.

The April 30, 2010, issue of the *Wall Street Journal* reported that ten percent of Americans controlled 75 percent of the wealth in this country:

> New calculations by Edward Wolff, the New York University economist and an expert on U.S. wealth statistics, show that the top 1% actually held onto its share of national wealth in the crisis, and may have even gained a bit. Meanwhile, share of national wealth held by the bottom 90% fell to 25%....."[12]

A 2007 report on Medicare long-term care, issued by the Government Accountability Office, stated the following:

> the services that are provided formally and funded by these programs as well as those that are provided informally by many Americans who are family members and those they care for and about, account for a big impact on the overall healthcare cost burden in this country. After all, these are the individuals who have the most serious healthcare needs. They're the individuals who often have the hardest time navigating our current healthcare system, getting from one setting to another, really testing the limits of our current healthcare system, in terms of its gaps in coordination of care, dealing with transitions of care, and dealing with evidence-based opportunities to prevent complications of chronic conditions.[13]

The National Alliance for Caregiving in Collaboration with AARP published a study in November 2009 called *A Focused Look at Those Caring for Someone Age 50 or Older.* Their study estimates there are at least 43.5 million caregivers age 18 and over, which is equivalent to 19% of all adults, who provide unpaid care to an adult family member or friend who is age 50 years or older.[14]

It is tempting to look at this research data and see the potential market for geriatric care management services, as well as other elder-care services such as private-duty home care, assisted living facilities, and seemingly hundreds of Web-based services that offer advice and support to elders and family caregivers. While writing this chapter, a Google search for "elder-care services" returned 535,000 results. "Caring for aging parents" returned 689,000 Web pages, and the search term "assisted living services" produced more than 19 million results.

Some of these websites mislead the caregiver or consumer by promising to send them free information if they agree to provide personal information including their address and phone number. In many cases these Web-based companies are nothing more than lead-generation companies that offer no services to elders and instead sell the addresses and phone numbers to elder-care professionals, assuring those gullible enough to pay for them that these are qualified leads that will bring in new business.

The National Family Caregiver Support Program (NFCSP), established in 2000 by the US Administration on Aging (AOA), provides grants to states and territories based on their share of the population aged 70 and over, to fund a range of support that assist family and informal caregivers to care for their loved ones at home for as long as possible.

The NFCSP offers a range of services to support family caregivers. Under this program, states provide five types of services:

- Information to caregivers about available services
- Assistance to caregivers in gaining access to the services
- Individual counseling, organization of support groups, and caregiver training
- Respite care
- Supplemental services, on a limited basis

These services work in conjunction with other state and community-based services to provide a coordinated set of supports. Studies have shown that these services can reduce caregiver depression, anxiety, and stress and enable them to provide care longer, thereby avoiding or delaying the need for costly institutional care.

Because of the combination of federal and state budget deficits cited earlier, and the fact that existing entitlement programs such as Medicare, Social Security, and state pension funds are seriously underfunded, available public funding for elder-care services will continue to shrink even as the population of older Americans who need such services continues to grow until at least 2030. For example the NFCSP has seen steady declines in its funding in recent years.

Funding for family caregiver support services during the past 4 years is as follows:

- Fiscal year (FY) 2006: $156,060,000
- FY 2007: $156,167,000
- FY 2008: $153,439,000
- FY 2009: $154,220,000[15]

Need vs. Demand for Geriatric Care Management Services

It appears that a large number of entrepreneurs, both for-profit and not-for profit, have based an elder-care business model, at least in part, on the well-documented needs of elders and family caregivers and expect that their elder-care business will soon be busy and profitable. After all, isn't the basic formula for building a successful business "Find a need and fill it?"

Although "Find a need and fill it" sounds like a logical approach to a prospective market niche, it is not a sound revenue model for an elder-care business. It's clear that the need for elder-care services is huge and growing rapidly. But to survive as independent business owners, GCMs and other elder-care professionals must look more closely at the data and embrace a more realistic philosophy. *Need* doesn't pay the bills, demand does. The mythology surrounding how long-term care is paid for presents an obstacle to the independent, for-profit, elder-care professional.

The tradition of having most long-term care paid for by third parties has created an expectation that has become firmly established in the American psyche. The prevailing attitude about payment for long-term care services, whether provided in a facility or in the community, has been that long-term care should be paid for by somebody else, regardless of the family's income and assets.

Only those with substantial financial resources can afford to pay privately for care at home, assisted living facilities, continuing care retirement communities, and other expensive discretionary health and preventive services, not paid for with public funds.

Because demand and *not* need determines the success of an elder-care business, this fundamental fact of life must be taken into consideration when developing a business plan for a for-profit, fee-based, elder-care business. The target market for such a business is not the 39 million families who need geriatric care management services, but the much smaller subset of those families who can afford to hire a GCM, are willing to pay for the services GCMs and other for-profit, elder-care enterprises provide, and can actually find their way to the fee-based provider. Raising awareness of the availability of private pay alternatives is a major challenge to bringing in new business, especially when most small business owners have very limited marketing budgets.

Frail elders and family caregivers with sufficient resources to pay for care can afford to hire a private care manager. Because of their knowledge and experience of the complex maze of care alternatives, care managers can often save caregivers and care recipients money by using this knowledge to find the best care and show families how to access that care in the most cost-effective way. However, those who can afford to pay privately for care management, home care, and care in the best facilities represent a much smaller percentage of those who need elder-care services. A report by the Brookings Institution confirms this: "Despite the estimated cost of paying for LTC [long-term care] services and the strain it puts on retirement savings, very few people in or approaching retirement have private resources or sufficient public benefits to protect them from long-term care costs."[16]

In addition, another barrier to setting up a geriatric care management services business that relies on care recipients to pay for services from private resources is the mythology of long-term care, which consists of the four following beliefs.

The Entitlement Mentality

This is the widely held view that the federal or state government should pay for long-term care, rather than requiring those who have income and assets to pay for their care for as long as possible. The tradition of having most health-care-related services paid for by an employer during a person's working years and then by Medicare when the person retires has created an expectation for free care that has become firmly established in the American psyche.

Resistance to Paying Privately for Care The resistance to paying privately for care has been so strong in this country that often even those with income and assets that place them in the middle and upper economic classes have used laws designed to help the poor to avoid paying for care or the care of a family member. It is this practice of becoming artificially poor by placing assets that could otherwise be used to pay for long-term care services that prompted the passage of the Deficit Reduction Act of 2006, mentioned earlier in this chapter.

Stephen Moses, president of the Seattle-based Center for Long-Term Care Reform, has written and spoken extensively on the issue of federal entitlements, especially federal and state funding that pays for care even when the person needing care has sufficient income and assets to pay for that care. "The solution to a looming long-term care crisis is in consumers taking personal responsibility, not in more government programs." says Moses.

With 77 million baby boomers near retirement and about to collect Social Security benefits, Moses sees a fiscal crisis at hand. He believes that the public is in denial because of a system that has seen the federal government shoulder most long-term care costs for decades. Medicaid is the biggest payer of these costs. Moses says that more of that burden is about to shift to individuals, saying "You're going to be responsible, so you better plan." More seniors will probably have to use some of the $4.2 trillion that is tied up in home equity to pay for care, perhaps through such financial tools as a reverse mortgage.[17]

This deeply ingrained entitlement mentality, even among those with assets and income to pay for care, makes the move to become an independent provider of elder-care services through nurses, social workers, and other elder-care professionals a risky business venture.

The federal government's own website, Medicare.gov, talks about the limits of publicly funded long-term care coverage, saying that generally, Medicare doesn't pay for long-term care. Medicare pays only for medically necessary skilled nursing facilities or home health care. However, you must meet certain conditions for Medicare to pay for these types of care. Most long-term care is needed to assist people with the activities of daily living, such as dressing, bathing, and using the bathroom. Medicare doesn't pay for this type of care, which is called custodial care. It may also include care that most people do for themselves, for example, diabetes monitoring. Some Medicare Advantage Plans (formerly Medicare+ Choice) may offer limited skilled nursing facilities and home care (skilled care) coverage if the care is medically necessary.

> Medicaid is available only to certain low-income individuals and families who fit into an eligibility group that is recognized by federal and state law. Medicaid is a state administered program and each state sets its own guidelines regarding eligibility and services . . . certain requirements must be met. These may include your income and resources (like bank accounts, real property, or other items that can be sold for cash); and whether you are a US citizen or a lawfully admitted immigrant. The rules for counting your income and resources vary from state to state and from group to group.[18]

The growing importance of private financing of long-term care services for American elders is reflected in an article by Howard Gleckman, Senior Research Associate at the Urban Institute, which was published in the *Kaiser Foundations' Health News* in August 2009. Gleckman points out that Medicaid was never intended to pay for long-term care, does a very poor job of managing long-term care services, and is rapidly becoming fiscally unsustainable. Gleckman says to "get Medicaid out of the long-term care business."

> Not only are the frail elderly and disabled at the mercy of increasingly desperate governors and state legislators, but they have to jump though incredible hoops to get the care that is most appropriate for them. For example, many frail elders suffer from multiple chronic conditions. More than almost anyone, their care needs to be carefully coordinated. Ideally, the medical system would make sure they could move seamlessly from acute care to long-term care, either at home or in a nursing facility. Despite that tragic lack of coordination, Medicaid now spends nearly one third of its total budget on long-term care services and half of its funds on medical and personal care combined for those frail elderly and adults with disabilities who are jointly eligible for Medicare and Medicaid.[19]

I'm Not Old Enough to Worry About That Now

The need for long-term care can occur at any age. An accident, a chronic illness, or an injury can result in the need for long-term care. According to the National Center for Health Statistics, nearly half of the population in the United States will need some type of long-term care in their lifetime. Forty percent of the population of people with disabilities who need long-term care are working-age adults. Unfortunate events that prevent a person from working can happen at any age, not just in old age.

It Will Never Happen to Me

Many Americans continue to mislead themselves into thinking they are not likely to need care. Furthermore, they are under the false impression that long-term care is something that is primarily a need of the very old, when in fact, 40% of those needing assistance with daily living tasks are younger than 65. Senator Russ Feingold of Wisconsin has been an outspoken advocate of long-term care reform in his 20-plus years in the US Senate. Feingold served as Chair of the Senate's Long-Term Care Working Group in 1994. In a speech from the floor of the Senate in July of 2009, Senator Feingold spoke about long-term care.

> Of the 10 million Americans needing long-term care, 40% were working-age adults or children who have become disabled or too ill, to live independently. As for the 60% of older Americans and senior citizens needing long-term care, who theoretically might have had time to save for these medical needs, financing long-term care on their own is simply too expensive. Not only is the cost of long-term care growing at twice the rate of inflation, seniors are using long-term care supports and services earlier and more often. And families are feeling the strain. Studies estimate that over 85% of long-term care is provided by family and friends, but the cost of providing care and forgoing earnings elsewhere is not included in projections of long-term care spending. Long-term care reform is not an issue of making people be more responsible, save earlier, or save more— it's needed because the system, on a fundamental level, is strained to the breaking point.[20]

My Family Will Take Care of Me

Historically, in the United States, women traditionally cared for their aging parents and other relatives. With the rise over the last several decades of the two-income household, working women can no longer serve as full-time caregivers. Many women start families later, meaning they're busy raising their own children, just as their elders need help. In addition, elders often live hundreds or thousands of miles away from potential family caregivers.

"Family cohesiveness is a tall order at any time of life," according to a *Wall Street Journal* article.[21] But as parents grow frail, brothers and sisters often encounter new obstacles to togetherness at precisely the time they most need to rely on one another. Sibling rivalry can emerge or intensify as adult children vie, one last time, for a parent's love or financial support. And even as parents grow dependent on children, the desire to cling to old, familiar roles can create a dysfunctional mess.

With the economy and household finances in disrepair, such strains become more pronounced. According to a recent report by the National Alliance for Caregiving and AARP, about 43.5 million Americans look after someone 50 or older, which is 28% more than in 2004. In comparison with 2004, a smaller percentage—41% versus 46%—are hiring help. And more—70% versus 59%—are reaching out to unpaid help, such as family and friends.[21]

As long as most Americans continue to embrace the prevailing mythology of long-term care, these myths will continue to create a barrier to operating a profitable elder-care service business that is based on fees paid by the care recipient or a family member.

Elder-Care Entrepreneurs Need to Become Experts in the Complexities of Financing Long-Term Care

As elder-care professionals who provide services largely paid for from private funds, GCMs have a vested interest in raising the level of awareness of the US public about the various private funding resources available to pay for geriatric care management and other elder-care services that GCMs incorporate into the care plans they develop for their clients. Care managers and other for-profit elder-care professionals must also become active advocates of the importance of planning ahead before an elder-care or disability care crisis occurs. We need to raise awareness of the undesirable consequences that will transpire if people continue to hold on to the mythology of long-term care.

■ BASING A PRIVATE ELDER CARE BUSINESS MODEL ON DEMOGRAPHICS: THE REALITY OF A NEED- VS. DEMAND-BASED REVENUE MODEL

We've all seen the data—America is growing older. The population of persons age 85 years and older is the largest in history and will keep growing for the foreseeable future. There are also 78 to 80 million baby boomers, the oldest of whom started turning 60 in 2004. Many elder-care entrepreneurs enter the private, fee-only market with a business plan that is based on these demographic projections.

It is tempting to create a business plan to serve the growing population of elders in need based on the demographic projections of an aging society. However, as noted earlier in this chapter, such naive thinking must be tempered by the harsh reality of many who have ventured into the private market and failed. Those who build an elder-care business model based on the number of elders who need care will sooner or later go out of business.

The fundamental rule in estimating the real market for private, fee-based elder-care services, as stated earlier, is that need doesn't pay the bills, demand does. This rule is simply a reminder of the first basic principle taught in any Economics 101 class. Economists call it supply and demand. If you're in the business of providing elder care that is paid for by your client's or customer's private resources, you'd better focus on the fact that a much smaller percentage of those in need of elder services can afford—or are willing—to pay for those services. That smaller group is the demand portion of the growing population of elders.

Because the vast majority of GCMs come to the private sector of elder-care services from a human services, health, or educational background, it is often hard to accept that many of those who seek out geriatric care management services can't afford to pay for them. However, to stay in business, GCMs simply can't afford to provide services to those in need who don't have the resources to pay. Only those who can pay our fees from their own resources can keep GCMs in business.

In his invaluable new book *How to Start a Home-Based Senior Care Business* (Global Pequot Press, 2010), author James L. Ferry addresses all aspects of setting up a small elder-care business, provides indispensable guidance on legal and ethical issues, and shows a small and solo elder-care entrepreneur how to become and stay profitable.

Ferry, a successful geriatric care manager for nearly 20 years, addresses the income realities of a start-up elder-care entrepreneur as follows.

> A major challenge for the aspiring senior care entrepreneur is being able to afford your current lifestyle while you plan and execute the numerous tasks that are necessary before you serve that first client. Additionally, you will need to invest financial resources in order to get your business established. Entrepreneurship, done right, requires tenacity and resilience. At times, it means servicing clients at the expense of leisure and time with family and friends. Entrepreneurship involving service to clients in need requires a new orientation toward your work—to some extent you are always "on call" and in the roles of practitioner, marketer, and manager.[22]

Independent practice professionals who previously worked in settings that were third-party funded had an infrastructure that pro-vided them with an office (or a cubicle), supplies, and overhead costs, such as reimbursement for travel and continuing education costs, along with health insurance and a predictable income. As Ferry states in his book, if a GCM wants to become an independent business owner, he or she must learn very quickly that to replace the amenities previously provided by a hospital, nursing home, home health agency, or other employer, the GCM must charge fees to those whom they provide services. The fees must be paid out of the pocket of the consumer rather than from a third party.

Even many of those who can afford geriatric care management services and who aren't eligible for subsidized services cling to the long-term care myths cited earlier, and are reluctant to pay GCMs out of their own funds. More than any other factor, the private, fee-based nature of independent geriatric care management practice, in the context of a widely held attitude opposed to paying directly for such services, is a barrier to operating a profitable business.

In developing a business plan for a fee-based, elder-care services business such as a geriatric care management business, it's important for GCMs to have a basic understanding of all likely sources of income, private and public, that are available to pay for the expanding range of long-term care services. A detailed list of eight alternative resources to cover the costs of long-term care appears later in this chapter.

Not only will state and federal government officials continue to slash Medicaid budgets and further limit care options for those who rely on public funding for their care, but the pool of workers in the labor-intensive, long-term care industry will continue to shrink due to these limited budgets. This happens as the number of frail and disabled elderly steadily grows at an ever-increasing pace.

To plan for their future long-term care needs properly, Americans must understand that the quality of care and the options available depend on whether they can pay the bill from private funds or rely on government funding to pay for care. The evidence is overwhelming and undeniable; the choices and the quality of care provided to those who rely on public funding are very limited and will only become more so as the aging population grows.

Those who are dependent on Medicaid and other sources of public funding receive poor care, very little care, or no care at all. It is a well-documented fact that nursing homes that rely on Medicaid funding are seriously understaffed, and their personnel are often poorly trained. Unfortunately, the situation is expected to worsen instead of improve.

Many needy elders and other disabled adults languish for months on waiting lists for publicly funded community care programs, even when they meet the eligibility guidelines. When service finally becomes available, it is typically much less than is needed. The publicly funded case manager is likely to be someone with little training or experience, carrying a caseload that often exceed more than 90 people with complicated needs and few resources.

The New York Nonprofit Press, (NYNP) a monthly publication covering 4000 nonprofit human service agencies throughout the New York metropolitan area, provides a graphic description of the deterioration of publicly funded elder services. According to NYNP, New York City's Bloomberg administration began a massive modernization program of its services to community-based elders in 2008. The stated goal of streamlining its system of senior services was to bring down costs and expand the numbers of individuals the system can serve in the future. Taken at face value, this would seem to be the right move at the right moment in time.

Unfortunately, the NYNP reported the following:

These seemingly well-intended initiatives now appear to be having precisely the opposite effect. The combination of service system consolidations and repeated cycles of across-the-board budget cuts now threatens to destabilize—rather than strengthen and expand—the city's senior services infrastructure.

Department for the Aging (DFTA) and its nonprofit service provider partners have been subject to a total of $16.6 million in funding reductions. . . . Complete service systems have been eliminated including the Social Adult Day Program, which allowed seniors with Alzheimer's to live in the community, and the Intergenerational Program, which brings youth and seniors together for mutual support.

Mayor Bloomberg's Budget for FY 2010 would more than double these cuts—reducing DFTA's budget by another $21 million. It would reduce funding for senior centers by another $5 million, Case Management by $1.1 million and Home Delivered Meals by $1.4 million. Elder Abuse Prevention services would be eliminated entirely.

Individual case managers are carrying caseloads ranging from 65 to as high as 145. As a result, they are unable to take on new cases or even provide services for existing case management clients. An estimated 900 seniors who had been receiving case management services prior to the transition have yet to be assigned to a new case manager. These "unassigned" clients are awaiting a potential crisis before they can receive services.[23]

It sometimes seems that the general public isn't paying attention to the growing crisis in long-term care for the elderly, but the press cannot be blamed for not trying to get the message out. It seems that almost daily, newspapers and other national and local media outlets publish articles that highlight the growing severity of what has already become one of the major problems facing an aging America in the 21st century.

UNDERSTANDING THE FUNDING SOURCES TO PAY FOR LONG-TERM CARE

There are 10 basic sources of funding to pay for long-term care services:

1. Medicare
2. Medicaid
3. Private savings and other liquid assets (including funds from adult children)
4. Private long-term care insurance (LTCI)
5. Blended life and LTCI policies
6. Long-term care annuities
7. Life settlements
8. Reverse mortgages
9. Collaborative professional networks
10. Community Living Assistance Services and Support (CLASS) Act

The health reform legislation passed in the House in March 2010 contains numerous provisions related to long-term care.

Medicare and Medicaid

As already noted, probably the most erroneous belief about paying for long-term care held by both elders and family caregivers is that when an older person needs long-term care, the government will pay for it. Despite the fact that this has never been true, the availability of universal coverage for acute care needs under the Medicare program fosters this myth even today.

GCMs know that long-term care refers specifically to a person's need for assistance with the activities of daily living (ADLs). These ADLs include six specific functional needs: assistance—hands on or through cueing—of another person with bathing, dressing, feeding, transferring from a bed or chair, ambulation, and bowel or bladder inconti-

nence. Assistance with ADLs is not considered by Medicare to be a skilled service. Because Medicare only pays for skilled services, most long-term care needs will not be paid for by Medicare. Medicare will pay for the following services.

Medicare in a Nursing Facility

Medicare covers some skilled care in an approved skilled nursing facility. A minimum 3-day prior hospital stay is required. The patient must enter a facility within 30 days after discharge from a hospital. The patient must continue to show improvement.

Medicare in a Home Setting

The patient must be confined to home and under a doctor's care. Medicare covers part-time skilled nursing care or physical therapy, speech-language therapy, and home health aide services. The patient's condition must continually improve. Examples of skilled care under Medicare include short-term intravenous lines or tubing, physical or speech therapy, and dressing bedsores.

Even when the skilled care requirement is met, Medicare funding is often limited. For example, once a Medicare-eligible patient is in a skilled nursing facility, the maximum amount of time Medicare will pay for care is 100 days. If it is determined that the patient can no longer benefit from skilled services such as physical therapy after 30 or 60 days, payment for care ceases.

Consumer Confusion about Medicare vs. Medicaid

Because both programs have similar sounding names and operate with public funds, elders and family caregivers frequently confuse the two programs. Despite their similar names, Medicaid and Medicare are two completely separate—and very different—programs.

Medicare provides certain health benefits only to Americans who are at least 65 years old. It is completely administered by the federal government. On the other hand, Medicaid is a healthcare assistance program for poor Americans of all ages. Funding comes from both the federal government and state governments. Within limits, the federal government allows the states some degree of leeway in how they run their own Medicaid programs. Medicaid payments can be used to cover the cost of nursing home care. With a federal waiver, Medicaid funds can also be used to pay for home health care. However, in reality, the availability of Medicaid-funded home care services is severely limited. While there have been recent moves to shift Medicaid spending in several states, the overwhelming share of Medicaid payments for long-term care goes to fund care in nursing homes.

Age has nothing to do with whether a person can qualify to receive Medicaid benefits. Instead, each state, within broad federal guidelines, sets its own eligibility requirements. There are limits based on the maximum amount of income a person has made and the amount of assets the person has. In addition, Medicaid requires a 5-year look-back assessment to prevent people from giving away assets ahead of time for the purpose of meeting the Medicaid eligibility requirements.

Private Savings and Funds from Family Members

Despite the fact that the costs of long-term care pose a substantial financial risk to most Americans, most will be required to pay for these costs from personal savings or other family resources until they have exhausted income and assets and become eligible for the Medicaid program. The average cost of long-term care in nursing homes and assisted living facilities continues to increase faster than the rate of inflation. As the Genworth study of 2009 revealed, the costs of nursing homes, assisted living, and in-home care are rising more sharply.

The Genworth study reports that as the first wave of America's 77 million baby boomers head into retirement, it becomes more critical for Americans to seriously evaluate how they will maintain their lifestyles, as we are living well into our 80s, 90s and beyond. The fact remains that most American households remain unprotected from the costly health challenges that come with greater longevity.

Private Long-Term Care Insurance

The LTCI industry began in the late 1980s when policies consisted mainly of nursing home coverage marketed to consumers in their late 60s, 70s, or 80s. Today, comprehensive coverage is most widely sold to protect against the high costs of a nursing home, an assisted living residence, and in-home care. Due to slower than expected sales and a substantial consolidation of carriers in the mid- to late 1990s, the number of companies selling this insurance declined sharply during the 1990s and has dwindled to fewer than a dozen major carriers.

The target market for this product is no longer those past the traditional retirement age of 65. The preretirement baby boomer who is looking at LTCI as a retirement planning element rather than as a financial product to add to his or her retirement portfolio is now the insurance industry's major target.

Still, LTCI has been a hard sell. Only an estimated 8% of the potential market of eligible consumers has been penetrated.

Blended Life and LTCI Policies

One reason many consumers give for not buying long-term care insurance (LTCI) is that if they die and never need to use the benefits, they will not receive a refund of the premiums they paid.

Genworth Life Insurance Company, Nationwide Financial Services, Lincoln Financial, and others offer a comprehensive insurance solution that merges the features of life insurance and LTCI into a single product. This approach helps consumers control their assets, protect their beneficiaries, and have access to long-term care benefits.

These new, so-called blended insurance products provide benefits such as the following:

- Policies can provide a death benefit or payment of benefits for long-term care expenses—or a combination of both. By choosing a single insurance product to meet multiple needs, customers can free up assets for other uses.
- The complete return of the initial premium is another potentially accessible feature if the policy is terminated by the customer in the first 15 policy years.
- A limited death benefit that is payable even if the entire benefit amount has been allocated to a customer's covered long-term care expenses.
- Inflation protection options are in place to help the customer keep pace with the rising cost of long-term care.
- A comprehensive set of benefit options is available, including a lifetime coverage option.

Long-Term Care Annuities

This approach to financing the costs of long-term care uses a single-premium deferred annuity to address the "what if I pay premiums and never file a claim" concern and also to provide a vehicle for those who are declined coverage through LTCI because of health problems. Consumers can set aside a specified amount of money to pay for long-term care expenses if needed. A higher interest rate is credited to withdrawals when the withdrawals are used to pay for long-term care. Because the annuitant is, in effect, self-funding a portion of his or her long-term care risk, it becomes the equivalent of a very large deductible. As a result, the insurer is able to

take a more liberal approach to underwriting and the consumer is able to obtain coverage for care for which he or she otherwise might not be eligible. If the funds in the annuity are not needed to pay for care, they are passed on to the beneficiary.

The Pension Protection Act of 2006 includes a section that provides a federal income tax exemption on an annuity's proceeds starting January 1, 2010, if the proceeds are used to pay for long-term care coverage. That means that the chronically ill or disabled will no longer have to rely solely on a regular long-term care insurance policy or Medicaid to fund their medical and nonmedical care.

Life Settlements

Some geriatric care clients likely purchased life insurance policies many years ago that no longer meet their needs. When clients arrive at this conclusion, the common response is for them to stop paying the annual premium, terminate the policy, and recover any cash value that may have built up. What they—and typically their financial advisor—may not realize is that they can recover significantly more cash by selling the policy to third-party investors.

Life settlement firms target policyholders with impaired health but not terminal illnesses. This typically includes seniors 70 years or older with no-lapse universal life insurance policies with face values of $250,000 or higher.

Reverse Mortgages

According to an AARP housing survey, the most important issue facing those who need long-term care is remaining in one's home. However, the costs of staying in one's home can be overwhelming. Many older Americans are trying to meet those costs with limited income and assets.

Until recently, many older homeowners were faced with selling the home they had worked hard for because they could not afford to live there any longer or could not afford the daily cost of home health care, which is often more expensive than nursing home care. But a new type of loan, called a reverse mortgage, has given homeowners the option of keeping their home and solving their financial dilemma.

A reverse mortgage is a special type of loan for homeowners over the age of 62. The loan does not have to be repaid for as long as the homeowner continues to live in the home. Reverse mortgage income may be used to finance living expenses, home improvements, home care costs, or any other need. As the name suggests, with this type of loan the payment stream is reversed; the lender makes payments to the borrower, rather than the borrower making monthly payments to the lender. And, unlike traditional mortgage loans, there are no income or credit requirements for a reverse mortgage.

The amount of money for which a borrower can qualify is based primarily on age, meaning the older the homeowner, the more funds available. Interest rates and lending limits can also affect this calculation. Because the federal government insures reverse mortgages, under no circumstances will the borrower (or the borrower's estate) ever have to repay more than the value of the home, which is the sole source of repayment for this type of loan. Lenders cannot force borrowers to leave the home if they lend them more money than the home is worth. Nor can lenders lay claim to other assets or the assets of the borrower's heirs.

Elders and their caregivers also need to be aware of other benefits of reverse mortgages. All payments received from a reverse mortgage are tax free, and the proceeds from a reverse mortgage do not affect eligibility for Social Security or Medicare. Also, most of the closing costs associated with a reverse mortgage can be financed, thereby limiting the amount of cash required from a borrower.

A study by the National Council on Aging, funded by the Centers for Medicare and Medicaid Services and the Robert Wood Johnson Foundation, shows that more than 13 million Americans can use reverse mortgages to pay for long-term care expenses at home. In this way, many can stay independent and live in their homes longer.

Participating in National Elder-Care Professional Provider Networks

Geriatric care managers can retain their independent business status while participating in national provider networks. For example, several major insurance companies that sell long-term care insurance policies use care managers to conduct home visits to gather functional and healthcare information, which helps them make underwriting decisions before issuing coverage to applicants.

One potential source of fee-based income for care managers is the workplace. Because of the aging workforce and the increasing percentage of workers with aging parents, some employers now provide support services for working caregivers. These services have been around for more than 20 years but, as yet, have not resulted in a significant source of business for most care managers.

According to a study conducted by the MetLife Mature Market Institute, there is substantial evidence that caregiving for older family members creates significant stress for many employees and has an impact on the profits of caregivers' employers.[14] Several studies have documented the costs of caregiving to business in lost productivity on the part of the employed caregiver, as well as management and administrative costs based on the time supervisors spend on issues concerning employed caregivers. According to one study, caregiving costs an individual upward of $659,000 throughout their lifetime in lost wages, Social Security benefits, and pension contributions because of time off taken, loss of job entirely, or compromised opportunities for training, promotions, and good assignments.

There are also organizations such as employee assistance programs, and so-called work-life companies that offer child and elder-care services to large employers. Others offer a broad range of elder-care consultation, referral, and caregiver support services to national organizations such as labor unions, religious groups, and other membership organizations who want to offer this service to their members.

One example is the Elder Life Planning for Organizations (ELPO) service, a nationwide program that serves employers, insurers, and membership associations. Local elder-care professionals are paid to provide such services as presenting on-site caregiver support seminars and providing individual consultations to those eligible for the ELPO program while remaining independent.

The Community Living Assistance Services and Support (CLASS) Act

This act was originally introduced by the late Senator Edward Kennedy and is contained in the Patient Protection and Affordable Care Act passed by Congress and signed by President Obama in early 2010. The CLASS Act will make long-term care insurance available to all Americans, who will be automatically enrolled with the choice to opt out.

Individuals will begin paying a premium immediately and, after 5 years, those with functional limitations have the option of receiving a cash benefit of around $50 per day that can be used to offset the cost of long-term care services.

MacKenzie Kimball writes the following about the CLASS Act in *Health Leaders Media,* in March 2010:

> The CLASS Act will help offset the high cost of long-term care services for aging and disabled populations. In particular,

these funds will allow individuals flexibility to receive services in their homes and potentially prevent admissions to nursing homes. The overarching goal of healthcare reform is to make health care both more accessible and affordable in the United States. Long-term care expenses, particularly in aging populations, are among the most costly to Medicare and Medicaid today. By providing insurance, there is a real opportunity to reduce costs in this sector.[24]

These revenue sources are reviewed in the following sections along with a discussion of the still small but growing demand for services from employers who are beginning to recognize the need for caregiver support for their aging workforce.

Long-Term Care Carriers Recognize the Value of GCMs

Insurance companies began to use care managers early on in the development of these policies. During the initial application, or underwriting stage, care managers have been used to help determine whether an applicant is an acceptable risk. Nurses and social workers with experience in long-term care have been retained, on a fee-for-service basis, to conduct interviews with selected applicants, usually those over age 70. Using a variety of functional assessment instruments, case managers help underwriters get a picture of how independent a potential customer is prior to approving the application.

When claims are filed, insurers use case managers to expedite the claims process. A GCM is retained to go to the home or the facility where the claimant is receiving care. Using ADL-based functional assessment tools, the care manager prepares a report that helps claims specialists confirm that the claim is valid.

GCM roles in LTCI will also continue to expand. Most major insurance carriers now see care managers as a cost-effective, value-added benefit for policyholders as care coordinators. As policyholders' age and claims activity both increase, the care management and care coordination role will grow steadily.

The services of GCMs are also used to help policyholders develop a plan of care that makes the best use of their policy benefits. The care coordination benefit was initially offered as an option for which the insured paid an additional premium. Today, newer LTCI products include care coordination as part of the basic benefit package at no additional cost.

Some insurers require that the case manager must be a participating member of that insurer's preferred providers network. Increasingly, the option to choose a GCM is left up to the policyholder or the family caregivers.

Most LTCI policies are issued with a deductible or limitation period. This limitation period, during which no benefits are paid, typically ranges from 20 to 100 days, a choice the insured makes when the policy is purchased. More policies now waive the limitation period for care coordination benefits and allow payment to the care coordinator as soon as the claim is approved.

■ TARGETING SPECIFIC GROUPS AND RESOURCES TO GROW A PROFESSIONAL PRACTICE

One way private care managers have found to reach those in need and those who can benefit from their services is to target specific groups. Private practice professionals have found, for instance, elder-law and estate planning attorneys, bank trust officers, and financial advisors who manage the resources of affluent clients can be excellent sources of referrals that can help GCMs build an independent practice.

To succeed, the private care manager must spread a message with three important components:

1. Eventually, you or a member of your family may need specialized professional attention because of aging or disability. Finding the services needed to help can be difficult, time consuming, and frustrating, so planning ahead is a good idea.
2. A high-quality alternative to the publicly funded long-term care delivery system is available if you want to pay for it.
3. The services of a geriatric care manager are well worth the price.

If GCMs fail to get this message across to consumers, it will be difficult for them to operate a profitable business. GCMs must be diligent and effective in spreading this message and raising awareness about geriatric care management as an effective alternative to the chaotic and underfunded public long-term care system. Otherwise, the consumer, who has been conditioned to expect that most if not all long-term care services will be covered by Medicaid or private charity, is likely to balk at having to pay fees for geriatric care management services.

A variety of ways exist in which GCMs can be paid for their services. One way is to seek reimbursement from private LTCI policies. At intake, care managers should ask whether the client owns a LTCI policy. The care manager should review any insurance policies to determine exactly what benefits for long-term care may be available. If necessary, the GCM can contact the insurance carrier or third-party administrator who manages the coordination and payment of claims. Since the mid-1990s, the inclusion of specific clauses in privately purchased LTCI policies that provide for the services of a care coordinator (also referred to as the personal care specialist, case management agency, or personal care advocate in various policies) have become the norm. Older policies may not contain a specific clause providing for reimbursement of the care coordinator, but it is worth calling the company that issued the policy and asking whether the services of a care manager can be reimbursed under the policy. Even if the services of a care manager are not specifically defined as reimbursable, a phone call to the benefits administrator, explaining how care management services may be cost-effective, can elicit a response that may result in payment for at least some services. In some cases, having the insured's family member contact the claims administrator and request compensation for care management services can be more effective.

Because the sale of LTCI policies has yet to achieve the market penetration expected for these products, insurance carriers are looking for new ways to raise awareness and visibility of their LTCI products. One way to achieve this is for insurance carriers to proactively offer care manager information and referral services or on-site educational seminars on caring for aging parents, combined with an LTCI employee benefit.

GCMs can also form joint ventures and alliances with other elder-care professionals to grow their practices. The appeal of operating one's own business, free of the restrictions and compromises imposed by working for highly regulated, wholly funded, public or nonprofit agencies, is very seductive for the independent-minded professional. However, the development of a small business is never as easy as it appears. Becoming an independent healthcare professional is no exception—the hard realities of managing and growing a small business soon become evident. Getting the message out about the availability of a GCM's services requires mounting a marketing and networking campaign that can be both expensive and time-consuming, and it is difficult for newer businesses to compete with other companies that have more capital. Many independent professionals first starting out find that the resources of both money and time are in short supply.

With the rapid growth of large social networking sites such as Facebook and LinkedIn, elder-care professionals have discovered that you can form or join specialty subgroups on these social networking sites. Some examples of these online groups include Make Elder Care Entrepreneurs, Family, Healthcare and Pastoral Caregivers of Older Adults, The Elder-Law Attorney Practice Group, Assisted Living Professionals, Elder Care Issue Resolutions Group, and Mature Market Experts.

After realizing that an individual or small group practice has its limitations, some care managers have begun to explore the idea of developing affiliations with other elder-care professionals in what are sometimes referred to as virtual partnerships. Individual care managers or small businesses can consider experimenting with such ideas as pooling their resources or banding together with related professionals to launch a cooperative marketing effort. Elder-law attorneys, independent home care providers, LTCI companies, or financial advisors are natural alliances for private care managers to cultivate. Each member of the group can maintain an independent business while jointly developing marketing materials, websites, and Internet marketing campaigns, as well as planning and cosponsoring joint educational programs in the community.

■ CONCLUSION

This chapter discusses a variety of ways care managers in the private marketplace can fund and grow their businesses while providing prospective clients more attractive alternatives to care management than can be provided by publicly funded sources.

Despite the growing awareness of the crisis that is looming in the nation's long-term care service delivery system, GCMs have had difficulty educating the public about the fact that a private-sector alternative exists and can be far more effective and desirable. Even 20 years after the formation of the National Association of Professional Geriatric Care Managers, most consumers are still unaware that this alternative exists.

Along with a well-versed knowledge of the various alternatives available to pay for elder care, it is critical to the success of your practice to produce a consistently high quality level of services and project an image of collaborative, rather than competitive, professionalism.

Paying privately for highly skilled professional services is nothing new in the American marketplace. When consumers seek the services of an attorney or architect or accountant or a financial advisor or even a carpenter or plumber, they are well aware that they will be expected to pay for services rendered. Because of the well-established precedent of elder-care services being paid for by taxpayers, charities, or third-party insurance sources, consumers have different expectations about elder-care services than they do about other fee-based services in the marketplace.

Care management entrepreneurs who stay abreast of the constant changes in the marketplace, especially changes that can directly or indirectly affect revenue and referral sources, have a far better chance of being successful than those who don't. Care managers who continue to believe that the revenue base will always be growing because the aging population is growing are likely to miss out on the real private elder-care marketplace, which is a much smaller subset of the aging demographic.

■ REFERENCES

1. CBSNews.com. $1 trillion more in debt since Obama took office. August 3, 2009. Available at: http://www.cbsnews.com/8301-503544_162-5209497-503544.html.

2. Congressional Budget Office. August 19, 2010. The budget and economic outlook: an update. Available at: http://www.cbo.gov/doc.cfm?index=11705.

3. Sanger DE. Deficits may alter U.S. politics and global power. *New York Times,* February 1, 2010. Available at: http://www.nytimes.com/2010/02/02/us/politics/02deficit.html.

4. Senate Budget Committee. 2008. Transcript of remarks by Senate Budget Committee Chairman Kent Conrad (D-ND) at press conference on President Bush's FY 2009 budget. Available at: http://budget.senate.gov/democratic/statements/2008/stmt_bushfy2009budget conradpressconftrans020408.pdf.

5. Powell M. The state budget disaster. July 1, 2010. Available at: http://economix.blogs.nytimes.com/2010/07/01/the-state-budget-disaster.

6. Pollack H. Guest graph: the future of Medicaid. June 19, 2009. Available at: http://voices.washingtonpost.com/ezra-klein/2009/06/guest_graph_the_future_of_medi.html.

7. Wilensky GR. The growing challenge of Medicare. *Healthcare Financial Management.* 2005 (April);34. Available at: http://findarticles.com/p/articles/mi_m3257/is_4_59/ai_n13621272.

8. Stefanacci RG. Reimbursement politics. *Clinical Geriatrics.* 15(2);2007. Available at: http:// www.clinicalgeriatrics.com/articles/Reimbursement-Politics.

9. Murphy JB. As growing shortage of geriatricians looms, geriatric medicine considers a redefinition of its scope. *Clinical Geriatrics.* 17(1);2009. Available at: http://www.clinicalgeriatrics.com/articles/As-Growing-Shortage-Geriatricians-Looms-Geriatric-Medicine-Considers-a-Redefinition-Its-Sco.

10. Data from the U.S. Bureau of the Census. Census 2000 counted 79.6 million U.S. residents born in the years 1946 to 1964, inclusive. That number is higher than the 76 million births because net immigration (the number of people coming into the United States from other countries, minus those moving the other way) more than outweighed the number of deaths. The flow of immigrants greatly increased after passage of the Immigration Act of 1965, just as the baby boom was ending.

11. Genworth Financial. 2010. 2010 cost of care: long-term care survey. Available at: http://www.genworth.com/content/products/long_term_care/long_term_care/cost_of_care.html.

12. Frank R. Top 1% increase their share of wealth in financial crisis. Washington Post, April 30, 2010. Available at: http://blogs.wsj.com/wealth/2010/04/30/top-1-increased-their-share-of-wealth-in-financial-crisis.

13. United States Government Accountability Office. Medicaid long-term care: few transferred assets before applying for nursing home coverage; impact of Deficit Reduction Act is uncertain. [Document GAO-07-280.] March 2007. Available at: http://www.canhr.org/reports/2007/GAO-07-280.pdf.

14. Aaron HJ. Children and the elderly: not children or the elderly. Brookings Institution, December 2009. Available at: http://www.brookings.edu/opinions/2009/1201_children_elderly_aaron.aspx.

15. National Alliance for Caregiving. A focused look at those caring for someone age 50 or older. National Alliance for Caregiving. 2009. Available at: http://www.caregiving.org/data/FINALRegularExSum50plus.pdf.

16. Brookings Institution. Health care reform and older Americans. December 1, 2009. Available at: http://www.brookings.edu/events/2010/0128_older_health_care.aspx.

17. Moses S. Center for Long-Term Care Reform, 2009. Available at: http://www.centerltc.com.

18. Centers for Medicare and Medicaid Services. Overview Medicaid program. Available at: https://www.cms.gov/MedicaidGenInfo. Accessed January 25, 2011.

19. Gleckman H. Get Medicaid out of the long-term care business. *Kaiser Health News.* August 3, 2009. Available at: http://www.kaiserhealthnews.org/Columns/2009/August/080309Gleckman.aspx.

20. Feingold R. Statement of U.S. Senator Russ Feingold on why congress should look to Wisconsin as model for long-term care reform. Available at: http://feingold.senate.gov/record.cfm?id=315564.

21. When siblings step up. *Wall Street Journal,* March 27, 2010.

22. Ferry JL. *How to start a home-based senior care business.* Guilford, CT: Global Pequot Press; 2010.

23. A graying NYC threatened by cuts and consolidations. *New York Nonprofit Press,* April 28, 2009.

24. Kimball M. Healthcare reform will impact long-term care. Available at: http://www.healthleadersmedia.com/content/LED-248406/Healthcare-Reform-Will-Impact-LongTerm-Care##. Accessed January 25, 2011.

Chapter 18

Care Management Credentialing

Monika White and Cheryl M. Whitman

■ INTRODUCTION

Care management continues to play a major role in the complex health and social services delivery systems. Advances in medical technology, medications, and other interventions have extended life expectancy and increased the numbers and types of consumers who need care management services. Older people, individuals with developmental disabilities, people with chronic mental illness, and others benefit from care management. Furthermore, care management has been increasingly encouraged by legislative and funding actions that have included it as a means of addressing the demographic, medical, and social challenges that create the need for ongoing, multiple services. For example, care management was a specific component of the Developmental Disabilities Act of 1975. During the 1980s, care management became a prominent feature of the Medicaid waiver programs and workers' compensation programs. Private practice care managers also emerged as resources for older adults and their caregivers. The growth of managed care in the 1990s and the emergence of long-term care insurance further established the need for care management.

In the late 1980s and early 1990s, numerous professional associations—including the National Association of Professional Geriatric Care Managers, the National Council on Aging, the National Association of Social Workers (NASW), and the Case Management Society of America—began to promote standards for care manager practice. Funded by a grant from the Robert Wood Johnson Foundation, Connecticut Community Care, Inc. (CCCI) established and convened the National Advisory Committee on Long-Term Care Case Management. The work of these national experts culminated in the 1994 publication *Guidelines for Case Management Practice Across the Long-Term Care Continuum*. Finally, efforts to certify individual care managers began in the early 1990s as the demand for care management staff expanded prior to the development of academically based curricula. In 1999, the American Accreditation Health-Care Commission/URAC, now known as URAC (Utilization Review, Accreditation, and Certification), established standards for care management organizations.

All of these developments demonstrate a broad-based consensus that care management has become a useful and important component of the health and social services delivery systems. Despite apparent agreement on the value of care management, there is little to guide individual or corporate purchasers about who should do it, under what circumstances, for whom, and through which funding mechanisms. This has created confusion among consumers, funders, policymakers, and even personnel.

Many professions use credentialing to establish criteria for quality and competent services. Credentialing is a form of recognition or acknowledgment that a standard body of knowledge and the skill set has been met. Because care management has evolved as a transdisciplinary field, it is important to delineate the functions, roles, values, and ethical perspectives of a competent care manager that may or may not correspond with the standards of the so-called parent profession.

Businesses and organizations providing rehabilitation, managed care, acute care, long-term care insurance, and chronic care increasingly request or require care management certification as a condition of employment, and healthcare professionals in these settings are obtaining certification by the thousands. At the same time, there has been little demand for care management certification in nonmedical settings. Many care managers from the proprietary and nonprofit community-based service and long-term care arena rely on their educational degrees and professional licenses and do not perceive a need to add another credential. Yet interest in credentialing programs continues to grow, as does the number of programs offering certifications.

This chapter addresses credentialing in general, and for care managers specifically. After a section on the motivations behind and history of care management credentialing, the chapter provides an overview of selected credentialing and certification organizations. A discussion of some current and upcoming issues concludes the chapter.

■ WHAT IS CREDENTIALING?

According to the National Organization for Competency Assurance (NOCA), credentialing is the umbrella term that includes the concepts of accreditation, licensure, registration, and professional certification. Credentialing is used by an entity to acknowledge that a standard has been met; that is, the body of knowledge and the skill set that enable the practitioner to perform the job tasks of a specific field of practice have been acquired. Credentialing confers an occupational identity and serves a number of purposes, such as the following:

- Protecting the public
- Establishing standards for professional knowledge, skills, and practice
- Meeting the requirements of government regulators
- Assuring consumers that professionals have met specific standards of practice
- Regulating a profession
- Assisting employers, insurers, practitioners, and the public in identifying individuals with certain knowledge and skills
- Advancing the profession
- Acknowledging the attainment of knowledge and skills by a professional
- Providing the certificant with a sense of pride and professional accomplishment
- Demonstrating a person's commitment to the profession and lifelong learning

Professional certification is described by NOCA as the "voluntary process by which a nongovernmental entity grants a time-limited recognition and use of a credential to an individual after verifying that it has met predetermined and standardized criteria."[1(pp 4–5)]

Interest in licensing care managers has gained some popularity in recent years. As noted by Bartelstone, "Certification is often the precursor to actual licensing and regulation of a profession."[2(p10)]

■ MOTIVATION

In addition to validating education and experience, people are motivated to earn care management certification for several reasons. Among them are the following:

- Informed consumer choice
- Consumer protection

- Marketing
- Insurability
- Education
- Research
- Self-regulation
- History

The following sections discuss each rationale.

Informed Consumer Choice

One of the primary reasons for the development of a credential is to enable the consumer to make a discriminating choice about the type of care manager who should be hired for a given circumstance. For example, an acute medical setting might warrant the employ of a nurse or other clinical technician with in-depth experience with a particular diagnosis. In a community-based setting, a care manager with a background in social work, psychology, or mental health might better serve a client, such as a grieving widow or individual with chronic mental illness. In other situations, an expert with a background in both medical and psychosocial fields might be most appropriate. There might also be differentiating circumstances based on the specific population whose needs are to be met. A care manager with a gerontological background might better serve an older adult, just as an individual with human immunodeficiency virus or acquired immune deficiency syndrome would need the expertise of someone knowledgeable about that specific disease process, treatment, needed services, and emotional impact. Rosen and colleagues note that certification could provide some consensus about expectations for service delivery.[3]

Consumer Protection

The consumer also needs protection from an individual who might call him- or herself a care manager but who has neither training in the care management process, roles, and functions nor an understanding of health and social services systems and psychosocial dynamics. Because no licensing or other regulation currently exists, the consumer has no guidelines with which to shop for services. The professional certifications, then, are very important mechanisms for guiding the consumer. They provide protection for other well-trained, appropriately experienced managers who are competing, perhaps unfairly, with individuals of lesser capacity, who charge lower fees—often for inferior services.

Marketing

Most healthcare and social services providers today seek a competitive advantage in the individual, corporate, and nonprofit markets. Credentialing of individual employees on the basis of their competency becomes a selling point, especially when providers are looking to broaden their markets and when there is a likelihood of passing along risk. Network providers of all types look to affiliate with organizations and individuals that meet industry standards for practice. Care managers can use the professional certification as a marketing tool to distinguish themselves from those who are not certified and as proof of core competency for network affiliation or membership.

Insurability

Another rationale for credentialing is the ability to be covered by malpractice insurance and to receive payments from third-party insurers and other reimbursement sources. Although reimbursement for care management is still limited, it is expected to increase as care management is more fully recognized and funded, especially in the social services arena. An insurer that is considering a malpractice policy for care managers or care management organizations needs to be able to identify whom it is insuring, for which job functions, in which settings, for what populations, and with what decision-making or fiduciary responsibilities. Without this knowledge, it would be impossible for an insurance company to develop such a liability policy. With the growth of care management networks that require insurance coverage, there are indications that certification may become the norm in the future.

Education

Educating care managers within a defined body of knowledge is another rationale for providing a credentialing process. As previously stated, care management did not evolve from an academic program within the nation's college or university systems, but developed in response to consumer need. For a field of practice or a discipline to become professionalized, there must be a defined and determinate body of knowledge, so it can be taught with uniformity and consistency.

Care management degrees and certificate programs are being offered or are under development in a number of universities. Many schools of nursing and social work have well-developed care management courses, specialty areas, or clinical tracts. Courses in care management can also be found in gerontology schools, undergraduate human services departments, and continuing education programs. In the last 5 years, the number of certificate programs at colleges, large companies, and online have increased significantly. Knowledge-based, curriculum-based, and attendance-based certificate programs are training programs focused on a specific topic such as care management. They typically require completion of course work and may require demonstrated attainment of course objectives. A credential is not usually given at the end of a certificate program.

Research

Credentialing of care managers enables research that defines specific outcomes and accountabilities as a result of the process of providing care. Outcomes need to relate to health status, quality of care, cost of care, and efficient use of systems to coordinate services. Outcomes must also be defined in terms of client goals. Such goals might include quality of life, knowledge about needs, increased ability to participate in or maintain care, ability to better use systems of care to meet needs, and better social and emotional functioning of the consumer and the consumer's support system. Again, most outcome measures currently in use come from medical settings. In psychosocial areas, outcomes tend to be anecdotal. Their value is limited because they are self-reported and self-selected by the provider organization.

Limited empirical research exists in these areas, especially in consumer-defined outcomes, but the body of research is growing. For example, Geron and colleagues have developed client satisfaction measures to determine consumer perceptions of home care and care management services. These measures are already in use by several states and agency programs and provide hope that the quality and success of care management will be more easily quantified in the future.[4]

Self-Regulation

Self-regulation is an essential aspect of any professional field. Just as it is in the best interest of consumers to be involved in defining and creating the systems that work for them, it is in the best interest of care managers to be involved in defining appropriate regulation for their work. Only in this way will accurate expectations for the individual practitioner or care management system be developed. Government-imposed guidelines often miss the essential ingredients of the value system, nature, and realities of the profession. It is important for care managers to participate in development and implementation of standards and guidelines, in research studies, in legislative and policy activities, and in available and relevant professional associations.

History

The disability movement of the 1970s spurred the development of several professional organizations focused on the rehabilitation needs of the individual. The more specific move toward credentialing of care managers began to gain momentum in the late 1980s and early 1990s with the emergence of a number of professional organizations focused on care management services for various populations in diverse settings. These organizations recognized that they had both competing and mutual interests that could best be served by finding consensus in the role played by care managers in the evolving health and social services environments.

A meeting of these organizations was held in 1991 and resulted in the formation of a National Case Management Task Force, which appointed a steering committee to address the issues of philosophy, definition, and existing standards of practice. There were 29 organizations involved in this task force. In 1992, the steering committee proposed the development of a voluntary care management credential.

An interim commission was incorporated as an independent credentialing organization, and in July 1995, it was renamed the Commission for Case Manager Certification (CCMC). The CCMC continues to be responsible for the certified case manager (CCM) credentialing process. To be eligible to be a CCM requires that an applicant "hold an acceptable license or certification (see the *CCM Certification Guide*) based on a post-secondary degree program in a field that promotes the psychosocial or vocational well-being of the persons being served."[5] This means that the CCM is effectively an advanced practice credential.

Although the interim commission included representation from the Certification of Insurance Rehabilitation Specialists Commission, later renamed the Certification of Disability Management Specialists Commission (CDMS), it is important to note that this group maintained its individual identity. It was instrumental in creating the new certification, and there was apparently no sense that this was a further fragmentation of the care management field.

In 1993, two other organizations began a second set of discussions about credentialing care managers: The National Association of Professional Geriatric Care Managers and the Case Management Institute of CCCI. Both viewed the CCM as medically oriented and focused primarily on rehabilitation and acute care management. Furthermore, the eligibility criteria for the CCM excluded most of the staff employed in the home- and community-based, long-term care, and social services programs serving clients through various nonprofit and publicly sponsored programs. It left out many of the frontline staff who provide direct client services through the Area Agencies on Aging, vocational and rehabilitation services, substance abuse programs, peer counseling programs, and other grassroots organizations. Such organizations rely on both formally and informally trained and supervised staff, including those with many years of hands-on care management experience.

For these reasons, an independent credentialing organization was formed in 1994 called the National Academy of Certified Care Managers (NACCM). The credential, offered since 1996, is the Care Manager Certified (CMC), given for meeting education and experience requirements and the successful completion of a standardized, validated examination that tests the skills, knowledge, and practice ethics needed to serve consumers. The NACCM exam is focused on the core care management functions of comprehensive face-to-face assessment, care planning, care implementation, monitoring, management, reassessment, termination, and professional issues and ethics.

Throughout the field's history, there have been formal discussions held between the various stakeholders in care management. In 1992 and 1993, six professional organizations came together as the National Coalition of Associations for the Advancement of Case Management. These associations represented more than 20,000 health and social services professionals and were hoping to influence the healthcare reforms that were part of the President's Task Force on National Health Care Reform, chaired by Hillary Rodham Clinton. A variety of organizations met throughout the 1990s and began the process of developing consensus about defining care management and its role in ensuring quality care and efficient use of resources. This process led to care management organizations taking an expanded role in defining needs and solutions and acting as a change agent within the system. In a 1994 paper published by the Foundation for Rehabilitation Certification, Education, and Research, Michael J. Leahy found that the most frequent settings in which surveyed CCMs worked were as follows:

> independent case management companies (23.8%), followed by hospitals (11.7%), independent rehabilitation or insurance affiliates (11.0%), and health insurance companies (8.0%). The most frequent job titles of respondents include case manager (45.9%), registered nurse (19.8%), rehabilitation counselor (10.9%), and administrator or manager (7.6%).[6]

Two important meetings were held in 1997 and 1999 under the auspices of the Foundation for Rehabilitation Education and Research and the National Association of Professional Geriatric Care Managers. These meetings were identified as the Care and Case Management Summits I and II. Sixteen associations and organizations participated in discussions about care management definitions, existing credentialing options and their ethical standards, and the domains of knowledge of the various definitions and options. According to the Summit II minutes, participants expressed interest in forming a coalition to continue discussions.[7] Although this particular group did not meet again, many of its members participated in the establishment of the Case Management Leadership Coalition in the early 2000s. This coalition met in 2002 and 2004 and continues to be active (see www.cmlc.org for more information). Membership is predominantly in the medical and rehabilitation arenas.

■ OVERVIEW OF SELECTED CREDENTIALING AND CERTIFICATION ORGANIZATIONS

There are many credentialing and certification organizations, and they each offer something slightly different. The number of programs has grown since the initial publication of this book. Care managers must be aware of the variety of programs, the difference between credentialing and certificate programs, and what will be most appropriate for their practice setting. Table 18–1 describes the credentials recognized by the National Association of Professional Geriatric Care Managers. Some of the other credentials that professionals may earn are listed in Table 18–2. These credentials are associated with nursing and rehabilitation and are institution oriented.

Commission for Certified Care Managers

The CCM designation has been available since 1993. The Commission for Case Manager Certification (CCMC) has defined case management as "a collaborative process that assesses, plans, implements, coordinates, monitors, and evaluates the options and services required to meet the client's health and human service. It is characterized by advocacy, communication, and resource management and promotes

Table 18-1   Overview of Eligibility Criteria and Examinations for Credentials Recognized by National Association of Professional Geriatric Care Managers (Alphabetical Order)

	Education	Experience	Prerequisite (license or other)	Exam Content (partial list)	Recertification
Commission for Case Management Certification *Certified case manager* (CCM) (847) 818-0292 http://www.ccmcertification.org	Postsecondary program in physical, psychosocial, and vocational and well-being	12–24 months full time as case manager or supervisor, 12 months under CCM or 24 without CCM	Valid license or certification	Coordination, service delivery, physical and psychological factors, benefit systems, case management concepts, community resources	Every 5 years 80 CEUs total
National Academy of Certified Care Managers, Certified Care Manager, Certified (CMC) (800) 962-2260 http://www.naccm.net	1. Master's (field related to care management) 2. Bachelor's (field related to care management) 3. Associate degree in field related to care management, or RN diploma or bachelor's or higher degree in non-human services field	1. 2 years as supervised care manager 2. 2 years as supervised care manager + 2 years direct client care in human services field 3. 2 years as supervised care manager + 4 years direct client care in human services fields	NA	Comprehensive assessment, care plan development, coordination, service delivery systems, monitoring, termination, ethical and legal issues	Every 3 years Continued care management practice or supervision of care managers + 45 CEUs total
National Association of Social Workers *Certified advanced social work case manager* (C-ASWCM)	Master of social work (MSW) degree	One year supervised, post MSW, direct case management	ACSW or DCSW or state SW license or passing score on ASWB exam *and* NASW membership	No exam	Every 2 years, 20 CEUs total, Maintain ACSW-, DCSW-, or MSW-level state licensure *and* NASW membership
Certified social work case manager (C-SWCM)	Bachelor of arts in social work (BSW)	One year supervised, post BSW, direct case management	ACBSW or current BSW level state license or passing score on ACBSW exam *and* NASW membership	No exam	Every 2 years 20 CEUs total Maintain ACBSW- or current BSW-level state licensure *and* NASW membership

CEU, continuing education unit; RN, registered nurse; ACSW, Academy of Certified Social Workers; DCSW, diplomate in clinical social work; ASWB, Association of Social Work Boards; NASW, National Association of Social Workers.

Table 18–2   Additional Credentialing Organization (Alphabetical Order)

	Education	Experience	Prerequisite (license or other)	Exam Content (partial list)	Recertification
American Case Management Association (ACMA) *Accredited case manager (ACM)*	1. RN 2. BSW or MSW or social work license	2 yrs full time hospital/health system case management	Valid RN license License if no BSW or MSW	Screening, assessment, care coordination and intervention, evaluation	Every 4 yrs 40 contact hrs
American Institute of Outcome CM *Case manager, certified (CMC)*	1. BA, MA, PhD 2. Associate or Diploma RN	1. 36–60 mo full-time 2. + professional license	License at associate level	Clinical, customer service, management/supervision, quality improvement, legal/risk aspects, payer, utilization review, employer and provider orgs, resources	Every 2 yrs 7 certification points
Certification of Disability Management Specialists Commission *Certified disability management specialist (CDMS)*	A bachelor's degree in any discipline or a current RN license	12 mo full time, paid	RN license	Job placement, vocational assessment, case management & disabilities, rehab services & care, disability legislation, forensic rehab	Every 5 yrs 80 contact hrs total
Commission on Rehabilitation Counselor Certification, *Certification rehabilitation counselor (CRC)*	MA or PhD in rehab counseling or related field (including 600 hrs of internship)	0–5 yrs depending on status of other requirements + 12 mo of supervision under a CRC	NA	Job placement, vocational assessment and services, individual, family and group counseling, medical, functional and environmental aspects of disabilities; health care and disability systems	Every 5 yrs 100 contact hrs total
National Board for Certification in Continuity of Care, *Continuity of care certification, advanced (A-CCC)*				No new certificants; those with A-CCC certification can continue to renew.	Every 5 yrs 50 contact hrs total or other eligible activities
Rehabilitation Nursing Certification Board, *Certified rehabilitation registered nurse (CCRN)*	RN	2 yrs in rehab or 1 yr in rehab nursing and 1 yr advanced study in nursing	RN license	Rehabilitation, rehab nursing, models and theories	Every 5 yrs 60 contact hrs total or retake exam + minimum of 2 yrs rehab RN nursing experience

quality and cost-effective interventions and outcomes."[8] The commission considers case management as an advanced-practice area within an already licensed or certified profession. Hence they have specified the following experience criteria:

- **Category 1:** 12 months of acceptable full-time case management employment supervised by a CCM
- **Category 2:** 24 months of acceptable full-time case management employment without supervision by a CCM
- **Category 3:** 12 months of acceptable full-time case management employment as a supervisor of individuals who provide *direct* case management services.

In 2008 CCMC moved to an online application, computer-based testing (CBT), and annual 3-week-long testing windows.[9]

National Academy of Certified Care Managers

The NACCM defines care management as "a service that links and coordinates assistance from both paid service providers and unpaid help from family and friends to enable consumers with functional limitations to obtain the highest level of independence consistent with their capacity and preferences for care."[10] Eligibility criteria reflect a biopsychosocial approach to care management in long-term, chronic, community-based, health, social, and mental health settings. The higher the educational level of the candidate, the fewer years of care management experience are required. (See Table 18–1.)

According to NACCM, *care management experience* must include all of the following tasks: a face-to-face comprehensive assessment; problem identification; goal setting; care plan development, implementation and monitoring; reassessment; and quality evaluation. Care management is done with individuals, not communities. Care managers follow clients across settings and work with staff and professionals in a variety of facilities and programs serving them. The comprehensive assessment must be face to face and include all of the following domains: health, function, social life, emotion, cognition, environment, spirituality, support system, and finances.

According to NACCM, *supervision and consultation* is defined as individual, group, or peer review of performance; use of clinical skills and core care manager functions; record review; peer consultation; and case review or case conference in the amount of 50 hours per year for 2 years.[11]

These criteria are more inclusive and reflective of the experience of care managers in the social services system, as differentiated from the health delivery system. The CMC designation has been offered since 1996, following a 2-year process creating a standardized, valid, and reliable examination. Periodic role and function surveys and analysis is done with CMCs to maintain the relevancy of the exam and credentialing process. NACCM began with computer-based testing (CBT) and currently offers the exam in two testing windows each year: March 1–April 30 and September 1–October 31.

National Association of Social Workers

The NASW Credentialing Center establishes and promotes credentials, specialty certifications, and a continuing education approval program required for excellence in the practice of social work. NASW specialty certifications and other professional credentials provide recognition to those who have met national standards for higher levels of experience and knowledge, and they are not a substitute for required state licenses or certifications. NASW defines case management "as a method of providing services whereby a professional social worker assesses the needs of the client (and the client's family when appropriate). The case manager arranges, coordinates, monitors, evaluates, and advocates for a package of multiple services to meet the specific client's complex needs."[12] One year of supervised direct case management experience is required for the NASW certified social work case management designation as C-ASWCM for those with a master of social work degree and C-SWCM for those with a bachelor of social work degree. Additional prerequisites and supervision are tied directly to NASW membership and designations as well as state-specific social work licenses. (See Table 18–1.)

National Board for Certification in Continuity of Care

The NBCCC administered the Continuity of Care Certification, Advanced. This certification was open to people from multiple disciplines, including nurses, social workers, therapists, dietitians, and physicians.[13] This certification evolved from the area of discharge planning within a number of institutional settings. The NBCCC no longer takes applications for new certificants. Professionals with the CCC-A may continue to renew their certification through the NBCCC.

Rehabilitation Nursing Certification Board

The Rehabilitation Nursing Certification Board administers the Certified Rehabilitation Registered Nurse (CRRN) certification. Applicants for the CRRN examination must have a current, unrestricted RN license and have completed at least one of the following requirements at the time of application. Applicant must within the 5 years preceding the examination have completed 2 years of practice as a registered professional nurse in rehabilitation nursing, or within the 5 years preceding the examination have completed 1 year of practice as a registered professional nurse in rehabilitation nursing and 1 year of advanced study (beyond a baccalaureate) in

nursing.[14] This process then is limited to those within the nursing profession and does not address the inter- and transdisciplinary nature of care management.

Certification of Disability Management Specialists Commission

The CDMS Commission administers the CDMS certification. This commission was originally developed in 1984 as the Certification of Insurance Rehabilitation Specialists Commission and was changed to the current name in 1996. This certification started with four different categories within which a candidate may qualify. The new criteria is less complicated: a bachelor's degree in any discipline or a current state RN license and a minimum of 12 months of full-time employment providing direct disability management services to individuals with disabilities receiving benefits from a disability compensation system.

Commission on Rehabilitation Counselor Certification (CRCC)

The CRCC administers the Certified Rehabilitation Counselor (CRC) certification. This certification also allows people multiple ways of meeting the eligibility requirements. There are at least 10 categories and several subcategories, seven of which have very specific course requirements. The reader is referred to the commission for more specific details. This credential defines care management as an advanced practice field, making the credential similar to the CCM.

Contact information for these certifying entities is shown in Exhibit 18–1.

■ CURRENT AND FUTURE ISSUES

To date, there is no unified approach to care management; there remain diverse views and even controversy in a number of areas. This section highlights some of the major issues that continue to be discussed:

Exhibit 18–1 Contact Information for Selected Certification Entities

1. American Case Management Association
   www.acmaweb.org
   (501) 907-2262

2. Certification of Disability Management Specialists Commission
   www.cdms.org
   (847) 944-1335

3. Commission for Certified Care Manager Certification
   www.ccmcertification.org
   (847) 380-6836

4. Commission on Rehabilitation Counselor Certification
   www.crccertification.com
   (847) 944-1325

5. National Academy of Certified Care Managers
   www.naccm.net
   (800) 962-2260

6. National Association of Social Workers
   www.socialworkers.org/credentials/
   (202) 408-8600

7. National Board for Certification in Continuity of Care
   www.nbccc.net
   (888) 776-2023

8. Rehabilitation Nursing Certification Board
   www.rehabnurse.org/certification
   (800) 229-7530

- Philosophical approach
- Training and multiple disciplines
- Supervision
- Specialty credentials and levels of credentials
- Organizational versus individual credentialing
- Implications for policy development and reimbursement

Philosophical Approach

Many philosophical questions are related to care management, including several that are posed here.

Is care management a social, medical, integrated, or coordinated service model? Traditionally, the social and medical models have been considered separate largely because of the diverse funding sources for each. In addition to reimbursement and funding differences, the fragmentation in legislation, authority, and standards in health, mental health, and social services programs have made it nearly impossible to develop a unified holistic or integrated model of care. There is increasing recognition on both health and psychosocial sides of the debate that there is a need for greater crossover and flexibility to allow the integration of these components. However, the structural and financial issues have yet to be resolved. Ideally, future public policy makers will look at the needs of the population and provide funds to be used for any social, mental health, or medical service needed by an individual or family at any given moment. Private insurance policies might likewise be integrated. The role of care managers would be to triage clients to help determine the most appropriate level of intervention and to monitor client status and service delivery.

Does the care management process cut across the continuum of care or can it be performed within a single setting? There is growing consensus that care management services cut across a variety of service settings. This is supported by a modification in the CCM eligibility criteria which now requires provision of services across a continuum of care to assure that the ongoing needs of clients are being met.

This does not change the fact that funding remains tied to particular settings and is not typically portable to other parts of the continuum of care. Long-term care insurance policies that include services beyond skilled nursing care often offer care management services as an integral part of the benefit or as an additional rider to the policy.

Is there a value to maintaining an individual patient at a level of functioning, or is the goal rehabilitation? There is a growing sense that there is value in ensuring that a level of functioning is maintained. Perry's study concluded that delaying institutional care through a program of maintenance would save the government $5 billion in healthcare and custodial costs in just 1 month.[15] Other studies suggest similar savings. The National Alzheimer's Association estimated that the annual cost of Alzheimer's to US businesses is at least $33 billion. Families and people with Alzheimer's pay an estimated $3.7–6.5 billion for the medical costs of Alzheimer's.[16] These costs are not borne by the general public. The implications for empowering caregivers and focusing on the quality of life are enormous.

Is care management considered a profession, a practice field within a primary profession, or a role that does not require professional sta-

tus? In 1964, Carr-Sanders and Wilson provided a model of professionalization that includes the following characteristics:

- Attracting practitioners on a full-time basis
- Having acquired support from foundations and large governmental sponsors
- Having a growing body of literature supported by academic journals
- Having numerous university training programs
- Having accreditation of academic programs
- Practitioners receiving a fee for services
- Being successful in influencing public policy
- Having a professional association with conditions for entrance
- Having registration or licensure requirements for practice[12]

According to this definition, care management has not quite reached professional status because of the lack of accredited educational programs to prepare individuals for practice as well as the lack of regulation to govern the field. Care management has been added to the curricula of many education programs such as nursing, social work, and continuing education departments.

Is the role of the care manager inherently that of a gatekeeper and resource allocator? The care manager's approach to service provision is best addressed in light of the practice setting. There are major differences in the ability to authorize, distribute, and use resources within a health maintenance organization, a state waiver program, or a private practice. Although all aspects of care management include some resource allocation, it is not always the duty of the gatekeeper. Furthermore, in times of scarcity, use of resources becomes an ethical matter, regardless of the source of funding or reimbursement. It is clear, however, that the way a care manager views this role will affect decisions related to the type, number, and length of services provided.

Training and Multiple Disciplines

Who should do care management and what core knowledge is needed to perform the essential tasks and activities within a given setting or specific population? These have long been topics of debate and discussion. Because the practice of care management developed from within the field rather than from an academic program, there is little consensus about the required body of knowledge, nor is there a unified set of core skills for care managers. Further complicating this issue is the lack of common standards for continuing education of care managers. The various credentialing organizations listed in Table 18-1 have different criteria for what continuing education credits will be accepted, what those credits should consist of, and who should have provided those credits.

There is great disparity as well among practicing care managers about what their core training should be. The backgrounds and training of social workers, nurses, psychologists, gerontologists, counselors, and therapists vary widely. Increasingly, practitioners are also coming into care management from other fields because of changes in demographics, corporate downsizing, midlife career decisions, and technology. Some come into care management as a result of their own experience in dealing with an aging loved one or other person with a catastrophic or chronic illness. Others enter from such diverse venues as the long-term care insurance field, law, financial planning, life planning, retirement planning, accounting, and recreation. This great diversity helps explain why some of the credentialing organizations require a prior license or certification.

Supervision

As Table 18-1 and the preceding text make clear, several credentialing organizations require an individual to have been supervised.

An individual care manager's professional training and degree may already include or require supervision to practice at the independent level. Supervision is one of many tools the professional has to ensure the quality of service delivery. The purpose of supervision includes but is not limited to the following:

- Ensuring compliance with internal and external policies and regulations
- Enhancing professional practice skills
- Ensuring the quality of service delivery to consumers
- Ensuring client outcomes
- Providing objective feedback and fresh ideas for interventions
- Complying with professional practice standards
- Clarifying ethical issues

Supervision and peer consultation is particularly important in care management because care managers work within the constantly changing health and social service delivery systems and must work with the intensely diverse dynamics of each family system, often with complex needs, preferences, values, faith traditions, and resources. Although a sophisticated practitioner may be experienced in working with a multitude of these complex systems, the specific details of each client situation remain unique. These challenging factors affect care management practice and necessitate periodic review to ensure high-quality and ethical service delivery.

This raises the question of who is qualified to provide supervision. The desire for supervision in the work setting is largely a result of the lack of practicum experience focused on care management, the lack of available credentialed supervisors, and the desire to ensure that the knowledge base of the care manager is successfully transferred to the client. For some credentialing organizations, the supervisor must be an individual who already holds the care management credential. Other organizations have a broader interpretation to include anyone in a supervisory capacity that can attest to the candidate's successful performance of care management functions. Even the most experienced independent practitioner benefits from a supervisory or consultative process. For the solo practitioner, burnout is a particular hazard. The opportunity for consultation and supervision in solo practice can be essential for maintaining an objective approach, working out ethical issues, and staying up to date with new interventions and services.

Specialty Credentials and Levels of Credentials

Another distinction that might be made among the various credentials is a determination of the level of practice and an area of specialization. The credentialing bodies that require another license or certificate might characterize the care management credential as a form of advanced or specialty practice. Several of the credentialing organizations that do not have such prerequisites might also consider this a specialty credential, but not an advanced credential. NACCM, for example, characterizes its examination as a test of *core* knowledge of the care management process and anticipates that workers will specialize based on their work with a specific population or setting. The specialty or advanced credential requires the differentiation of knowledge, skills, interventions, and outcomes from those of the general or non-advanced credential. This is a controversial area and one that is only now beginning to come to the forefront of credentialing activities.

Organizational vs Individual Credentialing

With the recent publication of the URAC standards for credentialing care management

organizations, a new question appears: should organizations, individuals, or both be credentialed? As provider organizations have carved out service specialties and the incidence of risk sharing has increased, credentialing of organizations has become important as part of risk management protocols. The question remains whether this credentialing has a tangible impact on quality or is just an additional cost to providers with little or no benefit to the consumer. It would be premature to speculate on the answer at this early stage. However, the burden imposed and the potential for positive outcomes should be carefully examined as organizational credentialing becomes more widespread.

Implications for Policy Development and Reimbursement

The failed attempts to reconfigure the healthcare delivery system in the early 1990s demonstrated how difficult it is to make revolutionary changes in an established set of services where so many individuals appear to have conflicting interests. Over the past decade, there have been dramatic changes in the healthcare delivery system because of a combination of administrative changes, regulatory modifications, economic changes, and the growing recognition of the needs of populations with chronic conditions. Typically, change has continued to be incremental and, therefore, fragmented. This has hampered the ability to integrate or coordinate the funding and delivery of health, mental health, and social services. Although a fully integrated system is a distant vision that may not be shared by the majority of policymakers, for this vision to become reality, it will be necessary to address many emerging issues, such as the following:

- How care management will be funded
- Under what auspices care management will be provided

- Who the care managers will be
- How the impact of particular programs' goals will be measured
- Who will be served by care management, how long they will be served, and what level of service they will receive

In addressing these issues, policymakers will need to be cognizant of different approaches and philosophies so programs can be sculpted to meet the particular needs of each setting and population. This potentially means that there is a need for recognition of different skill sets in different environments that still come within the commonly defined process of care management. It also means that all funded programs need to have a research component so outcome data can be obtained to answer these questions. Research design will be critically important if it is to enable the comparison of different care management models across programs and professions.

■ CONCLUSION

The growth of care management over the past few decades has been significant. Virtually every human services setting in the country provides some form of care management regardless of the population served. The growth of geriatric care management has also been noteworthy, especially in the private practice arena. The move toward credentialing is an effort to control quality by requiring those who want to do the work to meet established criteria and standards and to set some agreed-on level of consumer and professional expectations. Geriatric care managers can play an important role in both developing credential mechanisms and by becoming certified themselves.

Because there are many types of care and case management, individuals seeking credentialing need to determine which type of certification to obtain and which certifying entity is the best fit. This decision should be based

not only on background and discipline, but also on the care manager's current or planned practice in terms of population, setting, and specific condition. (See "Suggested Reading" section following the references.)

■ REFERENCES

1. Durley CC. The NOCA guide to understanding credentialing concepts. Washington, DC: National Organization for Competency Assurance; 2005. http://www.noca.org/publications/publications.htm. Accessed September 18, 2009.

2. Bartelstone R. History of care management credentialing. *J Geriatric Care Manage.* 10(2);2009:8–10.

3. Rosen AL, Bodie-Gross E, Young E, Smolenski M, Howe D. To be or not to be? Case/care management credentialing. In: Applebaum R, White M, eds. *Key Issues in Case Management Around the Globe.* San Francisco, CA: American Society on Aging; 2000.

4. Geron SM. Measuring the quality and success of care management: developments and issues in the United States, England and other countries. In: Applebaum R, White M, eds. *Key Issues in Case Management Around the Globe.* San Francisco, CA: American Society on Aging; 2000.

5. Commission for Case Manager Certification. FAQs. http://www.ccmcertification.org. Accessed February 15, 2010.

6. Leahy MJ. Validation of essential knowledge dimensions in case management. Rolling Meadows, IL: Foundation for Rehabilitation and Research; 1994.

7. National Association of Professional Geriatric Care Managers. Care/Case Management Summit II minutes. Tucson, AZ: National Association of Professional Geriatric Care Managers; March 1999.

8. Commission for Case Manager Certification. Definition of case management. http://www.ccmcertification.org. Accessed February 15, 2010.

9. Mullahy C. The CCM credential. *J Geriatric Care Manage.* 2009;Fall:21.

10. Geron SM, Chassler D. *Guidelines for Case Management Practice Across the Long-Term Continuum.*

Bristol, CT: Connecticut Community Care; 1994.

11. National Academy of Certified Care Management Candidate Handbook 2010. http://www.NACCM.net. Accessed August 2, 2010.

12. Oliensis-Torres M. NASW Certifications in Case Management. *J Geriatric Care Manage*. 2009;Fall:19.

13. NBCC. Eligibility. http://nbccc.net/eligibil.htm. Accessed March 28, 2010.

14. Association of Rehabilitation Nurses. Certification criteria. http://www.rehabnurse.org/certification/criteria.html. Accessed March 28, 2010.

15. Perry D. Aging research: keeping older Americans health. *Healthy Aging*. 1977.

16. Koppel R. Alzheimer's disease costs business $33 billion a year in caregiver loss, medical expenses. Presented at: Washington National Press Club for the Alzheimer's Association; September 1998; Washington, DC.

■ SUGGESTED READING

For a good discussion of types of care and case management, please see White M. Case management. In: Evashwick C, ed. *The Continuum of Long-Term Care: An Integrated Systems Approach*. 3rd ed. Clifton Park, NY: Thomson Delmar Learning; 2005.

Chapter 19

Preparing for Emergencies

Liz Barlowe, Erica Karp, and Angela Koenig

■ AN OVERVIEW

No one wants to imagine horrible things happening to people, but as they say, bad things happen to good people. Hurricanes, tornadoes, blizzards, terrorist attacks, epidemics, earthquakes—the list of possible disasters is overwhelming. Disasters are not the only emergencies that can befall a professional geriatric care management agency. The absence of key personnel can also occur suddenly for a variety of reasons, causing a disruption in service and business. Nevertheless, we can prepare ourselves and our agencies to navigate safely through an emergency. The key is to plan, plan, and plan more. Our colleagues who have experienced sudden illness, the events of 9/11, or one of the recent hurricanes, have taught us much about what worked, as well as what should have and could have been done to make a bad situation better.

We also know that, in any emergency, the geriatric and disabled client is particularly at risk. Preparing a professional geriatric care management agency for a disaster means having twin primary concerns: one for the agency and one for its clients. These concerns are inextricably tied together. The approach for securing your business and clients in a disaster must include planning, implementing, and recovery. This chapter provides necessary procedures to consider in developing a successful emergency plan. In this chapter, we consider a number of emergency scenarios as well as practical guidelines, checklists, procedures, and resources to enable care managers to develop useful emergency care plans for their businesses and their clients.

■ PREPARING THE AGENCY: ASSESSING YOUR COMPANY'S RISK

Absence of Key Personnel

The ability of an agency to function despite an emergency is critical. Informal procedures in a business, especially a smaller business, can appear to be an element of a family atmosphere, and it is easy to get into the habit of informality. However, if illness, accident, or some other unforeseen event overtakes an owner or manager, these habits can become a huge liability. Every professional geriatric care manager should have a formal, written backup plan that dictates action should a disaster or emergency arise. It is necessary to assess your company's risk of temporary or permanent service disruption if a disaster or emergency is experienced. This may seem an overwhelming task at first, but when you break it down into pieces, it becomes workable.

First review your policies, procedures, and job descriptions. Ensure specific procedures are written so anyone can do the task if need be. Next designate a person to assume control in an emergency (an agent for the authority figure) and give that person documented authority to sign checks and contracts, and conduct day-to-day business. Be sure to check with your attorney to anticipate any legal problems. Even if the agent has already filled in for the principal, a blueprint will be essential for the agent to run the business in a way the owner wants. The best way to ensure this is to create an emergency plan for the agency operation.

Documents: Company Emergency Plan

The emergency plan should contain specific policies and procedures, which are written out and made explicit. It should include directions that the owner or manager would like followed in emergency circumstances. The emergency plan should be signed and dated by both the owner and the manager, reviewed periodically, and updated as policies and procedures or circumstances change. This emergency plan will be your first line of defense when an emergency or disaster occurs.

The chain of command as well as a backup chain of command should be included. This will help the staff know who has decision-making authority given a disaster or absence of the owner or manager. Company policies and procedures should be kept in the emergency plan as well. These should be specific and include guidelines for an emergency, in addition to each team member's job description. The plan should also include a list of all employees and their contact information. Employees should be asked to provide contact information in the event of their own personal emergency during business hours.

Communication will be imperative in an emergency or disaster and could be disrupted for days or longer. We have learned from past disasters that text messaging appears to be the last mode of communication to be interrupted. Ensure that employees are proficient at texting before an emergency arises and have other means of charging their cell phones besides electricity (e.g., car charger, portable battery charger). Consider including an emergency number in another state in the event only local communication is interrupted.

Copies of your business's insurance policies and license(s) must be included, such as the agency's worker's compensation, professional liability, employee practice liability, and commercial business license. Include a written inventory and photo catalog of all business equipment and furnishings in your office. You may need this information to continue to pay your employees (check with your payroll company or bank on how payroll can be reoccurring given an emergency that doesn't allow for your approval) or to secure repairs to your offices. Include copies of any contracts with other services, such as emergency transportation or facilities willing to accept evacuated clients. Finally, a list of your clients and their disaster plans should be included.

In addition to paper copies, it is important the agency have documents loaded onto a memory stick, as well as make disaster plans accessible online. Many agencies will have documents loaded on their server to which employees have remote access, but if the server is housed in the office, all could be inaccessible or destroyed. Equally critical is having online authority outside of the disaster area established that houses necessary company information.

The emergency plan should be available in several locations. The plan should be accessible at the company office(s), as well as posted on the employee-only section of the company's secured website. The company owner and manager should have a copy at all times, both on paper and electronically. You never know when a disaster will occur, or where the key personnel will be when disaster strikes.

It is imperative you know how to act if a disaster or emergency occurs without warning. This will allow for direction rather than reaction in the midst of a disaster, which can be costly and time consuming.

Emergency Preparedness Meetings

Each business should have regular meetings scheduled during which the staff members are encouraged to think the unthinkable and prepare themselves to negotiate an emergency. An emergency is not only a disaster or an illness; it can be a fire, an epidemic, a lengthy power outage, or workplace violence. In fact, the emergency preparedness meetings should be a place to brainstorm possible scenarios. Just as fire drills teach everyone the quickest and safest way out of a building, contingency plans for responding to other emergencies can be rehearsed. This is also a good time to discuss emotional issues. Thinking about the possible absence of a colleague or any other emergency may trigger emotional issues, particularly sadness and fear. Insecurities and emotions can be addressed and acknowledged in these meetings because simply planning for such occurrences can give rise to issues around trust and relinquishing control. Another task of the emergency preparedness meetings is to evaluate the status of a client in the event of a disaster. Which clients will need immediate attention, which will be attended to as soon as possible, and which ones may be expected to function for a short time on their own?

Brainstorming with other companies in your area offers opportunities to develop relationships that allow for collaboration in the event of a disaster. Competition aside, a disaster is about responding efficiently and restoring functions as soon as possible. Set aside competition and plan for interagency collaborations. Exhibit 19-1 is an example of minutes from a care management disaster alliance meeting.

■ PREPARING FOR DISASTERS: AN OVERVIEW

Recent occurrences have shown that disasters come in many forms. Hurricanes, terrorist attacks, and earthquakes may grab the headlines, but blizzards and floods can also obstruct the safe functioning of a professional geriatric care management agency. Recent disasters have made it painfully clear that the elderly and disabled are dreadfully at risk in an emergency. Each disaster creates circumstances that have specific dangers and problems we should examine. However, there are some general precautions that can be categorized and looked at first. Professional geriatric care management agencies must foresee the worst to prevent it. Again, the keyword is planning. Planning, and engaging staff, caregivers, and clients in the planning, goes a long way toward forestalling potential injury and loss of life.

Most natural disasters are confined to particular regions. Hurricanes bedevil the southeastern and Gulf States, earthquakes are most likely to occur along the fault lines of the West Coast, and tornadoes are more frequent in the Midwest. The regional nature of potential disasters enables a level of predictability in planning for them. Evacuation routes and shelter sites, for example, can be identified long before an actual hurricane threatens. The professional geriatric care management agency should identify which types of disasters are most likely to occur in its area. Again, identifying likely types of emergencies will raise awareness when such emergencies are discussed during emergency preparedness meetings. Preparations can be put into two main categories. First, prepare the agency; second, prepare clients and caregivers.

Exhibit 19–1   Care Manager Disaster Alliance: Sample Meeting Minutes

---

Minutes of Care Manager Disaster Alliance (CMDA)   **Date:** December 10, 2010

Call to order: An initial disaster drill planning meeting of the CMDA was held in Clearwater, Florida, on December 10, 2010. The meeting convened at 8:30 a.m., N. Smith presiding, and M. Mackintosh, secretary.

Members in attendance: Care managers from local companies.

Approval of minutes: Motion was made by R. Barker to convene local care managers in the Tampa Bay area with the goal of creating a disaster response team serving the needs of seniors and disabled clients mutually during a disaster. **Motion carried.**

Officers' reports:

- President: M. Shannon discussed the scope of the alliance, and presented overall goals.
- Vice president: S. Jules presented needs assessment results, and outlined the committee groups that needed to be formed as a result of the assessment.

Committee reports: Not yet established.

Unfinished business: Committee selections from group members. Time was given for members to review and commit to the committee/s of their choice or expertise. Committees needed are: Technology Committee, Phone Tree/Communication Committee, County Lead Committee, Evacuation Coordination Committee, Response and Recovery Committee, Review Committee, Disaster Day Committee.

New business:

- Disaster Drill Day: April 1, 2010, was set for implementing a Disaster Drill Day, prior to the June 2010 hurricane season.

  Motion: Moved by S. Thompson that Disaster Drill Day be set for 4/1/2010, with monthly committee meetings to establish, evolve, and implement committee goals. Bi-monthly meeting for general membership to discuss and review. **Motion carried.**

Announcements: Emergency Operations Centers will be invited to the next general meeting for input, January 29, 2010. Committee meetings set for January 11, 2010.

Adjournment: The meeting was adjourned at 11:55 a.m.

M. Mackintosh   *12/10/2010*
Secretary   Date of approval

Source: Reprinted with permission by Julie Scott, 2010.

Preparing a Professional Geriatric Care Management Agency for an Emergency

The first step to protecting the agency is to preserve the files and the equipment. Vital information is stored as hard copy and on computers, such as insurance policy numbers and insurance agent information, bank account numbers and accountant phone numbers, attorney phone numbers and legal documents, and phone numbers and addresses for the relatives of clients—this is only the tip of the iceberg. All of this information needs to be backed up regularly, with backup hard copies stored at a secure, off-site location. In this day of computerization, information can be electronically filed, but there should still be a plan for salvaging paper files and office equipment if possible. Power outages can last for weeks, or even months. Designate a staff member to oversee continual review of emergency procedures, perhaps on a rotating basis so everyone becomes familiar with the process.

Staff safety is important, of course, but setting priorities ahead of time can result in everyone functioning more safely as well as keeping the agency working. Find an alternate location for the staff to work from for an indefinite amount of time in case of a lengthy, major disruption. An invaluable aid is to have a sister agency in another region to turn to, an agency that hopefully would be unaffected by the disaster. An alternate location with a compatible business may offer the best working solution for a backup location (e.g., a home health agency, a senior living community). While preparing the agency for an emergency, don't forget to take basic precautions at the office. Stock emergency supplies just as you would for a residence. Provide necessary equipment to work remotely wherever possible.

Sister Agencies

Partnering with another agency enables both agencies to have a backup for storing files and for relaying communications in an emergency. A hurricane is unlikely to occur simultaneously with an earthquake, so sister agencies work best if located in separate regions. At least one of them can be counted on to have access to computers. Perhaps the most important role the sister agency can play in an emergency is serving as an information center. The families of professional geriatric care management clients often live far away from their elderly relatives, and they will be understandably anxious; if they can call the sister agency, the families can be apprised of whatever information is available. In the likely event of power loss during an emergency, computers, cell phones, BlackBerry devices, and all the elec-

tronic conveniences that we rely on may cease to function. However, landline telephones often continue to work when other means of communications fail. Thus, the sister agency becomes invaluable as a hub for relaying information in and out of the affected area. Establish these relationships long before the need arises, and periodically practice the accessibility and feasibility of the relationship so you both know what to expect.

Preparing Clients and Caregivers

Preparing individual clients, their families, and their caregivers for disasters can be broken down into three simple steps: (1) basics, (2) emergency supplies, and (3) a personal plan.

The client, depending on his or her level of ability to function, should be encouraged to participate in preparations as much as possible. This is not only useful for the preparations but will go a good distance toward alleviating some stress if the emergency situation does arise. Remember to include any pets in the emergency preparation. Many evacuation vehicles and shelters will not allow pets, and the need to abandon one can cause considerable distress.

All the information gathered regarding a client's decisions and needs in preparation for an emergency should be filed and reviewed regularly. Put this information in each client's file, and also in a master document covering all clients. Exhibits 19–2 and 19–3 are samples of master documents that should be stored both as hard copy and electronically.

Basics

Knowing the basics begins with learning what types of disasters are particular to a professional geriatric care management agency's area. Earthquakes happen suddenly, whereas hurricanes give at least some warning. Some locations may have community preparedness plans that are essential for a professional geriatric care management agency to take into consideration. Federal Emergency Management Agency (FEMA) and Red Cross services

Exhibit 19–2   Homebound Client Disaster Plan   Year _____

Client Name: _____   Client Number: _____

Phone: _____

Address: _____

Evacuation Zone: A   B   C   D   E   Non-Evac   *All mobile home residents must evacuate, regardless of location.*

Will client evacuate? Yes   No

If yes, where will client evacuate? _____

Facility: Have you reserved client respite bed in a facility? **Yes   No**

Name and address of facility: _____

Have necessary admission forms been completed and signed by the doctor? **Yes   No   On file**

Daily rate of facility: _____ Will room be furnished? **Yes   No**   *Refer to checklist for add'l items to bring.*

Will client need assistance with packing? **Yes   No** Person responsible for packing: _____

Will client need transportation to facility? **Yes   No** Person responsible for transport: _____

Type of transportation needed: _____

Does client have a pet? **Yes   No** If yes, plan is _____

Family/friend: Have they confirmed their willingness to provide necessary assistance? **Yes   No**

Name, address, and phone: _____

Will client need assistance with packing? **Yes   No** Person responsible for packing: _____

Will client need transportation to facility? **Yes   No** Person responsible for transport: _____

Type of transportation needed: _____

Does client have a pet? **Yes   No** If yes, plan is _____

If no, please notify the local emergency services for your county and review the following safety measures with your client:

- Safest area in the home is an area with no windows, like a closet, hall, or bathroom.
- If possible utilize a space with no exterior walls and stock the area with supplies.
- If there is no power, use flashlights (never use candles).
- Do not use generators or grills inside.
- If there is a "boil water" warning, do not even brush your teeth with the water.
- Home will be secured by: _____. Person responsible for securing: _____
- Enough supplies for 2 weeks/per person. Person responsible for supplies: _____
- Please have client sign "Refusal to Evacuate Letter."

Is client receiving any home care services? **Yes   No** If Yes, what is their policy regarding services:

- Up to the time of the disaster: **Yes   No** Service will cease as of: _____
- During the disaster: **Yes   No** Caregiver remaining with client is: _____
- After the disaster: **Yes   No** Service will resume on: _____

_____   _____

Care Manager Signature   Date   Client/Responsible Party   Date

Please review annually or upon change in physical, cognitive status, or residency.

Source: Aging Wisely, LLC, © 2010, www.agingwisely.com.

Exhibit 19–3   Facility-Based Client Disaster Plan   Year _____

Client Name: _____   Client Number: _____

Facility Name: _____   **ALF   SNF   Other**

Phone: _____   Administrator/Contact: _____

Address: _____

Evacuation Zone: A   B   C   D   E   Non-Evac

Request to review facilities comprehensive emergency management plan (CEMP), which is required by state law, and ask the following questions:

1. Is the facility to be used as a shelter for other evacuating facilities? **Yes   No**

2. If this facility is required to evacuate, what is the location where the residents will be evacuated?
   _____

3. Secondary evacuation location? _____

4. What is the procedure for notifying families/responsible parties that the facility is being evacuated?
   _____

5. Facility responsible ER contact: _____ Phone: _____

6. What are your provisions for 24-hour staffing on a continuous basis? _____

7. When was the most recent facility staff disaster training? _____

8. How often are staff members trained in disaster preparedness? _____

9. Do you have an emergency power system (generator/s)? **Yes   No**

10. If yes, what is the capacity of the system, that is, what items will it power?

    a. _____

    b. _____

    c. _____

    d. _____

11. How many "hot" outlets do you have for oxygen concentrators, nebulizers, etc., available on generator power? _____ Location of outlets _____

12. What is your emergency means of transportation, and do you have a back up?
    _____

_____   _____

Care Manager Signature   Date   Client/Responsible Party   Date

Please review annually or upon change in physical, cognitive status, or residency.

Source: Aging Wisely, LLC, © 2010, www.agingwisely.com.

should be researched to see what plans are in place as well as consulting the local police, fire department, and city planning agencies for emergency plans. Exhibit 19–4 lists several websites that should be researched for useful information from experts. If at all possible, the professional geriatric care management agency should advise local agencies to make them more responsive to the special needs of the aging and disabled person.

Exhibit 19–4   Disaster Preparedness Website Resources

General Disaster Preparedness

http://www.disastercenter.com
The Disaster Center website offers information on a wide array of threats.

http://www.fema.gov/areyouready
"Are You Ready" is a booklet developed as an in-depth guide to preparing for potential disasters that can be downloaded or accessed online.

http://www.hhs.gov/disasters/index.shtml
Department of Health and Human Services. Information about responding to health crises during and after various types of disasters, particularly about stress issues following an emergency

http://www.fhwa.dot.gov/webstate.htm
State transportation websites. Information regarding transportation issues affecting your state, along with possible evacuation routes in case of a disaster

http://www.equipped.com/disastertoc.htm
Variety of disaster preparedness kits for purchase or ideas to prepare your own kit

http://www.safetyproof.com
Specialty disaster products and services with emphasis on earthquake preparedness

http://www.nhc.noaa.gov/HAW2/english/disaster_prevention.shtml
The National Hurricane Center website provides preparedness information for disasters related to tropical storms and hurricanes.

http://www.disasterprep101.com/tornadoes. htm
The six keys to safety in a tornado.

Business Preparedness

http://www.ready.gov/business/index.html
Department of Homeland Security in collaboration with Ready Business helps owners and managers of small- and medium-sized businesses prepare their employees, operations, and assets in the event of an emergency.

http://www.sba.gov/services/disasterassistance/disasterpreparedness/index.html
Resources related to disaster preparedness from the U.S. Small Business Administration

http://www.sba.gov/services/disasterassistance/businessesofallsizes/applyforloan/index.html
Checklist for Small Business Administration Disaster Recovery Loan

Disaster Response Organizations

http://www.redcross.org
American Red Cross website includes information on disaster preparedness, disaster response activities, and training.

Recovery

http://www.fema.gov
The Federal Emergency Management Agency website with information on planning, recovery aid, and rebuilding after a disaster.

Health Insurance Portability and Accountability Act (HIPAA) and Disaster Response

http://www.hhs.gov/ocr/hipaa/decisiontool
Disclosures for Emergency Preparedness—A Decision Tool

Physician Preparedness and Response Planning Resources

http://www.bt.cdc.gov
Variety of preparedness topics and links from the Centers for Disease Control and Prevention (CDC).

Disaster Planning for Persons with Mobility Impairments

http://www2.ku.edu/~rrtcpbs/powerpoint
The Nobody Left Behind disaster preparedness project of the University of Kansas, including power point presentations

Another basic essential is evaluating the client's residence. If the client still resides at home, the safety of the house needs to be assessed. How much of a storm can it withstand? Does it have safe areas inside for riding out a storm? Where are the gas connections that need to be shut down after an earthquake? How is this done? Who will do it? Where are the water and electrical outlets? In addition to the residence itself, learn who the neighbors are and (with the client's permission) exchange basic information with them, such as phone numbers, family names, and other helpful contacts. The professional geriatric care management agency should encourage the client's caregivers to constantly monitor the residence and assess it for potential risk. A group home also needs to be evaluated for safety. What emergency plans does the residence have in place? What kind of shelter does it provide? Does it have a generator, and what does the generator power? How long can it function without power?

Deciding whether to evacuate in an emergency and where to go is also part of basic planning. An evacuation plan should take into account not only the prospective shelter, but what transportation will be available and what routes to take. Will family members be available or will the client be dependent primarily on the professional geriatric care management agency? Is the best place to go another home, an independent living or assisted living community, or a medical facility? Some families have given professional geriatric care management agencies open-ended plane tickets so clients can leave the area entirely. The choice of where to evacuate must take into account special needs of the client, such as whether he or she needs dialysis or oxygen.

Emergency Supplies

The goal of keeping emergency supplies on hand is to be able to survive until help arrives or basic utilities are restored. Clients who decide to stay in place through a disaster should sign a document stating that they have refused to evacuate to demonstrate they understand the risk of the decision. (See Exhibit 19–5.) A supply of food, water, and medicine that will last for several days is essential. Drinking water for 3–6 days is estimated to be a gallon of water per person per day. Store a supply of food that won't spoil or require cooking because power most likely will be unavailable. A hand-operated can opener is a must.

Medical preparation for the professional geriatric care management client is of utmost importance. In addition to prescription drugs, the client may need oxygen or infusion. It is possible to have an emergency supply of these necessities available in areas where sudden disasters may be the highest risk. Special arrangements need to be made for clients who need dialysis. In the case of prescriptions, keep a list of medications, prescribing physicians, prescription numbers, dosages, and purchase dates with the emergency supplies. This information should also be kept with the emergency information on file at the professional geriatric care management agency office and online. Attach a copy of the prescription to the back of the list. If the doctor agrees, an emergency supply of medications can be added to the supplies. Every time a prescription is filled, put the new medications in with the emergency supplies and then use the medications that are being replaced so the emergency supply will not expire.

In addition, the emergency supplies should contain a flashlight, a battery-powered radio, a supply of spare batteries, and light sticks. Candles should be avoided as an open flame can pose a serious risk for fire. For an extensive list of supplies appropriate for your area, access your county's website or one of the websites listed in Exhibit 19–4.

If evacuation is necessary, have an evacuation bag packed and on hand to grab going out the door. A number of things from the stay-at-home supplies can be kept in the emergency evacuation bag, especially copies of important papers such as medication needs, a contact list with names and phone numbers,

Exhibit 19–5   Refusal to Evacuate Form

I, _____ have been informed of the imminent need to evacuate my residence due to the potential dangers, including injury and death, posed by the current emergency and choose to remain in my home against the advice of my care manager.

_____
(initial)

I understand that when I am ready for assistance it may be too late for a care manager to assist me in the evacuation process. I understand that they will not be able to come to me until the emergency passes, and that they may not be available by telephone until the emergency has passed. _____
(initial)

I understand that once a state of emergency is in place it may not be possible for the Emergency Medical Service (9-1-1) to provide me services, and the local police may not be able to assist me until the emergency passes. _____
(initial)

I understand the risks involved in this decision and accept all responsibility for my decision. I confirm that I have refused to consent to all care and assistance with evacuation. _____
(initial)

_____   _____
Client Signature   Date

_____   _____
Responsible Party Signature   Date

_____   _____
Care Manager's Signature   Date

If client refuses to sign, please indicate so by marking here.

Copy of completed form provided to client: _____
                                                                           Date

Copy of completed form provided to responsible party: _____
                                                                                          Date

Source: Aging Wisely, LLC, © 2010, www.agingwisely.com.

insurance policies, and other vital documents. Other items for the evacuation bag are a change of clothing, personal hygiene necessities, comfortable shoes, an extra pair of glasses, and a blanket or sleeping bag. Be realistic because this bag should be in place and ready to easily carry or roll at a moment's notice.

Personal Planning

Every client has unique needs and the professional geriatric care management agency should establish an emergency plan for each client. This plan should be placed in a file that includes emergency checklists and up-to-date assessments. Copies should be kept online on the agency's secure website, at the client's residence, and at the office. Caregivers should be encouraged to periodically review the plan. If the plan includes evacuation, there should be a trial run, just like a fire drill. In some areas struck by hurricanes, or in the case of earthquakes, the usual landmarks may disappear. Street signs, buildings, trees, or any kind of familiar marker may be destroyed, so having already been to the designated shelter could prove to be invaluable. For clients who have disabilities, it may be possible to register with the local police or fire department so the clients can be put on a list of people to check up on in the event of an emergency.

Evaluate the kind of shelter that is most appropriate for a particular client. The county's shelters or a hotel should be the last places to recommend. County shelters are uncomfortable and often crowded; hotels often have no provisions for medical care or emergency food supplies. Consider an assisted living residence even for the most independent of clients. Someone with Alzheimer's disease requires a facility that serves that population. If the client needs a place equipped to provide special needs such as oxygen or dialysis, arrangements can be made. Again, involve the client and family as much as possible because this can help reduce some of the stress of an emergency. Remember, most injuries and deaths occur in the aftermath of a disaster such as a hurricane, so the more decisions made ahead of time, the safer everyone will be.

Recovery

It is appropriate that during and immediately following a disaster or other type of emergency professional geriatric care management staff and caregivers will secure their own safety and that of their families. However, as soon as possible, these personnel should contact the agency and let the staff member in charge know their status, their client's status if they are a caregiver, and their availability. Immediately following an emergency, the most important task is to locate everyone, assess their status, and respond to the most urgent needs. Information will become the most vital resource following an emergency, so this is when having a sister agency to coordinate information will prove invaluable. Locate the services that can provide you with assistance, and offer to help where possible. In a disaster, former competitors may be the most capable allies.

After securing the safety of persons, a property damage assessment is in order. Can the central office still function? Is the backup location available? Protect and preserve whatever equipment is still in operating order. Computers, files, possibly vehicles, even the building itself will need to be checked for potential hazards and operational suitability. Begin the application process for relief resources from the appropriate agencies, such as insurance or FEMA, as soon as possible.

Remember to acknowledge the services of staff and caregivers. Later, when there is time for a full debriefing and for considering the emotional aftermath of experiencing a disaster, a greater acknowledgment can be made; however, immediate consideration and encouragement will go a long way to help everyone negotiate the crisis.

Preparing a professional geriatric care management agency for an emergency is a serious responsibility. As was mentioned earlier, seniors are very much at risk in any kind of disaster. In an emergency, something unexpected will always occur, but a little foresight will pay off in huge dividends. Planning, vigilance, and researching available resources are the keys to successful emergency preparedness.

Chapter 20

Geriatric Care Management: Working with Nearly Normal Aging Families

Anne Rosenthal and Cathy Jo Cress

■ INTRODUCTION

Eugene O'Neill's play *Long Day's Journey into Night* tells us the wrenching tale of a dysfunctional family, marked by strained relationships and unresolved conflicts. Most aging families are healthy, not dysfunctional, but are knocked off balance by losses sustained when older family members decline or die. Dysfunction can also result from caregiving taking up huge blocks of family members' time or when significant family relationships and continuity disappear. These losses can disrupt even a healthy family. A *nearly normal* aging family can be righted if they have historically been compatible, cohesive, productive, and stable.

This chapter discusses the work geriatric care managers (GCMs) do with healthy aging families who at times are challenged, caught in the vise grip of an elder's deterioration. It covers many hurdles healthy aging families face in supporting a progressively disabled older relative. This chapter gives the GCM maps to guide families, who are challenged by the exhausting overload of long-distance caregiving, to identify and relieve caregiver overload, to work as part of a team to help the older person, and to navigate through family meetings among baby-boomer siblings who, 50 years later, may be still chafing over who a parent loved best.

■ DIFFERENTIATING BETWEEN THE HEALTHY AGING FAMILY AND THE CHALLENGED FAMILY

Although in the spectrum of aging families, there will always be a blur between healthy families and difficult families, GCMs can differentiate between the two. You can refer to two sections in Chapter 21, Difficult Families: Conflict, Dependence, and Mutuality, to help distinguish between the truly difficult family and the healthy, challenged family. You can evaluate family interaction to distinguish between a difficult family and a healthy family. You can also use the guide *How Difficult Families Present* to assess whether the aging family served by the GCM is dysfunctional or challenged.

■ GERIATRIC CARE MANAGEMENT WITH FAMILIES

A recent survey by the National Alliance for Caregiving and the American Association of Retired Persons found that 22.4 million US households, nearly 1 in 4, are providing care to a relative or friend aged 50 years or older or have provided care during the previous 12 months.[1]

GCMs often find themselves assisting family caregivers. What are these caregivers providing? Typically, they spend 18 hours a week taking the person they care for to physicians, managing the older person's finances, helping with grocery shopping, and providing hands-on personal care. Two thirds of the caregivers also are employed. Of these, slightly more than half have had to make workplace sacrifices, such as arriving late, leaving early, dropping back to part-time work, or even passing up promotions, to provide elder care. How can GCMs assist families dealing with the conflicting demands of jobs, families, and caregiving?

There is much GCMs can do to offer families direct and indirect assistance. It behooves GCMs not only to be experts on community resources but also to be adept at understanding and communicating effectively with many different types of families, especially families that are in crisis.

In other words, GCMs are experts in knowing how to save families' time and money and prevent situations from taking an emotional toll on family members. Some of the areas where these resources can be conserved are through home care services, community-based programs, and facilities. GCMs can also help families keep their finances in good shape through options such as long-term care insurance and publicly funded programs.

From GCMs, families also learn more about the illnesses with which their family members cope. GCMs are familiar with the symptoms and course of chronic diseases such as Alzheimer's and vascular dementia as well as stroke, Parkinson's disease, and arthritis. Families will benefit from GCMs' suggestions about what adaptive equipment can make the older person safer, the most effective ways to communicate with a distressed, demented individual, and other matters.

Frequently, families contact a GCM during a point of crisis. For instance, Mrs. L came with her adult son and daughter to the office of a GCM to discuss a possible placement for Mr. L. Mr. L had been recently hospitalized for a debilitating stroke and was ready to be discharged from the hospital. The daughter and son wanted to see their father cared for at a skilled nursing facility, but their mother wanted to care for her husband of nearly 50 years at home. The adult children expressed an objection to the home arrangement primarily because their mother had always been extremely dependent on her husband.

Mr. L had been a successful businessman, active in the community and civic affairs. His wife, coming from an earlier generation of women, knew little of managing anything outside the home, let alone managing the team of home health staff (nurses, a physical therapist, an occupational therapist, and a speech therapist) that would be caring for her husband. Mrs. L could not arrange for the durable medical equipment (i.e., a hospital bed, a wheelchair, and a commode) that he would need to remain at home. In fact, Mrs. L had never even written out a check.

The GCM met with the family together to discuss each member's concerns. The GCM assessed Mr. L's aptitude for making judgments, his reasoning ability, his memory, his orientation, his cognition, and his motor skills. The GCM also assessed whether the home was safe for someone with limited mobility who was using a wheelchair. The GCM was able to assure the family that it was feasible to have Mr. L remain at home. Although he had some recent memory deficits, he seemed to be able to make sound judgments on his own behalf. He clearly expressed his desire to remain in his own home. Because the house had stairs, the GCM recommended that a ramp and strategically placed grab bars be put in and some area rugs be removed.

Together, the GCM and family were able to agree on a plan of care. The home care agency best equipped to care for Mr. L was contacted. It was Medicare certified, and Mr. L qualified for home services that would not have to be paid for out of pocket. The family members were grateful for the savings in time and cost.

A coordinated schedule of care that supported Mr. L at home was established. His wife was pleased with the experienced help.

The adult children were able to return home to their jobs and families, knowing that the GCM would be monitoring the home care, following up with any additional matters that arose, contacting them regarding any change in their parent's status, and keeping them updated on the situation at home. The physician was able to obtain details from the GCM, which helped him in treating Mr. L.

Although Mr. L eventually died peacefully at home in his sleep, the story does not end there. His wife continued to live in the same home. The GCM counseled the wife regarding her grief over the loss of her husband. After a period of mourning, she became interested in becoming more independent. She was supported and assisted in learning how to write out checks and take more control of her daily life. She has taken three cruises and regularly travels to see her family.

Recently, Mrs. L was hospitalized. The adult children, all of whom have busy professional schedules, contacted the GCM to assist with their mother's care. The GCM visited Mrs. L in the hospital. The GCM offered assurances that the GCM would take care of whatever was necessary to settle Mrs. L back in at home. In addition, the care manager met with the hospital nurses and discharge planner to understand Mrs. L's condition more fully. The GCM remained in close contact with Mrs. L's family members to ensure that they agreed to the recommendations made for the assistance Mrs. L would need once she returned home.

The family saved time and money. The GCM was able to identify services for which Mrs. L would qualify under her insurance program. Mrs. L, who always prided herself on her cooking skills, reluctantly agreed to receive home-delivered meals. Later, she admitted to being grateful for the nutritious meals and for the friendly volunteer who brightened her day.

A caregiver would come during the week to do light housekeeping, to stand by while Mrs. L took a bath, and to run errands until Mrs. L's strength returned. Mrs. L would soon be able to resume her visits to her family, enjoying new grandchildren. The family members know that when Mrs. L returns home, the GCM will be only a phone call away.

Adult children commonly face many problems, such as the three following examples. In each case, a GCM steps in to help the adult children solve the problems.

CASE STUDY

An older woman fell and broke her hip. She was hospitalized for hip replacement surgery, and she is now ready for discharge to return home. The woman's daughter is panicking because she is scheduled to leave for a trip to Europe in 2 days and she doesn't know how her mother can manage without her. She calls a GCM to ask for help.

The GCM asks the following questions:

- Does the mother want to return to her home or go to a care facility to recuperate?
- Can the mother complete activities of daily living (e.g., dressing, eating, toileting, bathing) on her own safely?
- How are the mother's cognitive functions? Is she oriented to time, place, and person?
- How are her executive functions such as writing out checks and paying bills?
- How is the mother's judgment and reasoning ability?
- What is the mother's living environment like? Are there hazards (e.g., stairs, bathroom adaptive equipment, rugs) that should be addressed?

The GCM talks to the hospital discharge planner regarding the following matters:

- What will Medicare cover if the mother is at home? What will Medicare cover if the mother is at a care facility?
- What will the GCM do if the mother returns home? Should the GCM determine the amount of home care required and recruit home care workers?
- What will the GCM do if the mother transfers to a care facility? Should the GCM locate a facility and arrange for admission?
- How will the GCM help the mother to deal with her questions, anxiety, and planning during her daughter's absence?
- What support system can be put in place during the daughter's absence? Is there a local family who can offer support? What will the GCM do if the daughter would like to retain ongoing care management services?
- What will the GCM do to communicate with the daughter, monitor the mother, and communicate with the mother's hired caregivers during the daughter's absence?

CASE STUDY

A working professor has concerns about his mother, who lives out of state. The mother is in an assisted living facility, appears quite depressed, and is now displaying some paranoid ideations. He is the only relative and is 3000 miles away. He thinks he should relocate his mother to live with him, but he is not sure. He asks for the advice of a GCM.

The GCM explores with the son the quality of his mother's living situation. Is she happy where she is? What is the quality of the care she is receiving? Are there other levels of care available in the facility? Should she request a higher or lower level of care?

The care manager visits the mother in her facility and has more discussions with the son to determine answers to the following questions:

- Who visits the mother now?
- What is the son's home situation like? What kind of social stimulation is available for the mother there?
- What has been the quality of her visits to his home in the past?
- If the mother moves to his home, what modifications would be necessary for her safety?
- What are the financial aspects of the two options being considered (i.e., relocation to the son's home or remaining in the care facility)?
- Are there facilities to be considered in the son's area in case the home arrangement turns out not to be feasible?
- What about the mother's paranoid ideations? Does she have a history of emotional disturbance? What is the nature of the psychiatric intervention she received at the care facility? Could that intervention be improved? If the mother relocates to the son's residence, can the mother's emotional problems be adequately addressed?
- How does the mother feel about her son's wish to relocate her to his home? Is she comfortable with the idea?
- What are the son's motivations for wanting to initiate the move?

Are there other family members to consider?

- If the mother remains where she is, what could be done to improve the quality of her life?

CASE STUDY

An older divorced woman with a history of dementia secondary to alcoholism is addicted to buying items from a home-shopping channel. The older woman is indiscriminately ordering hundreds of dollars of items each week. She has a live-in attendant who helps with personal care. The older woman's sister calls a GCM because she is concerned there will be no money left to use for the older woman's long-term care.

The GCM asks the following questions:

- What is the attendant's role with regard to the impulsive shopping? Can she be enlisted to intervene?
- What seems to trigger the older woman's impulse to make phone purchases?
- Can the older woman be diverted?
- Is the older woman cooperative?
- Does the older woman lack the capacity to consider the consequences of her actions? If she does lack this capacity, should a conservatorship or a guardianship be considered?

What do these three problem situations have in common? In all three, families are facing problems and GCMs provide assistance using their problem-solving skills and understanding of short- and long-term planning. All three families benefit from a GCM's assistance. In each case, the GCMs assess the situa-tion, learn what the family's preferences are, make appropriate recommendations based on what is feasible, implement the recommendations once the family members approve them, follow up and monitor the situation, and adjust services and GCM involvement as the family's needs change.

■ WORKING WITH LONG-DISTANCE CAREGIVERS

Families continue caring for older family members even if they live long distances apart. Nearly 7 million Americans are responsible for the care of an older family member who lives an average of 300 miles away.

Why are there so many long-distance care providers in the United States today? Baby boomers move frequently with their jobs. We are a mobile society and many of us have moved away from our birthplace, where our parents still live. Many parents of baby boomers retire to warmer climates (e.g., Arizona, Florida) while their adult children live far away with their job and family.

What Can a GCM Do for a Long-Distance Family?

Long-distance family members spend an overwhelming amount of time caregiving. They spend time caregiving over the phone and more time flying and driving to give care for older family members. The GCM can save the long-distance family member both time and money by taking over many of the care-giving tasks for the family. The GCM can also save the long-distance caregiver more money by assuming some of the adult child's duties. Many times, long-distance family caregivers are employed. They are leaving work early, getting to work late, and drop-ping back to part-time hours to deal with the burdens of long-distance caregiving; thus, they are losing money and productivity. Oftentimes, they exhaust their vacation days or family leave time to care for long-distance family members.

The GCM's involvement with long-distance family members and their aging relatives can save caregivers from being overcome by their daunting task. Long-distance caregivers, like all caregivers, are sandwiched between the needs of their aging parents, their teenagers, their own adult children, work, and caregiving. This is an explosive combination that can result in mental and physical problems for the long-distance caregiver. Depression and anxiety can result from the stress of long-distance caregiving; these dedicated adult children can end up with weakened immune systems that may lead to physical illness.

The stress of long-distance caregiving can also result in spousal and child abuse, troubled marriages, and divorce. The intervention of a GCM in a long-distance caregiving situation can be an incredible win–win opportunity for the long-distance caregiver, older family members, and the whole extended family.

Adult children living at a distance from their older relatives face complex emotional and logistical issues. How do they know what to look for if they suspect their parents are having problems? Exhibit 20–1 describes some red flags that should be raised for the long-distance caregiver when he or she visits an older relative.

You, as a GCM, can alert long-distance family members to these warning signs. If they observe these red flags on a long-distance visit with their older family member and then ask you to begin services, you have many excellent options to offer the family. Your first step is to complete a psychosocial and functional assessment (see Chapters 3 and 4 on psychosocial assessment and functional assessment). Administering a mental status questionnaire is also suggested to assess cognitive functioning. Your next step is to report these findings to the long-distance family

Exhibit 20–1   Alarm Bells List for Visiting Long-Distance Relative

- Unpaid bills
- Missed appointments
- Clutter in a home that was once always neat
- Weight loss
- Memory loss, change in short-term memory
- Poor grooming by a person who was once meticulous
- Getting lost
- Wandering
- Refusing to go with friends on outings or to religious services
- Refusing any suggestion or conversely agreeing to everything without consideration
- Mood swings, getting angry quickly
- Refusing to go to medical providers
- Can't take care of activities of daily living: cooking, bathing, dressing, housekeeping, etc.
- Entering contests, credit card maxed out on shopping channels

member, request that you be able to make an appointment with the older person's primary physician, and take the older person to the appointment. It is a good idea to call ahead to the office and explain your geriatric care management role to the physician's assistant and fax in a summary of your assessment findings so the physician or nurse can read them before the appointment.

Next Steps for the GCM Assisting Long-Distance Family Members

The next step is to find out, after the initial assessment, if the long-distance caregiver wishes you to monitor the older family member weekly, monthly, or at all. Ask if the family members want you to be on call for emergencies. Both monitoring and on-call service are a good idea. If they agree and they want to hire you, help them understand that there are many tasks for which you could offer assistance.

Work with the long-distance family members and older client to map out a plan in the event the older family member is hospitalized. This is sometimes best done in a family meeting with the GCM present or with just family members present. This plan starts with deciding which hospital the older person wants to use. This appears basic, but sometimes a person can favor one hospital over another, or one hospital may be better equipped than another. The discussion should include where the older person might go after hospitalization. Does the older person want to go home with care providers if needed? If care or rehabilitation is required after hospitalization, does the older family member want to go to a skilled nursing facility for recovery or go home using Medicare-covered physical therapy, occupational therapy, and paid home care? Would the adult children prefer to have the older person come to their home to recover? If the older person needs to move permanently because of disability, where does the person want to move? Does the person want to downsize to a smaller home? Would the person move to a nursing home? Would he or she move to one of his or her adult childrens' homes? (See Chapter 7 on moving.) Having a plan like this in place cuts down on crisis management and replaces it with preventative maintenance for the client and family.

Find a neighbor, old friend, or nearby family member who is willing to check on the older person on a regular basis, report regularly to you, and notify you of any change in the client's condition. This sets up a monitoring network and safety net through the elder's continuum of care. You can also implement an emergency response system, if there are no caregivers nearby. You should be the emergency contact in addition to the long-distance family members. Your value as a GCM is that you are there while the long-distance family members are far away.

Create a care plan for the older person (see Chapter 5 on geriatric assessment and writing a care plan). You can also help the family hire ongoing care providers if needed, monitor household maintenance problems, and generally manage the older family member for the long-distance family.

Additional ways you can help long-distance family members and give them peace of mind are shown in Exhibit 20-2.

The National Association of Professional Geriatric Care Managers has an excellent binder available in the GCM store on their website called *Caregiver Planner: A Notebook to Organize Vital Information,* written by Betsy Carey Evatt. It has most of the tabs mentioned in Exhibit 20-2, and the family member can add more.

You can also coach family members by having a conference call or a family meeting to decide how to share tasks. Delegate responsibilities so that one family member is not doing it all. You can also charge long-distance family members with doable responsibilities they can achieve without increased stress. See Exhibit 20-3 for some examples.

You can encourage the long-distance care providers to make good use of their time when they visit their parent. They should make an appointment with the elder's physician during their visit and establish a relationship with the doctor, if they do not have one already. On a visit to the older family member, they should also meet with an elder-law attorney to discuss estate planning and ensure there is a durable power of attorney, POLST (Physician's Orders for Life Sustaining Treatment) form, living will, and all appropriate legal documents in place.

Exhibit 20–2   Assisting Long-Distance Family Members

- Arrange regular visits from religious groups if appropriate.
- Telephone or e-mail or send a monthly report to long-distance family.
- Arrange services from the community such as meals on wheels.
- Accompany older person to all medical appointments.
- Monitor neighbors or friends or anyone who might take advantage of the older person, carry out any sweetheart scams, or exert an undue influence.

Creating a caregiver binder: If the long-distance family members want to manage the care and monitoring of the older person, suggest they make a binder containing information about the older family member, much like the client data book that you may have on each client in your GCM office.

Suggest including the following sections in the binder:

- Emergency contacts: Make a list of all the person's emergency contacts—telephone numbers, e-mail addresses, addresses—such as for neighbors, friends, and family members.
- Physician information: Complete information including name, address, telephone number, e-mail address, and specialty of older person's physicians.
- Pharmacy information: List the name of pharmacy, address, telephone number, exact meds, dosage, over-the-counter medications, vitamins.
- Religious information: List the person's clergy contacts if he or she has religious or spiritual connections.
- Local support agency information: List local agencies involved in the person's care, including names and contact info, such as meals on wheels or home care agency.
- Neighbor information: List the neighbor's name, address, phone number, and e-mail address.
- Friend information: List information on any old family friends in the area, including name, address, phone number, and e-mail address.
- Emergency plan for household

CASE STUDY

A working daughter became concerned because her mother, who lives across the country, began phoning her frequently through the day and night, sometimes up to 15 times per day. The daughter suggested that her mother come live with her or find a companion, but the mother refused to discuss the subject. The worried daughter contacted the employee assistance division of her company and was given the name of a GCM in her city as well as the names of several GCMs in her mother's town.

The daughter first contacted the GCM in her own city. That GCM gave the daughter information about the nature, depth, and scope of geriatric care management services. The GCM also provided the daughter with a guideline statement called *How to Find a Qualified Geriatric Care Manager* (see Appendix 20–A).

Shortly thereafter, the daughter flew out to see her mother. She had made appointments to interview four GCMs using the guidelines she had been given. She met with each GCM at her mother's residence, introducing the GCM to her mother as someone who specialized in helping older people live as independently as possible.

The daughter hired the GCM who responded to the guideline questions

Exhibit 20–3   Long-Distance Care Provider Tasks

- Take home a copy of the yellow pages from the area where the parent lives for reference.
- Find all legal documents, take them home, and put them in a binder. (If these include original signed documents, scan into a computer document, make copies, and put originals in a safe deposit box or safe place.) Key legal and financial documents might include the following:

  - Legal documents
  - Birth certificate
  - Social security card
  - Divorce decree
  - Will

- Set up a filing system (paper and/or electronic) at the long-distance caregiver's home for the older person and include all pertinent documents involving the older person.
- Have all mail forwarded to one of the long-distance caregiver's addresses and manage mail for the older person.
- Set up online chat room, Skype, or conference call where family members can discuss the older person's issues.
- Manage round-robin letter if family members choose that form of communication.
- Be a relief care provider—stay with the older person on a regular basis (once a month, once every 6 months)—to give the primary caregiver respite.
- Invite care receiver to your home for visit or respite.
- Gather all insurance information, and take it to a financial planner or SHIP program to make sure policies are current and appropriate:

  - Auto
  - Homeowners
  - Medicare
  - Medicaid
  - Medigap
  - Long-term care
  - Disability

most thoughtfully and competently and to whom her mother responded most favorably. This GCM was also the most proactive. For instance, the hired GCM was the only one who asked the mother what she thought she needed to make her life better. The mother was able to state that she would like to have someone live in her spare bedroom. The GCM assessed the mother and her home and made recommendations for household adaptations such as a railing, improved lighting, and an address that was clearly marked outside the house. Additionally, the GCM recruited a caregiver who was sensitive to the mother's habit of calling her daughter.

The incessant calls to the daughter gradually ceased as the mother became comfortable with her new caregiver. The GCM visited the mother on a regular basis, offering activity suggestions to the companion. For instance, the mother was very fond of dogs. Per the GCM's suggestion, the mother and her companion visited the local dog park, borrowed books from the library on dogs, and subscribed to a dog magazine. The

GCM was even able to arrange visits on a regular basis from a GCM assistant with a calm and responsive dog.

Other tasks provided by the GCM to this long-distance family on a direct and indirect basis included the following:

- Phoning the daughter regularly to provide status reports and to respond to the daughter's ongoing concerns about her mother
- Arranging for weekend relief help and other relief help when the regular caregiver needed time off
- Making appointments to meet with medical specialists, dentists, podiatrists, optometrists, and psychiatrists as needed
- Replacing a broken washing machine and a torn window dressing
- Locating a bill-paying service
- Locating an audiologist and reputable hearing aid specialist
- Arranging for plumbing and gardening services
- Arranging for volunteers to call regularly and arrange for intervention should any health or home care situation warrant follow-up
- Arranging for the installation of new technological home monitoring system that help older people age in place safely (see Chapter 11, Assessing and Supporting Aging in Place Through Technology)
- Arranging for an emergency response system to allow an older person who falls and is injured to push a button, leading an automatic dialer to contact a central system that can then contact the person or responsible parties

Some public utilities and the US Postal Service offer gatekeeper and home observation programs in which service people who visit the home regularly are trained to notice anything unusual or any indication of need and report it, so someone may investigate and take action.

It is not uncommon for a GCM to contact a GCM in another town (where either the out-of-town relative or the older person lives) to coordinate efforts or to provide background information (with the permission of all parties), so the other GCM can provide services.

■ HELPING ADULT CHILDREN AND FAMILIES MANAGE THE OVERWHELMING DEMANDS OF CAREGIVING

Middle-aged people, usually women, who are balancing family, work, and caregiving responsibilities, are likely to report feeling stressed, frustrated, and sometimes even angry. Because they often care for children and parents simultaneously, these adult children have sometimes been referred to as the sandwich generation. They feel squeezed between the needs of so many people that they are vulnerable to anxiety, depression, and weakened immune responses. Caregiving can also stress even the happiest of marriages.

GCMs are able to help with practical suggestions regarding placement, referrals, and medical needs as well as some very specific recommendations that can assist caregivers in reducing their stress. For instance, GCMs may recommend that caregivers join support groups or otherwise alleviate caregiver overload.

Support Groups

Support groups can be of help if the participants are focused on a particular problem. The following is one family's experience with a support group.

CASE STUDY

Mrs. R's husband was away on business when he suffered a debilitating stroke. Until this time, the Rs were actively enjoying their golden years. Mr. R's stroke rendered him unable to speak. He could still manage most of his daily living activities and attended speech therapy three times per week at a local rehabilitation center. However, his inability to communicate placed a tremendous burden on Mrs. R, who continued to work outside the home.

Mr. R continued to be as good-natured as ever, but Mrs. R was exhausted from worry and on the verge of mental collapse. The hospital social worker recognized the wife's fragile mental state and referred her to a private GCM. The GCM met with the wife in the hospital and, after recognizing her overwhelming situation, recommended that she join a support group for spouses of stroke victims. Mrs. R reluctantly joined the group and was immediately relieved to know that there were others who shared her experience. Through the support group, she made new friends and learned about new resources to help her.

In addition to the sense of camaraderie found in support groups, there is a cathartic effect that frequently takes place because it is only in a milieu of peers that some people can share their feelings. Support groups have been developed for various kinds of geriatric issues. There are support groups for spouses, adult children, those who have family members with an Alzheimer's diagnosis, those who have a diagnosis of early Alzheimer's, dementia, stroke, diabetes, Parkinson's, ALS, and others. Support groups are frequently organized through nonprofit entities such as family service agencies (e.g., Jewish Family Services,

Catholic Family Services) or the Family Service Association. Long-term care facilities also frequently offer support groups to the community at large. The local Area Agency on Aging, county department on aging, and senior centers offer support groups directly or can recommend support groups. Academic institutions, especially universities with medical and gerontological programs, offer support services. The Alzheimer's Association and Family Caregiver Alliance are also excellent sources for group support. You should develop a list of these support groups for use in practice.

Alleviating Caregiver Overload

Because many adult children take the I-can-do-it-all approach, they frequently become overwhelmed with unrealistic caregiving expectations. GCMs are in a position to point out the need to make compromises and assist adult caregivers with adjusting their expectations of the care receivers' deteriorating ability to function when they are distressed over the burden of caregiving. One helpful approach is to assist caregiving family members in setting limits on their time and energy; to assist them in knowing to what extent they are able to be directly involved and when they can rely on hired help or services to ease the burden of caregiving.

Even after family members set limits on their time, they may tend to push these limits. If this occurs, family members need to be encouraged to look at why they are uncomfortable with the limits they have established. Family members may be advised to be alert for signals that they have overextended themselves. Exhibit 20–5 lists signs of caregiver overload. Exhibit 20–6 suggests some strategies that a GCM can suggest to family caregivers experiencing caregiver overload.

Frequently, family members will express a sense of relief that they have found a GCM, someone on whom they can call to help with problem solving and to listen to frustrations.

Exhibit 20–4   Checklist of Brain Impairment Problems

Please check one box for each problem, indicating how often these problems have occurred *in the past week.*

Problem	Very Often	Somewhat Often	Never	Comments
1. Asking the same question over and over	❑	❑	❑	_____
2. Having trouble remembering recent events (e.g., items in the newspaper or on TV)	❑	❑	❑	_____
3. Having trouble remembering significant past events	❑	❑	❑	_____
4. Losing or misplacing things	❑	❑	❑	_____
5. Forgetting what day it is	❑	❑	❑	_____
6. Starting but not finishing things	❑	❑	❑	_____
7. Having difficulty concentrating on a task	❑	❑	❑	_____
8. Destroying property	❑	❑	❑	_____
9. Doing embarrassing things	❑	❑	❑	_____
10. Waking up others at night	❑	❑	❑	_____
11. Talking loudly and rapidly	❑	❑	❑	_____
12. Appearing anxious or worried	❑	❑	❑	_____
13. Engaging in behavior that is potentially dangerous to him- or herself or others	❑	❑	❑	_____
14. Threatening to hurt him- or herself	❑	❑	❑	_____
15. Threatening to hurt others	❑	❑	❑	_____
16. Being verbally aggressive toward others	❑	❑	❑	_____
17. Appearing sad or depressed	❑	❑	❑	_____
18. Expressing feelings of hopelessness or sadness about the future (e.g., "Nothing worthwhile ever happens," "I never do anything right")	❑	❑	❑	_____
19. Crying and being tearful	❑	❑	❑	_____
20. Commenting about the death of him- or herself or others (e.g., "Life isn't worth living," "I'd be better off dead")	❑	❑	❑	_____
21. Talking about being lonely	❑	❑	❑	_____
22. Commenting about feeling worthless or being a burden to others	❑	❑	❑	_____
23. Commenting about feeling like a failure or about nor having worthwhile accomplishments in life	❑	❑	❑	_____
24. Arguing, being irritable, and complaining	❑	❑	❑	_____
25. Being unable to communicate	❑	❑	❑	_____

Source: Reprinted with permission from L. Teri et al., Assessment of Behavioral Problems in Dementia: The Revised Memory and Behavior Problems Checklist, *Psychology and Aging,* Vol. 7, pp. 622–631, © 1992, Linda Teri, Ph.D.

Exhibit 20–5   Signs of Caregiver Overload

- Sleep disorder—Depression, overexertion, and nighttime caregiving may prevent caregivers from getting adequate sleep.
- Marital problems—Marriages can be strained because of caregiving responsibilities.
- Reduced employment—Caregiving demands may force family members to curtail their hours or quit a job, adding financial stress.
- Social withdrawal—Family caregivers may become lonely, lamenting diminished contacts with friends and fewer social activities.
- Depression—Caring for a physically or cognitively impaired individual may leave the caregiver feeling helpless and hopeless.
- Guilt—Caregivers may begin to wish the care recipient was the way he or she used to be or that someone else would take some of the responsibility. They may feel guilty about having these thoughts.
- Anxiety—Family caregivers may begin to feel edgy or nervous. Regardless of their efforts, they may have a sense of falling behind.
- Physical problems—Increased physical and emotional stress may decrease the caregiver's resistance to sickness. Family caregivers may complain about frequent colds, headaches, or backaches.
- Fatigue—Caregiving is physically and emotionally hard work and may lead to exhaustion.

Exhibit 20–6   Strategies for Solving Caregiver Overload

Following are some strategies that a GCM can suggest to family caregivers experiencing caregiver overload:

- The GCM can help family members to begin setting realistic expectations of themselves as caregivers.
- The GCM can encourage family members to explain to employers that flexible scheduling at certain times may be needed to help parents keep physicians' appointments. The GCM can also offer suggestions for making up the work. If comprehensive caregiving is required, the GCM can suggest that the Family Leave Act may be used.
- The GCM can encourage caregivers to talk with other family members about feelings and ask family members for their suggestions. Caregivers can ask children what they need (e.g., help with homework, a special shopping trip) and ask for their help in making it happen. Caregivers can also try to include children in caregiving responsibilities by asking them to run errands, fix a meal, or simply sit and visit with the older person.
- The GCM can encourage caregivers to plan some time for spouses, explaining personal stressors and asking the spouse to share personal stressors as well. Spouses can work together to make some changes in the partnership that will help accommodate the caregiving responsibilities.
- The GCM can encourage caregivers to seek out and use community resources. Most people are surprised at the wealth of community resources that are available at no cost. Public libraries, Area Agencies on Aging, and local senior centers have information about community resources.
- Most important, the GCM can encourage family caregivers to make time for themselves. Unless caregivers stay physically and mentally healthy, they will not be any good to themselves or others.

GCMs can also use an assessment tool to measure caregiver burnout. (See Chapter 3 on psychosocial assessment.) Exhibit 20-7 is the Zarit Burden Interview that can be used to assess a caregiver's response to caregiving.

Family Support Assessment

It is a good idea to suggest to a family, whether long-distance or local, that they sit down with the older family member and complete a family support assessment (see Exhibit 20-8). This assessment should be completed in a relaxed family meeting at the parental home. What you are really encouraging is that the family plan for incapacity, and ask the older person how he or she wishes the family to help should the person's health decline. This type of assessment and planning helps everyone have a map

Exhibit 20-7   The Zarit Burden Interview

Do you feel:

1. That your relative asks for more help than he/she needs?*
2. That because of the time you spend with your relative you don't have enough time for yourself?
3. Stressed between caring for your relative and trying to meet other responsibilities for your family or work?
4. Embarrassed over your relative's behavior?
5. Angry when you are around your relative?
6. That your relative currently affects your relationship with other family members in a negative way?
7. Afraid of what the future holds for your relative?
8. Your relative is dependent on you?
9. Strained when you are around your relative?
10. Your health has suffered because of your involvement with your relative?
11. That you don't have as much privacy as you would like because of your relative?
12. That your social life has suffered because you are caring for your relative?
13. Uncomfortable having friends over because of your relative?
14. That your relative seems to expect you to take care of him/her as if you were the only one he/she could depend on?
15. That you don't have enough money to care for your relative in addition to the rest of your expenses?
16. That you will be unable to take care of your relative much longer?
17. You have lost control of your life since your relative's illness?
18. You wish you could just leave the care of your relative to someone else?
19. Uncertain about what to do about your relative?
20. You should be doing something more for your relative?
21. You could be doing a better job in caring for your relative?

Overall, how burdened do you feel in caring for your relative (not at all, a little, moderately, quite a bit, extremely)?

* Items 1–21 are measured as never, rarely, sometimes, quite frequently, nearly always.

Source: Reprinted with permission by Steven H. Zarit.

Exhibit 20–8   Family Support Assessment

- Which child do you want to be your main caretaker? Why?
- How can your children divide tasks so they can meet your needs?
- Will nieces and nephews be a part of care supports?
- Will friends or people in the community be a part of your web? If so, who?
- Will a rabbi, minister, or spiritual leader be part of your support system? If so, who?
- If children live a long distance away, how can they contribute to your future care needs?

to follow as the parent ages. Family members will know which child will be the lead care provider and which other members of the family or community will have a role in the supportive and caregiving tasks.

Family Meetings

A family meeting is a meeting held with family members to discuss a problem, large or small, involving an older relative. These gatherings are often led by an outside party who can remain objective and keep attendees on track.

Reasons to Hold a Family Meeting

There are many reasons you may suggest holding a family meeting. If families are having difficulty sharing tasks, a family meeting is an opportunity for you to coach family members to divide tasks and delegate responsibilities so no one person is doing it all.

Family meetings are an excellent way to help families plan for the older person's disabilities, manage incapacity, or solve a crisis involving the older person, including decisions such as whether a person be put on life support or move out of his or her home of many years because upkeep is a problem. Family meetings are a great way to do general problem solving with a family. It is inevitable that when you arrange a family meeting in which hard decisions must be made that adult children will revert back to their childhood personas and dredge up old hurts and

angers while trying to solve here-and-now problems. Many families are dysfunctional in some way. These family systems may be the most challenging you deal with. (See Chapter 21, Difficult Families: Conflict, Dependence, and Mutuality.)

Who Should Moderate a Family Meeting?

You can moderate the meeting if you are a seasoned GCM and have skills and experience as a mediator. Five years of experience as a GCM is a good benchmark to assess whether you can mediate a family meeting. If you do not have this experience, find a licensed clinical social worker, licensed marriage and family therapist with a background in aging, or a mediator with experience in aging. Family meetings can be a brutal tug-of-war.

Setting Up a Family Meeting

If the family agrees to hold a family meeting, you and the moderator can plan the family meeting. Plan an agenda for a successful meeting. Before the meeting, ask all family members, especially long-distance members, to list their concerns and the tasks they are willing to do and to mail or e-mail this list to you. Integrate these concerns and agreements into your agenda, and hold the meeting at a neutral site. See a suggested list of family meeting agenda items in Exhibit 20–9 and pick items from the list that work for the agenda of any family meeting you set up for a care provider, or add others you may need.

Exhibit 20–9 Agenda Items for a Family Meeting

❑ Divide up tasks if one family member is doing caregiving directly.
❑ Break caregiving into manageable tasks. For example:
  ❑ Long-distance son pays for caregiving.
  ❑ Out-of-town daughter gets all mail, pays bills; teenage son sorts it for her.
  ❑ Local niece visits aunt on a regular basis; grandchildren send cards weekly.
❑ Coach adult children to ask for flexible hours at work.
❑ Help adult children who provide direct care to plan time alone with spouses.
❑ Encourage adult children caregivers to make time for themselves.
❑ Encourage adult children caregivers to go to support group.
❑ Help adult children members set realistic expectations.
❑ Decide who will check into all legal documents.
❑ Coach family members to share tasks.
❑ Delegate responsibilities so no one person is doing it all.
❑ Help adult children set realistic expectations.
❑ Decide who will be in charge of house repairs.
❑ Decide who will pay bills.
❑ Decide who will take parent to doctor's appointments if not the GCM.
❑ Arrange a schedule for all family members to call older person regularly.
❑ Decide who will be in charge of arranging for care.

❑ Decide which family member will respond to emergencies.
❑ Decide which family member will be main spokesperson to GCM.
❑ Arrange for long-distance family regularly to send cards, videotapes of family.
❑ Decide who will introduce new care providers to older adult.
❑ Decide who will contact all new possible services in continuum of care.
❑ Decide who will sign contracts for services.
❑ Decide who will have right to approve expenses and budget.
❑ Decide to whom all mail will be forwarded and who will manage mail.
❑ Decide who will set up an online chat room so all family members can communicate and share information.
❑ Decide who will manage round-robin letter if family chooses that form of communication.
❑ Arrange for family members to be relief care provider—stay with parent on some regular basis to give primary caregiver respite.
❑ Arrange for family members to have care receiver stay at their home for visit/respite on regular basis, if appropriate.
❑ Moderate and discuss problems with siblings not doing their share.
❑ Help siblings appreciate each other.
❑ Coordinate all family members writing regular notes to primary caregiver saying how much they appreciate what the person is doing and how hard it is.

During the Family Meeting

During the meeting, be certain everyone has an opportunity to express feelings, voice preferences, and offer suggestions. Focus on the positive. Identify something each person can do. Recognize each person's limitations (e.g., medical illness, long distance). Create a feeling of trust and support. Keep the meeting on current concerns rather than past conflicts (e.g., "Dad paid for college for you but not for me!"). Address the needs from each family member's point of view (usually siblings). Be certain everyone has an opportunity to participate.

Although the reason for the meeting may be to solve one major crisis or problem, it is a good idea to integrate many of the items listed in Exhibit 20–9 into the meeting, if they haven't already been addressed.

After the Meeting

In a family meeting, you or a moderator can help the family strike a balance. Following the family meeting, draw up the plan that was decided in the meeting of what each family member will do and when each person will do it. Send the plan to all family members for them to sign off on.

Improving Family Communication

Setting limits or boundaries is important in all clinical settings. It may be necessary to set limits with the family, when you work with them. Some family members may want to engage you in their arguments or may want you to share information that you are not comfortable sharing. In these instances, you can model ways of showing concern without rejecting family members, while also being sensitive to boundaries.

What should you do when you find yourself trapped in a mistake, such as getting involved in a family's argument? One approach might be to say, "You know, I realize that I have been trying to change your mind on something that you have some definite feelings about. Could you excuse me for this and explain the situation to me once more?" Another approach might be, "Although I didn't mean to, I think I've been arguing with you, instead of listening to you. Could you help me out by explaining it to me again, while I pay closer attention?"

Families who are having difficulties working as a cohesive system may benefit from guidance from a GCM. Family caregivers can be helped to recognize and prioritize their problems so they can become empowered to develop their own solutions.

Some things for you to consider are how the family seems to be functioning. What is the family caregiver's own attitude toward aging and an older person's particular illness (e.g., Alzheimer's disease)? If the caregiver has the attitude that older people are supposed to

become demented, then the older person's behavior will not be seen as a problem that requires consideration. What motivates the family to care? If a caregiver has a full load with a job, marriage, and children, he or she may not be looking for additional stress and deny the problem. How does the family work? Do the family members address problems together, or do problems split them apart? Is there domination from a single family member? Are abuse and threats, implied or real, used to control others? What is valued by the family? Will the family be receptive to suggestions?

If the family is receptive to suggestions, you can help improve how a family communicates by modeling the following communication techniques:

- Do not interrupt family members until they have finished speaking.
- Show each member that he or she has value in the family.
- Show each member that his or her views are valid.
- Acknowledge to each member that his or her experience of a situation is valid.
- Encourage family members to work together to make the load easier for all to bear.
- Realize that family members will make mistakes and that mistakes are acceptable as long as the family members learn from them.
- Remind family members that it is acceptable for one member to express that he or she has reached their limit of time, emotion, or stress.
- Encourage family members to ask each other for help.
- Allow family members to decide whether they can be helpful.

Helping Families Develop Solutions for Their Needs

Professionals should look beyond actual medical care and understand the caregiving dynamic of an older person's family to help ensure that both the older person and the caregivers have an adequate support system. Two older people can have exactly the same needs, but two caregivers will perceive the degree of burden very differently.

The following strategies can help the GCM assess the needs of family caregivers and counsel them to develop appropriate solutions for their individual needs.

Dealing with a Caregiver's Denial

Denial is a common defense mechanism, especially when an individual is under stress. To deny or ignore a problem allows the individual time to temporarily adjust to the idea of the problem or may serve to permanently keep the troubled thought or problem out of conscious awareness. Caregivers wait an average of 3 years from the onset of symptoms of Alzheimer's disease or vascular dementia before bringing an older person to be evaluated, usually following a dramatic event, such as setting the stove on fire. Caregivers in denial are restless and inattentive. Their ability to process information may be impaired. They may be exhausted from trying to control a situation and resisting the intrusion of the reality of the loss. They may report that they do not have time to exercise, or they may overeat. The coping strategies are not to think, not to feel, and not to do. Professionals need to repeat information, perhaps over a period of a year or more, until they know caregivers are assimilating it.

Dealing with a Caregiver's Emotions

Caregivers frequently attempt to control their emotions, particularly anger and anxiety, so they are not overwhelmed by them. That anger surfaces when an adult daughter looks at a mother who is falling apart physically and sees herself or when she looks at someone she has never really liked very much, such as an alcoholic and abusive father, and realizes she has to care for him or her. What motivates the caregiver may not be love but rather a sense of responsibility, ethics, and morality. Caregivers facing such predicaments struggle with a complex array of emotions. There may be a desire to be absolved from responsibility, but the family caregiver feels bound to the parent because he or she is a dutiful daughter or son and has a sense of filial responsibility. You can help with this by sorting out the emotions, clarifying feelings, and finding support for those feelings, including psychotherapy.

Helping Caregivers Build a Partnership

You can encourage caregivers to talk with older relatives without being controlling. Caregivers can work with the older person to develop a list of questions before a physician's appointment, for example, rather than monopolizing the discussion with the physician during the appointment. Partnerships are difficult to achieve when individuals have not always had a caring, loving relationship. When older people are not cooperative, caregivers can be accepting without attacking the person or becoming hostile. Family caregivers must be helped to recognize that they cannot always be the most effective change agents. Perhaps someone else within the family system can be the catalyst.

You can work with the family physician, neighbors, or clergy, who may be able to get the older person to see the world differently. The following story illustrates how a GCM can help a family build a partnership.

CASE STUDY

Mrs. D was always, according to her four children, a controlling mother. As a result, all of her children became successful professionals in their fields; Mrs. D would not have it any other way. However, when Mrs. D turned 87, she suffered a series of strokes that would have incapacitated most individuals. Mrs. D's determination overrode her frailty. Her adult children, with the help of her physician, who they believed was one of the few people in her life for whom she had high regard, finally convinced her to stop driving. Her life at home was quite marginal because it could not be adapted to meet all of her disabilities, which included losses in vision, hearing, and mobility. Her children were convinced that the only solution was for her to move to a care facility, but Mrs. D refused to discuss it. The GCM helped Mrs. D's children form a partnership with her physician, who fully agreed with her children that it was not safe for her to be in her home. Throughout several months of medical visits, Mrs. D's physician would bring up the subject of relocation, Mrs. D would agree to consider it, and the discussion progressed at each medical visit. When Mrs. D asked her physician where he thought she should move, he suggested her children be included in the discussion of relocation. Mrs. D finally agreed to make the move, especially because she convinced her physician to make her his only home-visit patient.

Building Partnerships with Professionals

GCMs work as part of a professional team. GCMs can offer a full-service package to their client families by developing alliances with allied professionals such as elder-law attorneys, certified public accountants, conservators, fiduciaries, trust officers, nurses, and geriatric psychiatrists and psychologists. This team approach is advantageous for several reasons: it streamlines the services offered to older clients, ensuring continuity of care; it makes for a more efficient delivery-of-services pathway; and it avoids duplication of services.

You can be at the fulcrum of the service matrix by recommending the types of services and the extent of service required, based on an initial evaluation of the client and adjusting the recommended services as the client's needs change. The following case study shows how a GCM can use his or her professional partnerships to the advantage of the client.

CASE STUDY

The chronically ill single son of an older client contacted a GCM to assist with concerns he had for his mother, Mrs. H. Mrs. H was living alone and seemed to the son to be losing weight, forgetting medical appointments, and unable to keep track of bills that needed to be paid. Mrs. H had several falls but no resulting injuries. The son stated that his mother had always been a private and self-sufficient woman, and this new behavior was very much out of character. He had had a recent medical emergency and was concerned about who could look after his mother in the event he was unable to do so. He said his mother had not yet drawn up a will.

The GCM arranged to meet with the son and his mother at the mother's residence the following week. The GCM wanted to assess Mrs. H in her home. During the course of this first meeting, the GCM was sensitive to Mrs. H's need for privacy and independence and yet was able to establish enough rapport with her that Mrs. H confessed to the GCM that she was worried about herself. She was aware that she wasn't managing as well as she once had. The GCM used this time as an opportunity to ask the mother if she was at all concerned about her memory. "Oh, yes, indeed," she replied. "I know my memory isn't what it once was because I can no longer do my New York Times crossword puzzles." The

GCM asked Mrs. H whether she would like to know how her memory was, that perhaps it was not as poor as she thought. The GCM explained that she could administer a short memory quiz and they could determine in just a few minutes whether there should be further concern about her memory. The GCM used the Short Portable Mental Status Questionnaire. The GCM administered a 10-question mental status evaluation. Mrs. H missed 3 out of 10, scoring within normal limits. She missed the questions related to the presidents and the math calculation. The GCM also noted that the home was quite cluttered and dusty. As a result of the first meeting with Mrs. H, the GCM identified several areas where Mrs. H's quality of life could be improved. With her son's and Mrs. H's approval, the GCM would proceed with the following suggestions:

- Although Mrs. H's memory showed only mild impairment, the GCM recommended that she see a neurologist for further testing to rule out any treatable conditions such as thyroid disorder, diabetes, dementia, or depression. The GCM offered to be available for these appointments.
- The GCM recommended having a home attendant to see that Mrs. H's house was cleaned up and to keep track of medical appointments. The GCM would recruit an attendant through the best home care agency. She would provide instructions to the attendant, introduce the attendant to Mrs. H and her son, supervise the attendant, and follow up with any necessary adjustment in the care provided.
- For some appointments, the GCM would individually make sure that Mrs. H got to the appointment, accompanying her on occasion if there was important information that should be relayed to the physician. On other occasions, the son would transport his mother for routine appointments, such as dental exams, or the attendant would accompany Mrs. H using public paratransit or transportation for the disabled.
- The GCM recommended a physical therapy evaluation to determine the reason for the recent falls.
- The GCM recommended finding a bank trust officer to handle the estate in the event Mrs. H's son was not able to manage his mother's financial affairs at a later date.
- The GCM recommended having an elder-law attorney draw up a current will and help Mrs. H identify an individual who could act as a surrogate executor in the event her son was incapacitated.
- The GCM would make regular visits to Mrs. H, address any new needs that arise, and make referrals and adjustments as required.
- The GCM would be in regular contact with the son, apprising him of the results of her efforts, and noting any change in his mother's condition. Likewise, the son would advise the GCM of any progression or other changes in his mother's symptoms.

As the preceding example illustrates, the GCM can be at the fulcrum of the service matrix, recommending the types of services and the extent of service required based on an initial evaluation of the client and adjusting the recommended services as the client's needs change.

Helping Caregivers Diffuse Conflict

The GCM can help caregivers manage conflict. Creative resolutions emerge out of conflict. Caregivers can be made aware of their conflict management skills and deficits. They must learn to think before they talk or act. Instead of escalating conflict, they can practice deflecting the negative emotions that stir conflict. Family caregivers can be reminded that an aging person with dementia may not be aware of what he or she says to a caregiver. The following story illustrates how a GCM helped a caregiver diffuse conflict.

CASE STUDY

A demented woman with a history of psychiatric disturbance was very hostile to her daughter-in-law and criticized how she dressed, prepared meals, and kept the house. The adult son and wife came to the GCM for assistance regarding managing the mother. They also disclosed during the course of the assessment that their marriage was under considerable strain because of the husband's mother's interference and criticism. The GCM was able to help the daughter-in-law deflect the criticism by framing it in the context of her mother-in-law's history of mental difficulties. The son was able to set limits with his mother. The daughter-in-law was gradually able to disregard the criticism and tolerate her mother-in-law to a greater extent.

Helping Caregivers Establish Good Communications

Some families work well together and develop a kind of partnership, where each member

assumes a certain role. Other families do not want to work together at all. If two siblings were not a close part of each others' early life, it is understandable that they may not care to work together to help with the care of an aging parent. For example, a 45-year-old son relocated from Delaware to assist his mother in Oregon, who was becoming increasingly withdrawn, depressed, and confused. He contacted a GCM, who assessed the mother, found psychiatric assistance for her, and offered support to the son, who was a recovering alcoholic and substance abuser. The son had not abused alcohol or drugs for 10 years. The mother had another son who lived in California, but this son expressed resentment toward his mother and chose not to become involved in her care. However, when the brother in Oregon assisted his mother with her financial and estate planning, the brother in California was outraged and asserted that his brother could not be trusted with their mother's estate matters due to his former alcohol and drug habits. The brother in California could not bring himself to become constructively engaged in his mother's care. Blaming his brother for his history seemed to be the only way he could remain involved, albeit negatively. The GCM worked with the brothers to help build trust and establish a working alliance where the division of labor was comfortably defined. For example, the brother in California managed the finances for their mother, while the brother in Oregon took care of her instrumental activities of daily living, such as transportation to medical appointments and meal shopping and preparation. The brothers did not develop a close relationship but were able to work together for the benefit of their mother.

Encouraging Families to Communicate Their Needs

The GCM should assess the caregiving situation from the perspective of each family member. Solicit opinions from each family member, from youngest to oldest. Tasks should be identified and plans formulated. Caregivers can become overwhelmed when there is one problem after another. Breaking caregiving into manageable tasks is important. For instance, can spouses or teens in the family help with errands or phone calls? Can out-of-area siblings offer monetary support? The following story illustrates how a GCM encouraged one family's members to communicate their needs.

CASE STUDY

One son and two daughters were concerned about their widowed mother, who was becoming increasingly forgetful. The mother had remained in the home where she had raised her family. One local daughter lived close enough to check in on her mother, do grocery shopping, and stand by when the mother took a bath, but this daughter was facing surgery and had a chronically ill husband. The other two adult children lived out of town.

The adult children came to see the GCM for guidance. The local daughter was inclined to have her mother placed in a local assisted living facility. However, the other two siblings did not like the idea. The mother was willing to be placed in a facility to relieve her daughter of "the burden of my care."

The GCM helped the family organize a system that would help the mother remain at home and not overburden the local daughter. The GCM helped the family caregivers strike a balance by making several suggestions for manageable tasks the adult children could handle:

- The GCM was told that the son was financially solvent. She therefore suggested that the son finance home care so that the main work

and personal care would be done by attendants. The son agreed.
- The daughter who lived out of state arranged to have her mother's mail sent to her address and engaged her teenage son to sort the mail. Bills to be paid were forwarded to the brother. The daughter maintained close contact with her mother and attendants and ordered groceries and household items on the Internet, arranging for their delivery to her mother's home.
- The local daughter was able to visit her mother when she felt up to the task. Her visits were primarily social. The older mother was most pleased with this new arrangement and lived in her home until she died 2 years later.

Helping Caregivers Strike a Balance

Juggling the demands of an aging parent, a spouse, children, and a job is at the heart of the caregiving dilemma. Professionals are in a position to provide caregivers with models of balance. What is a well-balanced caregiver? According to Donna Cohen, PhD, director of the Institute on Aging at the University of South Florida in Tampa, and Carl Eisdorfer, "It's someone who knows herself; what she can and cannot do. She's aware of the impact she has on others, can accept weakness in herself and others, and can identify strengths in others."[2(p130)] A happy caregiver can live with imperfections in him- or herself, his or her home, and his or her loved ones.

One of the single greatest challenges of caregiving is resisting doing everything. It is preferable to be a coach and delegate responsibility; professionals and caregivers alike can benefit from this advice. GCMs can assist family caregivers in striking a balance between doing it all and feeling guilty that they are not doing enough. Most family members are receptive to suggestions that they consider other individuals and service providers who can lighten their burden. For example, a GCM who is working with a caregiver who has siblings in other states can suggest a family meeting or conference call where each adult child and possibly older grandchild is able to offer a way to lighten the load of the local family caregiver. Some family members might offer to come into town to stay with the older parent on a scheduled basis to give respite to the local family caregiver. Other family members may be in a position to send financial support to hire help at the parent's home. Older grandchildren may be able to provide visits or household help themselves. Some older people are stable enough to split their residence, living part of the year with one relative and then returning to live with another relative. This option is feasible only if the older person likes the arrangement and is well enough to do so. Caregivers might consult with a family physician if a change of residence is being considered.

Helping Families Divide Up Family Treasures

Sometimes one of the most wrenching things a family of an aging parent does is to divide up family treasures. *Nontitled property* is a term that refers to personal items that do not have a legal document (such as a title or deed) to indicate who officially owns the item. These personal possessions may have monetary worth, or they may be cherished primarily for their sentimental value. Nontitled property can include such items as the following:

- Furniture
- Dishes
- Pets
- Collections
- Sporting equipment
- Photographs

- Books
- Family documents
- Linens and needlework
- Musical instruments
- Guns
- Jewelry
- Tools
- Toys

Resolving who in the family gets personal belongings, the nontitled property, is often more lacerating than determining the division of titled property or financial wealth. Dividing nontitled property can cause friction between siblings that can fast-forward through their lifetime. Many times, this is brought about by old wounds from childhood ("You are the baby, and you always got what you wanted, like you are doing with Mom's good doll collection.").

Aging parents have personal belongings such as a father's 49ers shirt collection, a mother's salt and pepper shaker collection, or the old cracked plate set that sat on the ledge in the kitchen and reminded everyone of how great it was to have breakfast together. Family items contain meaning to family members beyond money. Going through all these articles and distributing them when a father moves or a mother or father dies happens to everyone. This transfer of family treasures affects aging families regardless of income level or cultural background.

Possessions can be divided at many stages in an older person's life. The underlying value of a parent's possessions in many cases is the memories they hold. Counsel families to talk about how possessions are to be divided before anything is given to anyone. It is critical to check a parent's will and have an attorney review the will or trust before anything is divided.

Splitting up possessions when a loved one dies can lead to bitter words: "You took Dad's stamp collection, and it's just like when we were kids and Dad favored you because you have his eyes." There are ways to gracefully divide family items loaded with sentiment. Every family has horror tales about how the goodies were divided when a grandparent moved to a nursing home or when a parent died.

In one family, Grandma's engagement ring was passed on to her daughter, then to her granddaughter. When a grandson and his fiancé walked into a room full of his relatives, three aunts stared at the fiancé's ring finger and cackled miserably to the engaged woman, "How did you get Mom's engagement ring?"

In another family, five granddaughters couldn't decide who should get the grandmother's set of valuable sterling silver. Eventually, it was agreed it would be shared: each woman would have it for a year, then pass it along to another. However, there was so much stalling on passing the silver to the next sister, after 5 years, they had a family meeting and decided to hold a drawing to determine permanent ownership.

Who gets personal property is frequently ignored until a crisis occurs, like the death of a parent or a parent moving. At the zero hour, when family members are grieving, selling the home they grew up in, or facing the increased dependence of an elder, adult children can have a hard time making fair or equitable decisions.

Few families have planned ahead enough to decide who should get what personal belongings. If there is no will or no separate listing identifying the wishes of the property owner, family members are sometimes left with a fractious relationship and only old hurt feelings to guide them in dividing an elder parent's personal possessions.

When they must divide family treasures, you can suggest families use a great tool called "Who Gets Grandma's Yellow Pie Plate?" (see www.yellowpieplate.umn.edu) developed by the University of Minnesota.* It is a format to help families divide up nontitled property and to help them take time to make the process worthwhile. It helps the families tell stories, listen to both each other and the stories, and remember the past. It is designed to make dividing assets a positive experience. The University of Minnesota researchers who developed "Grandma's Yellow Pie Plate" have identified five factors that adult children should consider as they plan to transfer the property:

1. The adult children and aging parent, if alive, need to understand the sensitivity of the issue of transferring nontitled property. This means that, for example, a Menorah is not just an item but something that reminds all five children of the happy moments during Hanukah celebrations. If the mother dies, then the father remarries, and after his death the Menorah goes to the stepmother's kids, the adult siblings may be terribly bitter—not about the physical Menorah, but about someone who was never at their Hanukah celebrations getting their memories.

2. The family should determine what they want to accomplish in the transfer. Does the older family member want to find family members who will lovingly care for their beloved (though not valuable) Santa collection? Do the adult children want to carry out family traditions, such as only the firstborn daughter in the family gets Grandma's engagement ring?

3. The family should decide what is fair in the context of the individual family and

---

*For more information about "Who Gets Grandma's Yellow Pie Plate? Transferring Non-Titled Property," call the University of Minnesota Extension Service at 624-4900 or 1-800-876-8636 between 8 a.m. and 4:30 p.m. Monday through Friday. A packet of information (order number EP-6686-MST) costs $8, and a video (VH-6692-MST) is $30, plus shipping and sales tax. To arrange for someone to speak to a group about the transfer of nontitled property, call Marlene Stum at the extension service at 612-625-4270.

how that family wants to pass nontitled items along. Is it fair that the firstborn daughter gets the engagement ring, or should the firstborn daughter pick names from a hat to see who gets it, or should sons get a chance to get it also? Sometimes it is impossible for families to be fair. For example, three adult children may want the baby cereal bowl with Little Red Riding Hood on the bottom. Because there is no fair way to decide among themselves, except to break the bowl into three pieces, they may just have to work together to see who gets it or give it to the next born baby or grandchild.

4. The family and adult children should understand that belongings have different meanings for different individuals. When a mother moves, the oldest adult child may have a loving memory of a valuable silver tea set, not for its monetary value but for the tea parties the mother had with her when she was a toddler. The mother may have been too busy to have those tea parties with the other children, and they may value the set only because of its monetary value.

5. Consider distribution options and consequences. You can help the family agree to manage conflicts before they arise and avoid common obstacles before the items are divided.

GCMs and Dividing Family Items

You can be helpful to the family by researching this issue and utilizing the knowledge before an older person moves. You could guide the family by giving suggestions on how to manage conflicts over distributing family items and by offering even to be present at a family meeting about dividing treasures. If you have the skills, you can mediate or counsel at the family meeting. You can be helpful to the family by suggesting that the issue of distributing nontitled property be brought up and discussed. Oftentimes, family members think this is too sensitive an issue and never discuss it. A GCM who helps the family to plan ahead may really solve the problem.

Another thing you can do is to encourage family members to tell the stories that go along with the family items to be passed on. Before a client moves or after the death of a family member, you can facilitate a gathering of family members, especially the older family members, and have them pass on the stories that go with the items. A grandmother may believe that everyone knows that the mahogany rocker with the worn seat is where she nursed all her babies, but grandchildren who will inherit the rocker may have no idea. You can also facilitate recording these stories so that they can be passed down through generations. Having the story for posterity is a gift to the family member by itself.

You can encourage the family to take time while dividing up assets to tell family stories, listen to each others' stories, and find joy in remembering. You can help the family make dividing up assets a positive experience.

Teaching families how to hold discussions about nontitled property and options for dividing personal property, such as by using family meetings and the Grandma's Yellow Pie Plate methods, is a good geriatric care management skill. You can also counsel older clients to express their wishes about nontitled items and, through their attorney, add them to their will or trust. For example, a client may say, "I want my second son John to get my gun collection." You can counsel families dividing nontitled property on ways to divide items if there is no legal direction. For example, a 20-year-old may really need the microwave, but a 40-year-old may not need but want the battered teapot because its whistle woke him up every summer morning when he visited his grandmother. You can help families by giving them guidelines that can avoid complaints of favoritism and misunderstandings. Encourage family members to put their wishes about wanting family items in writing and send these wishes to the entire family, instead of making phone calls. In this way everyone gets the request in writing at the same time.

ASSISTING SPOUSAL CAREGIVERS AND WORKING WITH COUPLES

When people are married long enough, one spouse is likely to have to care for the other eventually. Spouses of the chronically ill are constantly reminded of a relationship that is no longer the same. They have stated that healthcare providers often overlook their needs. Almost all cultures place great value on caring for the sick, and yet caregiving can continue for more decades than many marriages used to last, and without the benefit of an extended family.

A spousal caregiver may be a depressed, lonely, isolated, fatigued, anxious individual who may have physical problems, a sleep disorder, and reduced employment. Spousal caregivers experience feelings they view as negative or unacceptable: they feel anger and resentment at the partner for being sick, they feel jealousy at always being second, and they feel deprived of pleasure because they have to do too much work. GCMs can help spousal caregivers considerably. Many of the suggestions discussed in the previous sections apply to spousal caregivers, too. Spousal caregivers face many of the same issues that other caregivers face, but spouses also have some special issues of their own.

Principles of Intervention with Spousal Caregivers

How can GCMs assist couples in managing the often overwhelming demands of spousal caregiving? Experts say that spousal caregivers need both the lifeboat and the oars; both the

support and the skills to do the job. These experts believe that caregivers are driven by five primary forces: love, morality, equity, ethics, and greed. Other factors affecting the caregiving process include family dynamics, divided loyalties, an understanding of age-related medical and psychological problems, physical endurance, the marital relationship, and the ability to communicate.

In *The Good Marriage,* Judith Wallerstein and Sandra Blakeslee cite four basic types of marriage: romantic, rescue, companionate, and traditional.[3] Although some may argue that this paradigm oversimplifies a most complex union, for the sake of examining caregiving styles, it may be useful.

Wallerstein gives case examples of couples who develop patterns that she deems good. For example, partners in a successful romantic marriage have at their core a lasting, passionately sexual relationship. The common bond the couple in a romantic marriage share is the sense that they were destined to be together.

Partners in a successful rescue marriage had early experiences that were traumatic. The comfort and healing that take place during their life together become the central theme of their relationship. Should one partner become frail and require caregiving, it might not upset the equilibrium as much as it might in another type of marriage, such as a companionate or traditional marriage.

A companionate marriage, which may be the most common form of marriage among younger couples, has at its core friendship, equality, and the value system of the woman's movement, with its corollary that the male role, too, needs to change. A major factor in the companionate marriage is the attempt to balance the partners' serious emotional investment in the workplace with their emotional investment in the relationship and the children.

The fourth type is the traditional marriage, where the stronger, more dominant spouse (usually the husband) is the breadwinner. Should the breadwinner become incapacitated and aphasic as a result of a stroke, for example, the system in this type of marriage would be profoundly upset. Changing dependencies, hostility, and the unspoken wish for escape all redefine the nature of affection in this relationship.

The style of spousal caregiving is determined in large part by a person's coping style, practical abilities, and marital relationship. Consider the following examples:

- A husband devotes himself for years to caring for his wife, who has Alzheimer's. Then he murders her. What might a GCM have done to prevent this tragedy?
- A wife cares for her chronically ill husband, quits her job, and neglects herself. Her adult children want her to spend more time with her grandchildren and have a more normal life. She says it is her choice and she would not have it any other way. How would a GCM counsel the family?
- A husband who is caring for his wife with Alzheimer's states that she instructed him to call Dr. Kevorkian when she no longer recognizes him. He has told a GCM of this directive. How should the GCM react?

How can GCMs help emotionally vulnerable clients to develop new coping styles that will be necessary to spare them further stress? How much preventive intervention can care managers offer? Is it possible to prepare spouses for the often inevitable spousal caregiving responsibilities they will face? Can advance directives or a durable power of attorney for health care play a role in this?

Mr. and Mrs. H believed so. They had been married for 50 years and were grateful for their many blessings. They had good, open communication and agreed to state in the advance directives that under no circumstance would one spouse be expected to sacrifice his or her physical or emotional health at the expense of the other. Both had experience with chronically ill parents and recognized the toll caregiving can take.

They agreed to purchase long-term care policies that included home health care as well as institutional care and to implement these policies as necessary at the discretion of the well spouse. The couple said that it was a tremendous relief to know that each of them could be cared for, not necessarily by the other, and still feel that the spousal devotion was intact.

Problematic Relationships

What about a situation in which a couple has not openly discussed caregiving preferences, and one spouse becomes chronically impaired both cognitively and physically? How can a care manager help the well spouse achieve a relatively satisfying life while caring for the ill spouse? A case in point occurred when a GCM was facilitating a support group for well spouses of the chronically impaired. Two of the well spouses approached the GCM for her opinion. They were interested in dating each other but were very conflicted. Both members of the support group had been caring for chronically ill spouses. Both of the ill spouses were impaired to the extent that they no longer recognized their well spouses.

The GCM counseled the two group members separately and together over a period of several weeks. They both expressed an overwhelming sense of devotion and guilt. Through counseling, the care manager was able to help the couple resolve the conflict. The result was that the well couple was able to define the parameters of the relationship in a way that would not conflict with the marriage vows and was comfortable. They shared a meaningful relationship and offered tremendous emotional support to one another.

What does the codependent caregiver look like? According to Melodie Beattie, the guru of codependency issues, that person is taking responsibility for others; too often not taking responsibility for him- or herself.[4] Codependent caregivers take inappropriate responsibility for the feelings, thoughts, behaviors, problems, choices, and life course of others. Codependent caring makes people feel used, victimized, unappreciated, and unsuccessful in their efforts. Codependent caring makes them feel controlled by the other's needs while simultaneously feeling that the caregiver's own needs are not being met.

In the context of clinical intervention for codependent spousal caregivers, GCMs might ask themselves the following questions:

- What is the caregiver's own attitude toward aging?
- What is the motivation to care?
- Is the caregiver denying the spouse's issues and his or her own?
- Can the caregiver be helped to deal with his or her emotions?
- Can the GCM help the caregiver build a partnership with the spouse and helping professionals?
- Can the GCM help the caregiver manage conflict?
- Is it possible to help the caregiver to establish good family communication?
- Can the caregiver be helped to strike a balance between the need to care and his or her own needs?

General Principles for All Types of Spousal Caregivers

True helping and healthy giving are good, and they are different from caretaking. The following guidelines are summarized from the National Council on Aging's "Caregiving Tips Series."[5] They may be useful for you to suggest to stressed spousal caregivers.

- Encourage spousal caregivers to admit their feelings. Feeling tired, isolated, helpless, angry, or scared can be an indi-

cation that they are trying to handle too much without the help and information they need. Such feelings, though difficult, are natural.

- Encourage spousal caregivers to talk to their family and friends about what they feel rather than keeping everything inside.
- Encourage spousal caregivers to set reasonable expectations and not to reproach themselves for failing to be a superwoman or superman.
- Encourage spousal caregivers to admit to themselves and their friends what they want and need and what they can and cannot do for themselves. Knowing their limits is an important part of taking care of themselves.
- Encourage spousal caregivers to seek help when they need it, looking to professionals and service agencies as partners who can provide guidance and counseling. Help caregivers realize that there is nothing wrong with asking for help.
- Encourage spousal caregivers to ask questions. If they do not find the answers right away, they should continue to search for people who can answer the questions.
- Suggest that spousal caregivers take care of themselves physically; eat regular, balanced meals; exercise as part of their daily routine to maintain fitness and ease tension; use relaxation techniques such as meditation, deep breathing, and massage; and maintain a sense of humor.
- Remind spousal caregivers not to forget to take care of themselves when things are tough. This is the most important time for them to be good to themselves.
- Suggest that spousal caregivers avoid destructive ways of coping such as overeating, abusing alcohol or drugs, and neglecting or taking out their stress on others.

- Encourage spousal caregivers to maintain activities and social contacts that they enjoy and plan occasions for their own pleasure and renewal.

Sometimes the most helpful counseling is based on good listening and empathic responding. Help caregivers give themselves permission to take care of themselves, emphasizing that this is not selfish or uncaring but part of surviving. Caregiving is difficult work that involves not only doing, but coping.

Expressions of Sexuality

The need for closeness and intimacy does not diminish with age. But despite the sexual revolution, our culture still views some types of sexual behavior as inappropriate.

One of the greatest fears is that older people will develop inappropriate sexual behavior. Inappropriate sexual behavior is an infrequent problem with individuals with dementia. More common than actual inappropriate behavior is the myth that confused older people will develop inappropriate sexual behavior. However, should such an unfortunate incident occur, a matter-of-fact reaction without any more fuss than is absolutely necessary is what is called for. The caregiver's reaction may have more impact on the observer or the victim than the actual incident does. For example, removing the person from the situation and explaining simply that, "He forgets where he is" may be all that is needed.

Some people with dementia-type illnesses have an increased sex drive, while others have a decreased sex drive. If the individual has an increased sex drive, remember that it is a factor of the brain injury, not a reflection on the relationship. You can assist the couple in finding a balance of sexual activity that is comfortable for both. Referral to a clinician who specializes in dementia problems might be helpful. A university-based clinic could be a good resource.

Inappropriate Behavior

Occasionally confused people will expose themselves in public or fidget in such a way that reminds others of sexual behaviors. This can be upsetting, especially to family members. Family members may benefit from knowing that the problem will probably not worsen as the dementia illness progresses.

There may be reasonable explanations for seemingly sexual behaviors such as disrobing or handling the genital area. You may suggest a family meeting to identify some of the triggers, suggest explanations, and allow family members the opportunity to vent their feelings. Solutions may arise during the process. Here is a list of behaviors with possible explanations and interventions:

- Unbuckling belt buckle; feels clothing is too tight
- Unzipping trousers; needs to urinate, forgets where bathroom is
- Fidgeting with buttons on blouse; is too warm
- Making sexual advances to attendant; confuses the attendant with a spouse
- Making frequent requests for sexual relations; forgets the sexual relations that do take place
- Handling genital area; has a urinary tract infection (should be checked by a physician)
- Pulling off pants; feels uncomfortable in clothing, needs to use bathroom
- Disrobing; is too warm, is uncomfortable in clothing

Differential Diagnosis: Sexual Acting Out versus Medical Problem

An older woman was placed in a care facility's unit for people with dementia. Her family was informed by the nurse on the unit that the older woman was wandering into the beds of other residents, disrobing, and touching her genital area. After a thorough medical examination and a family meeting, it was revealed that the woman had a urinary tract infection; she also came from a large family and was recently widowed. After her urinary tract infection was treated and she was more regularly taken to social activities, the wandering and genital handling subsided. The staff of the care facility were asked to provide more evening one-on-one attention, which seemed to address this woman's need for companionship at night.

■ CONTINUUM OF CARE RESOURCES: WORKING AS PART OF A TEAM

Just as no person is an island, no GCM stands alone. A good GCM knows a staggering array of experts who can assist clients in areas where the GCM's expertise is lacking or where there could be a conflict of interest. For example, a middle-aged son came to see a GCM because his father, with whom the son lived, was beginning to require more care than the son could provide. The father was falling on occasion and appeared to be confused at times. The son traveled regularly on business. As the consultation progressed, it became apparent that the home was held in joint tenancy by the son and his father. There was another sibling who lived out of state who had a physical disability and was receiving public assistance. The father was beginning to show signs of dementia and had not yet developed a will or a general durable power of attorney, or a health care power of attorney.

The GCM suggested that the son contact an elder-law attorney to advise him regarding estate matters. A neurologist was recommended to evaluate the nature of the father's dementia and possible interventions. In addition, the father's physician was contacted to see about an order for home health care, physical therapy, and occupational therapy that would include an evaluation of the need

for adaptive equipment and other equipment to make the home environment safer.

The GCM asked about the father's typical day, and the son explained that his father was alone all day, ate poorly during the day, and waited for his son to arrive home from work, which was sometimes not until 7 p.m. The GCM suggested an adult day program that provided transportation, meals, and socialization. The father responded favorably to the social stimulation and improved diet.

While developing a will with the father, the attorney also set up a trust for the estate and a special needs trust for the son with a disability. The special needs trust would allow that son to receive an inheritance and monthly stipend without disqualifying him from receiving public assistance. The neurologist diagnosed the father with a pseudo-dementia that abated after regular participation in a social day program and an improved diet. Many of these kinds of dementia have depression and nutritional deficiencies as their underlying problem, both which can be easily reversed, if treated early. The father now resides in a local retirement facility recommended by the GCM, who assisted in his acclimation. The facility has several levels of care so that as the father's needs change, he can receive assistance without relocating. The local son visits his father regularly and knows that he can rely on the GCM to advocate for his father, especially during his frequent out-of-town business trips.

GCMs should think of the following additional professionals and service providers when assisting families with identifying resources:

• Services that may be covered by Medicare
  1. Adult day health care
  2. Assessment services
  3. Home health aide services
  4. Homemaker services
  5. Hospice services
  6. Medical social work

7. Mental health services
8. Occupational therapy
9. Personal care
10. Physical therapy
11. Physician care
12. Protective services
13. Respite care
14. Speech therapy
15. Transportation

- Services that may be covered at no cost through a public agency
  1. Care management
  2. Chore services
  3. Health insurance counseling
  4. Information and referral
  5. Legal services
  6. Supervision
  7. Telephone reassurance

- Other services
  1. Emergency response systems
  2. Home-delivered meals
  3. Paid companions and sitters

■ HELPING A FAMILY DECIDE IF A PARENT SHOULD LIVE WITH THEM

Some family members may consider having their older relatives live with them. This can be a short- or long-term arrangement. Its success depends on several factors. There are many issues to consider in coming to this decision, and GCMs can help families consider the issues.

It is often painful for adult children to admit that they cannot ask their mother or father to live with them. They may have practical reasons (e.g., inadequate living space, poor health, no settled home) or more personal reasons (e.g., personality clashes, adolescents who require emotional attention, marital strain). However, it is much more difficult to take such an irrevocable step, inviting a parent to live in one's home, and then find out that it does not work. The ensuing

aftermath and responsibility the adult child will feel for disrupting the parent's life is even more painful.

Sons and daughters who are considering inviting an older parent to live with them even though they are reluctant to do so may be comforted to know that other people share that reluctance. National surveys consistently show that the majority of young and old adults in the United States think it is a bad idea for older parents and their children to live together. One might assume that the strongest opposition to such living arrangements comes from the younger generation, but that is not true; the surveys show that the older the parents, the less likely they are to favor living with their children. Older people particularly do not want to be burdens.

Even if the older mother or father directly or indirectly suggests a common living arrangement, sentiment should not dictate the decision. Instead, the decision should be based on a careful analysis of the situation, the wishes of the other members of the immediate family, and the history of the relationship between the parent and the adult child. GCMs can aid the family in considering these questions:

- How does the spouse of the adult child feel about the common living arrangement?
- What kind of financial arrangements are being considered?
- What kind of living space will be available for everyone?
- Will the older person depend completely on the son's or daughter's family for companionship and entertainment?
- What about other friends, relatives, and contemporaries? What about recreational, cultural, and religious needs?
- Can the family honestly expect to live comfortably together? Do the personalities clash? How have previous visits been? How often did family members

have a migraine headache, ulcer flare-up, or other stress-related symptom during these visits?

- When the older person visited in the past, were the family members counting the days until the older person left?
- Can the older person allow the adult child to run his or her own household?
- Would the older person (because of temperament) feel comfortable in the home and with having friends visit there?
- Will the adult children be able to make sure the older person has ongoing, accessible, competent medical care?
- Will having the older person in the house violate anyone's sense of privacy?

■ CONCLUSION

This chapter focuses on how a GCM can effectively work with adult children, spouses, and other family members to improve the quality of life for older people and ease the burden of caregiving in various situations. GCMs can help all types of families, including long-distance families, dysfunctional families, overwhelmed families, and families who are considering facility placement. GCMs can also work with couples and work as part of a professional team.

The future of geriatric care management work with families will increasingly be tied to the Internet. The Internet will allow family caregivers to identify GCMs in their community as well as GCMs in their older relative's region. The Internet will also enable family members to identify resources, services, and products that will improve the quality of their lives. However, there will never be an electronic replacement for responsive, clinically astute, and empathetic GCMs who can be instrumental in improving a challenging family circumstance.

■ REFERENCES

1. American Association of Retired Persons. *Tomorrow's Choices: Preparing Now for Future Legal, Financial, and Health Care Decisions.* Washington, DC: American Association of Retired Persons; 1992.

2. Eisendorfer C, Cohen D. *Care for the Elderly: Reshaping Health Policy.* Baltimore, MD: Johns Hopkins University Press; 1989.

3. Wallerstein J, Blakeslee S. *The Good Marriage: How and Why Love Lasts.* New York: Houghton Mifflin; 1995.

4. Beattie M. *Co-Dependent No More.* New York: Fine Communications; 1997.

5. Cassel C, ed. *The Practical Guide to Aging.* New York: New York University Press; 1999.

Appendix 20–A

■ HOW TO FIND A QUALIFIED GERIATRIC CARE MANAGER

Caregivers should be aware that a growing number of geriatric care managers (GCMs) are now certified and known as Care Managers Certified. They are professionals, usually social workers or nurses, who are capable of conducting assessments and providing short- and long-term care plans for clients.

It is recommended that some or all of the following questions be asked by consumers who are considering retaining a GCM:

1. What are your credentials? A GCM should have an advanced degree in social work, psychology, or gerontology or should be a registered nurse with public health experience.
2. Do you have certification as a GCM?
3. How long have you worked with the frail elderly? How long in private practice? Care managers with more years of experience are likely to be better choices than care managers with fewer years of experience. Public agency experience working with the frail elderly helps.
4. Do you belong to the National Association of Professional Geriatric Care Managers? This association has ethics codes and standards of practice.
5. Are you available 24 hours a day, 7 days a week? If you get sick or go out of town, who backs you up?
6. How do you charge? If by the hour, do you charge for telephone calls? Travel time? What else? GCMs do much of their business by phone and legitimately charge for that time. Most ask half their usual fee for travel. Charges for other services should be spelled out in contracts or fee schedules.
7. If a service you recommended does not work out, what will you do about it? The GCM should promise in advance to correct any problem, and if that fails should arrange something new.
8. Can you provide references from clients as well as local organizations such as hospitals and senior centers?
9. Do you arrange for free, low-cost, or medically insured services when available and appropriate?
10. Do you personally provide any of the needed services?
11. Who screens the home care providers and what methods are used? Do you run a background check, and does it include criminal records?
12. Are you bonded, and do you carry professional liability insurance?
13. How often and by whom is each service monitored?
14. How frequently can I expect to hear from you? Are your reports written or phoned?

The recipients of care management service should feel comfortable with the GCM.

The National Association of Professional Geriatric Care Managers in Tucson, Arizona, publishes a list of its members. Additional information may be found on their website, www.caremanager.org.

Chapter 21

Difficult Families: Conflict, Dependence, and Mutuality

Emily B. Saltz

■ INTRODUCTION

No two families are alike. Every family is its own complex, unique, constantly changing system of important relationships. And each one, at one time or another, must deal with life's most important events and issues: birth and death, marriage and divorce, intimacy and distance, growing up and aging. Dealing with the aging process within a family is a complicated matter. It can be a struggle even for families that are close-knit, well integrated, and highly functioning, as previously described in Chapter 20, Geriatric Care Management: Working with Nearly Normal Aging Families. It can be overwhelming and even destructive for the so-called difficult family, meaning the family that is marked by strained relationships and unresolved conflict.

This chapter explores the strategies and techniques a geriatric care manager (GCM) can use when dealing with families who are dysfunctional and are considered *difficult*. The concepts of filial maturity and mutuality—that is, balancing the giving and accepting of care—will be explored as a way to reframe dependence in old age as a normal rather than pathological process. These concepts are addressed as a means to assist families in developing positive reciprocal relationships during later-life transitions.

Families often seek out a GCM when they are in crisis and feel hopeless about finding solutions to their elder-care problems. Caregiving is often a demanding, full-time job for which there is no job description and no training. Many of the families GCMs meet struggle valiantly to meet the demands of this job for which they may feel totally unprepared and unappreciated.

For elders, the transition to dependence involves a role change that is frequently accompanied by feelings of loss and inadequacy. For family caregivers, this same transition evokes powerful conflicts regarding dependence and independence, which are rooted in early parent–child bonds. For many adult children, the task of meeting the emerging dependency needs of their parents triggers a reexamination of how their own needs were or were not met.[1]

The ordinary aging processes are made far more challenging when a family has a history of dysfunction. As GCMs, we face some of our greatest challenges in working with these so-called difficult families. These are families who are not able to organize themselves effectively in the face of elder-care challenges and crises. Regardless of whether the family system has been healthy or dysfunctional, its members are under stress as they move from long-established roles into uncharted territory.

■ UNDERSTANDING AGING WITHIN THE FAMILY SYSTEM

The aging of a key family member presents complex familial challenges in all families. "Aging families must deal with the psychological and relational stress associated with loss."[2] The loss may be multifaceted, involving not just the familiar effects of physical and mental decline, but may also have significant emotional components. Loss of control, loss of continuity, loss of defined roles, loss of significant relationships, and loss of a sense of purpose; all of these effects may not have been fully anticipated.

These transitions can disrupt any family, even those that have had success in the past in sustaining family bonds, reaching consensus, and managing prior developmental crises or losses. An elder-care crisis often exaggerates unresolved family conflicts. Adult children may find themselves disagreeing over anything and everything: how much care is needed, who should provide it, who should decide, and who should pay. Long-standing parent–child conflicts over such issues as control, approval, nurturing, money, and support may suddenly resurface. The geographical location of the adult children can also become highly problematic, causing conflict and resentment between those who live close to the elder and those who live at a distance. The ability of any family to manage these disagreements is almost always sorely tested.

According to family systems theory, each family is an emotional unit, and behavior within that system is reciprocal and reactive. It is a living system of which each member is an interdependent part. The central tenet of systems theory is that a change in behavior in one part of the system begins to change the behavior of the whole.[3] A major life cycle crisis, such as the physical and cognitive decline of an aging parent, simultaneously causes and requires reorganization in the system.

The problem is that reorganization is difficult. A family system is homeostatic and inherently resistant to change. Families seek equilibrium, and as long as everyone sticks to familiar roles, the system remains stable. The very nature of aging means that the prevailing patterns will inevitably be disturbed. Change or stress affecting the elder within the family system will unavoidably affect the whole.

Evaluating Family Interaction

Mindful of systems theory, GCMs can more properly evaluate the quality of interaction and the roots of conflict among family members. Dan Blazer has set forth parameters that are useful in helping GCMs to assess family interaction:

- **Compatible vs conflictual:** Do family members easily come to an agreement over care issues, or do they argue constantly, even over relatively unimportant issues? Do old conflicts between siblings or between adult child and parent resurface during the crisis period?
- **Cohesive vs fragmented:** Does the family present as a unit, or do they contact the GCM individually with their problems? Do family members ask the GCM to keep conversations secret from other family members?
- **Productive vs nonproductive:** Can the family respond to the GCM's suggestions and take necessary action to create change in the elder's life? Are there individual family members who are unable to mobilize and feel powerless to act?
- **Fragile vs stable:** Has the family been stable over time? Is there a history of emotional cut-offs or distance on the part of one or more family members? Is there a pattern of divorce, remarriage, or other disruptions in relationships that changes the balance within the family system?
- **Rigid vs flexible:** How has the family handled previous crises? Did the members accept the need to change roles in those

times? Are members able to exchange or share important roles in managing family affairs? If one member is unavailable to provide care, can other members assume the caregiving role? Do family members respond readily to crises?[4]

It is important to remember that, at the point of intervention, the GCM is meeting the elder and the family at a single, finite point in time and that the elder has had a lifetime of experience, habits, preferences, and patterns. Indeed, the family system itself may be the product of patterns handed down from generation to generation. By acknowledging the breadth and depth of family history, the GCM has a greater likelihood of initiating or promoting necessary change within the family.

■ INTERGENERATIONAL RELATIONSHIPS

The GCM also needs to remember that, for the adult child, the act of caregiving means reengaging with the most profound and influential attachment of one's life: the parent. There are few models for negotiating the powerful parent–child bond in later life.[1] Intergenerational relationships between parents and adult children are often characterized by ambivalence. Positive feelings include love, reciprocal help, shared values, and solidarity. Negative feelings include isolation, conflict, abuse, neglect, and caregiver stress.[5]

Robert Karen stated, "We are dealing with two different sets of parents—the parent we grew up with, whom we struggle with internally, and the living parent of today. These internal parents have mythic dimensions—they may have adored us or wounded us, we may idealize them or demonize them, we may or may not have fully separated."[6] An adult child may hold on to an internal representation of the parent at an earlier stage, when the parent was more powerful or more engaged, whether for better or worse. Likewise, most parents, no matter how old they have become,

have a residual wish to care for their children, which may cause them to hold on to their own images from the past.

The task for adult children is to let go of the mythic parent so that, in the late stages of family development, we can see our mothers and fathers as actual people. Adult children need to grieve the loss of the past, the loss of the internalized early parent, so that as adults they can relate realistically to their parents in the present and provide care unencumbered by out-of-date motives and impulses.

Dependency and Loss

The task for the elder is, in some ways, even more difficult. The struggle to accept care within the intergenerational family can be even harder than giving it. We live in a culture that emphasizes youth, independence, autonomy, and self-control and, conversely, a culture that regards dependence at any stage of life as a weakness or personal deficit.[7] The transition to dependence for an older adult who has had a lifetime of self-reliance and self-determination involves a role change that is often marked by feelings of loss and inadequacy. Erlanger notes, "Loss occurs during all phases of the family life cycle, but it assumes a central role in the influences on later-life families."[8]

In the context of intergenerational family caregiving, this loss is experienced in different ways by the elder and the family members. The elder may be entering into the new paradigm of caring and giving with a disturbing sense of diminished physical or cognitive functioning, a feeling that is most poignant among elders who are aware of their declining capacities. In addition to personal decline, the elder often confronts the erosion of social networks, economic stability, and sense of purpose, power, and autonomy in the community and in the family itself. On the other hand, for the adult children, spouses, and other family caregivers, these changes of definition for the elder may be experienced as the loss of a central figure in their own lives.

According to Terry Hargrave, the psychological and relational stress on the family that is associated with the individual elder's role change is a primary issue that aging families must address to negotiate the later stages of family development successfully.[2] Indeed, families are frequently emotionally unprepared to deal with the raw power and significance of the intergenerational shift caused by the elder's personal and social losses. The result is often family dysfunction and crisis that emerges or deepens at the worst possible time. Furthermore, although prior stages of family life inevitably include transitions in roles and attitudes between parent and child, these earlier transitions are dissimilar to, and provide no real guidance for, the profound and difficult changes in the parent–child bond in later life. Unlike the more predictable, normative developmental process for children, the character and timing of events and patterns that occur in old age are highly variable and generally undesirable. The growing dependency of the elder is not always predictable, desired, or confined to a particular life phase.

CASE STUDY

Case Example: Nancy Narcissist

Nancy Narcissist is an 82-year-old widowed woman currently living in a traditional assisted living facility. She is widowed with one son, Devoted Dan, who is married with two children. Nancy has several health problems, including severe arthritis and hypertension. Because of her arthritis, she walks slowly and uses a walker.

Recently, Nancy has been experiencing cognitive decline, and she is having trouble managing her daily affairs. She has papers and stacks of unpaid bills piled all over her apartment, and she leaves sticky notes to remind herself what needs to get done. She is having a hard time walking to the dining room and frequently asks that a tray be sent to her room. The assisted living facility does provide personal care services, but Nancy has refused all offers of assistance. The facility has called Dan several times to express concern about Nancy's continued ability to stay in her apartment. They would like Dan to consider moving his mother to the memory impairment unit, but he is reluctant to broach this subject with her.

Nancy is, and has always been, very critical and demanding of her son. She calls Devoted Dan several times a day, often announcing a so-called crisis and insisting that he come right away. When Dan arrives, he must endure a litany of complaints about the food, the staff, and the other residents. The rest of Nancy's complaints are about Devoted Dan himself. She tells him that, if he really cared about her, he would find her a new apartment. Despite his frequent visits, Nancy complains that she does not see Dan or her grandchildren enough. When Dan offers to help his mother pay her bills or offers to hire a companion for her, she angrily refuses.

Eventually, Nancy falls in her apartment and is hospitalized with a fractured hip. From the hospital, she is transferred to a nursing home where she remains. Dan continues to visit her on a daily basis and endures his mother's ongoing complaints and criticisms. He feels pressured, overwhelmed, and very guilty.

In the case of Nancy Narcissist, the fundamental question that Devoted Dan faces is, "How am I supposed to meet the dependency needs of my mother when my own dependency needs have not been met?" This is a good example of a son who is trying desperately to manage the increasing care needs of his mother, despite his own feelings of guilt and worthlessness and his mother's neediness and emotional withholding. Interestingly, despite not having received the bedrock of nurturance and warmth that one would expect to find in a good caregiver, Dan remains a thoughtful and devoted son. Why?

Myth of Role Reversal

Margaret Blenkner was well ahead of her time when, in the mid-1960s, she challenged the commonly held notion that *role reversal* is a normal development in the aging process.[9] As conventionally understood, role reversal assumes that an inevitable shift of power and control occurs within an aging family whereby the adult child becomes the parent figure to the elder and the elder becomes the child figure in need of care and protection.

Although the activities of raising a young child and caring for an older adult share some surface similarities, there are fundamental differences that the original theorists of role reversal largely ignored. Caregiving activities at the beginning and at the end of life both involve protecting, worrying, and planning for the needs of a dependent family member. They both exact a high cost physically, emotionally, and economically. And they both require the caregiver's frequent, if not constant, attention and physical presence.

The differences, however, are more profound. The relationship between a parent and a young child is asymmetrical: the parent has passed through numerous developmental stages, while the child has passed through few, if any. Ultimately, the parent's goal is to guide the child toward independence, separation, and self-identity. By contrast, no matter how diminished or impaired by time or illness, the elder brings a lifetime of experience, habit, preference, belief, attitude, wisdom, autonomy, and personality that inevitably informs and transforms the caregiving rela-

tionship. No matter how much the elder declines, he or she will always be the parent within the family system.[10]

Filial Maturity

Instead of role reversal, Blenkner introduced the concepts of filial crisis and filial maturity as normative aspects of individual and family development. According to Blenkner, filial crisis arises when the parent in an aging family is no longer the rock of support for the family and may now need to lean on others for support and comfort.[9] In a healthy family system, the adult child is able to achieve filial maturity, which is a state of emotional readiness to relinquish earlier roles as the needy youngster and to begin to support and provide care for the elder without infantilizing the elder. Successfully accomplishing the filial task entails a new understanding and a different kind of love for the aged parent by the adult child. Lowy, among others, explores Blenkner's recognition that the adult child's resolution of the filial crisis sets the stage for the adult child to confront and eventually meet the challenges of his or her own aging process and mortality.[7]

CASE STUDY

Case Example: New Jersey Norm
New Jersey Norm is a 92-year-old widowed man who is living with his 88-year-old female companion in his own apartment in Pleasantville, New Jersey. He has one daughter, Boston Barbara, a 45-year-old married woman living in Boston, and another daughter, California Callie, a 50-year-old unmarried woman living in California. New Jersey Norm was recently diagnosed with normal pressure hydrocephalus (NPH), a condition associated with problems involving balance and gait, urinary incontinence, and dementia.

During the past year, Norm was hospitalized five times for problems related to NPH, and he recently had surgery to have a cranial shunt implanted. Despite the surgery, his condition continues to deteriorate. He is incontinent, has fallen several times, and cannot be left alone. Norm's companion feels she cannot handle his care and turns to his daughters for help.

Norm did not have a close relationship with either of his daughters. He was always an emotionally distant father who did not take a great interest in his children's lives. In fact, both daughters were aware that, for more than 30 years during his marriage, Norm was having an affair with his current female companion. Both daughters were close to their mother, and they are still angry with Norm and resentful toward his female companion. Despite these historical tensions, both daughters have accepted their new role as caregivers. Norm, however, tends to act in a passive-aggressive manner, and he is unappreciative of their efforts.

California Callie has told both Norm and her sister that she is willing to give up her career job and well-established life in California to care for Norm. She proposes that she move into an apartment upstairs from Norm and his female companion. Boston Barbara tries to dissuade her sister, but Callie insists, admitting that she never resolved her feelings of guilt and loss at not having been at her mother's bedside when she died. She sees Norm's current elder-care needs as an opportunity to make up for her absence in the past.

What is motivating California Callie to move back home to care for a father with whom she never felt close and has a very conflicted relationship? Is it a feeling of unconditional love despite his emotional distance and betrayal? Or is she driven by feelings of guilt over her prior absence during a critical family moment? To what extent is her unresolved guilt about her mother a legitimate motivation for moving back to New Jersey and accepting the daily burdens of her father's caregiving? Is the anger she feels at her father playing any role in her decision making and should it?

From the perspective of filial maturity, Callie appears ready to forge a new bond that she was previously unable to have with her now-dependent father. She seems prepared to let go of her unresolved feelings about her father and what he did or did not provide in the past. She is seeking to find a way to connect with him at the end of his life, an act of selflessness that may assist her in resolving her guilt feelings about her absence from her mother's deathbed. If her father succeeds in letting his daughter care for him, it would be possible for them to achieve a new and closer relationship.

Mutuality and Generational Maturity

In a fully realized caregiving relationship, there are, of course, at least two players—aged parent and adult child—who must complete important developmental tasks. In articulating a new model of normal behavior for the adult child as caregiver, Blenkner did not address both sides of the equation. Her theories of filial crisis and maturity focused primarily on the new role of the adult child as emerging caregiver. Later writers have considered the corresponding tasks of the aging parent. They have developed new models of "mutuality in older families"[11] and "generational maturity"[12] in which the child assumes more responsibility for the elder and the elder allows this shift in responsibility to occur. In these models, the task for the elder is to enter into a reciprocal caring relationship and to learn to accept care without abandoning self-esteem, dignity, or integrity. By accepting this task, the elder enables the adult child to enter a new phase of adulthood. The resulting mutual exchange requires both sides of the parent–child pair to redefine dependency in old age as normal behavior and to recognize that continued growth, both psychological and relational, occurs at all stages of individual and family development, including the final stages.[11] Within this framework, dependence is not seen as an indicator of decline but as a meaningful readjustment of the balance in a reciprocal care relationship between the aged parent and the adult child. By accepting the elder's dependence, both parent and child engage in a shared relationship involving new meaningful roles based on familial love and reciprocity, rather than decline and incapacity.[13]

CASE STUDY

Case Example: Mr. and Mrs. Manhattan
Mr. and Mrs. Manhattan are 89 and 85 years of age, respectively, and live in an apartment in New York City. Their only son, Phil, requested care management assistance to relocate his parents to an assisted living facility in Philadelphia, where he lives. Phil has been trying to convince his parents to move closer to him for the past 15 years, but they have steadfastly refused.

During the past several years, the Manhattans have both experienced a significant decline in health. Mr. Manhattan had a stroke, leaving him partially paralyzed. He is still independent in all activities of daily living and is cognitively intact. Mrs. Manhattan's memory has been declining for several years. She needs a hip replacement, which she has refused.

Mr. and Mrs. Manhattan are socially isolated because most of their friends have died. Mrs. Manhattan is the "boss"

in the relationship, while Mr. Manhattan tends to be more passive. Mr. Manhattan has secretly confided in his son that he is overwhelmed and stressed by Mrs. Manhattan's care needs, and he would like to move to an assisted living facility closer to his son. Mrs. Manhattan, however, has adamantly refused to move, and Mr. Manhattan is unwilling or unable to challenge her.

Phil feels powerless, particularly with his mother, whose dominating personality seems insurmountable. Despite her decline, he still feels like a child in the relationship. He has tried reasoning with his parents with little success. On several occasions, Phil arranged for Mr. and Mrs. Manhattan to come to Philadelphia to tour appropriate assisted living facilities, but in each instance his parents backed out at the last minute and the appointments have been canceled. He tried to hire a GCM and a homemaker in New York, both of whom his mother refused.

The GCM in Philadelphia meets with Phil and helps him to revise the unsuccessful strategies he has been using with his parents. She reaffirms the appropriateness of moving his parents to a more supportive environment and helps him to understand the dynamics of his parents' resistance, particularly his mother's. In view of his mother's cognitive impairments, the GCM suggests that Phil's continued resort to reasoning and logic will not work. Instead, she promotes the use of *therapeutic fiblets* as a strategy for making the transition possible.

With the GCM's encouragement, Phil begins to take a firmer, more direct approach with his mother, while continuing to provide gentle reassurance to his father. He is less intimidated by his mother's obstinate words, and he asserts a newfound sense of adult authority. With his father, he speaks more confidently that the family will be able to negotiate the necessary changes that are ahead. As a result, his parents begin to signal a shift in attitude. His father now accepts his assurances and becomes less anxious about the future, and his mother becomes less resistant.

Eventually, Mr. and Mrs. Manhattan move to an assisted living facility in the Philadelphia area. Shortly after completing the move, Phil organizes a birthday party for Mr. Manhattan at the facility. In the presence of Mr. Manhattan's new neighbors and friends, and with his wife at his side, Mr. Manhattan offers a public toast to his son, thanking him openly for enabling them to move into a new and happier phase of life. Mr. Manhattan's words—"Without my son we would not be here. We are so thankful"—resonate with Phil for a long time.

What are the power struggles occurring in this family system? What strategies does the GCM use to enable Phil to overcome his sense of powerlessness with his mother? Is Phil ultimately successful in achieving filial maturity? What is the significance of Mr. Manhattan's toast, in terms of generational maturity?

■ IDENTIFYING THE DIFFICULT FAMILY

The successful resolution in the story of Mr. and Mrs. Manhattan does not occur, of course, in all families. There are families with histories of violence, abuse, neglect, or even simple dysfunction for whom the resolution of filial crisis is not likely to occur. In these families, the adult child may be thrust unwillingly into the role of caregiver with a parent who may not have provided support or nurtured the child in the past. Achieving filial maturity in this context is vastly complicated. These difficult families are, generally, most in need of intervention, but for the GCM, they are often the most challenging to assist.

From the GCM's perspective, what exactly does it mean for a family to be difficult? Does it mean that the family does not listen to us or accept our recommendations? Does it mean that the family is unfairly critical of the GCM's work and complains that the GCM is failing to do the job correctly? Or is being difficult as simple as repeatedly failing to return important phone calls to the GCM? Or, conversely, calling numerous times every day?

How Difficult Families Present

GCMs will have no trouble in recognizing the common themes that quickly identify the difficult family.[14]

- *The family usually presents with urgency to get their needs met.* The difficult family usually calls in crisis and expresses a sense of urgency in having their issues addressed at once. They expect the GCM to respond immediately, even if the GCM does not consider the situation to be a crisis.
- *The family spends much time in contact with potential resources in an attempt to meet their needs.* The difficult family may call several GCMs, elder care agencies, or other professionals to request help and will often spend unproductive time researching options. Even after exhaustive research, the family will not be able to reach a consensus regarding whether to even retain a GCM.
- *Relationships with agencies and individuals are often conflictive.* The difficult family will easily disagree or find fault with professionals engaged in helping them.

- *Families are unreasonably demanding with a strong sense of entitlement.* The difficult family will unreasonably perceive its own problems as entitled to or requiring special attention from the GCM. This family does not respond well to limits and may expect the GCM or other institutions to "bend the rules" to meet their needs.
- *Families are overly sensitive to criticism and disappointment.* The difficult family feels easily criticized by the GCM and may become defensive regarding the GCM's recommendations. The family also becomes easily disappointed in the GCM if his or her suggestions do not have an immediate positive impact on the situation.
- *Families may have intense emotional reactions.* Different members of the difficult family may have intense reactions to the GCM's suggestions and to other members of the family. Family members will often disagree with each other about the extent of the elder's problems.
- *Families accept little responsibility for their actions and tend to blame others when things go wrong.* Difficult families tend to blame the GCM or other institutions when the elder's situation deteriorates or when the elder resists a plan. These families easily find fault with services or staff, and they become critical or angry without trying to discuss, understand, or resolve the perceived problem.
- *Families often have unrealistic expectations of their elderly relative.* Difficult families often feel that the elder can do more than the elder is capable of, either physically or cognitively. These families may have little patience or understanding for the resistance that elders commonly show to accepting services. They may deny the existence of cognitive problems or disagree over how to handle behavioral issues.

CASE STUDY

Case Example: Unrealistic Expectations
Mr. and Mrs. Homebody are 85 and 86 years old, respectively, and living in their own home. They have one daughter, Cathy Controller, who lives 3000 miles away and who is trying to organize her parents' care from afar.

Cathy Controller retains a GCM to assess her parents' care needs and implement a plan that would keep them safely at home. She insists that the GCM force her parents to accept the help that Cathy has concluded they need. She considers herself an expert and frequently rejects suggestions offered by the GCM. Cathy calls the GCM frequently, and it is not unusual for these conversations to last for an hour. However, she also tells the GCM that she is worried about running up the bill and that the family cannot afford to spend a lot of money on GCM services.

Some of the questions that a GCM should consider are: What is the impact on Cathy of the long-distance nature of her relationship with her parents? How does her distance affect her own anxiety about their needs? What strategies could the GCM use to diffuse the daughter's anxiety? How should the GCM handle Cathy's belief in her own expertise and sense of entitlement? How should the GCM handle Cathy's insistence that her parents accept help?

Individual Roles within the Difficult Family

In establishing a relationship with a difficult family in the throes of an elder crisis, the GCM will recognize familiar roles and characteristics that individual family members play. Blazer describes these roles in the context of families dealing with an elder suffering from emotional problems.[4] I have modified his descriptions to make them relevant to the GCM's work with difficult families:

- *The Preserver* is more comfortable with the status quo and resists getting help for the elder. He or she is content if the elder remains overly dependent on the family without access to needed intervention.

- *The Victim* perceives the elder's problems as a direct threat to his or her own needs or self-interest. The victim will see his or her own emotional needs as more important than the elder's. He or she will frequently contact the elder or the GCM, but the purpose of the contact will involve seeking attention for his or her own problems.

- *The Manager* tends to be calm, organized, and analytical during a crisis, but is unable to provide emotional support to the elder or to other family members. Often, the manager lives at a distance, which can cause tension with family members who are more directly involved in daily care.

- *The Martyr* has an innate need to nurture the elder, even when this comes at the expense of the martyr or the elder. The martyr's seemingly endless devotion can sometimes interfere with an appropriate care plan. Most commonly, he or she will insist on carrying out the elder's wish to remain at home beyond the point that is safe or appropriate. Despite complaints of exhaustion, the martyr will avoid opportunities for respite. He or she may be motivated by guilt or an unresolved relationship with the parent.

- *The Escapee* is typically an adult child who lives far away and has withdrawn or is entirely absent during a family crisis. Involved family members will resent the escapee, particularly when there is a history of family conflict. The escapee may withdraw from family problems in self-defense and resist being drawn back into a stressful relationship with siblings.

- *The Meddler* will interfere with an established care plan in an attempt to wrest control away from other family members, to compete with siblings, or to assert dominance within the family. The meddler needs to be involved in every decision that is made and is overly involved with details. The meddler will have frequent contact with the GCM to change or challenge recommendations.

The elder, of course, is the central figure in the drama of the so-called difficult family. The GCM must assess the elder's own role in the creation of family dysfunction resulting in the roles described here.

Emotional Patterns of the Difficult Family

Dysfunctional families display common psychological and behavioral patterns that quickly come to the foreground when the stress of caring for an elder becomes predominate within the family system. These patterns include the following:

- **Contentiousness:** In struggling over current elder-care issues, the dysfunctional family will often revisit disputes over events that occurred years ago. Family property and family money are commonly sources of substantial contention.

- **Denial:** Adult children are frequently reluctant to recognize or admit early signs of decline in an elderly parent, particularly when the decline involves changes in cognitive functioning. For example, rather than acknowledge behavior associated with dementia, the adult child will often attribute the elder's current behaviors to earlier personality traits that are, in fact, no longer dominant. Denial becomes dysfunctional when the adult child fails to seek necessary treatment or assistance for the elder or allows self-destructive behaviors on the part of the elder to go unchecked.

- **Anger:** Anger occurs normally in all families, but in dysfunctional families, anger may take the form of physical or emotional abuse.

- **Distancing and cutting off:** Distancing means pulling away from the family, either emotionally or physically. Cutting off refers to an individual member's disengagement to the point of having no involvement in family life at all.

- **Fusion:** Bowen first used this term to describe a blending of one person into another. The assumption is that in all emotional systems, people seek closeness. The person trying to fuse will pursue a relationship, while the person trying to maintain autonomy will distance. A frequent reaction to fusion is distance.[15]

- **Triangulation:** This is a family systems term, used to describe a particular pattern involving the interaction among three members of the system. When tension exists between two family members, one of them may try involving a third as an ally. Triangles often represent an attempt to avoid change or conflict. Although they do occur frequently in normal family functioning, triangles that occur over a long period of time can create rigidity within the family system and make it more difficult for families to adapt or transition to new roles.[16]

▪GCM's RESPONSE TO DIFFICULT FAMILIES

Over the course of many workshops I have conducted with GCMs, I have found the following terms are the descriptors most often used to describe GCMs' experiences with difficult families: overinvolved, underinvolved, unrealistic, in conflict, angry, resistant, in denial, demanding, hostile, passive-aggressive, needy, disagreeable, noncompliant, entitled, unappreciative, threatening, and unwilling to pay.

It is obvious that, when working with difficult families, GCMs experience strong negative feelings and intense reactions, just as these families create intense reactions in the institutional systems with which they come into contact. This experience is analogous to the countertransference phenomenon in psychoanalytic theory in which the therapist develops an intense emotional reaction to the patient.

It is important for GCMs to acknowledge and understand any countertransference reactions to develop an effective strategy for intervention. Which types of emotional reactions might a GCM experience in dealing with the difficult family? Felder mentions some familiar reactions:

- Intense dislike of family members
- Condescension toward client or family
- Impatience with family decision making
- Arguing with client or family members
- Avoiding necessary contact with client or family
- Becoming paternalistic, for example, taking over decisions that should be made by family
- Becoming passive-aggressive, for example, the GCM does not follow through with own recommendations[14]

To manage and overcome these counterproductive negative feelings, we need to use the same listening and reframing techniques we use when dealing with our elderly clients. With a resistant or difficult elder, we listen carefully and show compassion regarding the source of the person's fears and resistance. We acknowledge the person's losses. We affirm the person's basic dignity as a human. We also try to motivate the person to exercise control and maintain autonomy in his or her life. We need to use the same compassionate approach in dealing with and understanding the difficult family. We need to recognize the complexity of their own family system, the causes of the dysfunction, and the magnitude of the task ahead of them. The GCM must redefine the family task as "our" problem to solve, not "their" problem for which they are at fault.

■ INTERVENING WITH DIFFICULT FAMILIES

Perhaps the most important role the GCM plays in clinical practice with difficult families is as a change agent. The GCM enables families to reconnect with each other and to transform themselves into more effective units of giving and caring. In doing so, the GCM helps the family to move toward filial maturity and to redefine dependence in old age as a normal and expected development.

To be effective, the GCM must use both clinical and practical skills in assessing families and moving them toward change, despite internal barriers. We need to distinguish our clinical approach from our instinctive approach to push families who are stuck. We must examine our own feelings to safeguard against the perils of countertransference. We must always be cognizant of the parameters of our relationship: we are not literally the client's therapist, coach, or friend, but we necessarily forge personal and even intimate bonds in doing our work.

Indeed, there is often an almost magical moment that the GCM may experience in working with families when seeming transformation occurs; that is, the moment when the family and the client, who at the outset appeared desperate and hopeless, become empowered to move forward, resolve the immediate elder-care crisis, and make the changes that seemed so insurmountable. Such transformation is, often, the goal of our intervention.

As GCMs, how can we make transformation possible? We must remain emotionally available for our clients and diligently exercise the listening skills that are innate to our profession. We must explore options and possibilities where options and possibilities may often seem lacking. We must project trust and confidence in our own abilities as GCMs, thus enabling families to use us as a guide and, more importantly, as a role model in believing that change is possible, even within their own difficult family systems.

Components of Successful Intervention

In my view, there are at least four interrelated components of successful GCM intervention:

1. **Assessment:** A comprehensive and careful assessment is the basic tool of any effective care management. Chapters 3 and 4 address the traditional components of the GCM assessment, which includes an evaluation of the cognitive, physical, and emotional status of the elder client. As discussed earlier, the GCM must also evaluate the health or dysfunction of the overall family system.

2. **Identification of intergenerational roles and conflicts:** The GCM must identify existing power dynamics within the family, redefine responsibilities to achieve generational maturity, and realign roles and tasks for each family member. The GCM should encourage a new two-way nurturing relationship between the adult child and the parent that may not have previously existed. At the same time, the GCM must enable the adult child as caregiver to set limits that are appropriate to a mature relationship. The GCM emboldens the adult child to identify and remove himself or herself from triangulated, fused, or other destructive family patterns, as described previously.

3. **Caregiver support and education:** The GCM can be instrumental in helping adult children understand that ambivalence, stress, and fear are normal and

common aspects of the caregiving role. Furthermore, the GCM can reassure the caregiver that our own professional experience and expertise allow us to offer a measure of predictability where, for the caregiver, none appears. By identifying concrete options and developing a positive plan for action, the GCM enables the family to move forward.

c. **Use of self:** Perhaps the most powerful tool for the GCM is the *use of self*. The GCM provides to families what the author refers to as grounded optimism. We provide a vision of the future that is based not only on a desire for hopeful outcomes but one that is also well grounded in our own clinical knowledge, prior professional experience, and belief that change within the family system is indeed possible. By being direct, empathetic, and nonjudgmental, we become a holding environment for stressed caregivers, creating a place of safety, confidentiality, consistency, and support. Finally, we offer our clients a model of perseverance. By not giving up on the possibility of positive change and by exploring all options, the GCM enables families to feel that, regardless of the outcome, they have done all that they can to support the elder.

Role Conflicts for the GCM and Difficult Family

Every GCM–client relationship requires the GCM to consider who the client is and to examine what the GCM can realistically advocate for and accomplish on the client's behalf. With the difficult family, these questions can become very troublesome.

Who Is the Client?

GCMs are rarely retained directly by an elder; instead, families or third parties retain a GCM to directly advocate on behalf of the elder. This arrangement raises numerous questions: Is the elder the client? Or is it the concerned family member who initiated contact? What if another family member signs the fee agreement? Sometimes a GCM is hired by a lawyer or other professional acting as the elder's guardian or attorney-in-fact. Who then is the client? Regardless of the legal implications of the contractual relationship, the author contends that, in all instances, the interests of the elder should be placed ahead of other interested parties. That is not to say that we can disregard the interests or viewpoints of family members and paying parties. On the contrary, recognizing that the elder is a part of a larger family system means that we must consider the interests of all parts of that system. However, the needs of the elder and the wishes of the family may be in conflict, which causes tension in our dual role in advocating for the elder and addressing the concerns of the family.

CASE STUDY

Case Example: Mr. Homebody

Barry Burnout contacts a GCM for assistance with nursing home placement for his 87-year-old father, Mr. Homebody, who has Parkinson's disease. Pursuant to a fee agreement signed by Mr. Burnout, the GCM conducts an initial assessment and concludes that, with increased in-home care and careful monitoring, Mr. Homebody's strong preference to remain in his own home can be safely accomplished. When the GCM shares her recommendation with Mr. Burnout, he reacts angrily. He tells the GCM that, after 5 years of caring for his father, he is exhausted, and he thinks his father's desire is not realistic. Mr. Burnout reminds the GCM that he is the one paying for services and that he retained her specifically for assistance with nursing home placement.

This represents the classic dilemma: Is Mr. Homebody the client, or is the client his exhausted son Barry? This conflict can be avoided only through a careful discussion at the outset of the GCM's representation. The GCM needs to have discussed with Barry—prior to entering into a fee arrangement—exactly what the GCM's own role would be as a professional, independent evaluator of Mr. Homebody's care needs. The GCM should have also discussed the fact that her professional assessment would have to include consideration of alternatives to Barry's preference for nursing home placement. On the other hand, the GCM cannot responsibly neglect the burned-out feelings of the son. Any successful care management plan has to take into account Barry's own circumstances at this stage of family development.

Who Is Being Difficult?

GCMs often advocate for families that have already been branded as difficult by other institutions, such as nursing homes or assisted living facilities. These families often retain the GCM when they are in active conflict with the institution. In these circumstances, the GCM must walk a fine line between advocating for a family that has truly been wronged versus representing a family that is unrealistic and overly demanding in its expectations. The GCM's investigative and assessment skills must come into play, and the sensitivity with which the GCM reports his or her recommendations to the family will determine the success of any intervention.

CASE STUDY

Case Example: Mrs. Lovely

Mrs. Lovely recently moved to a memory impairment unit in an assisted living facility. She initially adjusted quickly to her new life, and her daughter, Caring Carrie, was very pleased with the facility.

A month later, Carrie visits Mrs. Lovely and finds her sitting at the window, unresponsive to Carrie's questions. Her mother was not dressed or bathed. Carrie quickly notices that her mother had not taken her time-sensitive medications that day.

When Carrie asks the staff about her mother's condition, no one can explain why her medications were not administered properly that day. Carrie is upset, and she requests a meeting with the facility's administrator. The administrator politely tells Carrie that, as far as he knows, his staff are doing their best. Furthermore, he tells Carrie that he thinks someone did check on Mrs. Lovely that day but that she refused to get dressed or take her medications. He suggests that Carrie consider hiring a private companion to provide Mrs. Lovely with the additional care that the facility does not provide.

Carrie feels it is the facility's responsibility to work with her mother's resistance and to notify Carrie when there is a problem. She is angry and frustrated, and she retains a GCM to contact the facility on her behalf. When the GCM meets with the administrator, he describes the daughter as overinvolved and anxious, and he feels that she does not fully understand the limitations of what an assisted living facility can provide.

Is Carrie overinvolved in her mother's care? Or is she advocating responsibly for her frail mother? The GCM must do a thorough investigation of the incident from all vantages: she must look at what Mrs. Lovely's actual needs are, what Carrie's expectations are, and what the facility is able to provide. If Carrie is unrealistic about either her mother's care needs or the facility's resources, the GCM needs to reestablish appropriate expectations and facilitate improved communication. On the other hand, the administrator's somewhat dismissive response to Carrie may be a red flag. Does the facility have established protocols for dealing with resistant residents on the memory impairment unit? Did the administrator adequately investigate Carrie's concern? What is the basis for his suggestion that Carrie is overinvolved? The GCM's investigation must account for these types of questions. But no matter what recommendation the GCM ultimately makes, he or she needs to acknowledge the daughter's anxiety and validate her concerns in the face of her mother's decline.

Setting Limits

The familiar boundaries between professional and client are easily tested when the GCM works with the difficult family. Limit setting, both as to time and professional involvement, are essential precisely because the effectiveness of the GCM can be compromised if the GCM becomes, in effect, a part or extension of the dysfunctional family system. Signs that the GCM is losing appropriate boundaries include the following:

- **Overidentification:** Although it is professionally necessary to understand and empathize with the emotional realities of the family or the client, it is not appropriate for the GCM to routinely share details of one's own emotional story or personal history. Whereas some sharing may be effective, the GCM should be on guard against overidentification.
- **Overconsolation:** As helping professionals, it is in our own nature to want to take away our client's pain. The GCM should guide and strategize with the client or the family, but should not expect—or be expected—to erase the difficulties they face. The GCM can alleviate, but not eliminate, the difficult family's burdens.

- GCMs cannot always please the client. The GCM needs to be honest and direct, and sometimes the GCM may have a recommendation that the family may not be prepared to hear. The manner in which the GCM shares his or her recommendation is a matter of clinical judgment, but the GCM should not withhold information to please a difficult client or prevent discomfort.
- **Overinvestment in strategy:** It is easy to become too invested in one's own strategy. The care plan is a dynamic intervention that must evolve as family circumstances change. The GCM should always remain flexible and resist the temptation to adhere to a favored, original strategy.
- **Overinvestment of time:** GCMs often make themselves available on a 24-hour basis for client crises. It is important to carve out personal time so that the GCM does not blend personal and work lives. Failure to honor the distinction can eventually lead to professional burnout.

■ CONCLUSION

It is intrinsic to geriatric care management that we intervene in family matters that are innately complex and emotionally poignant. Our intervention frequently occurs during a family crisis. Even a healthy family that is able to mobilize resources and work cooperatively faces daunting tasks in negotiating appropriate care for the elder while maintaining emotional balance. For the dysfunctional family that is less emotionally equipped for these tasks, the path to resolution is perilous.

This chapter has explored the concepts of filial maturity and generational maturity because they provide a useful framework for our active interventions with all families. By rejecting the notion of role reversal and, instead, emphasizing dependence as a normal and expected stage of late-life family development, we can help family members mature into new roles defined by filial reciprocity and mutual caring. In this way, the family supports the strengths of the elder, rather than focusing on the elder's fragilities or deficits. Recognizing the elder as a complete person who can provide and accept care will reward healthy and difficult families alike.

■ REFERENCES

1. Sandmaier M. Oldest rifts. *Fam Ther Network.* 1998;22:23–31.

2. Hargrave TD, Anderson WT. Finishing well: a context family therapy approach to the aging family. In: Hanna SM, Hargrave TD, eds. *The Aging Family.* New York, NY: Brunner/Mazel; 1997:61–80.

3. Kuttner R, Trotter S. *Family Re-Union.* New York, NY: The Free Press; 2002.

4. Blazer D. *Emotional Problems in Later Life: Intervention Strategies for Professional Caregivers.* New York, NY: Springer; 1998.

5. Fowler L. Understanding and strengthening healthy relationships between adult children and parents. August 2004. http://ohioline.osu.edu/flm99/fs04.html. Accessed June 15, 2005.

6. Karen R. *The Forgiving Self.* New York, NY: Doubleday; 2001.

7. Lowy L. Independence and dependence in aging: a new balance. *J Gerontol Soc Work.* 1989;13:133–146.

8. Erlanger MA. Changing roles and life-cycle transitions. In: Hanna SM, Hargrave TD, eds. *The Aging Family.* New York, NY: Brunner/Mazel; 1997:163–177.

9. Blenkner M. Social work and family relationships in later life with some thoughts on filial maturity. In: Shanas E, Streib G, eds. *Social Structure and the Family: Generational Relations.* Englewood Cliffs, NJ: Prentice Hall; 1965:46–59.

10. Shulman S. The changing nature of family relationships in middle and later life: parent-caring and the mid-life developmental opportunity. *Smith College Studies in Soc Work.* 2005;75(2):103–120.

11. Greenberg S. Mutuality in families: a framework for continued growth in late life. *J Geriatr Psychiatr Neurol.* 1994;27:79–95.

12. Silver M. Caring and being cared for in old age: the development of mutual parenting. In: Demick J, Burkik K. *Parental Development.* Hillsdale, NJ: Lawrence Erlbaum Associates; 1993.

13. Cox C. Families and the frail elderly. In: *The Frail Elderly: Problems, Needs, and Community Responses.* Westport, CT: Auburn House; 1993.

14. Felder R, Beauchamp D. Working with the problematic client. *Geriatric Care Manage J.* 1995;5(2):12–18.

15. Bowen M. *Family Therapy in Clinical Practice.* New York, NY: Jason Aronson; 1978.

16. Shulman L. *The Skills of Helping Individuals, Families, and Groups.* Itasca, IL: F.E. Peacock Publishers; 1992.

Chapter 22

Mediation and Geriatric Care Management

Dana Curtis

■ INTRODUCTION

The Purpose of This Chapter

The time will come when a GCM will encounter families whose conflict prevents decision-making altogether and despite the GCM's best efforts, it becomes impossible to serve the family. In other cases, a GCM will encounter conflict that casts the GCM in the role of trying to help the family as an *accidental mediator*. In the impossible cases, referring the family to a professional mediator who has been specifically trained to work with geriatric care issues—an intentional mediator—may enable the family to work more effectively with the GCM and with one another. This chapter explores both accidental and intentional mediation, to give the GCM a basic understanding of mediation theory, mediator skills, and a mediator's critical personal qualities. The chapter addresses the following purposes:

1. Enable GCMs to become more effective accidental mediators, who can understand and use basic mediator tools, and cultivate the critical personal qualities needed to better assist families in making important decisions.
2. Allow GCMs to recognize cases in which mediation is advisable and to make skillful referrals to professional mediators.
3. Explain how GCMs can become intentional mediators who offer professional mediation services to adult families that are distinct from their GCM services.

At the outset, it is important to emphasize what this chapter is *not* designed to do. Although it will provide information about mediation, it will not teach GCMs to become competent, professional mediators. As cautioned in Chapter 20, "Geriatric Care Management: Working with Nearly Normal Aging Families," becoming a competent, professional mediator who can work with geriatric care issues is serious business. The special expertise of the professional adult-family and elder mediator requires considerable training and experience in both geriatric care management and mediation.

The Accidental Mediator and the Intentional Mediator

Although becoming a professional mediator demands years of training and experience, life provides us all with opportunities to help other people with their conflicts: parents with their children and children with parents; teachers with students; and, apropos of this book, GCMs with adult family members. So the accidental mediator is born. A basic understanding of intentional mediation enhances the effectiveness of the accidental mediator when these opportunities arise.

Mediation Defined

Mediation is a voluntary process in which the parties, with the help of an impartial third party mediator, work together to resolve their differences or solve a problem they were unable to address satisfactorily without help. The mediation process is built on the following pillars:

- **Voluntariness:** Participation in mediation must be consensual.
- **Self-determination:** The parties themselves will determine the outcome.
- **Confidentiality:** Mediation is private, and in most US jurisdictions the conversations and any documents created for mediation may not be used in subsequent legal proceedings.[1]
- **Impartiality:** The mediator must truly sit in the middle, metaphorically, and does not have a stake in the outcome. The mediator does not influence the parties or the process by taking sides or advocating for a particular outcome.

■ CONFLICT IN THE AGING FAMILY

As Emily B. Saltz emphasizes in Chapter 21, Difficult Families: Conflict, Dependence, and Mutuality, all families are unique, including in their ability to collaborate on decisions as older family members transition from independence to dependence. In general, nearly normal families described in Chapter 20, Geriatric Care Management: Working with Nearly Normal Aging Families, are close-knit, well integrated, highly functioning, and sufficiently resilient. These family members can communicate well enough with a GCM's help that they can make wise decisions about complex problems. Nearly normal families accept differences of opinion as inevitable and a normal part of decision making or, in some cases, as opportunities to expand their individual thinking, thereby enabling them to make better-informed decisions. They lock arms to

address the problems they encounter, such as in Figure 22–1.

Difficult families, on the other hand, lack this capacity. As described in Chapter 21, they tend to have more of the following qualities:

- Conflictual rather than compatible
- Fragmented rather than cohesive
- Nonproductive rather than productive
- Fragile rather than stable
- Rigid rather than flexible

These families, at best, simply cannot collaborate and, at worst, actively compound an already difficult decision with intractable interpersonal conflict that creates additional difficulty independent of the decision that brought them together in the first place. Instead of viewing the decision as a problem to be solved together with locked arms, they pit themselves against one another, assume they are right and others are wrong and assume the roles of adversaries in their individual quests to solve the problem (see Figure 22–2).

The extent of a family's ability to collaborate on decision making about elders is the pri-

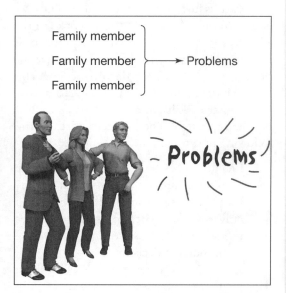

Figure 22–1　Family Members Lock Arms to Address Problems

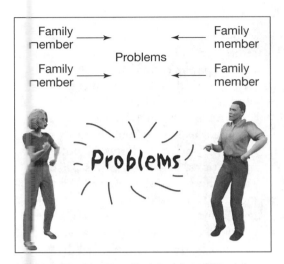

Figure 22-2   Family Members Pitted against One Another

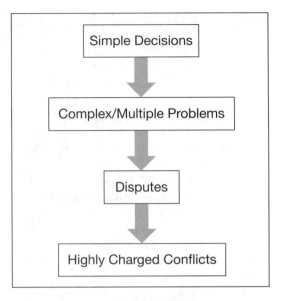

Figure 22-3   Complexity of the Problem and Intensity of the Conflict Continuum

mary variable in the equation of how much assistance a family requires. Additional important variables are the combined factors of problem complexity and the degree to which family members disagree (see Figure 22-3).

Clearly the degree of complexity of the problem and the degree of difficulty of the family are in direct proportion to the need for assistance of a mediator, as illustrated in Figure 22-4.

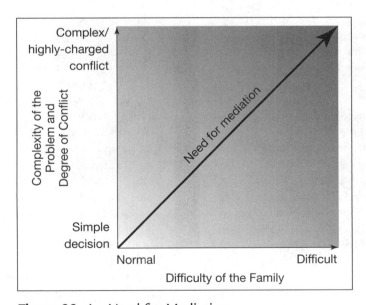

Figure 22-4   Need for Mediation

CASE STUDY

With this equation in mind, consider the Responsible and the Sniper families. Ruby Responsible grew concerned about her 88-year-old father, Richard, whose health and cognitive ability had declined during the past year, following her mother's death. She broached her concern with her brother Robert. Their parents had lived a healthy, safe, and independent life, so Ruby and Robert had no experience with elder care challenges. As they began to struggle with how to raise the issue with their father and assist him in determining what to do, a family friend suggested they consult a GCM to assess Richard and the situation and help the three of them to make this critical decision.

By contrast, in the Sniper family, Suzi grew concerned about her 88-year-old father, Steve, for the same reasons Ruby worried about her dad. Suzi concluded Steve could no longer live safely in the family home in San Francisco with her brother Sam, who was unemployed ("for the umpteenth time") and who was acting as Steve's caregiver. Attributing Steve's precipitous decline to his social isolation and poor nutrition, Suzi resolved to move him into her home in Utah, where, she believed, his interaction with her, her husband, and their three young grandchildren would lift his spirits and "keep him young."

Brother Sam, not surprisingly, balked at the idea. He felt he needed to be living with his father in the family home, where Steve would be happiest. He was in familiar surroundings, had access to his old friends and doctors, and was taken care of by his loving son Sam. After an initial angry outburst when Suzi informed Sam of her decision, Sam cut off all communication with Suzi. He

would not answer her telephone calls or return her many messages. After a week of no communication, Suzi drove to California, staked out at her father's house until Sam left, and then let herself in. She convinced her father to move to Utah to live with her. Before Sam returned, she packed Steve's clothing, medications, and a few of his personal effects and loaded him into the car, intending to drive him to Utah. As she was pulling out of the driveway, Sam returned. A screaming match ensued and ended when Steve told Sam he was in favor of the move.

Once in Utah, according to Suzi, Steve seemed happier. He and Suzi's family had numerous family outings and dinners at great restaurants. But rather than gain strength and mental abilities, his condition continued to deteriorate. After a couple of months, he had trouble paying his bills, so he added Suzi as signatory to his account. Within three months, he developed a respiratory infection. Suzi took him to her physician, who hospitalized him and thereafter discharged him to a convalescent hospital. The physician suggested Suzi consult a GCM to assess Steve and recommend appropriate placement and care going forward. Suzi called a GCM named Ms. Sortitout. (More to come about this consultation.)

In the meantime, Steve believed he was being discharged from the hospital to a nursing home and became enraged at Suzi for refusing to take him to her home. He called Sam and complained that he was miserable and desperate to return to San Francisco. He told Sam he would rather die at home than to waste away in an old folk's home. He also let on that he was worried about running out of money, telling Sam that at the rate he was writing checks to Suzi and paying her bills, he was afraid he would empty his bank account. He also intimated that Suzi was taking money from his banking and investment accounts and charging her household expenses to his charge cards.

Sam became increasingly worried about Steve's health and happiness, as well as Suzi's possible exploitation, if not financial abuse. Taking a page from Suzi's book, Sam swooped in, packed his father up, and drove him back home to San Francisco, without going through the facility's discharge procedures. In the rush to leave, Sam forgot Steve's medications. When the staff discovered that Steve was missing, they called Suzi and reported the potential elder abuse incident to Adult Protective Services (APS). Once APS came on the scene, what once appeared to be a straightforward, practical question of where Steve should live expanded into the following series of legal and medical issues:

- Did Sam kidnap Steve?
- Did Suzi kidnap Steve?
- Did Sam neglect Steve, and was he guilty of elder abuse?
- Did Suzi kidnap Steve, and was she guilty of elder abuse?
- Does Steve lack the mental capacity to make decisions about his care?
- Does he lack mental capacity to make decisions about his finances and property?
- Can Sam reside in Steve's home—and who can decide this issue?
- Did Suzi financially abuse Steve by borrowing money from him and using his credit cards to buy groceries and household items for her family, and was she criminally or civilly liable?

The following are reflection questions for you to consider about the Snipers and Responsibiles:

1. If the Responsibles had called you instead of Ms. Sortitout for GCM assessments and consultations, would you have had any reservations about working with either of them? Why or why not?
2. Would you have had reservations about working with the Snipers? How would you respond if Suzi called you, instead of Ms. Sortitout, during the following situations:
   a. When her physician suggested consulting a GCM?
   b. Before she took Steve to Utah to live with her?
   c. After Sam took him back to San Francisco?
   d. After APS became involved?
3. Do you think it would be appropriate for Ms. Sortitout to recommend mediation for the Sniper case at any of the above junctures? Why or why not?

■ MEDIATION BASICS

Mediation vs Facilitation

Although sometimes used interchangeably, the terms *mediation* and *facilitation* refer to different processes. Broadly stated, facilitation is a meeting management skill, while mediation is a process of assisting parties to resolve a conflict. In facilitation, a neutral facilitator enables a group to make decisions and accomplish a task by guiding them in effective communication processes. The facilitator maintains a collaborative and respectful environment that encourages full participation and helps the group overcome barriers to achieving its goals.[2]

GCMs frequently serve as facilitators of family meetings, assuming the role of meeting leaders. They may create agendas for meetings, ensure that all participants have the opportunity to be heard and to understand one another, and otherwise keep order so the family can come to a wise decision. Although differences of opinions are commonplace, which requires facilitation skills to keep the discussions on track, in most cases, family meetings do not require the skills of a mediator to address conflict. However, an aware GCM can incorporate some mediator techniques into GCM practice.

The Mediation Process

Mediation and Negotiation

At a fundamental level, mediation can be understood as a facilitated negotiation. We are required to negotiate whenever we are unable to get what we need without the cooperation of someone else. We negotiate with our neighbor to rebuild our garage after his tree fell on it, because we are unwilling to pay the entire cost ourselves. If we are unable to agree, we may suggest mediation, rather than hiring a lawyer to sue our neighbor.

Any successful negotiation unfolds through a well-defined process. The parties in a negotiation know the subject matter of the negotiation and at the outset exchange information about the situation, how they each see it, what is important or of concern to them, and what they need. They next identify available options and, if necessary, gather information about them. They evaluate the options, examining how well they meet their needs or address their concerns, and discuss the options to reach agreement on the best solution. Finally, they figure out how to implement their agreement.

To illustrate how a successful negotiation would proceed, consider the nearly normal Responsible family that needs to reach an agreement about Richard's care and living situation. Here's how the negotiation might unfold. Ruby expresses her concern about

Richard to Robert. Although initially Robert does not share Ruby's concern, he recognizes he may be missing some important information and becomes curious about Ruby's point of view. He also suggests they raise the issue with Richard directly, but after hearing that Ruby would like to seek the guidance of a GCM first, he agrees with her.

Ruby calls Ms. Sortitout, a GCM. In consultation with the GCM, they create a plan for talking with their father Richard. They first ask Richard to meet with Ms. Sortitout, who will assess Richard's abilities and needs. He resists at first, but relents once he understands how worried his children have become. At the meeting, the Responsibles exchange information about their perspectives and talk about their concerns and needs. They listen to Ms. Sortitout's analysis and suggestions about how to address their concerns. They also list the options they have considered—doing nothing, moving Richard into an assisted living facility, and hiring a caregiver. They also create some new options—making changes in Richard's routine, allocating responsibility for taking him on outings a few times a week, and looking into Meals on Wheels. They next discuss the options that seem most interesting and doable to them and analyze how well each option addresses their needs and concerns. Ultimately, they agree to investigate Meals on Wheels and services available at a local senior center. They also agree that Richard will have dinner with each of his children at least once a week. They agree that Ms. Sortitout will do a full assessment of Richard and his home, and the family will meet again in a month to hear Ms. Sortitout's report. At that time, they will see if their plan is addressing their concerns and meeting their needs and, if necessary, revisit the decisions they made. The thing to notice in this scenario is that Ms. Sortitout can apply mediator techniques long before deciding to recommend mediation.

The Structure of Mediation

As we will discuss more fully later in this chapter, the mediation process varies widely, depending on the mediator and the situation, but like skillful negotiation, mediation also follows a well-defined process. For the purposes of this chapter, we will present a generic mediation model that places a high priority on the parties' understanding one another's views and actively working together directly to resolve their differences. This approach to mediation divides the process into four phases:

1. Structuring
2. Understanding the problem
3. Focusing on solutions
4. Concluding

Each phase defines the sphere of the conversation, thereby creating a container for the parties' discussions. Each phase involves both process and content goals. Content, or substantive, goals consist of *what* the parties will want to accomplish, that is, the concrete matters they will address in each phase. Process goals relate to *how* they will work together.

Phase 1: Structuring the Mediation. Structuring focuses on the mediation process itself and agreements about working together. The mediator, in conversation with the parties, helps the parties decide on the best structure for the mediation, which will vary with every situation. Mediation's inherent flexibility makes it particularly useful for the wide variations in the needs of families. As part of the structuring phase, the parties and the mediator discuss the purpose of the mediation and the motivations of the parties, the roles of the parties and the mediator, the outline of the issues on the agenda for the session, how long the meeting will last, and any communication agreements the parties have made.

In terms of further process goals, an effective structuring phase builds the trust of the parties in the mediator, as well as of the parties in one another, and sets an optimistic tone by suggesting a positive outcome.

Phase 2: Understanding the Problem. Once the parties understand and agree on a structure for the mediation, they move to phase two, where the content goal is achieving understanding of the situation, both past (when relevant) and present; their feelings about it; and the impact it has on them. They also develop an understanding of the needs, interests, and concerns that are implicated in any decisions they will be making.

As for *how* they work together in phase two, the goal is for the mediator to demonstrate understanding, as described below in the section on empathy, and help the parties to do the same.

Phase 3: Focusing on Solutions. The content goals of phase three are to develop substantive and procedural agreements that will allow the parties to solve the problems that bring them to mediation. Agreements can be substantive (e.g., agreeing to hire a particular caregiver) or procedural (e.g., agreeing on a process the family will follow to hire a caregiver), such as delegating the responsibility to a family member or the GCM. The tried-and-true approach to finding solutions is brainstorming, which involves the following steps:

1. Identify and clarify options for potential solutions (without evaluating them).
2. Evaluate the options by analyzing how adequately they address the parties' needs, interests, and concerns that the parties expressed earlier.
3. Create procedural or substantive agreements that best accomplish the parties' goals and satisfy their needs, interests, and concerns.

Sometimes parties are not prepared to enter into agreements. They may need to think about the options, consult with other family members, gather additional information, or otherwise investigate further. In this case, they return to the structuring phase of mediation and adjust that structure, perhaps agreeing to allocate responsibility among the group or to consult with physicians, GCMs, or financial or legal experts before reconvening to resume their negotiation.

The process goals in this phase of focusing on solutions are to demonstrate understanding and, in addition, encourage participants to persevere, even when tension develops and no easy answer emerges. In other words, the mediator maintains optimism and patience and encourages the participants to trust the mediation process and the mediator in the search for solutions.

Phase 4: Concluding. Quality, clarity, certainty, and commitment are the fundamental goals of the concluding phase. Parties may be tempted to leave the mediation right after they agree on a solution, ignoring the tasks of this phase. Particularly in adult family or elder mediations, doing so is risky. These mediations often involve multiple issues. Given the normal challenging family dynamics and the often-flimsy level of trust, it is risky to leave without clarity about the substance of the agreement, timing of its implementation, and a plan for implementing it.

At a minimum, family members should put their agreements in writing at the conclusion of the session or ask the mediator to summarize the agreements for their review immediately following the session. There should be an understanding that they will each review the summary and work with the mediator until the summary is accurate from everyone's point of view.

Regarding process goals of the concluding phase, the mediator is aware of the quality of the parties' relationship and strives to achieve a level of generosity of spirit to the degree appropriate, given the circumstances.

The following chart in Figure 22–5 summarizes the mediation phases.

Mediation Tools

A masterful mediator spends hundreds of hours in training and an entire career gathering tools, refining the ability to use them, honing instincts for selecting them, and developing the fine art of timing for their use. Although the mediator toolbox eventually contains scores of tools, every successful mediator begins with three essential skills and relies on them consistently. Before describing them, let's consider a situation in which a GCM who is an accidental mediator may find them to be useful.

Francie Functional and her mother Flora have always had a close relationship, even though Francie moved 500 miles from Flora after graduating from college 40 years ago. Over the past several visits with Flora, Francie became increasingly concerned that Flora, becoming gradually more frail and forgetful, should no longer live by herself. Flora met Francie's efforts to initiate a thoughtful conversation about the situation with an uncustomary refusal to discuss the subject of moving. Francie called a GCM. Ultimately, Flora agreed to sit down with Francie and the GCM to discuss the situation.

Structuring. Mediators generally use the communication skill of *structuring* at the outset of the mediation process to paint a picture of how the mediation will proceed. Structuring as a communication skill is distinct from the structuring *phase,* which is the first stage in the mediation process. It is an in-the-moment communication technique for keeping any conversation moving forward in a clear, thoughtful, and understandable way. Mediators use the skill of structuring throughout mediation to introduce each new phase in the process and keep the discussions on track. Structuring serves the following purposes:

Phase 1: Structuring

Content:

Describe process: Mediator's role, parties' role, overview of session
Identify parties' goal(s): Purpose and motivation for participating
Establish ground rules: Confidentiality and communication guidelines

Process: Establish rapport and trust; set optimistic tone.

Phase 2: Understanding Different Views

Content:

Understand each participant's perspective:
- The situation, feelings, impact
- Needs, interests, and concerns

Process: Mediator and/or other participants demonstrate understanding.

Phase 3: Focusing on Solutions

Content:

Work on substantive or procedural agreements:
- Identify and clarify options for potential solutions (without evaluating).
- Evaluate the options in reference to the parties' needs, interests, and concerns.
- Create agreements that best address parties' needs, interests, and concerns in the future.

Gather additional information, if necessary: Options, finances

Process: Mediator practices patience and encourages participants to persevere; mediator and/or participants demonstrate understanding.

Phase 4: Concluding

Content:

Test agreements: Regarding goals and for stability, durability, and commitment
Summarize, clarify, and refine agreements.
Determine timeline for implementing agreements.
Determine next steps.
Oversee memorandum of agreement/understanding or follow-up in writing.
Conduct check-ins, scheduled or spontaneous.

Process: Notice feeling tone, encourage generosity of spirit.

Figure 22–5   Overview of the Mediation Process

- Educate participants about the process
- Build rapport and trust between the mediator and the participants
- Lower the participants' anxiety
- Enable the process to proceed efficiently

Structuring consists of the following three components:

1. Purpose: Summarizing the parties' objectives or goals for the mediation
2. Process: Providing a picture of how the meeting will proceed (along with the rationale), including:
   a. The roles of the mediator and the participants
   b. The agenda
   c. Communication guidelines
3. Agreement: Eliciting agreement to follow the structure.

Let's sit in on the beginning of the mediation between Flora and Francie Functional to see how Ms. Sortitout, their GCM and accidental mediator, employs mediator tools and structures the meeting.

1. **Purpose:** Ms. Sortitout: "Welcome. I am happy to be able to help you today to have this important conversation about Flora's living situation. I understand that by the end of this 2-hour meeting, you hope to make a decision about where Flora will live and the care she will need to give her the maximum control over her life, while keeping her safe and healthy. Is that right? Did I miss anything in this description? If you accomplish this goal, will both of you meet your expectation of a successful meeting?"

   Flora: "That's right. I have been a nervous wreck ever since this whole conversation started. I do want my freedom, but I also recognize I need to be safe, for myself and for Francie's peace of mind."

   Francie: "Yes, that is what we are here for. Mom, I want you to be happy, too, and I am glad we are having this conversation today."

2. **Process:**
   a. **The roles:**
   Ms. Sortitout: "Francie and Flora, you each have two equally important tasks during this meeting. The first is to say what is 'so' for you, to let each other know what the situation looks like from your vantage point, and, especially, to inform each other about what is important to you. The second is to listen for the purpose of *understanding* each other, even though you may not be *agreeing*. The quality of listening in mediation is unlike what we normally do when we have differences of opinion. We normally argue or try to convince the other person that we are right and the other is wrong. Here, I am asking each of you to work hard to educate each other, as opposed to debate each other.

   "I want to help you achieve your objective to reach a decision about Flora's care and living situation. I'll do this in a number of ways. I'll pay attention to whether we are following the agenda. I'll also help you listen to each other for the purpose of understanding, not debating. And, because you asked me to convey what I learned during my assessment of Flora, I'll share that with you. I'll also provide you with information about specific options you have identified as well as others that I have found during my research."

   Flora: "That sounds very helpful."

   b. **The agenda:**
   Ms. Sortitout next introduces the agenda:

   Ms. Sortitout: "Before we start, I would like to suggest an agenda. First, I propose the two of you, in turn, talk about what matters most to you. What do you want the other to keep in mind as you make decisions about Flora's living situation? What do you worry about? What do you need? What do you hope for? Next, I will tell you about my earlier assessment and answer any questions you have about it. Then, we can talk about options and, after that, discuss how well they meet the needs or address the concerns you expressed earlier. At that point, if you are ready to make a decision, you can do so, and then we will make a plan for implementing it. Did I leave anything out? Does that sound like a good way to work on this decision?"

Francie: "Yes, very good."

Flora: "I am fine with that."

Ms. Sortitout: "Good. Then let's get started."

c. **Communication guidelines:**

Ms. Sortitout: "Do you have any suggestions about how to ensure this is a good conversation? Do you have any requests of each other that will make it easier for you to say what is important to you or hear what each other has to say?"

Flora: "I just want Francie to listen to me. She has always been so good at listening until she started in on moving. Now, I feel like I am talking to a brick wall."

Francie: "That's interesting. I have been feeling the same way, like you aren't listening to *me*."

Ms. Sortitout: "So, it would be helpful for me to slow you both down and make sure you are really understanding each other? And perhaps an agreement that you let each other talk without interrupting? Do you agree?"

Flora and Francie: "Yes."

Ms. Sortitout: "It also seems like it would be a good idea to learn from each other what you are actually *hearing,* especially when you are speaking about what matters to you most. I can help you do that, too. What do you think?"

Flora and Francie: "Please do."

Ms. Sortitout: "And, just to be clear, may we all assume you are here because you want to learn more about each other, in addition to being able to talk about your own point of view?"

Flora: "Yes, I am."

Francie: "Me, too. I want Mother to know I care what she wants and what she thinks. And to do that I need to make sure I understand, so I will appreciate your help."

3. **Agreement to the structure:**

Ms. Sortitout: "Is there anything else? Are you okay with this plan? Are we ready to go?"

Flora and Francie: "Yes, let's begin."

Consider the following reflection questions on the use of the mediation skills you just heard.

1. How do you think Ms. Sortitout's structuring affected the tone of the meeting and the quality of the conversation between Flora and Francie that followed? Explain.

2. Do you think Ms. Sortitout accomplished the goals of structuring, outlined above, in this situation? Were some of the goals met more effectively or completely than others? For example, do you think structuring made for a more efficient meeting? Was it worth the extra time it took to have the structuring discussion?

3. What problems do you think Ms. Sortitout anticipated, and what did she do to prevent or minimize them?

4. Ms. Sortitout chose to have a conversation with Francie and Flora about their communication, rather than laying down ground rules (such as no interrupting). What are the advantages of having this conversation rather than setting ground rules? What are the disadvantages?

Empathy. Empathy, or the ability to understand the situational and emotional experience of another, goes to the very heart of conflict resolution. More than an essential tool, it is a mediator's power tool. And, it turns out, it comes naturally; we humans are hardwired for it. Our brains contain neurons designed to connect with the same type of neurons in the brains of others and mirror them, thereby enabling us to understand another person's experience.[3]

To use empathy as a communication skill and mediator tool, however, requires not only understanding the experience of another, but also demonstrating that understanding by listening carefully and then summarizing both the facts of the external situation and the feelings and personal meaning of the other person's experience. Merely saying, "I understand" or "I understand how you feel" doesn't unleash the power of empathy. Empathy requires the listener to restate *what* the listener understands. Empathy also differs from pity (e.g., "You poor thing.") and sympathy (e.g., "I am sorry your family is going through such a difficult experience."). These both focus on the *listener's* feeling (sorrow), rather than on what the listener perceives as the *speaker's* feelings.[4] A mediator's use of empathy is like an artist's use of paint. A mediator listens, then uses empathy to paint a word picture of what the mediator understands the speaker's experience to be. By showing that word picture to the speaker and listening to the speaker's reaction, the mediator learns if the listener painted the picture accurately. If not, the work on the word painting continues until the speaker is satisfied that the mediator understands.

Although empathy is a complex skill, requiring "a high level of cognitive and emotional maturity," and requiring study and unending practice, it is also straightforwardly simple.[5] To listen well, we need two ingredients: intention to understand the speaker's experience, and attention, which we focus entirely on the speaker.

Intention. The power of intention cannot be overstated. An essential Buddhist teaching holds that all action springs from intention. Negotiation theorists have identified stated intention as a powerful tool of persuasion, which they have named commitment and consistency bias. Research confirms that we are far more likely to do something if we have told someone else we will do it.[6] Car salespersons know this principle well. That is why one of the first things they do when potential buyers walk onto the lot is to confirm the buyers' intention to drive off the lot with a new car *today*.

In the context of listening, the intention to understand the experience of another enables us over and over to bring our attention back from the conversations in our head to the conversations in the room. Our intention can serve as our walking stick, helping us regain our balance and keep on the listening path when we stumble.

Returning to the Responsible family and the family meeting with Robert, Ruby, and Richard, we find them in phase two, understanding the problem, which unfolds as follows, when Ms. Sortitout makes skillful use of empathy:

Ms. Sortitout: "You agree that before making a decision about where Richard lives, it will help to understand the situation from each of your points of view: what is important to you, what you worry about, what you need, and anything else you think would help you all make a good decision. Richard, would you begin?"

Richard: "I just don't understand what all the fuss is about. I know I am not like my old self, but I have had a year of missing your mother. We were together for 50 years. You just don't get over a loss like this overnight. I admit that I am slower than I used to be, but that is what happens when you get to be 88 years old. I'm not supposed to be jovial and running all over the place under these circumstances and at my age. I am right where I should be. I hope there is never a reason I should go to a nursing home, but for damn sure it isn't now. While I appreciate your concern for my welfare, I'm upset that you don't seem to hear that I'm OK."

Ms. Sortitout: "From where you sit, Ruby and Robert shouldn't be worried about you. As you grieve the loss of your wife, your mood and subdued lifestyle are appropriate. Also, you are 88 years old, and understandably are slowing down. You accept the possibility that you may not be able to live alone forever, but that is not the case right now. You don't understand what Ruby and Robert are so concerned about, and you're upset with them for not listening to you. Is that right? Do you think I get it?"

Attention. To listen well, we need to be present, to focus our attention fully on the other person. Our ability to be present is compromised by both external and internal distractions. The external environment, where we are free from interruptions and disturbulences, is far easier to control than our internal environment. We can schedule a time, turn off the phone, shut the door, and create a quiet space for conversation.

Mostly, our inability to be present with another person is the result of the noise of our mind, the silent conversations we have with ourselves about whether I am doing a good job, how much I dislike (or like) the client, who is right or wrong, how I might fix the problem, how I can get the clients to do what is good for them (often, what I think they should do), what I don't know, what we are having for dinner, how worried I am about my children, and on and on.

We will never eliminate internal noise, but we can become more effective at managing it. Although it is beyond the province of this chapter, the study and practice of mindfulness meditation, which is a lifelong pursuit of many people, both as a spiritual practice and as a mind-training or stress-reduction tool, is so important to mediation that some commentators see it as essential to mediation mastery.[7]

Reframing. Reframing could be called "empathy plus." It is useful when a party makes a critical, threatening, blaming, or otherwise unproductive statement. As with empathy, the mediator must first grasp the meaning of the communication. However, rather than reflecting precisely the problematic statement using empathy, which could escalate the conflict and derail the conversation, the mediator recasts it into a statement that stands a chance of enabling the parties to move forward. The reframed statement helps the speaker, as well as the other party, look at the problem in a more constructive way. The intentional mediator has learned and practiced scores of ways to reframe, but Figure 22–6 gives a few reframing ideas for the accidental mediator who wants to help family members move their conversations in a positive direction.

Mediator Personal Qualities

As either accidental or intentional mediators, who we are *as people* is arguably more important than what we *know* about mediation or what we *do* in the process. In *Bringing Peace into the Room: How the Personal Qualities of the Mediator Impact the Process of Conflict Resolution*, co-editors Daniel Bowling and David Hoffman propose that "when we are feeling at peace with ourselves and the world around us, we are better able to bring peace into the room."[8]

Bowling and Hoffman emphasize the fundamental personal quality of presence, which they describe as including being centered; being connected to one's governing values, beliefs, and highest purpose; making contact with the humanity of others; and being congruent.[3] Presence, they assert, does not exist as a stand-alone quality, but arises from the integration of a constellation of interrelated qualities that together enable an individual to be "... fully in touch with, and able to marshal, his or her spiritual, psychic, and physical resources, in the context of his or her relationship with other people and with his or her

Now that Frieda, the widowed mother of Freddy and Fiona Fighting, is failing mentally and physically, the Fighting family has called a meeting with a GCM to resolve numerous issues about Frieda's care and living situation. Included is whether Freddy, the family black sheep, should move into the family home and become Frieda's main caregiver. We enter the family meeting just as the GCM has asked the family to talk about this issue and what matters to them. Teary-eyed Freddy said he wants this last chance to "give back," to take good care of Mom in her twilight years to make up for all of the grief he has caused her. Fiona shouts, "You have to be kidding me! You? Mr. Irresponsible? You want to take care of Mother? What a crock! All you have ever wanted is a chance to freeload, Freddy. There is no way I am going to let that happen!"

Reflection Exercise

Before reading further:

1. Without thinking about it, write down what you would say in response to Fiona.
2. How do you think Fiona would react? What about Freddy and Frieda?
3. Now, consider what you would like your response to Fiona to accomplish, and form an intention to accomplish it.

4. Next, write down what you would say. Was your response different from the initial one? If so, what role do you think intention played? What else allowed you to respond more skillfully?

Instead of empathizing, as in "It infuriates you to hear Freddy say he wants to take care of your mother, because you think Freddy has always been looking for a way he can be supported and taken care of himself. And you are adamant that Freddy will not be taking care of your mother," you could reframe your response in the following ways:

- **From the past to the future:** "You are skeptical about Freddy's motives. He needs to demonstrate that his present motivation is different from the past situations in which he was looking to be supported by your mother, not to support her."
- **From the person to the problem:** "The family's decision about your mother's care must be based on faith that her caregiver will be able to care for her and not require her to take care of the caregiver."
- **From position to interest:** "Before you entrust anyone with your mother's care, you need to know, without reservation, that person would have her best interests, and not his or her own, at heart."

Figure 22–6   Employing the Tool of Reframing

surrounding environment."[8] Numerous commentators have speculated on the most important qualities for a good mediation; the mediation literature and mediation training materials are replete with laundry lists of mediator qualities that read like qualifications for sainthood. Mediators William E. Simkin and Nicholas A. Fidandis, tongue in cheek, listed the following essential qualities:

1. The patience of Job
2. The sincerity and bulldog characteristics of the English
3. The wit of the Irish

4. The physical endurance of a marathon runner
5. The broken-field dodging abilities of a halfback
6. The guile of Machiavelli
7. The personality-probing skills of a good psychiatrist
8. The hide of a rhinoceros
9. The wisdom of Solomon[10]

Based on the thousands of mediations I have conducted, I have identified the following five qualities I believe to be key in mediation. Not coincidentally, they are as important to being a good person as they are to being a good mediator.

Ease with Uncertainty, or Not Knowing

Not knowing is paradoxically anxiety-producing and liberating. In the midst of the most difficult conflict and entrenched disagreement, there comes a moment when even the most experienced mediator wonders whether the parties will be able to find their way to resolution. If the mediator acknowledges the uncertainty and relaxes into not knowing, the mediator retains the ability to be present. But when *wondering* turns to *worrying,* the mediator's attention moves from the present moment to thoughts of the future. Anticipating a failed mediation, the mediator may try to control the outcome by forcing a particular solution or taking sides. Worrying about whether the parties will settle their dispute may also trigger irrational self-doubt: "If the parties don't work it out, it must mean I am not a very good mediator; my reputation will be damaged; I won't get any more mediation business. . . ." This internal conversation not only robs the parties of the mediator's attention, it robs the mediator of the other qualities I describe below that encourage resolution.

Tolerance of Conflict and Paradox

Whereas being at ease with uncertainty requires the mediator to relax about the substantive outcome—the *what,* or whether the parties will work it out—tolerance of conflict and paradox requires the mediator to relax about the process, that is, how the parties interact. Mediators who respect the upside potential of conflict as a catalyst for more creative, better-informed decisions and greater intimacy actually welcome conflict. On the other hand, mediators who worry about conflict sacrifice presence and conflict's positive effects. Mediators who are uncomfortable in the midst of conflict risk becoming self-focused, leading to interventions designed to

make the mediator more comfortable instead of furthering the parties' process.

Curiosity

Curiosity is the elixir of mediation: the cure for blame and judgment, the enabler of not-knowing. With curiosity, certainty becomes inquiry and "I know" becomes "I wonder." "I don't like you" becomes "What don't I understand?" Curiosity not only opens minds, it opens doors—to connection, ideas, and solutions.

Optimism

Optimism grows from faith—faith in the process, in ourselves, in the parties, and in the resources that are available to support them. Parties usually come to mediation as a last resort. Long before, they have given up hope. Any optimism they once had has turned not just to pessimism, but often to fatalism. The mediator is probably the only person in the room who is hopeful. If the parties can't muster optimism about the process, at least an optimistic mediator can encourage them to be optimistic about the mediator's determination to be optimistic. This attitude, along with the mediator's persistence, may help them stay in the room long enough to resolve their dispute.

Self-Awareness

Without the awareness that we are paying more attention to the conversations in our head than we are to the ones in the room, it is impossible to remain present. The absence of self-awareness also vitiates the other qualities that support presence.

In addition to returning us to the present moment, self-awareness provides the objectivity required to evaluate our own effectiveness in the process, to notice whether our actions are making things better or worse. When we see ourselves as a participant in the process, we can make decisions about our own conduct in a way that is similar to how we guide the parties.

■ MEDIATION AS A PROFESSION: BECOMING AN INTENTIONAL MEDIATOR

Before offering mediation services as an intentional elder and adult family mediator, we strongly suggest: 1) a minimum of 5 years of practice as a GCM; 2) 100 hours of mediation training; and 3) extensive in-session experience in mediation (as described below in the "Mediation Training" section). The training GCMs receive and their experience with older people and their families provide GCMs with essential ingredients that non-GCM mediators do not have and must acquire through study, specialized training, and hands-on experience. Highly developed elder and adult family expertise combined with mastery in mediation are a potent recipe for a successful elder mediation practice, an exciting alternative career or a powerful adjunct to a GCM practice.

Developing a mediation career begins by learning about the mediation process and exploring whether there is a potential fit between you and a mediation career. Cathy Cress's advice in Chapter 12, that a GCM career spring from "your passion, your competence, and market opportunity" also applies to becoming a mediator.[11] Once there appears to be a fit, the GCM looks forward to a long, fulfilling learning journey and the challenge of building a practice.

Mediator Aptitude

The discussion above about the personal qualities needed to become a mediator lists five essential qualities; in real life, however, most mediators develop those qualities over time and through much practice and focus on their personal development. In considering whether to become a mediator, make the decision based not only on the degree to which you currently embody those five essential qualities, but also whether you are interested in *developing* those qualities. In addition, consider what others say about you. Have you been told you are a natural born mediator? Do you have a knack for helping people resolve their differences? Are you are a good listener? Are you a calming presence? This sort of feedback indicates you may have the temperament of a mediator, which is a sign you could be a good mediator. However, there is more to it than personality.

Mediation is not for the faint-hearted. In addition to natural inclination to mediation, remember good mediators are at ease with uncertainty, tolerant of conflict and paradox, curious, and optimistic. Now add these items to that checklist: able to analyze and organize challenging and disparate topics and points of view; comfortable helping people resolve differences not by telling them what to do, but by helping them solve their own problems; and sufficiently self-aware to understand when they are getting in the way or becoming part of the problem.

Before investing in mediation training, in addition to reflecting on whether you have the personality and abilities to be a good mediator, GCMs should get real-life experience with mediation, to see firsthand whether the work suits them. Attend mediation sessions with clients, observe mediation sessions conducted by experienced elder mediators, serve as a consultant in mediations, and volunteer in community mediation programs (more on this later).

Mediation Training

We suggest at least 100 hours of mediation training and an additional 50 hours working with experienced mediators or under their supervision. Training should include at least one basic 40-hour mediation training course and advanced training courses in elder mediation and other relevant subject matter areas, such as advanced communication skills, mediating with adult families, dealing with difficult personalities, or working with emotional conflict.

Good mediator training also includes more individualized learning experiences, including observations or shadowing, with the opportunity to interact with the mediator during or after the session and comediation with experienced mediators, allowing time to prepare and to debrief the session. Peer supervision groups, sometimes called practice groups, are also an excellent learning container. These groups bring together beginning and experienced mediators to reflect on their mediations and gain insight from one another. The best groups are led by someone with extensive experience both as a mediator and a teacher.

Locating mediation training is simple with the Internet. Searching online for "mediation training" will bring up hundreds of programs. Websites associated with mediation, such as Mediate.com, offer lists of programs. Experienced elder and adult family mediators are also good referral sources.

Because elder and adult family mediation is a relatively new field, there are not as many classes, seminars, and workshops to choose from and training may require travel. Nevertheless, avoid shortcutting this phase of training with a 1- or 2-day course. The complex nature of this practice deserves more time—at least 3 days, preferably 4. Tips for shopping for mediation training appear in Figure 22–7.

Choosing from among the hundreds of available mediation training programs can be challenging. Below are some shopping tips for basic mediation training courses:

1. Check out the training program website and the credentials of the trainers. Make sure the trainers are:
   a. Experienced trainers with at least 5 years experience providing mediation training, preferably with some academic experience to give them a background in mediation theory. Also check out where the trainers were trained, both as mediators and as teachers.
   b. Experienced mediators with at least 5 years of full-time mediation practice, having conducted hundreds of mediations. Mediation trainers may be teaching mediation in lieu of practicing it and doing so as an adjunct to another profession, such as law or therapy practice. Make sure your trainer's mediation practice is longstanding and currently active. Working full-time as a mediator is a strong indication that they have sufficient skill and experience as a mediator to be able to provide solid training
   c. Bonus—Trainers who have experience mediating elder and adult family mediation will likely provide training in the basic skills that are most important

2. If the trainers are published authors, read their articles or books. If articles are not available on the training program website, ask the author to e-mail you a copy.
3. Review the description of the methodology, and if you do not find one on the website, request one from the trainer.
4. Effective mediation training is learning by doing and reflecting on what you do, not just reading, hearing about, or watching someone else mediate. Look for the following indicators the program is largely experiential:
   - Good training consists of 70–80% hands-on role play or small group exercises
   - The best programs provide experienced mediators and teachers who are trained in giving helpful feedback to supervise role plays.
   - Be wary of training programs that promise multiple or large "panels" of expert mediators, a sign there will be more talking than doing.
5. Examine a list of topics the course will cover or, better yet, an agenda, with times, to determine whether there is a balance between theory, skills, and personal qualities. The schedule will also indicate the allocation of time between lecture and experiential learning.

Figure 22–7   Mediation Training Shopping Tips

Many colleges and universities offer under-graduate and graduate courses and degrees in conflict resolution or mediation. In addition to academic courses, the most effective pro-grams also provide experiential learning courses, akin to nonacademic mediation train-ing programs. Certainly a 2-year graduate pro-gram (or a 4-year undergraduate program) focused on conflict resolution is a fantastic opportunity for mediator development.

Finally, one significant component of train-ing is not usually found within formal train-ing programs, but exists in the world of mediation, through shadowing and working with experienced mediators. Locating these opportunities takes effort, but worth the trouble. Tips for locating an elderly/adult mediator appear in Figure 22–8.

Regulation of Mediation

In most US jurisdictions, the profession of mediation does not require licensure. In Cali-fornia, for example, anyone at all can hang up a shingle as mediator, although private or court-connected mediation panels customar-ily impose requirements for training and experience. Some countries have imposed stringent requirements for mediators. Aus-tria, for example, demands that mediators have at least 200 hours of training to provide mediation services.[12] Aspiring mediators should contact professional mediation organ-izations within their jurisdictions for infor-mation about licensure.[13]

■ MEDIATION AS A RESOURCE FOR GCMS

This section offers GCMs guidelines for deter-mining when mediation may be appropriate and inappropriate, as well as suggestions for working with families to recommend media-tion and, once the process begins, supporting them to participate productively.

Indications that Mediation Is Appropriate

The warning signs of desperation—"I am out of ideas!," "These people are impossible!," and "Help! I give up!"—may prompt a GCM to consider a mediation referral, but waiting for the signal of hopelessness is not necessar-ily efficient or skillful. Depending on a GCM's level of tolerance for unproductive or coun-

---

1. Ask colleagues or lawyers about mediators they know and trust.
   - Specify, when asking, that you're seek-ing mediators who have experience in elder or adult family mediation.
   - A word of caution: Lawyers don't always fully appreciate the specialized expertise and training required for mediating con-flicts in the world of geriatric care.
2. Attend seminars and workshops on elder and adult family mediation.
   - Sometimes these are stand-alone events, and sometimes they are part of professional conferences.

- Follow up with a telephone call or lunch date with the presenter or other media-tors who attend the program (who, by the way, may be a good source of refer-rals to a GCM).
3. Read articles and books about elder and adult family mediation, and follow up with the authors in the same ways suggested in item 2.
4. Consult the Internet with a word search or exploration of specific mediation websites such as Mediate.com, where adult family mediators are listed.

Figure 22–8   Tips for Locating an Elder/Adult Family Mediator

terproductive conversation, precious time can be lost, relationships unduly damaged, and unnecessary pain inflicted on a parent by destructive behavior in family meetings. GCMs can learn to spot early warning signs. (See Figure 22–9.)

In some cases, GCMs can incorporate mediation from the outset. Mediation is almost always indicated when a high-conflict, difficult family faces complex high-stakes decisions, as discussed above and illustrated in Figure 22–4 previously. Developing the ability to assess conflict is the first step in addressing conflict for any purpose, including deciding whether to recommend mediation.

Assessing Conflict

Skillful conflict management requires the ability to assess the situation. In the midst of others' conflict, most people who want to help *react*, rather than *respond*. One impulse is to stop the conflict, to become a referee who pulls the parties apart, sending them to their corners to clean up their wounds and return for a cleaner fight. Another impulse is to fix their problem, to figure out a solution that may be an acceptable compromise and tell the parties what to do. Another approach is to declare the conflict impossible: to give up, particularly if the emotion is too high and the hurt is too deep. Ms. Sortitout, the GCM Suzi Sniper called for a consultation, may decide after the first few minutes of conversation with Suzi that the answer to the question "Can this family be saved?" is "No!" and leave the Snipers to muddle through their mess alone, under the watchful eye of APS or the court.

As indicated in Figure 22–4, the main factors in determining whether to recommend the services of a professional mediator are difficulty of the family, degree of emotional conflict, and complexity of the problem. Below are some early indicators that these factors weigh in favor of mediation in the earliest stage of GCM consultation, when high conflict appears.

1. **Family members are focusing on their own needs to the exclusion of their older family member's,** therefore requiring the GCM to be such a strong advocate for the older family member that the GCM cannot facilitate family meetings as a credible accidental mediator.

2. **The older person is unable to express her needs and preferences** due to any number of factors, including diminished mental capacity, fear of conflict, extreme dependency, behavior associated with adult dependency disorder, which, again, require the GCM early on to be the "voice"—or surrogate—for the older person.

3. **The presence of issues interrelated with the elder's care that exceed the GCM's subject matter expertise,** for example:
   a. Claims by family members that other family members are exerting undue influence or subjecting the older person to duress
   b. Claims of elder abuse, which may also involve reporting to the appropriate authorities, but can perhaps be addressed in mediation, as well
   c. Disputes about the extent of the older person's ability to make decisions regarding property or health care
   d. Disputes over who should manage the finances or healthcare decisions of the older person whose abilities are in question
   e. Trusts and estates disputes or decisions
   f. Hatred and/or viciousness between family members, particularly when it causes the older person's loyalty to be questioned

---

Figure 22–9   Early Warning Signs to Call In an Intentional Mediator

A more skillful approach is to respond, rather than react. Assess the situation and consider the family's options, one of which is mediation. To students of conflict, family fireworks are an opportunity to assess how functional or difficult the family is, how effectively family members communicate in conflict, and whether the GCM is competent to manage the situation. The process of assessing, or more deeply understanding the situation, is the GCM's first step in determining what to do. As discussed more fully below, assessment consists of four steps: 1) GCMs assess the conflict; 2) GCMs assess the parties; 3) GCMs assess themselves; and 4) GCMs assess the ethical implications.

1. GCMs Assess the Conflict. What is the source of the conflict? What is the family fighting about? How complicated is it? How divergent are the parties' perspectives? What is at stake if the family can't resolve the conflict? What could they gain if they do?

Applying this approach to the Sniper family, the source of the conflict is multifaceted:

- There are conflicting positions concerning Steve's best interest. Suzi thinks it is being near her; Sam believes it is living at home with Sam. Steve is back and forth.
- There are conflicting ideas about Steve's needs and concerns. On the surface, Sam thinks Steve needs to be in his familiar surroundings. Suzi worries her father is unsafe and too isolated living at home with Sam. She thinks he needs more social interaction, greater attention to nutrition, and the social interaction her active family can provide. Steve has expressed all of these needs and concerns.
- Suzi and Sam have conflicting needs and concerns. This is where it gets complicated. Although unstated, or not acknowledged, Suzi and Sam have their own needs and concerns. If Sam is right that Suzi is misusing Dad's money, she

may have a need to protect herself from legal action or to avoid the responsibility of repayment. If Suzi is right that Sam is a freeloader, then Sam needs a solution that takes into consideration his dire financial circumstances.

- There is conflicting data. Steve and Sam think Steve was sent to a nursing home to die. Suzi asserts he was sent to a rehabilitation facility to gain strength to enable him to return to her home.
- There are communication problems and relationship conflicts. It would be an understatement to say Suzi and Sam have exhibited an inability to engage in constructive discussions about the issues, nor, it seems, do they have a history of doing so in other circumstances.

Additionally all of these conflicts exist in the shadow of potential legal claims of financial elder abuse and elder abuse and neglect. On the scale of complexity of the problem and degree of emotional conflict, this family is off the charts.

2. GCMs Assess the Parties. It is also important for the GCM to assess the parties' ability to deal with the conflict. Is the family nearly normal or difficult? In the Sniper family, for example, how capable are the individual family members of communicating effectively? Are they willing to speak up? Can they express themselves without verbally abusing others? On the other side of the communication equation, are they capable of empathy? Are they at least willing to listen to the others, even if they disagree? Are they open to your suggestions and able to accept your help when they get themselves in trouble? Finally, are there cognitive barriers, substance abuse issues, or mental disorders that make it impossible for them to communicate effectively?

3. GCMs Assess Themselves. Stepping back emotionally and intellectually from conflict in a family meeting enables GCMs to assess honestly whether they are qualified to work with a family. This evaluation begins with, and in large part relies upon, accurate assessment of the conflict and the parties, but it ultimately rests on an honest self-assessment. Relevant inquiries include:

a. Am I just out of my comfort zone, which requires me to stretch, or am I out of my competence zone, which requires me to acquire significant expertise I do not presently possess? And should I refer the parties to someone who has it?

b. Is the family making progress or backsliding? Though meetings are challenging and difficult, is the family becoming more focused and directed or is the decision becoming more complicated, diffuse, and apparently unattainable?

c. Am I significantly more anxious than I normally am, both in the meetings and outside of them? Am I losing sleep, primarily because I doubt my ability to handle the situation?

d. If I answer yes to most of the questions above and I continue to mediate for the family alone, why is that? What am I afraid of that causes me to continue in an unproductive way? Am I trying to prove to myself I can do it, at the expense of the family? Am I extending myself because I don't think the family can afford mediation?

Not only is engaging in this analysis the responsible thing to do, it is also necessary to fulfill the GCMs' ethical obligation to provide only the services they are qualified to provide.[14]

4. GCMs Assess the Ethical Implications. In addition to judging whether they possess the conflict management expertise to work with a family in conflict, GCMs must also assess whether they can do so *ethically*. The Standards of Practice for Professional Geriatric

Care Managers anticipates that GCMs will work with families in conflict. Standard 1, Guideline A states: "In the event of conflicting needs within the client system, the goal of professional intervention should be to strive for resolution through a process of review and discussion among the parties, facilitated by the Professional Geriatric Care Manager." Yet, the GCM's duty of loyalty to the primary client, the older person, including the requirement to promote client self-determination may collide with the necessity to remain impartial to be effective in assisting a family to work out their differences.[15] There may come a point in a family meeting process when other members of the family or client system are so opposed in their positions concerning the elder's care that the GCM must choose between being an effective facilitator and being an ethical GCM. In these circumstances, GCMs may be pressured to sacrifice their neutrality in service of the greater GCM ethic of client loyalty, taking the side of the client to ensure a care plan is implemented that is aligned with the client's stated goals, or one that will enhance the decisions clients have made concerning their lives. In the midst of a family in conflict, how can the GCM at once act as a facilitator and advocate for the older person?[16] In this challenging situation, where the conflict is high and the family is extremely challenging, an experienced elder mediator can help the GCM resolve this ethical conflict.

The Option of Mediation

In the process of assessment, options emerge. However, when we are reacting, there are no options. There are only instinctive, knee-jerk impulses. Conflict assessment and reflection not only enable the GCM to understand the conflict, the parties, and themselves, it opens the mental space in which to consider, evaluate, choose, and implement those options. Mediation is just one of the many options available to help fighting families. However, because the focus of this chapter is mediation, we will not address the others.

When Mediation with an Intentional Mediator Is Appropriate

In general, mediation is appropriate any time the parties in conflict have the following characteristics:

- Willingness to participate
- Willingness to reach an agreement that works for the other parties, as well as themselves
- Ability, with help, to participate in the conversation, to say what is true for them and what they need, and to try to understand the other parties.

A GCM should consider making a referral to an intentional mediator if the family situation exhibits the following dynamics:

- Emotions are very high and communication is unduly challenging for the family.
- A difficult personality is preventing you from fulfilling your obligations as a GCM.
- Emotional safety and comfort of the older person is critical and the family is not able to respond as urgently as the situation requires.
- A care plan calls for a high degree of cooperation, but the family demonstrates a low degree of potential to implement it.
- There are pending or threatened legal claims (e.g., contested conservatorships, trust disputes, property disputes) that impede or sideline your work.

When Mediation May Not Be Appropriate

The rare instances in which a referral to a professional mediator may not be appropriate involve the absence of any one of the critical appropriateness factors described above, creating one of these resulting situations:

- One or more of the parties refuses to participate *and* the problem the family is dealing with requires the agreement of the unwilling party or parties.
- One or more of the parties will not entertain the possibility of an agreement that would work for the other party or parties, even after preliminary discussions with a mediator.
- One or more of the essential parties are incapable of expressing their perspectives and needs, even with help, perhaps due to adult dependency disorder, diminished mental capacity, fear of conflict, duress, undue influence, or some other form of intimidation.

Even when the situation initially looks like a dispute is inappropriate for mediation, a GCM or professional mediator may be able to work around the problems. Reluctant or intransigent parties, when they are educated about mediation and realize why it is in their interest to participate, may be willing to come to the mediation table and even to be flexible as long as they understand they have control over the decision.

In general, parties who cannot stand up for themselves or are afraid to do so are terrible candidates for mediation. An exception to this rule may be the older person whose decision-making authority has been delegated to a third party such as a trustee, conservator, or other person with power of attorney, who can work with older people to learn what is important to them. These third parties can make decisions on behalf of the older person that are in their interest and not subject to fear, intimidation, or undue influence. These situations are extremely delicate and may require the involvement of legal counsel, as well, but having this sort of assistance can enable mediation to go forward.

When the GCM, the professional mediator, the parties, and perhaps legal counsel have tried and failed to work around problematic circumstances that keep the parties from mediation, the GCM has a number of options:

- The GCM can wait and revisit the subject of mediation at a later point in time. With a little time to reflect, a resistant family member may change his/her mind.
- The GCM can suggest the family members seek legal counsel, who can ask the court or a private arbitrator to decide the controversy.
- If elder abuse is suspected, the GCM should report it to the appropriate authorities and seek assistance, as discussed in Chapter 6.

Once again, returning to the Sniper family, Suzi contacted a GCM named Ms. Sortitout after Sam took Steve from the rehabilitation facility. Based on the information provided, is this an appropriate case for mediation? Ms. Sortitout made a tentative decision to refer to Meredith Mediator, a professional mediator for the following reasons:

- In the first phone call, Suzi said her priority was keeping her father safe and that if she could accomplish that goal by having mediated discussions with her brother, she would be willing to do so.
- Although she was angry and upset, and spoke disparagingly of her brother, she did not express unwillingness to find an agreement that worked for him, too.
- Certainly Sam and Suzi could stand up for themselves in mediation, and Suzi was open to having Ms. Sortitout work with her father to assure his perspective and wishes would be brought to the mediation, through the GCM or Steve directly, depending on the mediator's suggestion.

Suggesting Mediation

Although mediation is commonplace in the family law and divorce context and, more recently, in litigated cases, elder and adult family mediation is a fairly recent development. Because it is not so much in the public awareness, the GCM may be the first point of contact the adult family has with the concept of mediation. The better the understanding of mediation, the more effectively a GCM can work with families to consider mediation as an option. The following approach can help the GCM work with a family to decide about mediation.

- The GCM should assess the situation, as discussed above.
- The GCM should describe the situation that is creating the need for mediation: "No matter what we do, you can't seem to find a solution, not simply because you have different perspectives, but because the level of trust is so low, and the emotions are so high."
- The GCM should propose and describe mediation: "You may want to consider working with a mediator. Do you know about mediation? In mediation you would work with an impartial third party to reach an agreement that is acceptable to all of you and that takes into consideration all of your needs. Mediators do not decide what you should do—you do that—but they are skilled at managing conflict and helping you have constructive conversations, especially when emotions are intense."
- The GCM should explain why he or she is suggesting mediation. To Francie and Flora, for example the GCM might say, "I can see you are highly motivated to solve this difficult problem and you want to do it quickly in the interest of getting your mother settled and keeping her safe. I also understand you are considering involving lawyers and litigating, which is an expensive, drawn-out proposition that will be stressful for all of you, especially your mother. It seems to me

you have little to lose by involving a mediator. The worst that will happen is you are in the same place you are now, having spent a few thousand dollars. In my experience with other families, mediation frequently leads to agreement."

- The GCM should describe how the mediator will work with the family in preparation for mediation. To do so, GCMs can interview mediators to learn how they approach their cases to explain these procedures to their clients. Experienced elder and adult family mediators generally hold a telephone conference with all of the family members who will be involved in the mediation to discuss and decide on logistical questions, such as timing, location, duration, and who will participate, as well as fees and the payment of them. In these calls, mediators may also address preparation for mediation, including whether the mediator will conduct private interviews with family members, how the agenda and ground rules will be presented, and they may make suggestions about how the participants can prepare to participate productively.

- The GCM should discuss the family members' questions and concerns.

- If they are amenable to mediation, the GCM should describe the steps in hiring a mediator, which consist of getting mediator names and contact information from the GCM or others, and interviewing and hiring the mediator (see Figure 22–9).

GCMs can also help parties streamline the hiring process by clarifying issues regarding payment of mediator fees (from a trust or other family assets or by individual family members and in what proportion) and discussing the logistics of mediator interviews (all parties together or separately and responsibility for arranging interviews).

GCMs who develop their conflict assessment skills and become educated about mediation can fine tune their referrals by matching the mediator to the dispute. Begin with an analysis of the obstacles to resolution, including the types of problems and the types of people involved, and an understanding of the personality and predilections of specific mediators. In making referrals, GCMs can consider whether the mediator's particular process skills and substantive expertise are sufficient. The mediator's personal qualities are critical. Particularly in a difficult case, as discussed above, this inquiry can be the most important consideration in choosing a mediator.

Let's go back to the Snipers and the conversation in which the GCM Suzi consulted discussed mediation.

Ms. Sortitout: "It seems like the situation with your father has escalated to the point that you really need some help. I want to talk with you about how I can be most useful, but before doing so, I want to suggest mediation as an option for you to consider. Have you any experience with mediation?"

Suzi: "I have heard of it, but don't know much at all."

Ms. Sortitout: "In mediation, you and your brother—and perhaps your father, if that is appropriate, and even a GCM—come together with the help of a professional mediator to discuss the problems you face and hopefully find a solution that meets everyone's needs and addresses all of the concerns you raise. Mediators are experienced with helping families address difficult problems, even when the emotions are high and conflict is intense, as they are for you and your brother right now."

Suzi: "Wow! That would be amazing, but I don't think my brother would ever agree to do that, and I have no idea how to find a good mediator."

Ms. Sortitout: "I can help you with the second problem. I will give you the names and contact information of several experienced adult family mediators, so you could call them. I could also talk with them with you, if you like. Or I could call them and explain the situation, see what they think and call you back. Regarding your concern that Sam wouldn't agree to mediation: once you find a mediator, the mediator can talk with you about approaching your brother, or the mediator can contact your brother and work with him to explore whether he might be willing."

Suzi: "That sounds great! Assuming we find a mediator and my brother agrees, how does it work?"

Ms. Sortitout: "Generally, the first step is for the mediator to meet with you and your brother, either in a conference call or in person, to talk about setting up the mediation and how you will work together. The mediator will want to get a brief idea of what the problems are and what you want to accomplish in mediation, and will work with you to plan the next steps in preparing for mediation. These steps generally include separate conversations with the participants, in this case with you and Sam and perhaps your father, privately and confidentially. The mediator will most likely prepare an agenda and communication guidelines for you to review and approve (or modify) before the mediation, so that when you come to mediation you know what to expect."

Suzi: "Sounds good. How much does it cost and who pays for it?"

Ms. Sortitout: "Mediators charge between $150 and $500 per hour. Some communities even have free services, and I can check on that for you. The difficulty is you will most likely not be able to choose the mediator, and you may be assigned to a mediator that has limited elder or adult family experience and who is not necessarily well suited to your particular case.

You, your brother, and your father will decide how to pay for mediation. Where the parents have sufficient resources, they usually pay the mediator's fee, or parties may share equally or according to their ability to pay. In any case, especially where there is the potential for litigation, as appears to be the case here, paying a single mediator, instead of separate lawyers, each of whom are charging fees equal to or higher than the mediator's fee, may make financial sense."

Suzi: "Gee, thanks. I would appreciate it if you would give me the contact information of some good mediators so I can get the ball rolling."

Ms. Sortitout: "I am happy to do so."

Serving as a GCM in Mediation

In addition to serving as accidental mediators in their own GCM cases and referring cases to mediation, GCMs may also be called upon to serve as consultants in ongoing adult family mediations. As the field of elder and adult family mediation expands and specialized training becomes more widely available, mediators are coming to understand the value of GCMs as resources in helping families with difficult substantive issues. To make wise decisions about elder-care issues, families need good information about older persons' needs, as well as their cognitive and physical abilities and limitations; about appropriate options for meeting the needs of all of the family members; about care-related financial issues; and about the myriad of resources and issues GCMs are trained in providing. Unless mediators are also GCMs or elder law lawyers, their knowledge is limited, and GCMs can fill this gap. As this awareness develops, GCMs will be called upon increasingly as resources for families in mediation.

GCMs can be involved in mediation in several ways: consulting privately with mediators concerning issues related to their particular cases; consulting with one or more family members who need information in preparation for mediation; and actually participating in mediation, with or without having met with the older family member or others before the mediation. As with any other consultation, it is important to be clear about the professional mediator's and family's expectations to consider whether those expectations are realistic and, if so, how you will work together.

When a GCM participates in mediation, it is especially important to get an understanding from the mediator about the timing, context, and purpose of any presentation the GCM may be called upon to make. Before presenting information in mediation, a GCM should reiterate the GCM's understanding of the information's purpose, meaning how it will help the family to make a good decision.

Let's return to the Sniper family. Sam agreed to mediation with intentional mediator Meredith. The family also agreed to hire Ms. Sortitout GCM to assess Steve and prescribe a temporary care plan to be in place until mediation concluded, hopefully in agreement, on an ongoing plan for Steve. Ms. Sortitout's plan for Steve provided that while professional mediation was pending Steve would stay put, but would have 24-hour care arranged by Ms. Sortitout.

Sam and Suzi had an initial call with Meredith Mediator in which they agreed to the following process:

1. Meredith would talk with Sam and Suzi each privately and then would meet in person with Steve at home to understand each of their perspectives on the situation, the issues that need addressing in the mediation, and their ideas for how to have a productive mediation.
2. Meredith would create an agenda and guidelines for the family's review and modification, resulting in an agreed agenda and guidelines for the mediation.
3. Suzi and Sam would meet, just the two of them, in an initial 3- to 4-hour professional mediation session with Meredith and follow-up mediation sessions, as necessary, during which they may

choose to involve Ms. Sortitout and Steve, if appropriate, until they reach agreement on all of the issues.

After the private calls, Meredith drafted a tentative mediation plan, including an agenda and communication guidelines, and worked with the parties until they all agreed. She then sent them the letter in Figure 22-10.

Thereafter, Sam, Suzi, and Ms. Sortitout met with Meredith. Despite the recent bad history and the extent of their anger, Meredith helped them to talk about what happened and to share their concerns and needs with each other on all topics. By the end of the first session, Sam and Suzi reached the following agreements:

1. At the suggestion of Ms. Sortitout, they would work with Steve to ensure that he sees a neurologist to determine the cause of his dementia.
2. Once Ms. Sortitout draws up a care plan based on this new information and her further meetings with Steve, Suzi and Sam will return to mediation to discuss the plan, agreeing ahead of time to cooperate in implementing it.
3. Regarding financial issues, they agreed to the following:
   a. At a future mediation session, they would exchange accountings of all financial contributions and gifts (including in-kind gift of free rent to Sam) from their father to each of them. Once they completed the accountings to the other's satisfaction, they would characterize these gifts as advancements of their inheritance to be deducted from their respective distributions of Steve's estate after his death.
   b. They would not request money or gifts from Steve in the future without the written consent of the other person to do so.

Meredith Mediator
Attorney at Law
MASTERFUL MEDIATION SERVICES
Marlborough, MD 33333

April 21, 2011

Mr. Stephen Sniper   Ms. Suzi Sniper
666 Snipe Lane   999 Snipe Street
Grenade City, GA 66666   Weaponton, WA 99999

Mr. Sam Sniper
666 Snipe Lane
Grenade City, GA 66666

Dear Stephen, Suzi, and Sam:

First of all, it was good to talk with you last week in preparation for mediation with Sam, Suzi, Stephen, and the GCM on April 12. The purpose of this letter is to propose a plan for the mediation. I also include suggestions to help Sam and Suzi prepare.

Statement of Purpose of the Mediation

You want to reach a resolution that (1) ensures Stephen's safety, health, and well-being; (2) enables Stephen to have ongoing contact with Suzi; (3) fosters respect, civility, and cooperation; and (4) provides a predictable, ongoing, collaborative procedure for working out any future issues regarding Stephen's care and finances.

Proposed Communication Guidelines

1. Treat one another with respect
   a. When the other is speaking, do not interrupt.
   b. Avoid disparaging one another.
   c. Avoid sarcasm.
   d. Bring your best intentions to the mediation, and trust the others to do the same.
2. Listen to *understand* one another's perspectives, recognizing you do not need to *agree*.
3. Express yourselves in a manner that stands the best chance of being understood by the others.

Proposed Agenda for April 30, 2011

1. Introductory remarks:
   a. Statement of the purpose of the mediation and suggestions for participating effectively
   b. Review of the communication guidelines
   c. Agreement on the agenda

continues

Figure 22–10   Mediation Plan Letter

2. Stephen's care
   a. General discussion
   b. Discussion of Suzi's, Sam's, and Stephen's needs, interests, and concerns
   c. Report from Ms. Sortitout
   d. Exploration of care options (Ms. Sortitout)
   e. Evaluation of care options
   f. Next steps—including involving Stephen in the discussions
3. Financial issues
   a. General discussion—Stephen's contributions to Sam's and Suzi's finances during the past 2 years
   b. Exchange of information and documentation all parties agreed to provide at mediation
   c. Identification of financial issues that need to be addressed, including additional information or documentation to be provided, if any, and areas of agreement and disagreement
   d. Planning next steps

Preparation Suggestions

1. I suggest you read Difficult Conversations, by Patton, Stone, and Heen.
2. Reflect on your contribution to the present difficulties between you.
3. Consider which, if any, of your own contribution(s) deserves an apology and consider how you might apologize.
4. Consider how you aspire to conduct yourself during the mediation.

Procedure for Finalizing the Mediation Plans

Please review this plan and let me know whether you agree to my proposed approach. If you have suggestions, please send them to me by return e-mail by replying to all of us. I would like to hear from you as soon as possible, but no later than this Friday. Feel free to call me if you would like to discuss these plans.

I look forward to working with you April 30.

With best regards,

Meredith Mediator

Meredith Mediator

Figure 22–10   Mediation Plan Letter (continued)

c. They would schedule a future mediation session where Steve, his trust and estate lawyer Ms. Lawful, Steve's accountant, Ms. Sortitout, and Sam and Suzi could address financial issues including the following:

   i. Management of Steve's finances in light of concerns about his mental capacity

   ii. A care plan and budget for Steve

   iii. The big picture of Steve's finances

In mediation, the Snipers, with the help of Ms. Lawful, the accountant, and Ms. Sortitout were able to resolve all of their conflicts to their mutual satisfaction, as well as to the satisfaction of APS that Steve would be safe. Along the way, Sam and Suzi were able to build their capacity to communicate effectively, which they would inevitably be required to do as Steve's condition worsened and circumstances changed. In addition, they were able to avoid litigation and its high costs emotionally and financially.

■ CONCLUSION

Mediation and geriatric care management are a marriage destined for a fruitful partnership. As complementary disciplines, they are great resources for each other. The expertise of GCMs helps mediation parties expand their options and better understand the consequences of their decisions, and the expertise of mediators allows families working with GCMs to deal with difficult dynamics and overcome obstacles to responsible, wise decisions concerning their aging family members.

GCMs who understand mediation make skillful referrals and also maximize opportunities to help their clients as accidental mediators. Experienced GCMs who become mediators can have fulfilling careers as mediators, and as referral sources for other GCMs and lawyers whose clients need help with conflict.

Conflict giving rise to chaos and destruction can make it impossible for family members to reach agreements about care, and even, at the extreme, require courts to intervene at great emotional and financial cost. Conflict can cause excruciating pain among family members, opening old wounds and inflicting new ones, resulting in permanent alienation extending into future generations. It can split children and parents or make life a living hell for an elderly parent caught between warring children. Although it is difficult to deal with the fallout of destructive conflict at any age, it is especially tragic when it comes at the end of life, a time when one of the deepest developmental needs is for integration and peace.

On the other hand, conflict can lead to connection and creativity. Nearly normal families quite readily realize these benefits as they struggle with decisions about an increasingly dependent parent, especially if their GCMs are skillful accidental mediators. For difficult families who have drifted apart or have been separated by miles or years of ill will, this experience does not unfold as elegantly. However, with the help of a professional mediator, even these families can pull together out of shared concern for a parent. A positive experience of working together may restore the respect that eroded years before. In addition to understanding one another more deeply, when family members exchange conflicting perspectives, needs, and proposals in a constructive fashion, together they can achieve more fully informed, creative solutions than any of them would have done independently.

Helping families as either accidental or intentional mediators enhances GCMs' already fulfilling careers. The transition parents make from independence to dependence is one of the most challenging and painful times in the life cycle of a family and is made far more so by conflict. At the very least,

GCMs who are skillful accidental mediators and sophisticated in referring clients to mediation can help families reduce the destructive potential of conflict. At best, GCMs can be conduits for families to reap the benefits of conflict, including growing closer, healing old wounds, and making better-informed, more creative decisions.

■ REFERENCES

1. For example, California Evidence Code Section 1119 provides:

   Except as otherwise provided in this chapter:

   (a) No **evidence** of anything said or any admission made for the purpose of, in the course of, or pursuant to, a mediation or a mediation consultation is admissible or subject to discovery, and disclosure of the **evidence** shall not be compelled, in any arbitration, administrative adjudication, civil action, or other noncriminal proceeding in which, pursuant to law, testimony can be compelled to be given.

   (b) No writing, as defined in Section 250, that is prepared for the purpose of, in the course of, or pursuant to, a mediation or a mediation consultation, is admissible or subject to discovery, and disclosure of the writing shall not be compelled, in any arbitration, administrative adjudication, civil action, or other noncriminal proceeding in which, pursuant to law, testimony can be compelled to be given.

   (c) All communications, negotiations, or settlement discussions by and between participants in the course of a mediation or a mediation consultation shall remain confidential.

2. Susskind L, McKearnan S, Thomas-Larner J, eds. *The Consensus Building Handbook: A Comprehensive Guide to Reaching Agreement.* Thousand Oaks, CA: Sage Publications; 1999:7–9, 207–208.

3. Fadiga L, Fogassi L, Pavesi G, Rizzolatti G. Motor facilitation during action observation: a magnetic stimulation study. *J Neurophysiology.* 1995;73(6):2608–2611.

4. Curtis D. Reconciliation and the role of empathy. In: Alfini J, Galton E, eds, *ADR Personalities and Practice Tips.* Washington, D.C.: American Bar Association; 1998:49–63.

5. Hocker J, Wilmot W. *Interpersonal Conflict.* New York: McGraw-Hill; 1995:39.

6. Cialdini R. *Influence: The Psychology of Persuasion.* New York: William Morrow and Company, Inc.; 1993:56–113.

7. Bowling D, Hoffman D, eds. *Bringing Peace into the Room: How the Personal Qualities of the Mediator Impact the Process of Conflict Resolution.* San Francisco: John Wiley & Sons, Inc.; 2003:277.

8. Bowling D, Hoffman D, eds. *Bringing Peace into the Room: How the Personal Qualities of the Mediator Impact the Process of Conflict Resolution.* San Francisco: John Wiley & Sons, Inc.; 2003:28.

9. Bowling D, Hoffman D, eds. *Bringing Peace into the Room: How the Personal Qualities of the Mediator Impact the Process of Conflict Resolution.* San Francisco: John Wiley & Sons, Inc.; 2003:27.

10. Bowling D, Hoffman D, eds. *Bringing Peace into the Room: How the Personal Qualities of the Mediator Impact the Process of Conflict Resolution.* San Francisco: John Wiley & Sons, Inc.; 2003: 17–18.

11. Cress C, ed. *Handbook of Geriatric Care Management.* 2nd ed. Sudbury, Mass.; 2010:127.

12. Trofaier MT. Mediation in Austria: the new Austrian Mediation in Civil Law Matters Act. *Croat Arbit Yearb.* 2004;11:99.

13. For example, California Dispute Resolution Council, http://www.cdrc.net.

14. See Standards of Practice for Professional Geriatric Care Managers, Standard 6, Guideline A: "The GCM should act only in the roles for which he or she has the appropriate skills, knowledge, and training. He or she should recommend consultations with specialists as needed." http://www.caremanager.org/displaycommon.cfm?an=1&subarticlenbr=282. Accessed February 15, 2011.

15. See Standards of Practice for Professional Geriatric Care Managers, Standard 2, "The GCM has a responsibility to identify and articulate the client's wishes, values, and preferences so that these can be incorporated into the plan of care to the greatest extent possible. . . ."; and Guideline A, "The Professional Geriatric Care Manager should involve the primary client and/or designated decision maker, to the great-

est extent possible, in decisions that impact his/her life regardless of the client's decisional capacity." http://www.caremanager.org/ displaycommon.cfm?an=1&subarticlenbr=282. Accessed February 15, 2011.

16 The Standards of Practice provide that, "[a GCM] should request assistance of peers, as needed, to help the client system find an acceptable solution when conflicts occur" (Standard 1, Guideline C). http://www. caremanager.org/displaycommon.cfm?an=1& subarticlenbr=282. Accessed February 15, 2011.

■ADDITIONAL RESOURCES

Selected Articles on Elder Mediation

Vanarelli DD. Keeping family peace through elder mediation. *Aging Well.* 2009(Summer).

Larsen R, Thorpe C. Elder mediation: optimizing major family transitions. *Marquette Elder's Advisor.* 2006;7(2):293–312.

Mariani K. Developing ethical standards for elder mediation: questions along the way. *BIFOCAL.* 2007;28(6):85–90.

Larsen R. Mediating a key estate settlement issue: dividing personal property. http://www. mediate.com/articles/larsenR1.cfm. Accessed June 18, 2008.

Jackson M. Mediators ease decisions on elders. *The Boston Globe,* December 3, 2006, Balancing Acts Section.

Rhudy RJ. Senior mediation: reaching the tipping point. *Maryland Bar Journal.* 2008;41(2):12–29.

Cooper MD. Elder mediation: an opportunity for professional geriatric care managers. *Inside GMC.* 2008;Fall.

Largent K. Addressing adult guardianship and conservatorship concerns through mediation. *ACResolution.* 2009;Summer.

Selected Books on Mediation and Conflict Resolution

Bowling D, Hoffman D, eds. *Bringing Peace into the Room: How the Personal Qualities of the Mediator Impact the Process of Conflict Resolution.* San Francisco: John Wiley & Sons, Inc.; 2003.

Cloke K. *Mediating Dangerously: The Frontiers of Conflict Resolution.* San Francisco: Jossey-Bass; 2001.

Cloke K. *The Crossroads of Conflict: A Journey into the Heart of Dispute Resolution.* Santa Ana, Calif.: Janis Publications; 2006.

Hocker J, Wilmot W. *Interpersonal Conflict.* New York: McGraw-Hill; 1995.

Cialdini R. *Influence: The Psychology of Persuasion.* New York: William Morrow and Company, Inc.; 1993.

Mayer B. *The Dynamics of Conflict Resolution: A Practitioner's Guide.* San Francisco: Jossey-Bass; 2000.

Moore CW. *The Mediation Process: Practical Strategies For Resolving Conflict.* 3rd ed. San Francisco: Jossey-Bass; 2003.

Stone D, Patton B, Heen S. *Difficult Conversations: How to Discuss What Matters Most.* New York: Viking; 1999.

Susskind L, McKearnan S, Thomas-Larner J, eds. *The Consensus Building Handbook: A Comprehensive Guide to Reaching Agreement.* Thousand Oaks, Calif.: Sage Publications; 1999.

Ury WL. *The Third Side: How We Fight and How We Can Stop.* New York: Penguin; 2000.

Selected Websites

American Bar Association, Section of Dispute Resolution: http://www.abanet.org/dispute

Association for Conflict Resolution: http://www. acresolution.org

Conflict Resolution Information Source: http:// www.crinfo.org

Harvard Program on Negotiation: http://www. pon.harvard.edu

Mediate.com: http://www.mediate.com

California Dispute Resolution Council: http:// www.cdrc.net

Index

C

F

M

N

O